Genetic Predisposition to Cancer

Second edition

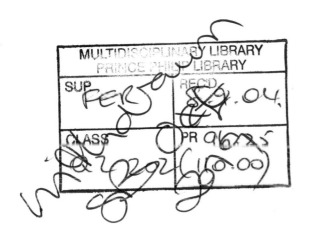
Edited by

ROSALIND A. EELES MA PhD FRCP FRCR

Reader in Clinical Cancer Genetics and Honorary Consultant in Cancer Genetics and Clinical Oncology, Institute of Cancer Research; and Royal Marsden NHS Foundation Trust, Surrey, UK

DOUGLAS F. EASTON PhD FMedSci

Director, Cancer Research UK Genetic Epidemiology Unit; and Professor of Genetic Epidemiology, University of Cambridge, Strangeways Research Laboratory, Cambridge, UK

BRUCE A.J. PONDER PhD FRCP FRCPath FMedSci FRS

Cancer Research UK Professor of Oncology; and Co-Director, Hutchison/MRC Research Centre and Strangeways Laboratory for Genetic Epidemiology, University of Cambridge, Cambridge, UK

and

CHARIS ENG MD PhD FACP

Dorothy E. Klotz Chair of Cancer Research; Professor and Director, Division of Human Genetics, Department of Internal Medicine; and Director, Clinical Cancer Genetics Program The Ohio State University, Columbus, Ohio, USA

A member of the Hodder Headline Group
LONDON

First published in Great Britain in 1996 by Chapman and Hall
This second edition published in 2004 by
Arnold, a member of the Hodder Headline Group,
338 Euston Road, London NW1 3BH

http://www.arnoldpublishers.com

Distributed in the United States of America by
Oxford University Press Inc.,
198 Madison Avenue, New York, NY10016
Oxford is a registered trademark of Oxford University Press

Whilst the advice and information in this book are believed to be true and
accurate at the date of going to press, neither the authors nor the publisher
can accept any legal responsibility or liability for any errors or omissions that
may be made. In particular (but without limiting the generality of the preceding
disclaimer) every effort has been made to check drug dosages; however, it is still
possible that errors have been missed. Furthermore, dosage schedules are
constantly being revised and new side-effects recognized. For these reasons the
reader is strongly urged to consult the drug companies' printed instructions
before administering any of the drugs recommended in this book.

British Library Cataloguing in Publication Data
A catalogue record for this book is available from the British Library

Library of Congress Cataloging-in-Publication Data
A catalog record for this book is available from the Library of Congress

ISBN 0 340 76254 3

1 2 3 4 5 6 7 8 9 10

Commissioning Editor: Joanna Koster
Development Editor: Sarah Burrows
Project Editor: Wendy Rooke
Production Controller: Lindsay Smith
Cover Design: Sarah Rees

Typeset in 10/12 pt Minion by Charon Tec Pvt. Ltd, Chennai, India
Printed and bound in the UK by Butler and Tanner Ltd.

What do you think about this book? Or any other Arnold title?
Please send your comments to feedback.arnold@hodder.co.uk

To those patients and their families who have led us to the discoveries of genetic predisposition to cancer that have resulted in prevention or early diagnosis in others.

Contents

Contributors

Colin F Arlett BSc PhD
Professor, Genome Damage and Stability Centre,
University of Sussex,
Brighton, UK

Yves-Jean Bignon MD PhD
Professor, Unit of Oncogenetics,
Centre J Perrin,
Clermont-Ferrand, France

Jillian M Birch PhD
Professor and Group Director,
Cancer Research UK Paediatric and
Familial Cancer Research Group,
Royal Manchester Children's Hospital,
Stancliffe, Manchester, UK

D Timothy Bishop PhD
Professor, Genetic Epidemiology Division,
Cancer Research UK Clinical Centre in Leeds,
St James's University Hospital, Leeds, UK

Susan K Boolbol MD
Breast Surgeon, Beth Israel Medical Center,
New York, USA

Norman E Breslow PhD
Professor, Department of Biostatistics,
University of Washington,
Seattle, Washington, USA

Philip J Byrd PhD
Cancer Research UK Institute for Cancer Studies,
Department of Cancer Studies,
University of Birmingham Medical School,
Birmingham, UK

Lisa Cannon-Albright PhD
Professor, Department of Medical Informatics,
The University of Utah,
Salt Lake City, Utah, USA

Pierre O Chappuis MD
McGill University Health Centre Research Institute; and
Departments of Medicine,
Human Genetics and Oncology,
McGill University, Montreal, Quebec, Canada

Mary Kay Dabney MS
Clinic Audit Coordinator, Guy's and St Thomas' NHS Trust,
London, UK

Timothy I Davidson ChM MRCP FRCS
Consultant Breast Surgeon,
University Department of Surgery,
The Royal Free Hospital, London, UK

Malcolm G Dunlop MD FRCS
Professor and Group Leader, University of Edinburgh,
Colon Cancer Genetics Group,
MRC Human Genetics Unit,
Western General Hospital,
Edinburgh, UK

Douglas F Easton PhD FMedSci
Director,
Cancer Research UK Genetic Epidemiology Unit; and
Professor of Genetic Epidemiology, University of Cambridge,
Strangeways Research Laboratory,
Cambridge, UK

Rosalind A Eeles MA PhD FRCP FRCR
Reader in Clinical Cancer Genetics and Honorary Consultant,
Cancer Genetics and Clinical Oncology,
Institute of Cancer Research; and Royal Marsden NHS
Foundation Trust, Surrey, UK

Charis Eng MD PhD FACP
Dorothy E. Klotz Chair of Cancer Research;
William C. and Joan E. Davis Professor of Cancer Research;
Professor and Director,
Division of Human Genetics,
Department of Internal Medicine;
Director, Clinical Cancer Genetics Program,
The Ohio State University,
Columbus, Ohio, USA

D Gareth R Evans MB BS MD FRCP
Professor, Department of Cancer Genetics,
Paterson Institute for Cancer Research,
Christie Hospital, Manchester; and
University Department of Medical Genetics and Regional
Genetics Service,
St Mary's Hospital,
Manchester, UK

Peter A Farndon BSc MD MB BS FRCP DCH
Professor of Clinical Genetics,
Consultant Clinical Geneticist,
University Department of Clinical Genetics,
Birmingham Women's Hospital,
Birmingham, UK

Susan M Farrington PhD
University of Edinburgh,
Colon Cancer Genetics Group,
MRC Human Genetics Unit,
Western General Hospital,
Edinburgh, UK

William D Foulkes MB PhD
Program in Cancer Genetics,
Departments of Oncology and
Human Genetics; and Department of Medicine,
McGill University, Montreal, Quebec, Canada

Alisa M Goldstein PhD
Senior Investigator,
Division of Cancer Epidemiology and Genetics,
Genetic Epidemiology Branch,
NCI/NIH/DHHS,
Bethesda, Maryland, USA

Shirley V Hodgson DC FRCP
Professor, Department of Medical Genetics,
St George's Hospital,
London, UK

Richard S Houlston MD PhD FRCP FRCPath
Reader in Genetic Epidemiology, Section of Cancer
Genetics, Institute of Cancer Research,
Surrey, UK

Pia AJ Huber PhD
Division of Genetics and Development,
Guy's, King's and St Thomas' School of Medicine,
King's College London, Guy's Hospital,
London, UK

Susan M Huson MD FRCP
Consultant Clinical Geneticist,
Department of Clinical Genetics,
Oxford Radcliffe Hospital, The Churchill Hospital,
Oxford, UK

William Isaacs MD
Professor, Department of Urology,
Johns Hopkins University School of Medicine,
Marburg 105 Brady Urological Institute,
Baltimore, Maryland, USA

Sarah Jefferies MRCP FRCR
Consultant in Clinical Oncology,
Addenbrook's NHS Foundation Trust,
Cambridge, UK

Kathryn M Kash PhD
Associate Professor,
Thomas Jefferson University,
Department of Psychiatry and Human Behavior,
Philadelphia, Pennsylvania, USA

Elsa Lanke MSc
Research Institute of the McGill University Health Centre; and
Departments of Medicine,
Human Genetics and Oncology,
McGill University, Montreal,
Quebec, Canada

Alan R Lehmann BA PhD
Professor and Chairman,
Genome Damage and Stability Centre,
University of Sussex,
Brighton, UK

Eamonn R Maher MD FRCP
Professor and Head,
Section of Medical and Molecular Genetics,
Division of Reproductive and Child Health,
University of Birmingham,
The Medical School,
Birmingham, UK

Somai Man PhD
Cancer Research UK Institute for Cancer Studies,
Department of Cancer Studies,
University of Birmingham Medical School,
Birmingham, UK

Christopher G Mathew PhD FRCPath FMedSci
Professor of Molecular Genetics,
Division of Genetics and Development,
Guy's, King's and St Thomas' School of Medicine,
Guy's Hospital,
London, UK

Christopher Mitchell PhD FRCP
Consultant Paediatric Oncologist,
The John Radcliffe Hospital,
Headington, Oxford, UK

Patrick J Morrison MB BCh MD FRCPCH MFPHMI
Professor,
Department of Medical Genetics,
Belfast City Hospital Trust,
Belfast, UK

Sue Moss PhD Hon MFPHM
Associate Director of Unit,
Cancer Screening Evaluation Unit,
Institute of Cancer Research,
Surrey, UK

Victoria A Murday BS FRCP
Consultant Clinical Geneticist,
Ferguson-Smith Centre for Clinical Genetics,
Yorkhill Division, NHS Greater Glasgow, Glasgow, UK

Aurelia Norton
Clinical Fellow in Paediatric Oncology,
Royal Marsden NHS Foundation Trust,
Surrey, UK

Gloria M Petersen PhD
Genetic Epidemiology,
Prevention and Control Program,
Mayo Clinic Cancer Center,
Minnesota, USA

Julian Peto DSc FMedSc
Cancer Research UK Professor of Epidemiology,
London School of Hygiene and Tropical Medicine,
London, UK; and Institute of Cancer Research,
Surrey, UK

Paul DP Pharoah PhD MRCP
Cancer Research UK Senior Clinical Research Fellow,
Department of Oncology,
University of Cambridge,
Strangeways Research Laboratories,
Cambridge, UK

Bruce AJ Ponder PhD FRCP FRCPath FMedSci FRS
Cancer Research UK Professor of Oncology; and Co-Director,
Hutchinson/MRC Research Centre and Strangeways Laboratory
for Genetic Epidemiology,
University of Cambridge,
Cambridge, UK

Trevor J Powles CBE PhD FRCP
Parkside Oncology Clinic,
Wimbledon,
London, UK

Kathryn Pritchard-Jones PhD FRCPE FRCPCH
Consultant Paediatric Oncologist,
The Royal Marsden NHS Foundation Trust,
Surrey, UK

Paul J Ross MRCP
Specialist Registrar,
The Royal Marsden NHS Foundation Trust,
Surrey, UK

Teresa Rudkin MD MSc
McGill University Health Centre; and
Department of Human Genetics,
McGill University,
Montreal, Quebec, Canada

Nigel PM Sacks MS FRCS FRACS
Consultant Breast Surgeon,
The Royal Marsden NHS Foundation Trust,
London, UK

Asher Y Salmon MD
Barclay Clinical Research Fellow,
Section of Cancer Genetics,
Institute of Cancer Research,
UK and Hadassah Medical Centre,
Jerusalem, Israel

Thomas A Sellers PhD MPH
Associate Director,
H Lee Moffitt Cancer Center and Research Institute,
Florida, USA

Rashmi Singh FRCS(Urol)
Clinical Research Fellow,
Translational Cancer Genetics Team; and Urology Unit,
Institute of Cancer Research; and Royal Marsden NHS
Foundation Trust, Surrey, UK

Tatjana Stankovic MD PhD
Cancer Research UK Institute for Cancer Studies,
Department of Cancer Studies,
University of Birmingham Medical School,
Birmingham, UK

Grant Stewart PhD
Cancer Research UK Institute for Cancer Studies,
Department of Cancer Studies,
University of Birmingham Medical School,
Birmingham, UK

Yousin Suh PhD
Department of Physiology,
University of Texas Health Science Center,
San Antonio, Texas, USA;
Formerly Department of Biochemistry and Molecular Biology,
Seoul National University,
College of Medicine,
Seoul, Korea

A Malcolm R Taylor MSc PhD
Professor,
Cancer Research UK Institute for Cancer Studies,
Department of Cancer Studies,
University of Birmingham Medical School,
Birmingham, UK

Deborah Thompson PhD
Statistician, Cancer Research UK Genetic Epidemiology Unit,
Strangeways Research Laboratories,
Cambridge, UK

Margaret A Tucker MD
Chief, Genetic Epidemiology Branch,
Division of Cancer Epidemiology and Genetics,
NCI/NIH/DHHS,
Bethesda, Maryland, USA

Jan Vijg PhD
Department of Physiology,
University of Texas Health Science Center and Geriatric
Education and Clinical Center,
South Texas Veterans Health Care System,
San Antonio, Texas, USA

Richard Wooster PhD
Senior Investigator
Cancer Genome Project,
Wellcome Trust Sanger Institute,
Hinxton, Cambridgeshire, UK

Ping Yang MD PhD
Associate Professor,
Mayo Clinic College of Medicine;
Consultant, Division of Epidemiology and
Mayo Clinic Cancer Center,
Rochester, Minnesota, USA

Berton Zbar MD
Chief,
Laboratory of Immunobiology,
Division of Basic Sciences,
National Cancer Institute,
National Institute of Health,
Frederick, Maryland, USA

Foreword by Sir Walter Bodmer

Cancer is essentially a somatic evolutionary process in which successive genetic or epigenetic changes are selected for their advantage to the outgrowth and progression of a tumour. It is mostly driven by environmental factors, which include a large element of chance. A significant subset of cancers is, however, clearly inherited. Knudson's famous hypothesis, put forward in 1971, related germline genetic changes to somatic changes. Thus he pointed out that, if a genetic change has already occurred in the germline that provides an advantage to an outgrowing tumour, this could be the basis for an inherited susceptibility to cancer. He furthermore suggested that this would involve a second genetic change in the tumour in the same gene, resulting mostly in the complete loss of the relevant gene's normal function. In its simplest version each of the two genetic changes, one in the germline and the other somatic, knock out the function of the gene, so that the effect at the level of the tumour is recessive, hence tumour suppressors. On the other hand the inheritance pattern due to the germline change is dominant. The implication is that if the gene that is mutated in certain inherited cancers is identified, then that gene may also be one that is commonly mutated somatically in sporadic cancers. The first clear success for this approach was the identification of the *RB* gene as the gene that is mutated in families with a history of retinoblastoma. This uncovered a key somatic pathway to carcinogenesis. With the development of genomic technology, and ultimately the whole human genome sequence, many other such discoveries have followed, including in particular the *APC* gene, mutations of which are responsible for the vast majority of cases of familial polyposis coli, again leading to the discovery of another major pathway in carcinogenesis. These results demonstrate once again how the study of rare exceptions – treasure them as William Harvey said – can lead to fundamental insights that are generally applicable.

There are however other possible bases for clear-cut inherited cancer susceptibility, such as the recessive DNA repair deficiencies, which in contrast to, for example, the *RB* and *APC* genes, are not found to be mutated or otherwise altered somatically. These particular genes seem to work largely by causing a general increase in the mutation rate, either spontaneous, or induced, for example by the ultraviolet in sunlight as in xeroderma pigmentosum.

Beyond the clear-cut inherited cases is the difficult question of identifying the basis for lower penetrance inherited susceptibilities that may sometimes be associated with quite common polymorphisms.

This book is a comprehensive multi author survey of these different aspects of cancer genetics, which inevitably is much changed since its first edition, given the rapidity of progress in this important area of cancer research. The editors are well known for their own contributions to cancer genetics and between them cover the spectrum from formal clinical genetics, through quantitative expertise, knowledge of the underlying molecular biology, and clinical experience. They are thus well placed to choose a wide range of excellent contributors and to oversee the editorial process from their own knowledge. The basics are first introduced, then there is comprehensive coverage, from population to clinic to laboratory, of clearly inherited cancer susceptibilities. This is followed by discussion of the less clearly defined problems of multifactorial inheritance. The book concludes with interesting contributions on questions such as how to set up inherited cancer clinics, approaches to screening and prevention in a genetic context, and psychosocial and ethical issues.

This will be a valuable reference work for any oncologist's or cancer researcher's shelves. In it you can find almost anything you need to know about cancer genetics at the family level, well and comprehensively described by experts in their respective fields.

Walter Bodmer FRS FRCPath
The Principal
Hertford College
Oxford
July 2004

Foreword by Sir Walter Bodmer

Foreword by Henry T. Lynch

The second edition of *Genetic Predisposition to Cancer* continues to assuage the thirst for new knowledge about hereditary cancer not only of those involved at the clinical and basic research level but equally of those at the clinical translational level. Clearly, this knowledge can be truly lifesaving. The authors have kept this tome updated and have continued to introduce fresh themes, particularly when demanded by the prodigious progress being made at the molecular genetic level in hereditary as well as sporadic cancers. Progress in molecular biology is also being made at the therapeutic level. For example, molecularly designed drugs, when shown to be efficacious, will one day replace chemotherapy for certain cancers. A recent example is STI571 (imatinib mesylate) and its dramatic efficacy in such highly fatal diseases as chronic myelogenous leukemia and gastrointestinal stromal tumor (GIST). Surgical practices will be revised when it is demonstrated that the lives of those *BRCA1* and *BRCA2* mutation carriers who undergo prophylactic mastectomy and/or oophorectomy will be saved. Women with *BRCA1/2* mutations will not only achieve the benefit of protection from metastatic ovarian carcinoma through prophylactic oophorectomy but, moreover, will receive protection of about 50 per cent against breast cancer. These issues are highlighted in this book.

The 32 chapters begin with Timothy Bishop's opening chapter, which depicts the three distinct sources of information about hereditary cancer. These are families with cancers that are rare in the general population but nevertheless show phenomenal increases in cancer in mutation carriers, families with 'common' cancers that occur in marked excess and manifest at an earlier age in the subject families than in the general population, and finally those at the population level where there is an increased empirical risk to relatives of cancer probands.

Certain classical hereditary cancer syndromes are given ample coverage, such as retinoblastoma and the *Rb* causal mutation in Chapter 6 by Christopher Mitchell, and neurofibromatosis types 1 and 2 and the respective *NF1* and *NF2* mutations in Chapter 7 by Susan M. Huson and Aurelia Norton. Charis Eng and Bruce A.J. Ponder provide an exhaustive coverage of multiple endocrine neoplasia type 2. Throughout the text, examples of hereditary cancer syndromes receive thorough coverage of the salient clinical, genetic, molecular (when pertinent) and screening/management issues.

Bringing all of this together, one might consider 'pattern recognition', which employs the cardinal principles of hereditary cancer; this can be effectively employed to aid in hereditary cancer syndrome recognition. It requires gathering a comprehensive cancer family history, including cancers of all anatomic sites and age of cancer onset, with emphasis on multiple primary cancers and the pattern of certain cancers such as carcinoma of the breast and ovary in the hereditary breast–ovarian cancer syndrome, carcinoma of the colon, particularly proclivity to the proximal colon, and endometrial carcinoma in HNPCC (Lynch syndrome), medullary thyroid carcinoma and phaeochromocytoma, often bilateral, in the MEN 2A and 2B syndromes. Distinguishing pathology findings, such as an excess of medullary features, aneuploidy, and a deficit of estrogen receptor positivity in *BRCA1* vs tubular-lobular histology excess in *BRCA2*, and the presence of a germline mutation will then constitute the diagnosis of a hereditary cancer syndrome.

Many confounders may obfuscate hereditary cancer syndrome diagnosis and thereby limit surveillance, management and control. One of the most important of these is the variable gene penetrance of many cancer-prone mutations. The presence of phenocopies may also confound the diagnosis of a hereditary cancer syndrome. In addition to these genetic uncertainties, the family history may be obscured by false paternity or other incorrect or incomplete family history information. Diagnosis can also be confused by the prolific phenotypic and genotypic heterogeneity which is characteristic of countless hereditary cancer syndromes. The authors carefully consider these issues.

We are likely to identify a potpourri of low-penetrant genes such as those comparable to the I1307K Ashkenazi Jewish mutation predisposing to colorectal cancer and the *MYH* gene which poses a recessive mode of colon cancer in FAP with colonic adenomas, or the *CHEK2* gene predisposing to a form of hereditary breast and colon cancer. Thus, in certain of these low-penetrant mutations, we may be compelled to initiate lifetime regimens of surveillance and possibly we may even wish to perform surgical prophylaxis on an individual with reduced penetrance of an otherwise cancer-causing mutation, who thereby may never manifest the cancer phenotype. This book carefully examines all of these issues.

This book is a 'must' for physicians, particularly medical, surgical and gynecologic oncologists, as well as genetic counsellors, molecular geneticists, medical social workers and basic scientists, particularly those dealing with molecular genetics and carcinogenesis. Indeed, it is difficult to find a specialty in medicine where this book would not be of benefit.

This text provides a good grounding in this subject for people of diverse disciplines. In this fast moving field, this is a good basis from which to go into more depth into the subject.

Henry T. Lynch MD
Professor and Chairman
Department of Preventive Medicine
Creighton University School of Medicine
Omaha, Nebraska
USA
July 2004

Preface

We are entering an era of genomic medicine in which conditions are starting to be defined by their underlying genomic changes. It is becoming increasingly clear that many diseases arise as a result of a genetic predisposition, either alone, or in conjunction with environmental changes which may exert greater effects on certain genetic backgrounds. Genetic predisposition to disease is also starting to have an effect on the type and efficacy of the treatment delivered. The practice of oncology is one of the mainstream areas of medicine where genomics will impact upon the care of a common condition. This book aims to inform health care practitioners in the field of oncology in the following areas: the basis of genetic predisposition, the cancer syndromes, the genetic basis of predisposition to the common cancers, early detection and management, and the ethicolegal and psychosocial issues surrounding the subject of genetic predisposition to cancer. We hope that this second edition of *Genetic Predisposition to Cancer* will be of interest to all those within the multidisciplinary team who work with cancer patients and their relatives.

Rosalind A. Eeles
Douglas F. Easton
Bruce A.J. Ponder
Charis Eng
July 2004

Acknowledgements

All the authors are grateful to the patients and families who have participated in studies that have informed this book, and to members of our laboratories and collaborators.

The editors' laboratories are funded by the National Institutes of Health, American Cancer Society, US Department of Defense, Susan G. Komen Foundation, Mary Kay Ash Charitable Foundation, V Foundation, The Prostate Cancer Charitable Trust, Cancer Research UK, the Monte Carlo Cancer Challenge, Hugh Knowles/Tony Maxse Fund, The Ronald and Rita McAulay Foundation, MRC UK, The Royal Marsden NHS Foundation Trust and the Institute of Cancer Research.

Professor Bruce Ponder is a Gibb Fellow of Cancer Research UK.

Professor Charis Eng is a Doris Duke Distinguished Clinical Scientist.

Professor Douglas Easton is a Principal Research Fellow of Cancer Research UK.

Dr Rosalind Eeles is a Reader at The Institute of Cancer Research, UK

Glossary

Allele	Alternative sequences at a locus (can be coding or non-coding).
Alpha (α)	The proportion of families linked to a particular locus.
Alternative splicing	Alternative forms of mRNA produced by splicing at different points in heterologous nuclear RNA.
Alu	A short interspersed repeat about 300 bp long homologous to 5' and 3' ends of 7SL RNA. Conserved across all primates.
Antisense	A nucleotide sequence complementary to the coding sequence (sense strand).
Apoptosis	Programmed cell death; an active mechanism of cell death in which DNA degradation and nuclear destruction precede loss of plasma membrane integrity and cell necrosis.
Autosome	A chromosome which is not a sex chromosome (X or Y).
Bayesian analysis	A method of calculating posterior probability from prior probability.
Candidate gene	A gene that is considered to be a contender for the cause of a disease.
cDNA	DNA complementary to RNA and synthesized from it by reverse transcription.
Centimorgan (cM)	A measure of genetic distance. One cM is the distance over which the probability of recombination is 1%.
Centromere	Specific DNA sequences at the joining of the p and q arms of a chromosome which attach it to the mitotic spindle.
Chromosome	Packages of chromatin in the cell nucleus that contain the DNA.
Cloning	The generation of multiple identical copies of a DNA sequence by replication in a suitable vector.
Codon	A triplet of nucleotides coding for one amino acid.
Constitutional	Present in every cell of the body.
Contiguous gene syndrome	A syndrome with several phenotypic features, which is due to an alteration (e.g. large deletion) affecting more than one tightly linked gene.
Cosmid	A vector that replicates like a plasmid but can be packaged *in vitro* into phage coats.
C-terminus	The terminus of the protein corresponding to the 3' end of the gene.
Cytogenetics	Analysis of chromosome structure.
Deletion	Loss of a segment of DNA.
Deoxyribose nucleic acid (DNA)	The building block molecule of genetic material.
Disomy	Two copies of a particular chromosome (also monosomy, trisomy).
Dominant	A disorder in which only one allele at a locus is needed for a phenotypic effect.
Dominant oncogene	An oncogene which only has to be altered in one allele at a locus to have an oncogenic effect.
Epistasis	Where genetic alterations at more than one locus are required to cause strong susceptibility ('gene–gene' interaction).

Exon	Transcribed sequence not spliced out of mature RNAs.
Frameshift	A deletion or insertion that results in a shift in the reading of sets of the three bases (codons). This usually results in a stop codon being created downstream.
Gene	DNA sequence that becomes transcribed and then translated into protein.
Genetic map	A representation of a chromosome in which the distances between loci are genetic distances (cM) rather than physical distances.
Genome	Genetic component of a cell.
Genotype	The hereditary information encoded by DNA: the combination of alleles or haplotypes at a given locus.
Germline	In the DNA of every cell and inherited from the parents.
Haplotype	The combination of alleles on a single chromosome at several linked loci.
Hardy–Weinberg equilibrium	The genotypic probabilities that occur in a random mating population.
Hemizygous	Only one parental copy of the gene is present (usually in a tumour).
Heterogeneity	Where several genes can each independently cause the same disease phenotype (locus heterogeneity) or where several mutations in the same gene can cause the same disease (allelic heterogeneity).
Heterozygous	The two alleles at a locus in an individual differ.
Homogeneity	A disease entity is only due to one gene.
Homologous	Areas of the genome that have similar sequences.
Homozygous	The alleles at a locus are identical.
Hotspot	A site in a gene that is commonly mutated.
Human Genome Project	An international effort to sequence the Human Genetic Code.
Hybridization	The basepairing of complementary single strands of nucleic acid that leads to a double stranded molecule.
Imprinting	Where parental origin affects the expression of a gene.
Intron	Transcribed sequences spliced out of mature RNA.
Karyotype	The chromosomal composition of a cell.
Kilobase (kb)	1000 bases.
Kindred	A family (also termed a pedigree).
Library	Collection of different cDNAs or genomic DNA fragments propagated in a cloning vector.
Linkage	Co-segregation of two genetic loci (because they lie close together on a chromosome) at a greater frequency than would be expected by chance.
Linkage disequilibrium	Association between a disease and a marker allele, or two marker alleles, owing to founder effects in closed populations.
Locus (pl. loci)	Position on a chromosome.
LOD score	A measure of the evidence for linkage. Logarithm to the base 10 of the ratio of the probability of the observed data given linkage divided by the probability of the observed data given no linkage. LOD score of >3 is often taken as convincing evidence for linkage.
Logistic regression	A method of statistical analysis used to evaluate the association by a binary variable (e.g. disease status) and one or more covariates (e.g. polymorphisms).
Loss of heterozygosity (LOH)	Loss of one allele at a heterozygous locus reducing it to hemizygosity.
Physical mapping	A map based on actual distances in base pairs between loci.
Genetic mapping	A map where distances between loci are based on recombination frequency.
Microsatellites	Runs of short repeat sequences, such as dinucleotide repeats (CACACA), tri- or tetra-nucleotide repeats.

Minisatellites	Runs of longer repeat sequences, such as VNTRs (variable number of tandem repeats).
Missense	A mutation where one base pair is replaced by another.
Mitotic recombination	Recombination occurring during mitosis.
Mosaic	The presence of different genotypes.
mRNA	Messenger RNA; the product of DNA transcription and splicing that serves as a template for protein translation.
Mutation	An alteration in DNA sequence.
Non-disjunction	Failure of chromatid sequences to separate during mitosis.
Nonsense	An alteration in DNA sequence resulting in the formation of a stop codon, which results in premature termination of translation into protein.
Northern analysis	Technique to identify RNA molecules to analyse gene expression.
N-terminus	The terminus of the protein corresponding to the 5′ end of a gene.
Open reading frame (ORF)	A sequence of translatable codons not interrupted by stop codons (codes for a polypeptide).
p arm	The short arm of a chromosome.
PAC	P1 artificial chromosome.
Pedigree	A family tree.
Penetrance	The chance that a disease will occur as a result of the presence of a predisposing mutation.
Phage	A virus that replicates in bacteria.
Phase	The ability to determine the pattern of inheritance of markers unambiguously.
Phenocopy	An individual who has the disease but does not have the disease-predisposing mutation (i.e. a sporadic case).
Phenotype	The physical or biochemical effect of the genotype (e.g. occurrence of a certain type of cancer).
Plasmid	A double-stranded circle of DNA capable of being anonymously replicated in bacteria.
Pleiotropy	Where several phenotypic features are caused by the same mutation.
Point mutation	Substitution of one base by another.
Polymerase chain reaction (PCR)	An *in vitro* method that uses enzyme synthesis to exponentially amplify DNA sequences.
Polymorphism	Alternative forms of a DNA sequence occurring naturally in a population.
Posterior probability	A probability where the prior probability is conditioned according to circumstances. For example, the probability that the person being considered in the pedigree will have the predisposing mutation given all the information available, including the age of the individual and number and type of affected relatives.
Prior probability	The chance that the pedigree has a predisposition gene.
Proband	The initially ascertained case in a pedigree.
Probe	A short specific DNA sequence with a marker label (e.g. radioactivity) that can be used to detect complementary sequences in 'test' DNA.
Pulse-field gel electrophoresis	Electrophoresis during which the orientation of the electric field is altered in time. It separates large pieces of DNA of up to 2000 kb.
Purine	Adenine (A) or Guanine (G).
Pyrimidine	Cytosine (C) or Thymine (T) (or, in RNA, Uracil (U)).
q arm	The long arm of a chromosome.

Recessive	A disorder in which the gene can only exert a phenotypic effect if both alleles are altered.
Recessive oncogene	Tumour suppressor gene; both alleles at a locus have to be altered to have an oncogenic effect.
Recombination	Crossing over at meiosis resulting in the formation of a different haplotype.
Restriction fragment length polymorphism (RFLP)	A polymorphism in the size of restriction fragments after cutting by a bacterial enzyme due to sequence differences between alleles at cutting sites.
Segregation	Co-inheritance, e.g. of a disease and a genetic marker.
SNP	Single nucleotide polymorphism.
Somatic cell hybrid	Formed by fusing the cells from two different species or by fusing the cells of one species with microcells of another that contain one or a few donor chromosomes. A cell line is then established which contains a set of donor chromosomes.
Southern analysis	A technique of fixing DNA to a nylon or other synthetic membrane. Usually the DNA is digested with a restriction enzyme and the DNA fragments are separated by electrophoresis, denatured and transferred by blotting on to a nylon membrane. A labelled probe will hybridize to a complementary sequence on the membrane.
Splice acceptor site	Boundary between intron and exon at the 5′ end of the exon.
Sporadic	A cancer case occurring in a person who is not a germline mutation carrier.
Stop codon	A codon that codes to end the translation of coding sequence into protein.
STS	Sequence tagged site.
Susceptible	An at-risk individual.
Telomere	Either end of the chromosome.
Theta (θ)	Symbol often used for the recombination fraction.
Transcription	Conversion of DNA into RNA.
Transition	Conversion of a purine base into another purine or pyrimidine into a pyrimidine.
Translation	Conversion of RNA into protein.
Translocation	The attachment of part of one chromosome arm on to another.
Transversion	Conversion of a purine base into a pyrimidine or vice versa.
Tumour suppressor gene	See 'Recessive oncogene'.
Vector	An independently replicated DNA molecule into which specific DNA sequence can be integrated and replicated.
Western analysis	A technique for analysing proteins.
5′	The end of the gene from which transcription starts.
3′	The end of the gene at which transcription ends.

Basic principles

Genetic predisposition to cancer: an introduction

D. TIMOTHY BISHOP

INTRODUCTION

Evidence that inherited susceptibility plays a role in the risk of malignancy comes from three separate sources of information. The sources are as follows.

1 The observation that, in some syndromes, which are rare in the general population, but which are clearly genetic, there is a dramatically increased risk of cancer in carriers of the mutation(s). Often these syndromes predispose to cancers that are especially rare within the general population.
2 The observation that, occasionally, families are found that contain a number of cases of 'common' cancers and, even though these cancers are prevalent in the general population, the number of such cases in these families far exceeds the number predicted by population rates. Often these cancers occur at ages earlier than seen in the general population, and family members have an increased occurrence of synchronous and metachronous lesions.
3 The observation that, on a population level, there is an increased risk of cancer to relatives of cases; in many cases, the relatives are at increased risk of the same cancer, although relatives may also be at increased risk of other cancers.

To make this list more precise by defining 'rare' vs. 'common' is not necessary, since there would doubtless be counter-examples to any 'rules'; the list is intended to define the nature of the observations. Each of these three categories requires further detail (which will be discussed in subsequent chapters for specific cancer sites), but broadly we can say that the clarity of the role that genetic susceptibility plays ranges from the most straightforward (category 1) to the most indirect (category 3). In the first category, rare inherited syndromes have been recognized where genes are obviously important simply by examining the pattern of occurrence of disease within families. By definition, these syndromes are rare, since it is the unusual occurrence of multiple cases in the same family that brings the syndrome to attention. In category 3, family aggregation alone could be attributable to genes shared by family members, exposure to the same non-genetic risk factors or the interactive effects of genetic and environmental exposures. The understanding of these risks to relatives is the focus of much current research. Syndromes from the first type of observation indicate the occurrence of genetic mutations, which produce an inordinate risk for a carrier, but, among the general public, few persons have that predisposition; the documentation of such syndromes indicates that they explain a fraction of a percent of all cancers. At the other extreme, the third category of observation leaves open the possibility that genes could play a role in the majority of cancer occurrence. The net result is that, while we can elaborate on the mechanisms of inherited susceptibility, it is impossible to say with any precision the extent of inherited susceptibility, i.e. to say the proportion of each cancer that is directly attributed to inherited susceptibility. Estimates usually provided are based on rare, highly penetrant predisposition.

Table 1.1 *Examples of the 'rare' syndromes associated with an increased risk of malignancy and their mode of inheritance*

Syndrome	Neoplasia or malignancy	Risk[a]	Frequency[b]	Mode[c]	Location and gene name	References
Neurofibromatosis Type 1	Plexiform		1/3000	D	17q *NFI*	6
	Neurofibroma	<4%				
	Optic glioma	<15%				7
Familial Polyposis Coli	Bowel cancer	~100%	1/8000	D	5q21 *APC*	8–10
	Cancer of duodenum	NA				
Von Hippel Lindau	Cerebellar		1/35 000	D	3p *VHL*	11
	Haemangioblastoma	84%				
	Retinal angioma	70%				
	Renal cell carcinoma	69%				
Ataxia Telangiectasia	Lymphoma	60%	1/40 000	R	11q22–q23 *ATM*	12
	Leukaemia	27%				
Multiple Endocrine Neoplasia 2A	Medullary carcinoma of thyroid	70%	1/300 000	D	10q11.2 *RET*	13 14
	Phaeochromocytoma	50%				15

NA, not available.

[a] Lifetime risk of neoplasia or cancer.

[b] The estimated population frequency at birth of individuals with this syndrome.

[c] Mode of inheritance is classified as 'autosomal dominant' (D) or 'autosomal recessive' (R).

Rare syndromes

Many rare syndromes predispose to cancer (Table 1.1). In his catalogue of inherited disorders, McKusick[1] lists several hundred that feature cancer susceptibility. We recognize that these syndromes are due to a mutated gene within each family because relatives are observed to have either the same type of cancer or one of a limited list of other cancers, even though this syndrome is rare in the general population. The genetic relationships of affected relatives to each other forms a recognizable 'pattern', which indicates the mode of action of the responsible gene. For instance, some rare syndromes have the following readily recognizable feature: one parent is affected and on average one half of all of the offspring of an affected parent also have the syndrome, but the precise number affected in each family is variable (some will have none affected, some will have all); grandchildren with an affected grandparent but an unaffected parent are less likely to be affected. Such a pattern suggests that the syndrome is due to a single gene in each family, since the relationship between affected individuals is consistent with a mutation in a gene (where the frequency of the mutation among the general public is rare) and where mutation carriers have an extremely high risk of the disease (and/or cancer). We call such syndromes highly penetrant (since carriers have a high risk of disease) dominant syndromes (since only a single copy of the mutated gene is required for the disease to be expressed).

In many instances, these syndromes have been identified because the syndromes lead to malignancies that are 'rare' in the general population and that, when observed in close relatives, are particularly noticeable. For instance, while childhood retinoblastoma is the commonest malignant ocular tumour, it affects only 1/20 000 children.[2] However, in retinoblastoma due to inherited susceptibility, about 90 per cent of gene carriers develop a tumour so, in such families, approximately 45 per cent of children of parental carriers of the mutation will also develop retinoblastoma (one half will inherit the mutation and, of these, 90 per cent will develop retinoblastoma). Multiple endocrine neoplasia type 2A, another dominant syndrome, is characterized by predisposition to medullary thyroid carcinoma and phaeochromocytoma.[2] These latter tumours develop in approximately one half of the patients and about 10 per cent of the lesions are malignant. Again the rarity of the tumours in the general population, but the increased prevalence in some families, provides evidence in favour of a genetic aetiology.

In other cases, there are other phenotypes associated with the syndrome that are particularly overt. The recognizable characteristic of the syndromes may itself be the indirect reason for susceptibility to malignancy. For instance, in familial adenomatous polyposis (FAP), a dominantly inherited disorder, carriers develop hundreds or even thousands of adenomas in the bowel. These are apparent from the second decade of life, and increase in number and size until eventually the bowel must be removed. Adenomas, while themselves benign, are thought to be the precursor lesion of most, if not all, colorectal cancers and carriers develop colorectal cancer, on average, during their fifth decade of life. Estimates of the prevalence of polyposis vary widely but, in one of the most respected studies, Bülow[3] calculated that the carrier frequency is 1 in 8000 live births.

Table 1.2 *A list of examples of syndromes associated with increased risk of malignancy where the major site associated with the syndrome is a 'common' cancer. For none of these sites are there currently precise estimates as to their frequency. The references refer only to the mapping and cloning of the genes, or the estimation of penetrance associated with the mutations*

Reference name	Malignancies	Risk of cancer[a]	Location	Gene name	References
Melanoma	Melanoma	67%[b]	9p13–p22	CDKN2A	16–18 (see also Chapter 17)
Breast/Ovary Syndrome	Breast and ovary	50–97%	17q21	BRCA1	19, 20 (see also Chapter 19)
		25–45%	13q12	BROA2	
HNPCC	Colon and endometrium	50–90%	2p2q	hMSH2	21–24 (see also Chapter 24)
			3p7q, 5q	hMLH1, MSH6	21, 25–27
Muir–Torre Syndrome	As HNPCC with skin lesions				28 (see also Chapter 24)
Li–Fraumeni Syndrome	Brain tumours	75–90%[c]	17p13	TP53	29 (see also Chapter 11)
	Early-onset breast cancer				
	Sarcomas				
	Adrenocortical carcinoma				

HNPCC, hereditary non-polyposis colorectal cancer.

[a] The risk is either the 'lifetime risk' as quoted in the referenced articles, or the 'risk to age 70 years' in those studies which have performed detailed age-specific calculations. Where possible, a per-site risk is given; in the absence of such figures, a 'syndrome' penetrance estimate is provided.

[b] Risk to age 80 years.

[c] 75% by age 60 in men; 90% by age 60 in women.

The implication of such syndromes is that, within each family, the inheritance of a single mutated allele is sufficient to predispose to the syndrome. There is a separate class of syndromes that should also be mentioned. These syndromes are characterized by failure to deal appropriately with DNA damage either through increased sensitivity to the damaging agent or through an inability to repair the damage. Many of these syndromes are recessively inherited, meaning that to be at increased risk of cancer, a person must carry mutations on both alleles of this gene. Recessively inherited syndromes also have a recognizable pattern of inheritance within families in that brothers or sisters of cases are particularly at risk of the syndrome while parents and offspring essentially never express it. Among such syndromes, ataxia telangiectasia is an autosomal recessive disorder, which has a frequency of about 1 in 40 000 live births. Persons with the recessive phenotype have a 10–20 per cent chance of developing malignancy. Often these malignancies are lymphoma or leukaemia, although there are increased risks later in life for epithelial carcinomas.[2]

Rare families showing aggregation to common cancers

We expect to find families containing several cases of 'common' cancers; such families must sometimes occur by chance. However, in some families, the excess is particularly noticeable, especially if the cancer onset occurs particularly early in life (as compared to the general population) or if bilateral tumours are frequently reported in family members. Observations in this area involve the recognition of families with an 'unusual' combination of cancers, the particular configuration of cancer cases being extremely rare under the age- and sex-specific rates of the general population. The identification of a number of such families, which show similar characteristics in terms of the spectrum of cancers recognized and the ages at which the cancers occur, suggests a 'syndrome'. In some families, family members seem to be predisposed to malignancies at the same site, while in other families, susceptibility applies to a number of different sites (Table 1.2). The two cancers that have received the most interest in this area are colorectal cancer and breast cancer.

For colorectal cancer, the work of Dr Henry Lynch and colleagues is particularly notable. Lynch obtained detailed family history information of cancer and followed 'interesting' leads. Many of these searches led to publications reporting extensive families, which showed evidence of dominantly inherited susceptibility to cancer extending over many generations (see e.g. Lynch[4]). Of course, many of the distant relatives within the families were unaware of each other's disease state or even of the existence of such distant relatives; this provides further evidence that genetic factors play a major role. Following families with a family history of colorectal cancer sometimes led to identifying previously unrecognized familial polyposis families, but also led to the observation of families with none of the characteristic phenotypic features of polyposis, but in which the average age of onset of colorectal cancer was similar. Observation of a large number of such families prompted Lynch to propose two characteristic patterns. In the first, labelled Lynch Syndrome I, predisposition is to colorectal cancer alone, while in Lynch Syndrome II, predisposition is predominantly to colorectal and endometrial cancer, although authors differ in their acknowledgement as to the other cancers contained under the definition. The generic term for both syndromes is 'hereditary non-polyposis colorectal cancer' (HNPCC), acknowledging the lack of the usual phenotypic marker associated with polyposis. Lynch Syndrome II is also often termed 'cancer family syndrome'.

For breast cancer, examination of families shows at least two types of families; in some, female gene carriers are at high risk (over 80 per cent over a lifetime) of breast or ovarian cancer, while in others only breast cancer is observed. There is still a debate as to whether such families truly represent a separate syndrome, or whether susceptibility is to both breast and ovarian cancers, but, by chance, no female relatives have developed ovarian cancer. Susceptibility is again due to a rare autosomal dominant mutation.

Population studies

Analytical epidemiological studies of cancer often involve the interviewing of cases with a particular tumour and controls (individuals with a similar age and of the same sex as cases but without a diagnosed tumour). The same questions are asked of the cases and the controls, and the answers of the two groups compared. A significant difference in response may suggest that the focus of the questions is involved in the disease process either as a risk factor or as a reflection of the disease state. Many of these studies have considered the question of family history by asking if 'the person being questioned has a relative with the same tumour'. Often attention is focused on first-degree relatives (parents, brothers and sisters, children) and the presence of a first-degree relative with the tumour is noted. A person has a positive family history if one or more of the relatives has indeed been diagnosed with a tumour at the defined site previously.

For cancer, the majority of such studies have indeed shown that cases more frequently have a positive family history than controls and often the ratio is between two and four (although there are notable exceptions outside this range). An alternative way of thinking about this ratio is to interpret it as the increased risk to relatives of cases as compared to relatives of controls; strictly speaking the equivalence of these two interpretations is not always exact but for the examples considered here, the similarity is sufficient.

Several general findings can be made for the common cancers. First, the absolute risk of cancer in the relative of a case is inversely proportional to the age of onset of the interviewed case. Thus, the earlier the age of onset of that case, the higher age-specific risk is observed in the relatives. For cases diagnosed around the median age of onset of that cancer or later, the increased risk to the relatives is usually minimal. For instance, in the Cancer and Steroid Hormone Study (CASH) performed in the USA during the early 1980s, almost 5000 women diagnosed with breast cancer before the age of 55 years were interviewed about their family history of cancer. The risk of breast cancer being diagnosed in sisters of cases diagnosed before the age of 55 years was estimated to be 3.7% by age 50 years as compared to 1.8% for the general female population. Second, the risk to relatives of cases depends upon the number of cases diagnosed in the family to date. Specifically, a family with two first-degree relatives affected leads to a considerably larger risk than when only one first-degree relative is affected. For instance, again in the CASH study, the risk up to age 50 years to sisters of cases diagnosed before age 55 years who also had an affected mother was estimated to be 12.2%.

As mentioned above, these studies are not able to resolve the reasons for the increased risk to relatives. We would suspect, on the basis of those families with obvious inherited predisposition, that some of the family aggregation must be due to one or more cancer predisposition genes. However, there are usually no simple methods for deciding the proportion of such cases due to a genetic cause.

IDENTIFYING GENES ASSOCIATED WITH RISK OF CANCER

There are two approaches to identifying genes that predispose to cancer. The first and simplest approach conceptually is applicable when a known gene is considered to be a likely candidate for being predisposing. This gene can then be sequenced in both affected ('cases') and unaffected individuals ('controls') and, if functional mutations are shown to occur more frequently in cases than controls, then this suggests that this candidate gene is actually involved in susceptibility. Practically, this approach is often not feasible unless mutations are easy to detect because of the resources required for mutation detection on a large scale but, in theory, the approach is straightforward. Such studies are termed 'case-control studies' or 'association studies'.

The second approach is applicable when there are no clues to the particular chromosome on which the disease gene lies. The approach is based on the knowledge that genes that are physically located on the same chromosome are not inherited independently of each other from one generation to the next, while genes that are located on separate chromosomes will be independently inherited. So, if a disease gene is located adjacent to another gene, and this correlation in inheritance is observed and we are aware of the genetic location of the other gene, then this will be sufficient to tell us the location of the disease gene. This approach has been enhanced greatly over the last 10 years with the identification of thousands of DNA sequences (some of which are part of genes, most of which are not), which have now been characterized so the degree of variation among the general population for that sequence is known as is the genetic location; we term such sequences 'DNA markers'. By screening large numbers of DNA markers until one or more that co-segregates with the disease is identified, we initially identify regions in which the disease gene does not lie until one in which it does lie is found. Such approaches, which are often termed 'linkage analyses', are also resource intensive, requiring the collection of DNA from families with multiple cases of cancer and often the typing of a large number of such markers. Molecular techniques involving the identification of genes adjacent to these DNA markers are subsequently applied to identify the precise gene involved.

ASSOCIATION STUDIES

While linkage studies are an efficient method of identifying genes with an high penetrance, they are much less efficient at finding genes in which one or more genotypes have risks which are only double or triple that of other genotypes. Association studies are particularly relevant for studies of genetic variants, which are common in the general population (e.g. more than 2 per cent of the general population carry the higher risk genotypes whose effect is to double a person's risk of cancer). Currently, such studies are limited to genes involved in pathways with apparent biological relevance for the cancer in question, for example, steroid hormone levels and prostate cancer, ability to detoxify tobacco smoke-derived carcinogens and lung cancer, or skin tone and melanoma. Such studies, which typically involve at least several hundred cases and a similar number of controls (persons of similar age, from the same geographical region and with a similar gender, racial and ethnic mix), investigate variants in the genes of interest. The distribution of genotypes among the cases is compared to that of the controls with significant differences taken as being indicative that the gene of interest may have a role in the aetiology of the cancer.

Such interpretations need to be treated with some caution, however. For instance, there are some concerns that, within the general population, there may be a number of genetically distinct groups or strata, which have differing genotype frequencies and inherently different risks of disease. Thus, a study that inadvertently collected cases that came from one group while the cases in fact came from a separate group would find evidence that the genes of interest differed in frequency between cases and controls. This observation would promote the interpretation of causality when in fact it simply reflected the genetic structure of the population. Racial and/or ethnic groupings are an obvious example of such genetic differences. However, recent evidence suggests that the differences within populations may be at least as great as those between racial or ethnic groups. The concern, therefore, is more that such genetic stratification exists within a population and has not been recognized. Such concerns have probably been overplayed within the literature as there are few objective data indicating that this is a real problem in practice.

A second issue with respect to interpretation is the evidence that the gene being considered is actually the causative gene. Genetic mutations arise on a single copy of a chromosome. If this mutation is associated with an increased risk of cancer so that it is found in a number of cases, then genetic variants at genes adjacent to the causative gene will also show the same association. The extent of this effect depends upon the number of generations since the mutation arose and the genetic distance between the gene under consideration as well as the frequencies of the differing alleles in the population. Genes in closer proximity will tend to show a larger effect; this is called 'linkage disequilibrium'. It is, therefore, not certain that the gene under consideration is actually the causative gene, so knowledge of the other genes in the proximity may be important. A third, more subtle issue may be the relevance of the actual mutation being assayed. The mutation may be the critical variant or it may be another mutation in linkage disequilibrium with that mutation. Such an issue can be an extremely difficult issue to resolve, as the actual critical mutation may be more difficult to identify, especially if it involves a mutation in the promoter region or a mutation that modifies splicing. Often such issues can only be resolved when the functional significance of the protein and its various mutations is known.

A final issue concerns the nature of the mutations being considered. Mutations in, for instance, BRCA1, which have been identified in multiple case families, are often protein truncating, indicative of a quantitative reduction in the availability of the full-length protein. Other types of mutations may be more difficult to interpret. For instance, point mutations in CDKN2A gene that predispose to melanoma.

MECHANISMS OF ACTION OF PREDISPOSING GENES

For many of these syndromes described in Part 2 of this book, the genes have usually been mapped and in many cases characterized. The identification of these genes has been important scientifically because mechanisms of carcinogenesis have been elaborated with the aid of these syndromes. For instance, retinoblastoma and familial polyposis represent mutations in tumour suppressor genes, genes that have the responsibility within the cell of suppressing growth or cellular proliferation. They are regarded as the 'brakes' of the system. Mutations within these genes are thought to inactivate the genes so that their slowing down effect is lost and less restricted cellular proliferation follows. Multiple endocrine neoplasia type 2 is caused by mutations in a proto-oncogene, a class of genes that play a role in the normal cellular growth and differentiation. In the mutated form, they act as 'accelerators' to the process. Germline mutations in either of these two classes are rare in the general population but somatic changes may be common in tumours that arise outside of the context inherited predisposition. For instance, somatic changes of the *APC* gene (mutations in which cause familial polyposis coli) are found in more than 60 per cent of all colorectal carcinomas.

COLORECTAL CANCER AS AN EXAMPLE

For some cancers, the three categories of observations have been made and produce interesting conclusions. In this section, we focus on colorectal cancer because evidence of predisposition can be made at each level. We have already described how some people have a germline mutation in the *APC* gene resulting in the proliferation of adenomatous polyps throughout the colon. This syndrome, termed 'familial adenomatous polyposis', is a rare autosomal dominant disease with a carrier frequency for the mutation of 1 in 8000 individuals. In a survey of colorectal cancer cases diagnosed under the age of 45 years, 4 out of 80 such cases were found to be due to familial polyposis coli (Hall, personal communication).

A second syndrome that predisposes to colorectal cancer is HNPCC. Recent linkage analysis has shown that there are at least six genes implicated; the majority is due to two mutations, either of which can produce HNPCC. One of these genes has been shown to lie on chromosome 2 and the other on chromosome 3. Subsequently, these two genes have been cloned and shown to be involved in DNA repair, so mutations in these genes are presumably important because such cells are unable to repair DNA damage efficiently. Genetic analysis suggests that, in the majority of families with the disease, HNPCC is due to one of these mutations. While the occurrence of the disease in the majority of the HNPCC families is due to these genes, we would like to estimate the proportion of all colorectal cancer cases that arise in the context of this syndrome. In a survey of 525 cases of colorectal cancer, diagnosed at any age, St John *et al.* identified four families with apparent evidence of HNPCC through a detailed examination of the family history of cancer occurrence in relatives of index cases.[5] They conclude that this syndrome accounts for perhaps 1 per cent of all colorectal cancer. This estimate may be a little on the low side because, by chance, families with a mutation in one of the HNPCC genes may not have produced a sufficient number of colorectal cancer cases to be identified in this way.

While these two syndromes are associated with highly increased risks of colorectal cancer, as can be seen from the population studies (assuming that the majority of polyposis coli patients will develop cancer before the age of 45 years), together they account for probably 2 or 3 per cent of all colorectal cancer. In the study performed by St John, cancers diagnosed in family members were verified as far as possible through medical and pathological records.[5] Examination of the risk of colorectal cancer in relatives showed that, overall, relatives had a 2.4-fold increased risk of colorectal cancer as compared to the general population. The risks for parents, and brothers and sisters of cases were similarly elevated, and the risk of colorectal cancer depended upon the age of onset of the interviewed case. Relatives of cases diagnosed before the age of 45 years had a lifetime risk of colorectal cancer of 12 per cent (to age 80 years), while relatives of cases diagnosed after the age of 65 years had a lifetime risk of 4 per cent, so that there is clear evidence that colorectal cancer still aggregates in families over and above these two syndromes.

This family aggregation of 'common' colorectal cancer could be due to inherited susceptibility, but the mechanism would be different from that presented by these two syndromes. These syndromes described previously are clearly due to rare mutations that have a major effect on risk of colorectal cancer; observation of families suggests that the lifetime risk of cancer for someone who has one of these mutations approaches 100 per cent from *APC* mutations. Such high risks associated with another mutation are not consistent with the data, but could be consistent with a more frequent mutation, which has a more moderate effect on cancer risk. One gene that is thought to be a candidate for playing a role in susceptibility is the *GSTM1* gene. Cytosolic glutathione S-transferases catalyse the conjugation of glutathione to a variety of electrophilic compounds, including carcinogens, and one of the four classes of this gene family is termed the mu family. Because of the function of these genes, they have been considered to be potentially functionally involved in risk determination. In a recent survey, colorectal cancer cases were shown to have a different distribution of genotypes than random controls. This distinction was most noticeable when only cases with tumours of the proximal colon were considered. Their figures would suggest that carriers of a common *GSTM1* genotype would have a 1.5-fold increased risk of colorectal cancer and that about 40 per cent of the general population would have this common genotype. On this basis, almost 60 per cent of all colorectal cancers would occur in this 'higher'-risk group. A meta-analysis has cast doubt on this result,[30] but if the results of this study were confirmed, then this would represent a gene that contributed to 'common' colorectal cancer rather than through the rare syndromes. Of course, interaction with the appropriate environmental exposures must be important within this class of genes.

CLINICAL MANAGEMENT OF THOSE PREDISPOSED

The knowledge of the specific genes involved in predisposition provides important information to assist in the understanding of carcinogenesis. Clinical management needs to take into account the potential breadth of disease, the potential impact of specific aspects of the disease and the potential for impacting on the natural history of disease to minimize the morbidity for the person. Opportunities for management include screening surveillance, such as mammography at young ages for women with a strong family history of breast cancer, prophylactic surgery to remove the at-risk organ and, potentially for the future, chemoprevention (taking of drugs or supplements to reduce cancer risk). These approaches require taking into account ages of onset of disease, the actual risk of disease and the variation in expression of disease.

Genetic testing is feasible in some families currently. Typically, these are families in which a mutation can be found; finding mutations in these genes remains technically challenging with significant numbers of families remaining with unrecognized mutations. Without a mutation, risk assessment is based on the 50:50 transmission of dominant inheritance; with mutations, the risk assessment can be changed essentially to certainty (for mutation carrier status, of course, or risk of disease, since non-carriers should have population risks of cancer). In such circumstances, management can be focused on those with the inherited predisposition.

SUMMARY

In this chapter, we have attempted to elaborate some of the concepts of inherited susceptibility to cancer. The majority of these issues will be discussed in greater detail throughout the book. Broadly, we can say that the three types of observations that implicate the genetic factors range from the recognition of rare syndromes, which are clearly genetically determined but account for small percentages of all cancers, through to evidence that relatives of cases of a particular cancer have an increased risk of the same cancer. This latter category of observations has been consistently made for essentially all of the common cancers; currently we are not in a position to judge the importance of genetic factors to the familial susceptibility.

KEY POINTS

- There is incontrovertible evidence that genes predispose to cancer in some families. This evidence comes from the observation that, in a few families, the pattern of occurrence of cancer among family members is consistent with the inheritance of a mutated gene and carriers of this mutated gene have a high risk of cancer.
- For a number of these syndromes, the responsible gene(s) have been identified.
- Within the population, we also find strong evidence for family aggregation of the common cancers, over and above that attributable to the rare syndromes.
- There is considerable speculation concerning the causes of this family aggregation and particularly the possibility that 'common' mutations (but in this case only associated with moderate levels of risk) are the explanation.
- The effect of these genes might be particularly evident in the presence of other genetic or environmental exposures ('gene–environment interaction').

REFERENCES

1. McKusick VA, Francomano CA, Antonarakis SE. *Mendelian inheritance in man: catalogs of autosomal dominant, autosomal recessive and x-linked phenotypes,* 10th edn. Baltimore: Johns Hopkins University Press, 1992.
2. Hodgson SV, Maher ER. *A practical guide to human cancer genetics.* Cambridge: Cambridge University Press, 1993.
3. Bülow S. Familial polyposis coli. A clinical and epidemiological study. *Lægeforeningens Forlag* 1986; 3–52.
4. Lynch HT, Watson P, Kriegler M, *et al.* Differential diagnosis of hereditary nonpolyposis colorectal cancer (Lynch Syndrome I and Lynch Syndrome II). *Dis Col Rect* 1988; **31**:372–377.
5. St John DJB, McDermott FT, Hopper JL, *et al.* Cancer risk in relatives of patients with common colorectal cancer. *Ann Intern Med* 1993; **118**:785–790.
6. Huson SM, Compston DAS, Harper PS. A genetic study of von Recklinghausen neurofibromatosis in south east Wales II. Guidelines for genetic counselling. *J Med Genet* 1989; **26**:712–721.
7. Lewis RA, Riccardi VM, Gerson LP, *et al.* Von recklinghausen neurofibromatosis: II Incidence of optic-nerve gliomata. *Ophthalmology* 1984; **91**:929–935.
8. Alm I, Licznerski G. The intestinal polyposes. *Clin Gastroenterol* 1973; **2**:577–602.
9. Bodmer WF, Bailey CJ, Bodmer J, *et al.* Localization of the gene for familial adenomatous polyposis on chromosome 5. *Nature* 1987; **328**:614–616.
10. Groden J, Thliveris A, Samowitz W, *et al.* Identification and Characterization of the Familial Adenomatous Polyposis Coli Gene. *Cell* 1991; **66**:589–600.
11. Maher ER. Genetic mechanisms in von Hippel–Lindau disease. *Lancet* 1991; **337**:1478–1479.
12. Johnson JA. Ataxia telangiectasia and other a-fetoprotein-associated disorders. In Lynch HT, Hirayama T (ed.) *Genetic*

epidemiology of cancer. Boca Raton: CRC Press, 1989: 145–147.

13. Eng C, Stratton M, Ponder B, *et al.* Familial cancer syndromes. *Lancet* 1994; **343:**709–713.

14. Saad MF, Ordonez NG, Rashid RK, *et al.* Medullary carcinoma of the thyroid. A study of the clinical features and prognostic factors in 161 patients. *Medicine* 1984; **63:**319–342.

15. Mulligan LM, Knole JBJ, Healey CS, *et al.* Germ-line mutations of the *RET* proto-oncogene in multiple endocrine neoplasia type 2A. *Nature* 1993; **363:**458–460.

16. Cannon-Albright LA, Goldgar DE, Meyer LJ, *et al.* Assignment of a locus for familial melanoma, MLM, to chromosome 9p13–p22. *Science* 1992; **258:**1148–1152.

17. Bishop DT, Demenais F, Goldstein AM, *et al.* Geographical variation in the penetrance of *CDKN2A* mutations for melanoma. *J Natl Cancer Inst* 2002; **94:**894–903.

18. Nancarrow DJ, Mann GJ, Holland EA, *et al.* Confirmation of chromosome 9p linkage in familial melanoma. *Am J Hum Genet* 1993; **53:**936–942.

19. Miki Y, Swensen J, Shattuck-Eidens, *et al.* A strong candidate for the breast and ovarian cancer susceptibility gene *BRCA1.* *Science* 1994; **266:**66–71.

20. Antoniou A, Pharoah PD, Narod S, *et al.* Average risks of breast and ovarian cancer associated with *BRCA1* or *BRCA2* mutations detected in case Series unselected for family history: a combined analysis of 22 studies. *Am J Hum Genet* 2003; **72:**1117–1130.

21. Fishel R, Lescoe MK, Rao MRS, *et al.* The human mutator gene homolog *MSH2* and its association with hereditary nonpolyposis colon cancer. *Cell* 1993; **75:**1027–1038.

22. Leach FS, Nicolaides NC, Papadopoulos N, *et al.* Mutations of a *mutS* homolog in hereditary nonpolyposis colorectal cancer. *Cell* 1993; **75:**1215–1225.

23. Anderson DE. Risk in families of patients with colon cancer. In Winawer S, Schottenfeld D, Sherlock P (eds) *Colorectal cancer: prevention, epidemiology and screening.* New York: Raven Press, 1980:109–115.

24. Peltomäki P, Aaltonen LA, Sistonen P, *et al.* Genetic mapping of a locus predisposing to human colorectal cancer. *Science* 1993; **260:**810–812.

25. Bronner CE, Baker SM, Morrison PT, *et al.* Mutation in the DNA mismatch repair gene homologue hMLH1 is associated with hereditary non-polyposis colon cancer. *Nature* 1994; **368:**258–261.

26. Lindblom A, Tannerg'a'rd P, Werelius B, Nordenskjöld M. Genetic mapping of a second locus predisposing to hereditary non-polyposis colon cancer. *Nature Genet* 1993; **5:**279–282.

27. Papadopoulos N, Nicolaides NC, Wei Y-F, *et al.* Mutation of a *mutL* homolog in hereditary colon cancer. *Science* 1994; **263:**1625–1629.

28. Hall NR, Murday VA, Chapman P, *et al.* Genetic linkage in Muir–Torre Syndrome to the same chromosomal region as cancer family syndrome. *Eur J Cancer* 1994; **30A:**180–182.

29. Malkin D, Li FP, Strong LC, Fraumeni JF Jr, *et al.* Germ Line p53 Mutations in a familial syndrome of breast cancer, sarcomas, and other neoplasms. *Science* 1990; **250:**1233–1238.

30. Zhang S, Wyllie AH, Barnes D, *et al.* Relationship between the *GSTM1* genetic polymorphism and susceptibility to bladder, breast and colon cancer. *Carcinogenesis* 1993; **14:**1821–1824.

2

Biological basis of cancer predisposition

YVES-JEAN BIGNON

INTRODUCTION

Cancer is a multistep genetic process that occurs when a cancer cell divides. Knowledge of the steps and errors in our genomic book, leading to cancer, is fascinating, but still incomplete. The biological 'Holy Grail' would be to know the very first event leading to the inexorable progression of a normal cell to a malignant cell, and then to a malignant tumour. One clue lies in the genes involved in hereditary predisposition to cancer, since the very early embryo can be considered as genetically normal, except for one inherited mutated gene, which will lead to an increased risk of cancer, sometimes decades later in the person's life. This is a fruitful quest, but the 'Holy Grail' is still hidden in a more complex cancer process, involving the effects of mutations in possibly multiple genes with or without environmental factors, which may be interacting. Nevertheless, the genesis and biology of a tumour cell is now better understood, largely due to the study of the function of cancer predisposition genes. This will also provide new hope for innovative molecular therapeutic tools.

The first germline mutations in inherited cancer predisposition genes were discovered relatively recently, in the late 1980s. Most of these genes have a high penetrance, but account for only approximately 5–10 per cent of all cancers. Moreover, their penetrance is almost never 100 per cent, and other acquired factors are still necessary for oncogenesis. Numerous other genes with low penetrance are also now thought to be involved in cancer predisposition. These latter genes may account for 10 per cent or more of cancers, or even to all of the currently so-called 'sporadic cancers', if we consider cancer as a multigenic disease, whose development is the result of interactions between genes and environment. In terms of public health, the low penetrance genes are probably the most important because they may contribute to a much greater overall burden of cancer, but they are poorly characterized at present and as yet have no medical implications in the follow-up of patients.

This chapter will focus upon the former high-penetrance genes involved in inherited predisposition to cancer. The goal of this chapter is to describe how molecular events effect the change of normal cells with an inherited genetic mutation into malignant transformed cells. After reminding us of some biological hallmarks of cancer and hereditary predisposition to cancer, this chapter will describe:

- the targets and the nature of the inherited genetic 'first hit'
- the secondary genetic 'hits', discussing their number and the nature of the 'second hit': is it a 'biological big bang' after the 'first hit', or is it a slow progressive pathological disorder?
- the final malignant tumour development, its clinical characteristics, and the biological comparison between 'sporadic' and familial tumours with an inherited germline mutation.

MAJOR BIOLOGICAL HALLMARKS OF CANCER AND HEREDITARY PREDISPOSITION TO CANCER

Cancer research has generated a complex body of knowledge hard to summarize in a few words. Nevertheless some hallmarks of the cancer biology process could be listed as follows.

1 Cancer is multistep disease that drives the progressive transformation of a normal cell into a malignant immortalized and invasive tumour cell.
2 Cancer is a clonal multigenic disease: a malignant cell, while dividing, always gives rise to two malignant cells. Genomes of tumour cells are invariably altered at multiple sites, which is a mark of 'genome instability'.
3 Genes have an effect only when they are expressed in a particular environment: cancer results from continuous interactions between genes and the macroenvironment/microenvironment throughout the life of the patient.
4 Two classes of genes are involved in malignant transformation of cells when they are mutated: oncogenes with dominant gain of function (usually one allele is mutated) and tumour suppressor genes (or recessive oncogenes) with recessive loss of function (both alleles are usually mutated). Mutations in cancer predisposition genes of both these classes may be acquired or inherited; germline mutations mainly affect tumour suppressor genes, although exceptions are the *RET*, *MET* and *CDK4* dominant oncogenes, which predispose to MEN 2 (see Chapter 8), papillary renal cell carcinoma (see Chapter 10) and melanoma (see Chapter 27), respectively. There is no known genetic mutation to date that predisposes to all forms of cancer. In order for loss of function (a mutation in a tumour suppressor gene) to cause tumourigenesis, the function of the normal allele of the gene, which normally protects against malignant transformation, has to be lost. In this event, both alleles need to be mutated, hence it follows a recessive model at the level of the cancer cell.
5 Cancer can affect humans from the fetus to old age, but most cancers exhibit an age-dependent incidence. Time is one of the major non-biological stochastic factors of oncogenesis (see Figure 2.1).
6 A fully developed tumour is highly heterogeneous with multiple cellular subclones, and can be considered as more or less unique for each patient with its specific molecular and cellular fingerprints. Microarray technology is beginning to show that complicated patterns of gene expression changes may be able to define tumours into different groups that have common behaviours (e.g. chemoresistance).
7 Cancer cells exhibit a specific panel of growth characteristics: self-sufficiency in growth signals, insensitivity to growth-inhibitory signals, evasion of programmed cell death (apoptosis), extensive replicative potential, sustained angiogenesis, and tissue invasion and metastasis.[1]

Cancer has the common features of monoclonality, immortality, growth autonomy and invasiveness. This implies that a network of genetic alterations/mutations is necessary for its development. When an inherited predisposition to cancer exists, at least one genetic mutation is identified from the very beginning of the conception of the patient and this can aid the understanding of the biological pathways followed by cells to reach a malignant status. Starting from this first event, we will try to trace the path.

THE INHERITED GENETIC 'FIRST HIT'

The concept of inherited risk or hereditary susceptibility to cancer has been known for a long time but was confined to rare situations, such as xeroderma pigmentosum (see Chapter 16), retinoblastoma (see Chapter 6), familial adenomatosis polyposis (see Chapters 24 and 25) or multiple endocrine neoplasia (see Chapter 8). It is only recently that the genetic risks of common cancers such as colon or breast cancer were clinically recognized in families, followed by molecular analysis (see Chapters 5, 17 and 30). In all cases, a genetic defect underlies the cancer risk and is considered as the 'first hit' in the genome of the affected individuals.

The targets of the 'first hit'

The 'first hit', by definition, is in the germline. This may either be inherited or occur *de novo* in the gamete cells. Almost all target genes are tumour suppressor genes whose functions are recessive at the cellular level. Only three syndromes have been attributed to germline-activating mutations in oncogenes (*RET, MET, CDK4*), which act dominantly in the cell.[2]

The proteins encoded by inherited cancer genes have been implicated in a diverse array of key cellular processes, including maintenance of genomic integrity, the cell cycle, apoptosis, differentiation, transcription or signal transduction. Anticipation is a phenomenon where the age of disease onset due to a genetic defect decreases throughout the generations. In diseases such as Huntington's chorea, this is due to expansion of genetic coding repeats as they are copied down the generations. Anticipation is frequently noticed in cancer families (familial breast cancer, colon cancer, leukaemia); however, no dynamic mutations have been observed and no triplet repeats are known to occur in inherited cancer predisposition genes. It is noteworthy that mutated inherited cancer predisposition genes never cause immortality of cells *per se*, and it is possible that non-functional mortality genes are lethal for the embryo.

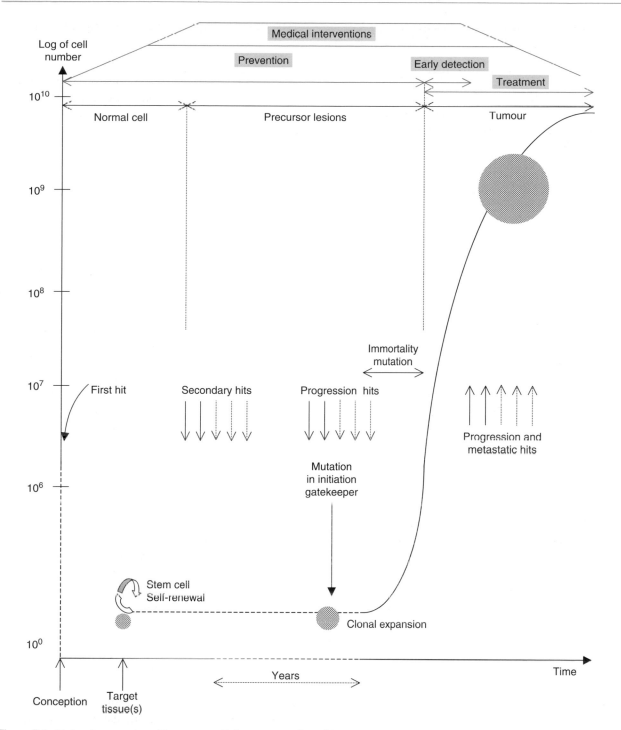

Figure 2.1 *Molecular genesis and tumour growth in cancer predisposition.*

It is noteworthy that immortality is one of the key features of a malignant cell and, therefore, should be acquired by the predisposed cells through additional gene mutations. This may explain why a single genetic mutation predisposes to a cancer only years or decades later, as other critical genetic events are needed first.

Whatever the target at the cellular level of the action of cancer predisposition genes, most of the inherited cancer syndromes show a dominant pattern of inheritance.

Several, rare, recessive cancer syndromes have been well described, usually resulting from inactivation of genes encoding DNA damage repair proteins in both alleles in the germline. In those cases, the 'first hit' has less or no cellular consequences, in terms of cancer risk. Nevertheless, in ataxia-telangiectasia, a recessive condition for the ataxia and telangiectasia (see Chapter 13), epidemiological studies suggest an increased risk of cancer in heterozygotes, and especially breast cancer in mothers of affected children.[3,4] This phenomenon raises the issue as to whether the cancer risks in a heterozygote population for other recessive traits could be increased and it could account for a significant proportion of cancer in the general population, but it is hard to diagnose without the presence of affected children (who are carriers of two recessive alleles, or homozygotes) in families.

In syndromes for which genetic heterogeneity (several genes predispose to the same disease phenotype) has been found, implicated genes appear to function in a common conserved pathway. Inactivation of *MLH1*, *MSH2*, *PMS2* and *MSH6* in individuals with hereditary non-polyposis colorectal cancer (HNPCC; see Chapter 24), alter the fidelity of DNA mismatch recognition and repair at various points in the repair pathway. Mutations in *p16INK4* (or *CDKN2A*) and *CDK4* in patients with inherited predisposition to melanoma alter the cell-cycle control at the G1/S transition through the phosphorylation of p105RB1. In other syndromes, proteins may interact directly together, such as BRCA1 and BRCA2 in patients with inherited risk of breast and ovarian cancers, or ATM and hMre11 in ataxia-telangiectasia.

The nature of the 'first hit'

An enormous variety of mutations has been found in cancer susceptibility genes: point mutations are the most common mutation event, but all kinds of mutations or epigenetic alterations are now described: base methylation, imprinting, large genomic and deletions/insertions. Nonsense mutations, deletions and insertions are the most frequent types of mutation, and are clearly loss-of-function mutations producing either an absent or a truncated protein product. An exception is *TP53*, where missense mutations are the most common event.[5] In the von Hippel–Lindau syndrome (see Chapter 10), both missense and truncating mutations exist.

Difficulties emerge when missense or splice site mutations are found, since these changes can also be normal variants. They then have to be distinguished from rare polymorphisms. This is effected by demonstrating co-segregation of the disease with the suspect allele, but this can be insufficient, especially if there are few affected individuals in a pedigree to test for the alteration. In most cases, functional tests are still needed to distinguish deleterious mutations from a polymorphism. (For example, the *TP53* gene, where a functional assay is available in a yeast system, which involves demonstrating that the resultant P53 protein is dysfunctional by looking at transcription of downstream genes. *BRCA* genes are one of the best examples where at present an easy functional test is lacking.) To add to the complexity, some common polymorphisms (e.g. in *TP53*) can influence oncoprotein interactions and tumour development.[6]

THE SECONDARY GENETIC 'HITS'

How do we explain that a single mutation present at conception induces a cancer decades later? Is it a 'biological big bang' or a slow progressive process?

The 'two-hits' Knudson and Comings model

In the Knudson model,[7] completed by Comings,[8] predisposed individuals inherit one mutant copy of a predisposing gene and need one additional somatic mutation in the second allele to initiate neoplasia. Sporadic tumours form in people with no germline mutation when both copies of the relevant gene become somatically mutated. Because the probability of acquiring a single somatic mutation is much greater than the probability of acquiring two such mutations, people with a hereditary mutation are at much greater risk of cancer than the general population. This model could explain why people with a mutation in a cancer predisposition gene more often develop cancer earlier in their life than the general population, the delay necessary for two mutations being longer than for only one somatic mutation. This also explains why people with a mutation in a cancer predisposition gene more often develop bilateral tumours, which are usually rare in the general population. In this model, cancers are not hereditary, only *predisposition* to cancer is hereditary, through one inherited mutated allele. It opens a window for medical interventions and prevention of cancer for people at genetic risk of this disease.

Usually the second genetic 'hit' inactivating the remaining allele occurs in the cancer cells via loss of heterozygosity (LOH), and is a larger molecular event than the 'first hit' and often includes adjacent genes.[2] Usually there is no direct relation between the two different 'hits' on the two alleles of one gene, with the exception of the *APC* gene. Patients with germline mutations around codon 1,300 tend to acquire their 'second hit' by allelic loss and to suffer more severe disease, whereas tumours with a mutation outside this region tend to harbour truncating mutations and have milder disease. Sometimes the second allele is lost through a 'third hit' by loss of the germline mutant allele (somatic deletion after germline point mutation).[9]

Knudson's model holds true for most cancer risks with autosomal dominant inheritance.[10] Interesting exceptions are nevertheless described. For example, the *RET* dominant oncogene is implicated in the autosomal dominantly inherited multiple endocrine neoplasia type 2 (MEN 2) syndrome and there is no LOH at the *RET* locus in the resultant tumours. Additionally, not all tumour suppressor genes invariably show LOH: *BRCA1* is mutated in the germline in breast/ovarian cancer families, but has no consistently demonstrated somatic mutation of both alleles, and many genes harbour somatic LOH without known corresponding germline mutations in the other allele. Finally, there are increasing amounts of data demonstrating that the 'second hit' on the remaining wild-type allele is not a prerequisite for neoplasia. Haplo-insufficiency and the recognition that Knudson's hypothesis does not preclude the 'second hit' occurring at a distinct but non-complementary locus in the genome, is changing our perspective of tumour suppressor gene function and regulation.[11] Haplo-insufficiency can induce imbalanced target protein levels, or have a dominant negative effect, or transcriptionally silence the wild-type allele.

Hereditary predisposition genes can be subcategorized into (1) 'gatekeeper genes', which directly control cellular proliferation; (2) 'caretaker genes', which maintain the integrity of the genome; and (3) 'landscaper genes', which modulate the microenvironment in which tumour cells grow and, therefore, promote the neoplastic conversion of polyclonal adjacent cells.[12,13] Each cell type would have one or few gatekeepers leading to a very specific distribution of cancer risk. Once the gatekeeper gene is inactivated (or activated if it is a dominant oncogene), clonal expansion occurs by a permanent imbalance of cell division over cell death. This cellular proliferation is followed by the accumulation of multiple somatic genetic events leading to the tumour. For example, the inherited mutations of the *RB1* (retinoblastoma), *VHL* (von Hippel–Lindau), *NF1* (neurofibromatosis), *PTCH* (patched) or *APC* (adenomatosis polyposis coli) genes lead to tumours of the retina, kidney, Schwann cells, skin basal carcinoma and colon epithelial cells, respectively (the gatekeeper gene for breast cancer is still unknown). In these cases, the Knudson model is adequate and both maternal and paternal copies of these genes must be mutated for tumour development.

In contrast, inactivation of a caretaker or a landscaper gene does not promote tumour initiation, rather it leads to genetic instability, which induces increased mutations of several genes, including gatekeeper genes. Once inactivation of a gatekeeper occurs, tumour progression is accelerated. In this case, individuals at increased cancer risk inherit a single mutant caretaker/landscaper gene from one of their parents. Three subsequent somatic mutations at least are required to initiate cancer: mutation of the normal caretaker/landscaper allele inherited from the healthy parent, and mutations of both alleles of the gatekeeper gene.[12] In sporadic cancers, four somatic mutations are required. We would, therefore, expect that the cancer risk in families with caretaker cancer predisposition genes is greater than in the general population, but to a lesser extent than for gatekeepers: one more mutation is still needed for the sporadic form of the cancer, but the background is different (three mutations vs. one mutation). Moreover, sporadic cancers due to caretaker genes would be expected to be less frequent than with gatekeeper gene-induced

cancers, but actually this is not the case. Known caretaker genes include, for example, the *MMR* (mismatch repair), and *BRCA* (breast cancer) genes responsible for the HNPCC and breast/ovarian cancer predisposition syndromes, respectively. As expected, the risk of cancer arising in families with *BRCA* or *MMR* mutations is high compared to the general population. However, since the background population risk is high, the four expected mutations in somatic cancers must occur more frequently than expected in gatekeeper genes for which cancer is rare where they are only due to two somatic mutations. Moreover, as already noted, somatic mutations of both alleles of the *BRCA1* caretaker gene are not observed (or not firmly demonstrated[14]) in sporadic breast cancers. This paradox means that other biological pathways seem to be used for common cancers, but these are still to be unravelled. One hypothesis would be that multiple genes can be mutated and converge to a common final effector leading to a highly frequent cancer.

The first gatekeeper concept described an initiation gatekeeper gene. It would be surprising if there were not subsequent 'gates' monitoring tumour progression or metastasis. In fact, Kinzler and Vogelstein subsequently qualified the 'gatekeeper' definition of tumour suppressor genes to include all direct inhibitors of cell growth.[13] Thus, the 'gatekeeper' class of tumour suppressor genes can be further subdefined as 'initiation gatekeepers', 'progression gatekeepers' or, indeed, 'metastasis gatekeepers'.

How many genetic 'hits' are obligatory for malignant transformation? (see Figure 2.1).

In tumours occurring in individuals with a genetic predisposition, one gatekeeper/caretaker/landscaper allele is mutated, and other acquired somatic mutations in many genes may need to be accumulated before mutation of the second gatekeeper/caretaker/landscaper allele occurs. This explains why decades are sometimes needed between the 'first hit' and tumour development. If identified, these precursor lesions could be of profound importance for physicians in preventing progression from precursor to malignant lesions[15] (Figure 2.1). In some instances, it is clear that two 'hits' produce only a benign precursor lesion and that other genetic events are necessary for malignancy (e.g. two 'hits' in the *APC* gene induce benign adenomatous polyps).

The questions are: how many genetic events are needed, and at what point do they have to intervene in the malignant cell transformation process? In inherited tumours due to mutations in gatekeeper genes, the event number is probably lower than those in tumours due to mutations in caretaker/landscaper genes, where hundreds of mutations are theoretically needed. Embryonal tumours presumably need fewer events than adult solid tumours. As the number of necessary events increases, the impact of the germline mutation diminishes.[10] It is not yet known if a somatic altered genetic background occurs before and/or after the 'hit' on the second allele of the cancer predisposition gene.

In all cases, environment (microenvironment of the cells and macroenvironment of the patient) plays a role (either by inducing mutations or by epigenetic changes) and should be borne in mind when considering the mechanism of malignant cell transformation. Epigenetic changes and mutations may be intricate. DNA methylation, for example, is an epigenetic modulator of gene expression and can inactivate tumour suppressor genes, but also induce chromosomal instability and genetic mutations.[16]

Are normal rates of mutation sufficiently high to account for the required mutations, or do premalignant cells have intrinsically high rates of mutation? This question has been debated for years without resolution. An answer to this question has been proposed in predisposition to colon cancer, where mutation rates in cells with an MMR gene deficiency, is twice to threefold higher than in normal cells.[17] Many papers report that the loss of function of ATM or BRCA1 leads to a decrease in DNA repair and thus an increase in genomic instability.[18,19] The earlier age of cancer onset in predisposed individuals argues in favour of a higher mutation rate in cells inheriting the first genetic 'hit'. This phenomenon is called the mutator phenotype hypothesis.

Most cancers exhibit an age-dependent incidence, which, when analysed statistically, implicates four to seven rate-limiting stochastic events.[20] However, this number is widely debated, and some recent experiments on experimental malignant conversion of normal cells have shed a new light on this. Normal cell conversion into a tumourigenic cell needs different genes in rodent and human. Primary rodent cells are efficiently converted by the co-expression of cooperating oncogenes,[21,22] while similar experiments failed with human cells. Conversion to malignant cells in humans requires the ectopic expression of the telomerase catalytic subunit (hTERT) in combination with two oncogenic products (the SV40 large-T oncoprotein and an oncogenic ras, H-ras V12) in epithelial and fibroblast cells.[23] Very similar experiments, using a different order of genes, failed to transform human fibroblasts,[24] therefore, specific molecular pathways are required in time. This landmark work demonstrated that three genetic events (which altered multiple biochemical pathways), including telomere maintenance, were sufficient to cause tumour growth. It is interesting to note that in no case were tumour suppressor genes necessary for in vitro malignant conversion. This implies that gatekeeper genes do not cause cellular immortality. Evidence for this is that some tumours, such as neuroblastoma, stage IV-S, can regress spontaneously; these tumours have no increased telomerase activity; it could, therefore, be hypothesized that

the gatekeeper is mutated, but immortality is not acquired in this tumour. This model raises the question: when do cells shift to immortalization? It is probably a relatively late event in the normal to malignant transformation process.

In vivo conversion appears more sophisticated and requires probably more genetic events involving other classes of genes. In vivo, cancer relies on the tumour's ability to evade the immune system, to attract its own blood vessels and to metastasize. Extrapolation from in vitro models to the multistep tumour formation in man cannot be assumed.

Animal models can be of help. Transgenic mice, which are mice deficient in one gene (null mice), are a close model to the 'two hits' in human cancer predisposition. For example, p53 inactivation in mice, acts as a mutation-rate modifier, accelerating the gate-pass events: stochastic modelling of the time pattern of tumour occurrence can help in this case to distinguish gatekeepers from caretakers.[25] The key gene for malignant transformation appears to be different from one tumour type to the other. In the mouse melanoma model, null for the tumour suppressor ink4a, oncogenic ras expression was shown to be crucial for the genesis and maintenance of the tumour.[26]

In an established tumour, it is more difficult to determine the molecular event number needed for malignant transformation. Indeed, gene alterations can be primary events in transformation or secondary (and epiphenomenal) and, therefore, intimately intricate and hard to distinguish. Molecular analysis of MSI+ (microsatellite instability) colonic adenomas estimate that they are nearly as old as the cancers they predispose to, and would have undergone as many as 2000 divisions (and potential mutations) since the loss of their MMR genes.[27] The latent period before visible neoplasia is, therefore, long, allowing a lot of time for the accumulation of mutations. DNA chip technology studies of cancer cells has identified hundreds of genes whose expression is altered.[28]

In conclusion, when we ask, 'is cancer predisposition a situation of a 'biological big bang', or a slow progressive pathological disorder?', it appears to be a mixture of both models, depending mainly on the target tissue, and the multiple somatic events acquired with time and environmental factors.

THE FINAL GENETIC PROFILE OF FAMILIAL MALIGNANT TUMOURS

The cancer risk consequences of the 'first hit'

In hereditary cancer syndromes, individuals carry a particular germline mutation in every cell of their body.

Nevertheless, only a few cell types undergo malignant transformation (mostly in adult tissues), even if the gene is ubiquitously expressed and has multiple key functions in cell biology.

With a few exceptions (e.g. medullary carcinoma of the breast associated with the *BRCA1* gene or medullary thyroid cancer associated with the *RET* gene), no histological subtype of cancer hints at the presence of an inherited predisposition to cancer; often the histology of the tumour types are the same as in sporadic cancers. This does not mean that the tumour behaviour is the same, however, and closer analyses have demonstrated differences (see later).

Once inherited, the mutated gene increases the risk of a limited number of cancer types. (There are exceptions, such as *TP53* in the Li–Fraumeni syndrome, which has a broad spectrum of tumours, although even within this setting, predisposition to some cancer types is still rare, e.g. ovarian cancer; see Chapter 11.) For example, *MLH1* induces colon, gastric and endometrial cancers, *BRCA1* induces ovarian and breast cancers in women, *RB1* induces retinoblastoma and osteosarcomas (rarely soft tissue sarcoma and melanoma). Why is there this spectrum? Answers may come from biological knowledge of the gene's molecular action (e.g. the tissue-limited expression of the *WT1* gene; see Chapter 9) or regulation of its mutated protein (such as BRCA1, whose regulation and level of action is partly via oestrogenic hormones), but a better knowledge of tissue–stem-cell differentiation at a molecular level and its implication in modulating the expression of the cancer predisposition gene will be important.

Complicating the clinical outcome, besides genetic heterogeneity, inherited cancer syndromes harbour a clinical heterogeneity. From one type of germline mutation, clinical outcome may vary within one family or between families. Some *RET* mutations can even induce benign disease such as Hirschsprung disease, whereas in other patients the same mutation induces a medullary thyroid cancer. The likelihood that an individual who carries a mutant allele of an inherited cancer gene will ultimately develop cancer is highly variable and unpredictable; this is the concept of incomplete penetrance and variable expression.

The genotype/phenotype relationship in inherited cancers

The connection between genetic heterogeneity and clinical heterogeneity increases the complexity of genotype/phenotype relationship. The likelihood that an individual who carries a mutant allele of an inherited cancer gene will ultimately develop cancer is probably dependent on other genes in the genetic background (modifier genes which can protect against or increase tumour development, or modify the target of cancer risk), and of poorly

understood, but important factors such as lifestyle factors, e.g. environment and diet.

In some cases, a good genotype/phenotype correlation exists that enables an improved medical management of the families. One of the best examples is probably the *VHL* gene where missense mutations predispose to phaeochromocytomas, whereas mutations inducing a truncated protein do not, and where the Tyr98His missense mutation does not induce risk of renal cancer.[29] This is also the case with the *RET* gene, where different mutation hot spots are correlated with MEN 2A or MEN 2B clinical presentations (but, alternatively, the *RET* genotype does not always account for the differences between MEN 2A and familial medullary thyroid cancer; see Chapter 8b), and familial adenomatous polyposis (FAP) where the mutation position in the gene is correlated with attenuated forms of polyposis (mutations at positions 78 and 157 or COOH-terminal to codon 1920 are associated with attenuated FAP) or retinal lesions (mutations between positions 413 and 1387).[2] Nonetheless, there may be considerable phenotypic differences among patients who inherit the same mutant *APC* allele (intestinal polyposis only, or Gardner syndrome, or polyposis and medulloblastoma). This suggests that modifier genes may have significant effect on the FAP phenotype, as demonstrated in the FAP mouse model.[30]

Usually the genotype/phenotype correlation is vague. Despite indications that *BRCA1* and *BRCA2* function in the same cellular processes, mutations in the two genes are associated with different cancer profiles. Women with germline *BRCA1* mutations exhibit principally breast and ovarian carcinomas, whereas germline *BRCA2* mutations predispose to female and male breast cancer as well as other cancer types, such as pancreatic or prostate adenocarcinoma. Even if some mutations in *BRCA1* predispose to a major risk of ovarian cancer,[31] the same mutation can induce differential breast or ovarian cancer risks through the generations of one family, and the individual risk is still unpredictable. The situation is the same in HNPCC families, where a given *MMR* gene mutation can predispose to either colon or endometrial cancer or both in individuals.

Biological comparisons between sporadic and familial tumours

Earlier cancer-age of onset in inherited cancer predisposition than in sporadic cases has already modified the medical management of such families by the offer of early detection of cancer in these families. Knowing specific biological hallmarks of familial cancers would be useful to improve management of patients. Are sporadic and corresponding familial cancers different or similar?

When considering the paradigm of the tumour suppressor gene model, described in the Knudson and Comings model, sporadic as well as familial tumours arise when two 'hits' of both alleles are mutated, the 'first hit' mutated either in the germline or somatically. The question is: is the 'first hit' identical in sporadic and inherited tumours? The answer is unknown, because the 'first hit' that occurs in a sporadic case has not yet been elucidated. Certainly, genetic changes have been found in extremely early precursor sporadic lesions. In sporadic retinoblastomas, or colorectal adenomas/cancers, reported data suggest that the 'first hit' could be in the *RB1* and *APC* genes, respectively, and therefore it is the same as that in the inherited form of the disease.[32] Somatic mutations in the *APC* gene are present in more than 70 per cent of all adenomatous polyps and carcinomas of the colon and rectum.[17] However, sporadic adenomas can persist for years before the appearance of sporadic colon cancer, whereas in HNPCC patients, the latent period before tumour formation is about 2–5 years.[27] Data suggest that a minority of MSI[+] cancers (from HNPCC or sporadic tumours) initiate tumourigenesis by mutations at a locus other than *APC*. As in FAP, the two *APC* mutations in sporadic colorectal tumours are not independent of each other and are not selected for simple loss of protein function.[9]

There is less evidence in other sporadic cancers that the first genetic 'hit' is the same as in the inherited form of the disease. In many cases, loss of tumour suppressor gene(s) has been regarded as a late event in malignant transformation.[33] Moreover, the mechanism of mutation seems to be different: deletions and insertions constitute 33 per cent of the somatic mutations of *p16^{INK4}* (or *CDKN2A*), whereas only 5 per cent of the germline mutations are of this mutation type.[5] Other genes such as *BRCA1* or *PMS2* have no known or very rare somatic mutations.[34]

There is the concept of initiation gatekeeper genes, where a tumour will develop once an initiation gatekeeper gene is inactivated (if a tumour suppressor gene) or activated (if an oncogene). This is the crucial molecular event, when this mutation occurs in normal (or dysplastic) cells with few previously acquired somatic mutations. A mutation in the gatekeeper gene can, therefore, be a relatively late event.

The paths that cells can take on their way to becoming malignant are highly variable and the composition of these pathways may not be crucial to know, if biological endpoints are ultimately shared in common by all types of tumours. Detailed histological comparison of inherited and sporadic tumours has found subtle differences in some cases, for example, in invasive ductal carcinoma of the breast, where *BRCA1*, *BRCA2* and non-*BRCA1/2* inherited tumours have significant distinguishable patterns of lesions usually corresponding to high-grade aggressive tumours in the former and more indolent cancers in the last of these three types.[35–37] Familial and sporadic colon cancers have

other clinical differences: sporadic cancers are mainly localized in the left colon with multiple losses of heterozygosity, whereas familial tumours can occur preferentially in the right colon with microsatellite instability. The repertoire of genes altered in inherited colon tumours would be different from their sporadic counterparts,[38] and it is suggested that colon cancer in HNPCC is the result of a more rapid transformation of a benign polyp into invasive cancer than in a sporadic situation. The same faster evolution of invasive breast cancer also occurs in some inherited disease (*in situ* cancer is exceptional in *BRCA1* patients[35]). In both these cases, this could be easily explained by the altered functions of caretaker genes.

In conclusion, familial tumours have a different biological profile from their sporadic counterparts. That means that the germline 'first hit' does have importance for the future biological and clinical characteristics of the tumour.

Prognosis of inherited cancers

Under the microscope, tumours associated with some of the most common inherited cancer-susceptibility genes appear aggressive. On the other hand, many familial tumours have a better prognosis than their sporadic counterparts, even accounting for a possible better follow-up of patients determined to be at a high risk of a second cancer.[39] This better prognosis is debated;[40] it is not the situation for all inherited cancers. It would be expected that some specific germline mutations will induce a more severe phenotype than those somatic mutations observed in sporadic cases. Familial and sporadic tumours have a different biological presentation and, therefore, would be expected to have a different prognosis.

Some of the inherited predisposition to cancers exhibits an increased host immune response with infiltration of lymphocytes into the tumour, such as colon cancer in HNPCC[41] or medullary breast cancer linked to germline *BRCA1* mutations.[35] The former have an improved prognosis compared with sporadic colon cancer, but the relative prognosis of medullary breast cancer in *BRCA1* carriers is uncertain. Moreover, microsatellite instability, which is largely, but not exclusively, observed in HNPCC, is predictive of a relatively favorable outcome and reduces the likelihood of metastasis in young patients with colorectal cancer.[42,43] It is noteworthy that mutations in DNA repair genes have pros and cons, they increase the cancer risk in the patient, but also increase the sensitivity to anticancer drugs,[44] which could modify the prognosis of such cancer patients.

Whether inherited forms of cancer are different enough from their sporadic counterparts to be classified as a 'different disease' remains to be demonstrated.

CONCLUSION

Inherited predisposition to cancer is an unusual situation, where often the very first genetic hit is known, leading to a high risk of cancer decades later. The challenge is to understand the intricate relationship between genes and environment, which progressively drives target cells to immortalized malignant transformation, through a multistep process and many additional genetic hits.

The first inherited genetic hit usually inactivates tumour suppressor genes, but rarely occurs in oncogenes. Secondary genetic hits are accumulated, and allow mutations of an 'initiation gatekeeper', which directly controls the cellular proliferation and induces clonal expansion. Gatekeeper genes fit into the 'two-hit' Knudson model, but cancer predisposition may also be linked to inherited caretaker genes (maintaining the integrity of the genome) or landscaper genes (which modulate the microenvironment in which tumour cells grow and promote their neoplastic conversion), which need more genetic hits to achieve malignant transformation. Immortality would occur eventually but, once initiated, it defines the development of a cancer cell, and shifts the medical intervention from possible prevention, to early detection and cancer treatment.

Cancer predisposition is a mixture of a 'biological big bang' from the first inherited hit, and a slow progressive pathological process. The likelihood that an individual who carries a mutant allele of an inherited cancer gene will ultimately develop cancer is highly variable and unpredictable (incomplete penetrance). Familial tumours have a different biological profile from their sporadic counterparts. Their prognosis would, therefore, be expected to be different, and some reports suggest a better prognosis in many cases, leading to hopes of better medical management of these cancer patients.

Research into the genetics of inherited cancer syndromes has provided fundamental insights into the cellular defects that subvert normal cell growth and lead to the destructive properties of cancer. Cancer is a genetic disorder, but not exclusively genetic, and the relationship between genes and environment will shed interesting light on the cancer process, in the near future. An important and still poorly understood area is the role of low-penetrance genes in cancer susceptibility. The official announcement in 2001 of the decipherment of the human genome should accelerate our knowledge of the malignant transformation molecular mechanisms of human cells. We expect that new 'chip-based' DNA technologies may accelerate and revolutionize genetic analysis (see Chapter 4).

The main goals for physicians are to use the molecular data to target those at high risk for early detection and prevention, and to offer tailored therapies to patients, based upon their molecular profile. It is possible that the cancers that have developed due to an inherited predisposition may require different oncological approaches.

KEY POINTS

- Cancer is a clonal, multistep, pathological process involving interaction between genes and environment.
- The 'two-hit' Knudson model is that predisposed individuals inherit one mutant copy of a cancer predisposing gene, and need one additional somatic mutation on the second allele to initiate neoplasia. Sporadic tumours form in people with no germline mutation, when both copies of the relevant gene become somatically mutated and inactivated. This model may now be too simplistic for all inherited cancer prediposition situations.
- Hereditary predisposition genes can be subcategorized as: 'gatekeeper genes', which directly control cellular proliferation; 'caretaker genes', which maintain the integrity of the genome; and 'landscaper genes', which modulate the microenvironment in which tumour cells grow and, therefore, promote the neoplastic conversion of polyclonal adjacent cells. Gatekeepers fit the Knudson model; caretakers/landscapers require more genetic 'hits'.
- The first genetic 'hit' never induces immortality to the cell. Immortality is the key-event for malignant transformation, but is probably late in the multistep process from a normal to a cancer cell.
- The likelihood that an individual who carries a mutant allele of an inherited cancer gene will ultimately develop cancer is highly variable and unpredictable; i.e. cancer predisposition usually shows incomplete penetrance of the inherited mutated gene. This allows for a window for preventative interventions.
- Genetic heterogeneity is seen in many inherited cancer syndromes.
- Low-penetrance inherited genes may subsequently be shown to be the cause of many apparently sporadic cases and, therefore, could be of importance to the overall cancer burden. They may also be involved in gene/environment interactions.
- Tumour biology of some sporadic tumours and tumours with an inherited predisposition are different, which may influence their prognosis.

REFERENCES

1. Hanahan D, Weinberg RA. The hallmarks of cancer. *Cell* 2000; **100**:57–70.
2. Fearon ER. Human cancer syndromes; clues to the origin and nature of cancer. *Science* 1997; **278**:1043–1050.

3. Swift M, Morrell D, Massey RB, *et al*. Incidence of cancer in 161 families affected by ataxia-telangiectasia [see comments]. *N Engl J Med* 1991; **325**:1831–1836.

4. Easton DF. Cancer risks in A-T heterozygotes. *Int J Radiat Biol* 1994; **66**(6 Suppl.):S177–S182.

5. Hussain SP, Harris CC. Molecular epidemiology of human cancer: contribution of mutation spectra studies of tumour suppressor genes. *Cancer Res* 1998; **58**:4023–4037.

6. Marin MC, Jost CA, Brooks LA, *et al*. A common polymorphism acts as an intragenic modifier of mutant p53 behaviour. *Nature Genet* 2000; **25**:47–54.

7. Knudson AG. Mutation and cancer: statistical study of retinoblastoma. *Proc Natl Acad Sci USA* 1971; **68**:820–823.

8. Comings DE. A general theory of carcinogenesis. *Proc Natl Acad Sci USA* 1973; **70**:3324–3328.

9. Rowan AJ, Lamlum H, Ilyas M, *et al*. APC mutations in sporadic colorectal tumours: a mutational 'hotspot' and interdependence of the 'two hits'. *Proc Natl Acad Sci USA* 2000; **97**:3352–3357.

10. Knudson AG. Hereditary cancer: two hits revisited. *J Cancer Res Clin Oncol* 1996; **122**:135–140.

11. Macleod K. Tumour suppressor genes. *Curr Opin Genet Dev* 2000; **10**:81–93.

12. Kinzler KW, Vogelstein B. Cancer-susceptibility genes. Gatekeepers and caretakers [news; comment]. *Nature* 1997; **386**:761, 763.

13. Kinzler KW, Vogelstein B. Landscaping the cancer terrain [comment]. *Science* 1998; **280**:1036–1037.

14. Papa S, Seripa D, Brando B, *et al*. Identification of a possible somatic *BRCA1* mutation affecting translation efficiency in an early-onset sporadic breast cancer patient [letter]. *J Natl Cancer Inst* 1998; **90**:1011–1012.

15. Sidransky D. Is human patched the gatekeeper of comm on skin cancers? [news; comment]. *Nature Genet* 1996; **14**:7–8.

16. Singal R, Ginder GD. DNA methylation. *Blood* 1999; **93**:4059–4070.

17. Kinzler KW, Vogelstein B. Lessons from hereditary colorectal cancer. *Cell* 1996; **87**:159–170.

18. Takagi M, Delia D, Chessa L, *et al*. Defective control of apoptosis, radiosensitivity, and spindle checkpoint in ataxia telangiectasia. *Cancer Res* 1998; **58**:4923–4929.

19. Foray N, Randrianarison V, Marot D, *et al*. Gamma-rays-induced death of human cells carrying mutations of *BRCA1* or *BRCA2*. *Oncogene* 1999; **18**:7334–7342.

20. Renan MJ. How many mutations are required for tumourigenesis? Implications from human cancer data. *Mol Carcinog* 1993; **7**:139–146.

21. Land H, Parada LF, Weinberg RA. Tumourigenic conversion of primary embryo fibroblasts requires at least two cooperating oncogenes. *Nature* 1983; **304**:596–602.

22. Ruley HE. Adenovirus early region 1A enables viral and cellular transforming genes to transform primary cells in culture. *Nature* 1983; **304**:602–606.

23. Hahn WC, Counter CM, Lundberg AS, *et al*. Creation of human tumour cells with defined genetic elements [see comments]. *Nature* 1999; **400**:464–468.

24. Morales CP, Holt SE, Ouellette M, *et al*. Absence of cancer-associated changes in human fibroblasts immortalized with telomerase. *Nature Genet* 1999; **21**:115–118.

25. Mao JH, Lindsay KA, Balmain A, *et al*. Stochastic modelling of tumourigenesis in p53 deficient mice. *Br J Cancer* 1998; **77**:243–252.

26. Chin L, Tam A, Pomerantz J, *et al*. Essential role for oncogenic ras in tumour maintenance. *Nature* 1999; **400**:468–472.

27. Tsao JL, Yatabe Y, Salovaara R, *et al*. Genetic reconstruction of individual colorectal tumour histories. *Proc Natl Acad Sci USA* 2000; **97**:1236–1241.

28. Ross DT, Scherf U, Eisen MB, *et al*. Systematic variation in gene expression patterns in human cancer cell lines. *Nature Genet* 2000; **24**:227–235.

29. Zbar B, Kishida T, Chen F, *et al*. Germline mutations in the Von Hippel–Lindau disease (*VHL*) gene in families from North America, Europe, and Japan. *Hum Mutat* 1996; **8**:348–357.

30. Cormier RT, Hong KK, Halberg RB, *et al*. Secretory phospholipase Pla2g2a confers resistance to intestinal tumourigenesis. *Nature Genet* 1997. **17**:88–91.

31. Neuhausen SL, Mazoyer S, Friedman L, *et al*. Haplotype and phenotype analysis of six recurrent *BRCA1* mutations in 61 families: results of an international study. *Am J Hum Genet* 1996; **58**:271–280.

32. Lamlum H, Papadopoulou A, Ilyas M, *et al*. APC mutations are sufficient for the growth of early colorectal adenomas. *Proc Natl Acad Sci USA* 2000; **97**:2225–2228.

33. Di Cristofano A, Pandolfi PP. The multiple roles of *PTEN* in tumour suppression. *Cell* 2000; **100**:387–390.

34. Ma AH, Xia L, Littman SJ, *et al*. Somatic mutation of *PMS2* as a possible cause of sporadic human colon cancer with microsatellite instability. *Oncogene* 2000; **19**:2249–2256.

35. Consortium BCLC. Pathology of familial breast cancer: differences between breast cancers in carriers of *BRCA1* or *BRCA2* mutations and sporadic cases. *Lancet* 1997; **349**:1505–1510.

36. Lakhani SR, Jacquemier J, Sloane JP, *et al*. Multifactorial analysis of differences between sporadic breast cancers and cancers involving *BRCA1* and *BRCA2* mutations. *J Natl Cancer Inst* 1998; **90**:1138–1145.

37. Lakhani SR, Gusterson BA, Jacquemier J, *et al*. The pathology of familial breast cancer: histological features of cancers in families not attributable to mutations in *BRCA1* or *BRCA2*. *Clin Cancer Res* 2000; **6**:782–789.

38. Olschwang S, Hamelin R, Laurent-Puig P, *et al*. Alternative genetic pathways in colorectal carcinogenesis. *Proc Natl Acad Sci USA* 1997; **94**:12122–12127.

39. Marcus JN, Watson P, Page DL, *et al*. Hereditary breast cancer: pathobiology, prognosis, and *BRCA1* and *BRCA2* gene linkage. *Cancer* 1996; **77**:697–709.

40. Narod SA. Host susceptibility to cancer progression. *Am J Hum Genet* 1998; **63**:1–5.

41. Graham DM, Appelman HD. Crohn's-like lymphoid reaction and colorectal carcinoma: a potential histologic prognosticator. *Mod Pathol* 1990; **3**:332–335.

42. Gryfe R, Kim H, Hsieh ET, *et al*. Tumour microsatellite instability and clinical outcome in young patients with colorectal cancer. *N Engl J Med* 2000; **342**:69–77.

43. Offit K. Genetic prognostic markers for colorectal cancer. *N Engl J Med* 2000; **342**:124–125.

44. Wei Q, Frazier ML, Levin B. DNA repair: a double-edged sword. *J Natl Cancer Inst* 2000; **92**:440–441.

From families to chromosomes: genetic linkage and association studies for finding cancer-predisposition genes

DOUGLAS F. EASTON

INTRODUCTION

The past two decades have seen rapid progress towards the mapping and identification of genes involved in inherited predisposition to cancer. Before 1987, no genes conferring a high inherited risk of cancer had been identified or even localized; at that time the only genetic loci known to be involved in cancer predisposition were the HLA system, where certain HLA haplotypes were known to predispose to Hodgkin's disease[1] and to nasopharyngeal cancer,[2] and the ABO blood group, where stomach cancer had been shown to be slightly more common in individuals with group A.[3] All of these associations are, however, quite weak. This situation was transformed in the 1980s by the development of techniques for typing DNA polymorphisms, which could be used for linkage analysis.[4] In 1987, the loci for familial adenomatous polyposis[5] and multiple endocrine neoplasia[6,7] were first localized, and, since then, genes for all the major 'inherited cancer syndomes' (i.e. those rare syndromes where evidence for Mendelian inheritance was apparent from clinical studies) have been identified (see Chapter 1).

Genetic linkage analysis has been the major technique by which these genes have been initially localized, although, in some cases, there were cytogenetic clues as to the location. In the 1990s, genetic linkage studies successfully localized a number of loci responsible for predisposition to common cancers, where the evidence for a single major gene was previously more equivocal. These include the localization of two genes responsible for colon cancer (or human non-polyposis colorectal cancer; HNPCC) families,[8,9] the *MTS1* gene on chromosome 9p responsible for familial melanoma,[10] and the *BRCA1* and *BRCA2* genes on chromosomes 17q and 13q, respectively, responsible for familial breast and ovarian cancer.[11,12] In each of these examples, mapping by linkage has led to identification of the gene itself by positional cloning (see Chapter 4).

In addition to being the first step in positional cloning of disease genes, genetic linkage analysis has several other uses in complex disorders such as common cancers. Perhaps most importantly, it provides conclusive evidence that the existence of certain families with a high risk of disease is due to genetic susceptibility. (Although evidence of major genetic effects can be strongly suggested by anecdotal high-risk families or segregation analyses, neither of these is definitive.) Secondly, it can provide information on the model of susceptibility underlying the disease, for example, whether the gene acts in a dominant or recessive fashion, and provide an estimate of penetrance (see section on 'Estimating penetrance' below). Once one gene is localized by linkage analysis, it becomes possible to evaluate whether there is evidence for genetic heterogeneity (i.e. the gene is only responsible for the high risk of disease in a subset of families) and, hence, whether there are other disease genes to be mapped. It may also be possible to define more precisely the phenotype associated with different susceptibility genes. For example, following the linkage of certain early-onset breast cancer families to chromosome 17q [11], it became clear that this gene (*BRCA1*) was responsible for most families with a high risk of both breast and ovarian cancer, but a lower proportion of breast cancer families without ovarian cancer.[13,14] Similarly, the high risk of male breast cancer in certain breast cancer families has been shown to be due (at least in part) to the *BRCA2* gene on chromosome 13q and, to a lesser extent, the *BRCA1* gene.[12,15] Finally, linkage analysis can be an important aid to genetic counselling, since it enables gene carriers and non-carriers in linked families to be identified with a high degree of certainty.

While linkage analysis is a powerful technique for mapping relatively high-risk susceptibility genes, it has much less power to detect variants conferring lower risks. It has become clear that, for many cancer types, much of the familial aggregation of the disease is likely to be due to variants of this type, and it will be impossible to collect sufficient numbers of families to identify the susceptibility genes by linkage. There has, therefore, been a growing interest in the use of alternative techniques, particularly association studies, which we discuss later in the chapter.

In this chapter, we describe the general principles of linkage analysis and association studies. For a fuller treatment of the statistical methods, the reader should refer, for example, to the textbook by Ott.[16] This chapter is primarily aimed at non-statisticians and the number of equations has been kept to a minimum. Some other statistical derivations are given as footnotes, which can again be ignored by non-mathematical readers.

LINKAGE ANALYSIS

The concept of genetic linkage was first recognized by Mendel, who noted that certain characteristics of his experimental plants tended to be co-inherited. The explanation for this phenomenon became clear once it was recognized that chromosomes contained the genetic material: two traits were linked if and only if the corresponding genes reside close together on the same chromosome. Loci that are located some distance apart on the same chromosome need not be co-inherited, owing to the process of recombination or crossover, which occurs at meiosis. In humans, there are typically one or two crossovers on each chromosome per meiosis, with about 30 crossovers in total over the human genome, but the actual positions of the crossovers vary from one meiosis to another. The probability that a recombination occurs

between two loci is known as the recombination fraction, usually represented by θ. Thus $\theta = 0$ indicates that no recombinations ever occur between the two loci, i.e. they are completely (or 'tightly') linked, as would occur if the two loci are very close together. At the other extreme, $\theta = 1/2$ indicates that the two loci segregate independently, i.e. they are unlinked; this would occur if the two loci are far apart on the same chromosome, or on different chromosomes. Thus, the recombination fraction is a measure of distance between two loci, with θ increasing as the two loci become further apart. The distance over which the probability of recombination is 1 per cent is known as 1 centimorgan (cM). Since the total physical length of the 22 human autosomes is about 3 billion base pairs, 1 cM equates, on average, to about 1 million bases (1 Mb). However, the genetic distance is not linearly related to physical distance, since there are known regions of high and low recombination per unit physical distance. In particular, centromeres are known to be regions of low recombination, whereas the telomeric regions tend to exhibit high recombination rates. The rate of recombination differs between male and female meioses; overall the female recombination rate is higher, but the pattern across each chromosome differs between the sexes and there are regions where the male recombination rate is higher.

Statistical analysis of linkage data

In experimental systems, the results of an experiment examining the genetic linkage between two Mendelian traits can be summarized straightforwardly in terms of the numbers of recombinant and non-recombinant events in informative backcrosses. Figure 3.1 illustrates a simple example in which there are ten informative meioses, generating the ten offspring of individual II-1. In nine of the meioses, alleles from the disease locus and the marker locus are co-inherited (D with A); in the tenth, generating individual III-10, the disease and marker alleles are not co-inherited, since individual III-10 gets the disease allele D from her affected father but the marker allele (B) on the opposite chromosome. Thus, a recombination between the disease gene and the marker has occurred. The estimated recombination fraction between the marker and disease loci is, therefore, $\theta = 1/10$. The probability of such a low rate of recombination occurring by chance if the loci are unlinked is $11/2^{10}$ (a simple one-tailed probability from a binomial distribution, the same as the probability of obtaining zero or one tails in ten tosses of a coin), or about 0.01, indicating strong but not overwhelming evidence of linkage. Note that the test for linkage is a one-tailed test because linkage implies values of less than 1/2 – values of greater than 1/2 have no biological interpretation.

Most linkage analyses in human pedigrees are, unfortunately, not this simple. Most human disease pedigrees

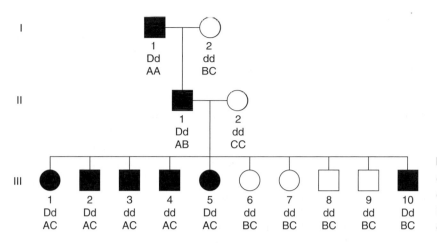

Figure 3.1 *An example of linkage analysis in an experimental backcross. D denotes the disease causing allele and d the normal allele at the disease locus. A, B and C are alleles at the marker locus.*

are not simple backcrosses and, moreover, one must also be able to allow for complexities in the disease, such as incomplete penetrance (where not all genetically susceptible individuals become affected) and sporadic cases (i.e. cases occurring in individuals who are not gene carriers), and other complications, such as individuals being untyped. The standard method for analysing linkage data in humans, which can handle all these complexities, is known as the LOD score method, first proposed by Morton.[17] The LOD score method is based on the following function:

$$LOD(\theta) = \log_{10}[L(\theta)/L(1/2)] \qquad (3.1)$$

Here L(θ) is the likelihood or probability of the observed pattern of marker and disease phenotypes within the family, given a recombination fraction θ between the disease and marker loci. LOD(θ) is thus the logarithm to base 10 of the ratio of the probability of the observed data given linkage at a certain recombination fraction to the corresponding probability in the absence of linkage (where θ = 1/2) or, more informally, the logarithm of the odds in favour of linkage. The values of LOD(θ) for different values of θ are known as LOD scores; below we give some examples of LOD scores computations in simple situations. First, we note three important properties of LOD scores that explain why they are so useful for summarizing linkage evidence. These are as follows.

1 Summing LOD scores across families. LOD scores can be added up across families. Thus, if, for example, linkage data are available for two families with the same disease, and the LOD scores at recombination fraction θ are LOD$_1$(θ) for family 1 and LOD$_2$(θ) for family 2, then the LOD scores for the two families combined, for different values of θ are LOD$_1$(θ) + LOD$_2$(θ). (This is a consequence of LODs being a logarithm of probabilities. Probabilities of independent events can be multiplied to give their combined probability, so logarithms of probabilities can be added.)

2 Estimating the recombination fraction. The value of θ between 0 and 1/2 at which LOD(θ) takes its maximum value provides a good estimate of the recombination fraction. (In statistical jargon, it is the maximum likelihood estimate and, hence, given a sufficiently large amount of data, will provide an unbiased estimate with the smallest possible standard error.) LOD scores can also be used to construct confidence intervals for the recombination fraction. These are given by those values of for which LOD(θ) is within some value k of its maximum.*

3 The maximum LOD score is a test of linkage. The maximum value of LOD(θ) over different values of θ can be used as the basis of a statistical test of linkage. The conventional critical value in linkage studies by genomic search is a maximum LOD score of 3.0. This corresponds, approximately, to a P value of about 0.0001.†

The reason for using such a stringent significance level is that the prior probability of linkage to any given marker is low – in a typical genomic search several hundred markers might be typed, almost all of which would be unlinked. Lander and Schork[18] have shown that, for an infinitely dense map of markers, the probability of achieving any LOD score greater than 3 by chance is approximately 0.09, and that the appropriate threshold for a 5 per cent genomewide significance level is 3.3. However, other authors have demonstrated that these criteria are unduly conservative for marker maps used in

---

* According to standard statistical theory, 95 per cent confidence limits are given by k = 3.84/2 log$_{10}$ e; however, it is also common to see confidence limits based on k = 1 (called 1–LOD confidence limits) quoted.
† In standard statistical terminology, the maximum LOD score is a log-likelihood ratio statistic, so that in large samples the statistical significance of the maximum LOD score can be derived by referring 2(log$_e$ 10)LOD(θ) to a chi-squared distribution on 1 degree of freedom. Thus, a LOD score of 3 corresponds to χ^2 = 13.82, or a one-tailed P value of about 0.0001.

practice, e.g. Sawcer *et al.*[19] Like any significance test, these thresholds are only a guide. If one is testing linkage to a marker that is tightly linked to a strong candidate susceptibility gene, then a lower positive LOD score (say 2.0) could be quite convincing. On the other hand, many linkage analyses in complex diseases make use of multiple analyses and demand a higher threshold. It is important to note that these *P* values are not necessarily a good approximation in small samples.[20] For example, a LOD score of 3 can be obtained using 10 scorable phase known meioses, if all 10 are consistent with linkage, which would occur by chance with probability $(1/2)^{10}$ or about 1 in 1000. If necessary, 'exact' *P* values can be obtained by simulation.[21]

Example of LOD score calculations

Figure 3.2 illustrates some examples of LOD score calculations in simple families. In Figure 3.2(a), the disease is assumed to be due to a rare autosomal dominant gene with complete penetrance (i.e. all individuals with the gene develop the disease). Individual II-1 receives allele A from his affected parent; therefore, the disease gene, if it is on the same chromosome as the marker, must be on the same chromosome as the A allele rather than the maternal allele in individual II-1. We describe individual II-1 as being of 'known phase', since the chromosome on which the mutated disease gene lies is determined. The three affected children of II-1 all receive the A allele from

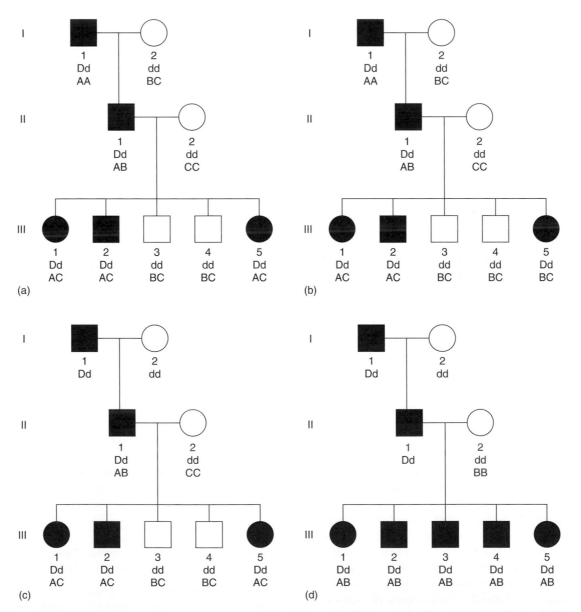

Figure 3.2 *(a–d) Some simple examples of linkage analysis with a single marker. D denotes the disease-causing allele and d the normal allele at the disease locus. A, B and C are alleles at the marker locus.*

II-1, whereas the two unaffected children receive the B allele, i.e. all five meioses are 'consistent' with linkage. The LOD score for this family is then:

$$\text{LOD}(\theta) = \log_{10}\{[(1/2)^5(1-\theta)^5]/[(1/2)^5(1/2)^5]\}$$
$$= 5\log_{10}(1-\theta) + 5\log_{10}2 \qquad (3.2)$$

This maximizes at $\theta = 0$, with a maximum LOD score of $5\log_{10}2$ or about 1.5. Thus, the best estimate of θ is 0, as expected. In Figure 3.2(b), the marker segregation is identical except that affected individual III-5 receives the B allele; thus, a recombination must have occurred in between the disease gene and the marker at meiosis. The probability of one recombinant meiosis and four non-recombinant meioses, given a recombination fraction θ, is $5\theta(1-\theta)^4$ so the LOD score is:

$$\text{LOD}(\theta) = \log_{10}\{[(1/2)^5 5\theta(1-\theta)^4]/[(1/2)^5 5(1/2)^5]\}$$
$$= \log_{10}\theta + 5\log_{10}(1-\theta) + 5\log_{10}2 \quad (3.3)$$

This maximizes at $\theta = 0.2$, with a maximum LOD score of about 0.42. In general, in a family with n children where the phase is known, and where r of the children are recombinant, the LOD score is:

$$\text{LOD}(\theta) = \log_{10}\{[(1/2)^n\,\theta^r(1-\theta)^{n-r}]/[(1/2)^n\,5(1/2)^n]\}$$
$$= r\log_{10}\theta + (n-r)\log_{10}(1-\theta) + n\log_{10}2 \qquad (3.4)$$

with the maximum LOD score occurring at $\theta = r/n$.

In Figure 3.2(c), all five children in generation III are again consistent with linkage. However, their affected grandparent I-1 is not typed, so it is not known whether the mutated disease gene in individual II-1 is on the same chromosome as the A allele or the B allele – each of these possibilities is, *a priori*, equally likely; in this case, individual II-1 is said to be of unknown phase. The LOD score computation must take account of both these possibilities:

$$\text{LOD}(\theta) = \log_{10}\{[(1/2)\theta^5 + (1/2)(1-\theta)^5]/[(1/2)^5]\}$$
$$= \log_{10}[\theta^5 + (1-\theta)^5] + 4\log_{10}2 \qquad (3.5)$$

This maximizes at $\theta = 0$ but with a maximum LOD score of 1.2. The effect of the phase being unknown is, therefore, to reduce the overall informativeness of the family, in this case by one meiosis.

In Figure 3.2(d), individual II-1 is untyped. Suppose the marker is known to have just two alleles, A and B. Given the marker typings in her offspring, her genotype at the marker locus must be either A-A or A-B; the probabilities of these two possibilities will depend on the frequencies of the A and B alleles in the population from which she is descended. A priori, the probabilities of an individual having genotypes A-A, A-B or B-B are

p_A^2, $2p_Ap_B$ and p_B^2, respectively, where p_A and p_B are the population frequencies of alleles A and B. [‡] The LOD score is then of the form:

$$\text{LOD}(\theta) = \log_{10}\{[p_A^2 + p_Ap_B(\theta^5 + (1-\theta)^5)]/$$
$$[p_A^2 + 2p_Ap_B(1/2)^5]\} \qquad (3.6)$$

If $p_A = 0.2$, say, then the maximum LOD score would be 0.60 at $\theta = 0$. If, however, p_A were small, say 0.001, the maximum LOD score would increase to 1.2, the same as in the example from Figure 3.2(c). (This is because if A is rare, the affected parent II-1 almost certainly has genotype A-B and is, therefore, informative for this marker.) Thus, as one would expect, the fact that the marker is less than fully informative substantially reduces the informativeness of the family.

Finally, suppose the penetrance of the disorder is incomplete. Then in the example from Figure 3.2(a), say, the LOD score will be:

$$\text{LOD}(\theta) = \log_{10}\{[(1/2)(1-\theta)^3[(1-t)\theta + t(1-\theta)]^2$$
$$+ (1/2)\theta^3[t\theta + (1-t)(1-\theta)]^2]/(1/2)^5\} \qquad (3.7)$$

where t is the penetrance. If $t = 0.5$, say, the maximum LOD score would be 0.60 at $\theta = 0.0$. Thus, again, the reduced penetrance decreases the informativeness of the family.

Notes on LOD score calculations

The computation of LOD scores by hand in the way outlined above becomes impractical for large pedigrees, particularly with complications such as missing typings and incomplete penetrance. Fortunately, a number of efficient computer algorithms exist for computing LOD scores in general pedigrees. A widely used program of this type is the LINKAGE package developed by Lathrop et al.[22] This is an extremely flexible program, allowing one to handle markers with any number of alleles, disease genes with penetrances that can vary between individuals according to covariates such as age and sex, and even quantitative trait loci. Computations can be performed on pedigrees of essentially arbitrary size using an algorithm known as *peeling*. More recent adaptions of this approach, implemented in programs such as FASTLINK and VITESSE,[23,24] provide faster computations.

To facilitate combining the data between families, it is usual to report LOD scores in the form of a table giving LOD scores at standard recombination fractions (often 0.001, 0.01, 0.05, 0.1, 0.2, 0.3 and 0.4). Table 3.1 gives an

---

[‡] These probabilities are strictly only appropriate for a random mating population, when the allele frequencies are said to be in Hardy–Weinberg equilibrium,[16] but this assumption is usually satisfactory in linkage analysis.

Table 3.1 *Two-point LOD scores for 11 Edinburgh breast–ovarian cancer families, for linkage between the marker D17S588 and the disease. (Reprinted from Cohen et al.[25])*

| Family | Recombination fraction | | | | |
	0.0	0.05	0.1	0.2	0.3
37	0.51	0.43	0.36	0.21	0.10
1	−0.81	0.22	0.21	0.21	0.07
11	2.08	1.85	1.60	1.11	0.63
2000	0.66	0.58	0.54	0.49	0.32
16	0.68	0.60	0.51	0.32	0.17
33	0.24	0.21	0.17	0.11	0.05
2	0.39	0.70	0.72	0.57	0.33
3	0.58	0.48	0.38	0.20	0.08
1021	−0.06	−0.05	−0.04	−0.02	−0.01
30	0.30	0.24	0.19	0.11	0.05
84	−0.06	−0.05	−0.05	−0.03	−0.01
Total	**3.83**	**5.21**	**4.59**	**3.28**	**1.78**

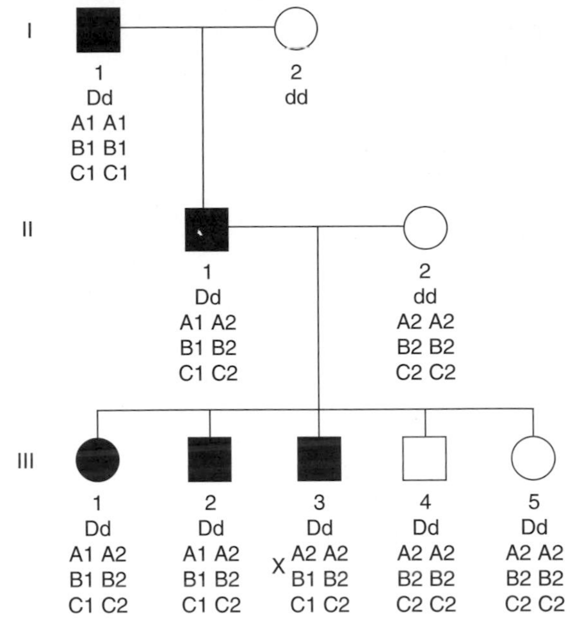

Figure 3.3 *The principle of multipoint linkage analysis. A, B and C denote linked marker loci in chromosomal order ABC, each with alleles 1 and 2. D and d denote the disease-causing and normal alleles, respectively, at the disease locus. 'x' indicates a recombinant event.*

example of a LOD score table summarizing evidence for linkage between breast and/or ovarian cancer and the marker D17S588 on chromosome 17q in 11 families.[25] Even though none of the families has substantial evidence for linkage on its own, the overall evidence for linkage is strong, a result confirmed by other studies.[13]

An important point about linkage calculations is that the computed LOD scores do not depend at all on the process by which the disease families came to be selected for study. Thus, it does not matter that families with multiple affected individuals might be extremely rare. It is perfectly legitimate (and usually essential) to select such families from a larger sample of families in order to increase the informativeness of the study; the recombination estimates and significance levels based on the maximum LOD score will remain valid.

Multipoint linkage analysis

Once a disease gene has been localized to a chromosomal region by linkage analysis, a more precise localization can usually be obtained by typing a series of markers in the region. This process is illustrated in Figure 3.3. In this example, the disease co-segregates with markers B and C, but not with marker A. Individual III-3 receives the A2 allele from his affected parent, whereas his affected siblings receive the A1 allele. This single observation suggests strongly that the disease gene (if located in the region of these markers) must be below marker A. If the disease gene were above A, at least two recombination 'events' would be required to explain the markers alleles inherited by individual III-3, which is unlikely in a small chromosomal region. If the disease gene were below A, only a single recombination is required, a far more likely

explanation given that the markers are relatively close together. This process can be formalized into multipoint linkage analysis, in which LOD scores can be computed for different locations of the disease based on the segregation of the disease and a number of marker loci. A number of programs including LINKAGE are able to carry out such computations. The results of such analyses are often presented in terms of a graph of LOD score against position along the chromosome. An example of such an analysis is given in Figure 3.4 which is taken from the linkage analysis of breast–ovarian cancer families with the 17q markers D17S588 and D17S250 conducted by the Breast Cancer Linkage Consortium.[13] The maximum LOD score is 20.79, which is obtained at a location between the two markers. This analysis, therefore, not only provides strong evidence of linkage to this region, but also provides a more precise indication of location than is possible with analyses involving a single marker; the maximum LOD scores in the intervals proximal to D17S250 and D17S588 are substantially lower (16.88 and 18.86) and these positions are, therefore, less likely. The evidence in favour of a particular location is usually expressed in terms of the 'relative odds' of a particular order, defined as the ratio of the antilogarithms of the maximum LOD score with the disease gene at the best location and the maximum LOD score in other possible intervals. In this example, the 'odds' in favour of

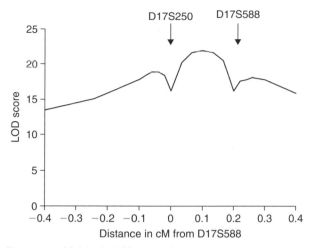

Figure 3.4 *Multipoint LOD scores from 57 breast–ovarian cancer families, for linkage between the markers D17S588, D17250 and breast and ovarian cancer.*[13]

a location between D17S588 and D17S250 are 86:1 over a location distal to D17S588 and 8050:1 over a location proximal to D17S250. A detailed discussion of the precise significance of these ratios is beyond the scope of this chapter, but odds of 1000:1 or greater are conventionally regarded as strong evidence.[16]

In addition to the improvement in localization, multi-point analysis can also improve the overall power to detect linkage (i.e. the expected maximum LOD score). This is because, by using several markers in the same region, the lack of informativeness of a single marker in a given family can be compensated by other neighbouring markers. For these reasons, multipoint analyses have to a large extent replaced two-point analyses in reports of linkage.

Unfortunately, the computational difficulty of such analyses increases dramatically as the number of loci increases, particularly in complex disease pedigrees, so that formal multipoint analyses using programs such as LINKAGE based on peeling are usually not computationally feasible with more than three marker loci and a disease locus. An alternative computational approach, first suggested by Lander and Green, allows much larger numbers of markers to be analysed simultaneously.[26] This approach does not attempt to subdivide pedigrees by peeling, but instead considers inheritance at each locus in the whole pedigree. Under the assumption of no interference (i.e. recombination at different loci occur independently of one another), inheritance at different loci along a chromosome behaves as a Markov chain. Data on each marker, therefore, can be added sequentially, with computations increasing only linearly with the number of markers. This approach has been implemented in the program Genehunter.[27] Since it allows all the markers across a whole chromosome to be analysed simultaneously, this approach is in widespread use.

One disadvantage of the Lander-Green algorithm is that, because the pedigree is analysed as whole, the computations increase exponentially with the number of individuals, so the approach is not applicable to large extended pedigrees. Current versions of Genehunter are typically limited to less than 30 individuals.[¶] A general approach that incorporates both the hidden Markov chain and peeling approaches, and would allow arbitrary numbers of markers to be analysed in general pedigrees, may be technically feasible, but has not yet been implemented. Alternative approximate approaches, based for example on Monte-Carlo Markov chains, have also been developed, but these are not in widespread use.[28,29]

Individuals such as III-3 in Figure 3.3 who show recombination with some markers in the region but not others are often described as 'critical recombinants'; identifying them often is a key process in localizing the gene to a small interval. Unless the disease is fully penetrant, the recombinant must occur in an affected individual (or in an obligate gene carrier) to be totally convincing, since an unaffected individual may or may not be a gene carrier. Even an affected individual in a linked family does not provide completely definitive localizing information in cancer families, since they may be a sporadic case. In this regard, phenotypic features of the case may be helpful in determining whether the case is likely to be a sporadic; for example, the familial risk of breast cancer is strongly related to age at onset[30] so that, in a breast cancer family, a case diagnosed at age 35 would be less likely to be a sporadic case than a 75-year-old case. A woman with both breast and ovarian cancer, or a male with breast cancer would be very unlikely to be sporadic, since such cases are so rare in the general population.

Another important step interpreting these critical recombinants is 'haplotyping' the marker alleles in the family correctly, i.e. assigning the alleles for a number of different markers on the same chromosome to the correct copy of the chromosome. In the example given, there is no ambiguity, but often several configurations of haplotypes are possible and these may lead to different interpretations of critical recombinants. Haplotyping can often be done by eye, although various algorithms for assigning marker haplotypes have been developed.[31] Haplotyping closely linked markers is helpful for identifying data errors, which will often be revealed as unlikely multiple recombinants.

Another related technique is to compare marker haplotypes between different linked families. If the disease gene is thought to be rare, it is quite likely that different families carry the same ancestral mutation. This is particularly likely if one is studying families from an isolated

¶ The limitation is actually on the value of 2 × (number of non-founders) − (number of founders). This generally has to be less than about 20 on most computers.

population. Since there may be a large number of meioses between different families, the region shared between different families could quite small, allowing precise localization of the disease gene. This has occurred, for example, in the case of diastrophic dysplasia in Finland.[32]

Types of genetic marker and laboratory techniques

Before 1983, very few important genes causing inherited diseases had been mapped to a particular chromosomal region. The reason for this was simply that very few genetic markers were available with which to detect linkage. The most important breakthrough in mapping disease genes came in the late 1970s with the realization that single base-pair DNA polymorphisms could be recognized by restriction enzymes and resolved by electrophoresis, using a technique known as Southern blotting.[33] This revolutionized the field by providing a much larger class of polymorphisms, which were numerous throughout the genome. These restriction fragment length polymorphisms (or RFLPs) became the basis of many successful linkage studies in Mendelian disorders, including cancer syndromes, such as familial adenomatous polyposis.[5]

Another major advance has been the development of DNA polymorphisms based on repetitive sequences. These were first recognized by Jeffreys et al.,[34] who noted that certain short DNA sequences were tandemly repeated and that the number of repeats was often highly variable between individuals. The variation in these 'minisatellite' polymorphisms (also known as variable number of tandem repeats or VNTRs) can also be detected by electrophoresis. The great advantage of these polymorphisms over RFLPS is that they are usually much more polymorphic. Almost all RFLPs have just two alleles and are often not particularly informative; for example, if an affected individual is homozygous for the marker, all their offspring are uninformative for linkage. In contrast, the 'minisatellite' polymorphisms often have large numbers of alleles so that most individuals are heterozygous, making the marker much more informative for linkage. The next important advance was the identification of dinucleotide 'microsatellite' polymorphisms by Weber and May.[35] These are based on repeats of dinucleotide sequences, most frequently repeated runs of the bases CA, or $(CA)_n$. Such sequences are extremely frequent throughout the genome: there are estimated to be 50 000–100 000 in total. Most sequences with at least ten repeats are polymorphic, and many have ten or more alleles. Many other short tandem repeat markers (or STRs) have also been identified, for example, based on trinucleotide or tetranucleotide repeats, e.g. $(GATA)_n$. These longer repeats are often easier to resolve than dinucleotide repeats owing to the larger differences in size between adjacent alleles. STR polymorphisms have now become the markers of choice in most linkage searches. Typing these markers relies on using the polymerase chain reaction (PCR) to amplify the repeat, using primers based on unique DNA sequences either side of the repetitive sequence.[36] Historically, different alleles were resolved by radiolabelling one of the primers, running the PCR product down an electrophoretic gel and autoradiographing. This approach has now largely been replaced by fluorescently labelled primers, with fragment lengths resolved on automated DNA sequencers. Standard panels of microsatellite markers for whole genome linkage searches are available, based on markers every 5 or 10 cM, and a number of laboratories provide facilities for genome searches.

Since typing of these markers relies on PCR, they can be typed using very small quantities of DNA. In particular, they have been typed successfully using DNA extracted from stored pathological sections of tumour. This is particularly useful in cancer families since it enables the markers to be typed on tumour material from dead affected individuals.[36]

More recently, there have been some developments in the use of single nucleotide polymorphisms (SNPs) rather than microsatellites in linkage searches. The advantage of using SNPs is technical; methods for typing large numbers of SNPs simultaneously (e.g. using chip technologies) have been developed, and these potentially allow typings to be completed more quickly, cheaply and, importantly, more accurately. SNPs have only two alleles, and the potential for miscalling their genotypes is much reduced as compared with resolving large numbers of slightly different fragment lengths. As with the earlier use of RFLPs, individual SNPs have poor information content for linkage, as compared with microsatellites, therefore, much larger numbers are required. It has been estimated that to obtain the same information as a typical 400-marker microsatellite map (i.e. with markers every 8 cM), a map of 1000–3000 SNPs is required.[37]

Genetic heterogeneity

In the linkage calculations discussed above, we assumed implicitly that all families were due to the same gene. However, many genetic diseases, including inherited cancer syndromes, can result from mutations in more than one gene. This situation is known as genetic heterogeneity. (A more accurate term is locus heterogeneity, to distinguish it from allelic heterogeneity in which different mutations in the same gene cause the same disease. Allelic heterogeneity does not complicate linkage analysis.)

Genetic heterogeneity introduces a major complication in linkage analyses because in any given set of families, the disease may be linked to one locus in some families and to a second locus in other families. A genetic marker linked to the first locus will then give evidence for linkage (i.e. positive LOD scores) in some families and evidence against linkage (negative LOD scores) in others, so that adding up the LOD scores from different families is not so helpful. (In fact, the maximum LOD score across all families is still expected to be positive, so that one should still detect linkage given a sufficiently large sample size, but the best estimate of θ will be larger than the true value.)

It is tempting to deal with the situation of apparent genetic heterogeneity by combining only the positive LOD scores, discarding those families with evidence against linkage. The maximum LOD score generated by such an approach would, however, be uninterpretable. The usual method for dealing with genetic heterogeneity into linkage analysis is based on the *admixture* model of Smith.[38] Under this model we assume that some proportion α of all families is due to the locus of interest, the remaining proportion 1 − α being due to some other gene(s). One can then construct a LOD score for a set of families under the assumption of heterogeneity, depending on both α and θ.[§]

The effects of genetic heterogeneity are illustrated by data from a study of HNPCC families.[39] Table 3.2 shows LOD scores for linkage to the marker D2S123 in 10 families. The maximum total LOD score is 3.79, maximizing at a recombination fraction of 0.20. However, inspection of the LOD scores indicates that some of the families (such as L7) show strong evidence against linkage. Using the admixture model, the maximum LOD score under heterogeneity is 4.92 at θ = 0.01, with α = 0.41 (i.e. occurrence of the disease in an estimated 41 per cent of families is due to a gene on chromosome 2p). The test statistic for heterogeneity is 5.16, which corresponds to a P value of about 0.01 indicating some evidence of heterogeneity. This is much closer to the truth, since families positive for linkage to 2p have been shown to be due to germline mutations in the *MSH2*, which is about 2 cM from D2S123.[40] Thus, neglecting genetic heterogeneity gives an exaggerated estimate of the recombination fraction. In fact, occurrence of the disease in a number of the families with evidence

Table 3.2 *LOD scores between D2S123 and the disease in 10 HNPCC families (Reprinted from Nyström-Lahti et al.[39])*

| Family | Recombination fraction | | | | | |
	0.0	0.01	0.05	0.10	0.20	0.30
L4	2.69	2.73	2.78	2.66	2.12	1.61
L7	−2.60	−2.61	−2.24	−1.48	−0.64	−0.24
L8	1.74	1.70	1.54	1.33	0.94	0.56
L621	2.64	2.60	2.43	2.18	1.60	0.94
L1933	0.29	0.30	0.34	0.35	0.30	0.18
L2516	−1.29	−1.08	−0.62	−0.33	−0.10	−0.04
L3106	−0.26	−0.16	0.09	0.25	0.31	0.20
L3427	−1.21	−1.11	−0.79	−0.52	−0.19	−0.03
B1	−1.97	−1.79	−1.30	−0.92	−0.45	−0.19
B2	−1.02	−0.82	−0.46	−0.27	−0.10	−0.05
Total	**−0.99**	**0.24**	**1.77**	**3.25**	**3.79**	**2.70**

against linkage to 2p has been shown to be due to the *MLH1* gene on chromosome 3p.[39,40]

Once evidence of heterogeneity has been established, the admixture model can be used to determine the probability that any given family is linked, given their linkage result (the so-called posterior probability of linkage).[**]

For some disorders, it is possible to define a useful subdivision of families on the basis of the observed clinical phenotypes, which may reflect the action of distinct genes. For example, selecting breast cancer families on the basis of the presence of male cases defines a set of families likely to be linked to *BRCA2*.[15] In this case, it will be more powerful to test for linkage by summing LOD scores within these phenotypic subsets rather than by using the admixture method.

In practice, detection of genetic heterogeneity can be quite difficult using data on a single linked marker, unless the families are quite large. The reason for this is that recombination between the disease and the marker in a small family could indicate a recombination event in a linked family or that the family is unlinked, so it is difficult to distinguish tight linkage in a small proportion of families from loose linkage in a high proportion. (In statistical jargon, α and θ are confounded.) However, it is usually possible to obtain much clearer evidence for or against heterogeneity with multipoint linkage.[41] This is because a multipoint analysis can determine a particular interval in which the gene lies (effectively restricting the possible range of the recombination fraction), so that strong evidence against linkage in a particular family may be obtained if affected individuals in the family do not share a haplotype across the interval in which the gene must lie.

[§] This is given by:[37]

$$\text{LOD}(\alpha, \theta) = \Sigma_i \log_{10}\{\alpha L(\theta \mid linked) + (1 - \alpha)$$
$$L(\theta \mid unlinked)/L(1/2)\}$$
$$= \log_{10}\{1 - \alpha + \alpha 10^{\text{LOD}_i(\theta)}\} \quad (3.8)$$

where $\text{LOD}_i(\theta)$ is the LOD score for family i at recombination fraction θ. Maximizing $\text{LOD}(\alpha, \theta)$ over α and θ provides estimates of these parameters, and a statistical test of heterogeneity is provided by calculating the statistic:

$$X^2 = 2 \log_e 10\{\text{LOD}(\hat{\alpha}, \hat{\theta}) - \text{LOD}(1, \tilde{\theta})\} \quad (3.9)$$

In this formula, $\text{LOD}(\hat{\alpha}, \hat{\theta})$, is the maximum heterogeneity LOD score, and $\text{LOD}(1, \tilde{\theta})$ is the maximum LOD score under homogeneity. Since this is again a log-likelihood ratio statistic, its significance is determined by comparison with a chi-squared distribution on 1 degree of freedom.

[**] This posterior probability is given by:

$$P_i = \alpha 10^{\text{LOD}_i(\theta)}/[1 - \alpha + \alpha 10^{\text{LOD}_i(\theta)}] \quad (3.10)$$

In addition to testing for heterogeneity, the maximum heterogeneity LOD score can also be used as an alternative linkage test statistic. Under certain circumstances it can provide a more powerful test than the standard (homogeneity) LOD score. Since the LOD score is maximized over two parameters rather than one, the appropriate critical value for declaring linkage must be increase. Chiano and Yates[42] have calculated that a heterogeneity LOD score of 3.44 will provide the same type I error rate as a homogeneity LOD score of 3. The correct threshold for multipoint analysis is less clear.

Although these statistical methods are helpful for detecting and estimating genetic heterogeneity, they cannot take away the fact that the power of any given set of families to detect linkage can be much lower under genetic heterogeneity than under homogeneity. To take a simple example, for a disorder caused by a single dominant gene, five families each with three fully informative phase unknown meioses could be sufficient to detect linkage, assuming a highly polymorphic marker tightly linked to the disease gene. If, instead, the disorder can be caused by either of two genes of equal frequency, then, on average, 22 such families will be required to detect linkage. This can be particularly serious for families with few affected individuals so, in general, it is better to collect families with many affected individuals than many small families if one suspects genetic heterogeneity.

Non-parametric methods of linkage analysis

One of the perceived disadvantages of classical linkage analysis, using LOD scores, is that performing the calculations requires one to specify in advance the precise genetic model underlying the disease, i.e. whether the gene is dominant or recessive, the gene frequency and penetrance, and the rate of sporadic cases. These parameters are usually known, at best, very imprecisely and, at worst, not at all. Fortunately, as discussed below, misspecification of the genetic model does not usually lead to a serious loss of power. Nevertheless, it is unsatisfactory for the results of a linkage analysis to be dependent on an arbitrary choice of genetic model. For this reason, many authors have considered methods for linkage analysis that do not depend on specifying a particular model. These methods depend on counting marker alleles, or haplotypes, shared between affected relatives, for example, affected sibling pairs. The principle is illustrated in Figure 3.5. At any locus, the two affected siblings may share either two, one or zero of the haplotypes they inherit from their parents. If the locus is unlinked to any disease susceptibility gene, the probabilities of sharing two, one or zero haplotypes based on Mendelian segregation are 1/4, 1/2 and 1/4. On the other hand, if the marker locus is linked to a disease susceptibility locus, these probabilities will differ from the values under no linkage. Therefore, evidence for linkage in a series of affected sibling pairs can be assessed by testing whether the proportions sharing two, one or zero haplotypes identical by descent differ significantly from the proportions expected given no linkage (for discussion of efficient tests for detecting linkage in sibling pairs, see Holmans[43]). This principle can easily be extended to other types of affected relative pair, such as uncle–nephew or cousin pairs.[44,45]

Where parents are not available for typing, it will not always be possible to determine unambiguously how many chromosomes are shared by the affected siblings pairs (since a shared allele may occur if there are two copies of the allele among the parental chromosomes). Instead, the distribution of the allele or haplotype sharing among affected siblings needs to be estimated, dependent on the marker allele frequencies. Programs, such as MAPMAKER/SIBS, are available to carry out these computations.

Allele sharing methods have been extended to families with more than two affected relatives. One method,

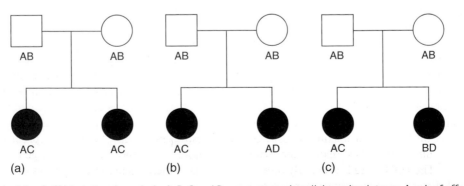

Figure 3.5 *The principle of affected sib pair analysis. A, B, C and D represent marker alleles or haplotypes. A pair of affected siblings may share two haplotypes as in (a), one haplotype as in (b), or zero haplotypes as in (c). These outcomes have probabilities 1/4, 1/2 and 1/4, respectively, if the marker is unlinked to any disease-causing gene. Deviation from these probabilities provides evidence for linkage.*

known as the affected pedigree member (APM) method, is based on counting the number of shared alleles between all possible pairs of affected relatives.[46] A statistic is generated by comparing the observed number of shared alleles with the number expected by chance, which will depend on the allele frequencies. An alternative method is based on estimating the number of alleles or haplotypes shared by descent (i.e. truly identical chromosomes) among affected individuals in the pedigree. This method, which generates a so-called non-parametric linkage (NPL) statistic, is implemented in the Genehunter program.[27]

Pitfalls in linkage analysis

Although the LOD score method of linkage analysis is an extremely powerful and flexible technique, it does have some drawbacks. The first is purely a presentational one. A table of LOD scores in a paper disguises the raw data and can be difficult to interpret. One cannot tell at a glance, for example, how many recombinant and non-recombinant affected individuals there are. Ideally, these raw data should be conveyed by displaying the actual pedigrees with marker typings, but this is not always practical. One compromise is to present, in addition to the LOD scores, a summary of the sharing of marker alleles (or haplotypes) between affected individuals. A second difficulty with the LOD score method is that the method requires one to specify the exact genetic model, including gene frequency, degree of dominance and penetrances, possibly age- and sex-specific, whereas in practice these will not be known with any certainty. In some cases, population-based family studies can be used to provide at least rough estimates of the genetic parameters, using segregation analyses. Unfortunately, such analyses have only been possible for a few cancers. Moreover, the results of such segregation analyses may not apply to high-risk families selected for linkage analysis. Fortunately, both theoretical studies and practical experience have shown that linkage analysis is fairly robust to misspecifying the genetic model. It can be shown that assuming the wrong genetic model has no effect on the type I error rate, that is, the probability of obtaining any specified maximum LOD score (e.g. greater than 3) when there is, in fact, no linkage. It is also true that, at least for two-point linkage analysis, the power to detect linkage is not seriously impaired by misspecifying the disease parameters. In particular, misspecifying the penetrance is known to have relatively little effect on the overall maximum LOD score, although it will result in a biased estimate of the recombination fraction.[47] The LOD score is also fairly insensitive to the assumed disease gene frequency. A more serious error is misspecifying the degree of dominance (i.e. specifying a dominant model instead of a recessive model or

vice versa), which can lead to a serious loss of power.[48] For this reason, LOD scores should be computed under both dominant and recessive models, if there is any doubt as to which is correct.

Multipoint linkage analysis is less robust to misspecifying the genetic model than two-point analysis. In two-point linkage analysis, misspecification of the model will lead to a biased estimate of the recombination fraction, but little change in the maximum LOD score. However, with multipoint analysis, the recombination fraction is not free to vary in the same way. This can lead to linkage being erroneously rejected from the whole region. Risch and Giuffra[48] have suggested that this difficulty can be overcome by assuming a common disease gene frequency (e.g. 0.05 for a dominant gene or 0.20 for a recessive gene). A similar problem arises with genetic heterogeneity. If genetic heterogeneity may be present, it is critical to conduct multipoint analysis allowing for heterogeneity, or the presence of unlinked families may lead to the region containing the true disease locus being rejected.

Although the LOD score method is robust to misspecification of the disease model, the same is not true of the marker allele frequencies. Allele frequencies have no impact on linkage analysis, if all the relevant individuals can be typed, but this is rarely possible in cancer families. Misspecifying marker allele frequencies can then easily lead to spurious evidence for linkage, if affected individuals share (by chance) a marker allele which is common in the population, but the allele is assumed incorrectly to be rare.[49] Ironically, this problem has become worse with the introduction of microsatellite markers. Although these markers can have a dozen or more alleles, it is typical for one or two alleles to be relatively common in the general population (occasionally 50 per cent or more). Since allele sizes may only vary by two base pairs, it is fairly easy to misread a common allele for a rare one. A further complication is that allele frequencies may vary substantially between populations. Fortunately, with the density of polymorphic markers now available, it should always be possible to resolve the problem of unknown allele frequencies by typing a number of markers in the region and developing haplotypes. With a haplotype of four or five microsatellite markers, for example, it becomes unlikely that any observed haplotype would have a frequency of, for example, more than 10 per cent. However, one should always be cautious of positive linkage results generated on the basis of a single marker. Another way in which a high probability of type I errors can be generated is by using multiple phenotypic end-points. This can lead to a serious multiple testing problem. This type of problem has been much more in evidence in psychiatric genetics (e.g. schizophrenia), where there are many ways of defining the disease, than in cancer, where the disease of interest is usually well defined. However, it can become an issue, if one is conducting linkage studies based on different types of cancer.

One rather common example of multiple testing is performing linkage analysis over a range of penetrance estimates, when the penetrance has not been previously estimated. In this case, an appropriate correction can be made by increasing the LOD score threshold.[50]

While the use of non-parametric methods avoids the need to specify a particular model, this advantage is something of an illusion. They may provide more power than a parametric model, if the model is a poor description of the true model, but conversely non-parametric methods will lack power relative to a parametric analysis under a reasonable model. Only for studies based on affected sib pairs, where allele sharing methods contain essentially all the information, are non-parametric methods routinely preferred.

Design considerations

Now that highly polymorphic markers spanning the entire genome are available, the main limitation in any linkage search is the availability of a sufficiently large set of informative families. The important question, therefore, in designing a linkage search is what constitutes a large enough sample of informative families. For a simple rare Mendelian disorder, such as familial adenomatous polyposis, the ideal family is clear, namely, a family with as many affected individuals as possible. (The number of unaffected individuals does not have much impact on the power to detect linkage, unless the penetrance is close to 100 per cent.) This is particularly important if there is genetic heterogeneity. More generally, the power to detect linkage using any given set of families can be estimated by simulation, using programs such as SLINK[21] or SIMLINK.[51] Marker data are simulated in each family under the assumption of linkage at a particular location and power can be determined by the proportion of replicates for the maximum LOD score that exceed the required threshold (e.g. 3). The informativeness of individual families is often expressed most simply in terms of the expected LOD score (or ELOD), which will be generated for a given marker at a given recombination fraction. ELODs can help to determine which families are worth including in a linkage search.

Most common cancers are not, of course, Mendelian. However, population-based segregation analyses have suggested that at least some of the common cancers do contain a subpopulation caused by a relatively rare autosomal dominant gene conferring a high risk; these include breast, colon, ovarian, prostate and melanoma. In order to detect these high-risk genes, one needs to identify those families that are most likely to be segregating the high-risk gene; this again implies families with as many affected individuals as possible. For many of these cancers, one should also try to select families with many early onset cases (e.g. in the case of breast cancer, cases diagnosed below age 50), since family studies suggest that these are more likely to be due to a high-risk gene than later onset cases.

At the opposite extreme from using large families is the affected relative pair design (i.e. two affected individuals per family). The power to detect linkage using a set of affected relative pairs is relatively straightforward to evaluate. If disease susceptibility is due to a single dominant gene, then the power to detect linkage depends only on the observed familial relative risk to first-degree relatives of affected individuals.[44] For example, if the observed familial relative risk is threefold, then about 60 affected sibling pairs would be required to detect linkage with 50 per cent power and a significance level of 0.0001 (equivalent to a LOD score of 3), assuming that a highly polymorphic marker (or haplotype) tightly linked to the disease locus is available. Sample sizes required in some other situations, including families with three or four affected individuals, are illustrated in Table 3.3. If the disease is due to a recessive gene, the power to detect linkage is dependent on the familial relative risk to both parents and siblings of affected individuals.[44] If disease susceptibility is the result of more than one gene, the power to detect linkage depends on the contribution to the familial risk made by each locus.[44] It also depends on how the different loci interact, for example, whether they act additively or multiplicatively (epistasis) on disease risk. Some examples of the effect of heterogeneity on the power of affected relative pairs are given in Table 3.3.

The major limitation of the relative pair approach is that the sample sizes required to detect linkage increase rapidly, if the familial relative risk due to the gene of interest falls to below about 2. Unfortunately, with some notable exceptions, such as testis cancer and thyroid cancer, the overall familial relative risk for most common cancers is only about 2.[52] A simple affected relative pair design is thus unlikely to detect susceptibility genes unless one gene is responsible for most of the familial risk. A more promising approach is to select the relative pairs based on a subset of cases with a higher familial risk. For example, the familial relative risks for several common cancers, such as prostate, breast and colon, are much higher at young ages,[52] so it makes sense to select relative pairs with early onset disease.

The optimal linkage designs for detecting relatively common low-penetrance genes are not as clear as for rare high-penetrance genes. As shown in Table 3.3, families with three or four cases are almost always more powerful than affected pairs. However, families with large numbers of affected individuals may be less efficient in this case for two reasons. First, because the disease gene is common, families with many affected individuals could be segregating more than one copy of the disease susceptibility allele. This could make the family uninformative for linkage, if the transmitting parent were homozygous at the disease locus. Second, if the disease can also be

Table 3.3 *Sample size requirements for various types of family and various genetic models (number of families required to give an expected LOD score of 3.0,[a] assuming a highly polymorphic marker tightly linked to the disease locus)*

Familial relative risk	One gene				Two genes[b]			
	3		2		3		2	
Dominant gene								
	0.001	0.05	0.001	0.05	0.001	0.05	0.001	0.05
Risk ratio	50.2	21.1	34.8	10.0	34.8	10.0	24.4	6.1
Affected sib pair	57	56	106	104	244	239	439	424
Three affected sibs	11	25	13	37	52	123	61	185
Four affected sibs	6	18	7	25	27	97	30	132
Avuncular pair (e.g. uncle–nephew)	53	53	122	125	219	222	495	499
Cousin pair	48	49	128	131	182	185	491	493
Sib pair + affected parent	17	42	20	75	74	200	90	337
Recessive gene								
	0.01	0.2	0.01	0.2	0.01	0.2	0.01	0.2
Risk ratio	289	26.0	203	14.7	203	14.7	143	9.3
Affected sib pair	13	26	23	45	51	100	88	175
Three sibs	3	15	3	19	10	61	11	83
Four sibs	1	15	1	18	6	61	6	73

[a] Strictly, the appropriate LOD score threshold under heterogeneity is >3, but 3 is used for simplicity.
[b] Genes acting additively on disease risk (as in a genetic heterogeneity model). These sample size estimates assume two genes each with identical allele frequencies and penetrances. If the two genes have different models (e.g. a rare gene and a common gene) the relative efficiencies of different family structure may be very different.[54]

caused by a rare high-penetrance gene or genes, families with many affected individuals are probably due to the high-risk gene. Goldgar and Easton[53] found that affected sib trios are a good strategy for detecting low-penetrance genes across a wide range of models.

Estimating penetrance

It is not always appreciated that, once linkage has been established, marker data in linked families can provide useful estimates of model parameters, such as penetrance. This is true even though the families may have been ascertained on the basis of a large number of affected individuals. Suppose, for example, that the disease is due to a rare dominant gene with uncertain penetrance. If the penetrance is high, most carriers will be affected, so the proportion of unaffected relatives who carry the marker allele linked to the disease will be low. Conversely, if the penetrance is low, the proportion of unaffected siblings carrying the linked allele will approach 50 per cent. This approach can be formalized into a procedure for estimating penetrance by maximizing the LOD score over possible penetrances[54] (sometimes referred to as the MOD score method[47]). A similar

approach of comparing LOD scores can be used to distinguish between different modes of inheritance, such as dominant and recessive.[55]

Penetrance estimates obtained by this approach need to be interpreted with some caution because many inherited disorders show variation in penetrance between families. The maximum LOD score approach is necessarily based on large families used for linkage, which will be the families due to the mutations with the highest penetrance. If there is variable penetrance, therefore, the method will provide an estimate relevant to the families with high penetrance, rather than an average penetrance over all possible mutations. Similar concerns apply if the penetrance can be modified by other genetic polymorphisms or familial risk factors.

PHENOTYPIC MARKERS

An alternate approach to the problem of detecting cancer susceptibility genes conferring only a moderate risk is to attempt to identify phenotypes associated with cancer risk that are themselves heritable. Many potential examples of such 'phenotypic markers' of susceptibility have been proposed. These include in particular a number of phenotypes that are precursors of cancer, such as adenomatous polyps of the large bowel, which are known precursors of colorectal cancer,[56] and atypic melanocytic naevi or large numbers of benign naevi, which are associated with a high risk of melanoma.[57] Recently, breast density as measured on mammograms, a strong risk factor for breast cancer, has been shown to be highly heritable.[58,59] Other promising phenotypes include sex steroid hormone levels (e.g. oestradiol),[60] insulin-like growth factor levels (a potential risk factor for multiple cancer types) and abnormal sensitivity to ionizing radiation.[61] More speculatively, it may be possible to develop novel quantitative phenotypes based on expression profiling.

The rationale for using these phenotypic markers in place of cancer in linkage (or association) studies is that the penetrance of a predisposing gene for the precursor trait is presumably likely to be higher than the cancer risk and, moreover, it will be expressed at an earlier age (perhaps at all ages). In many cases it may also be possible to score the phenotype on a continuous scale. Moreover, since one is not restricted to families with multiple individuals affected with the disease, it should be possible to collect much more informative pedigrees than are possible based on a cancer phenotype. Despite this, very little use has been made to date of such precursor phenotypes for linkage analysis, although this may change, as most of the obvious cancer syndromes have now been mapped and linkage analysis based on cancer as a phenotype becomes more problematic. The major drawback of the phenotypic markers is that the genetics of these phenotypes are likely to be complex. For example, segregation analyses of a large Utah dataset suggest strongly that benign naevi have a large inherited component but that this is almost certainly polygenic.[62,63] The power of a linkage search based on a quantitative trait is largely dependent on the proportion of the phenotypic variance due to one locus. Power calculations indicate that loci that explain 20–30 per cent of the variance should be mappable with reasonable numbers of families but, since the sample size is related to the inverse square of the effect size, the number of families rapidly becomes prohibitive for loci of small effect.[64] However, association studies based on quantitative traits may detect loci contributing 1 per cent or less of the variance. Another problem with many of the phenotypes proposed to date is that they are not easy to measure and there may be substantial inter-observer variability.

ASSOCIATION STUDIES

Association studies are based on a direct examination of whether a particular polymorphism is associated with

Table 3.4 *Association between BRCA2 N372H and breast cancer risk (Adapted from Healey et al.[65])*

	Cases	Controls	RR[a]	95%CI[a]	95%FCI[b]
NN	647	463	1.0	–	0.89–1.13
NH	451	381	0.85	0.71–1.02	0.74–0.97
HH	122	63	1.39	1.00–1.93	1.02–1.88

[a] Odds ratios in the paper are adjusted for strata and differ slightly from those presented here.
[b] Floating confidence intervals (see text).
CI, confidence interval; RR, relative risk.

disease, usually by comparing the frequency of genotypes in cases of the disease and matched controls. Thus, unlike linkage studies, they do not rely on the availability of multiple case families.

Table 3.4 summarizes the results of a large study of the *BRCA2* polymorphism N372H in breast cancer cases and controls.[65] We observe that the frequency of HH homozygotes is somewhat higher in the cases than in the controls. The statistical analysis of such data is, to a large extent, the same as for any other case-control study. We can assess the statistical significance of the association using a standard chi-squared test on the 3×2 contingency table. In this case, $\chi^2 = 9.34$ on two degrees of freedom, which corresponds to a *P* value of 0.009. An alternative is to test for a trend in risk with number of H alleles,[66] which gives $\chi^2 = 0.14$ on one degree of freedom, corresponding to $P = 0.71$.[††] This may be preferable, if homologous alleles are expected to have a additive or multiplicative effect on risk, but generally the standard two degrees of freedom test is probably preferable. In this case, the trend test shows no effect because only the HH homozygotes show an apparent risk. In addition to the significance level, one would also wish to present relative risk estimates (approximated by odds ratios) for each group and confidence intervals.[‡‡] In the example given, the odds ratio for the HH genotype, relative to the NN

[††] This test is equivalent to testing whether the *allele frequency* differs between cases and controls. A simple chi-squared test based on allele counts is, however, strictly valid only if the population genotype frequencies are in Hardy–Weinberg equilibrium, whereas the trend test does not require this.

[‡‡] Thus, if the following genotype counts are observed:

	AA	AB	BB
Controls	a	c	e
Cases	b	d	f

then we approximate the relative risk associated with genotype AB, relative to that AA, by the odds ratio ad/bc, and the corresponding relative risk for BB by af/be. Approximate confidence intervals on these odds ratios can be calculated straightforwardly, using the approximation that the standard error of the log of the relative risk (for AB) is given by $\sqrt{(1/a + 1/b + 1/c + 1/d)}$. Thus, the 95 per cent confidence limits for the odds ratio ad/bc are given by (ad/bc) $\exp[\pm 1.96 \sqrt{(1/a + 1/b + 1/c + 1/d)}]$. More accurate approximations are available if some cell counts are small.[67]

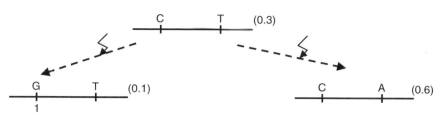

Figure 3.6 *Linkage disequilibrium. Two markers generated only three haplotypes unless there is recombination between them, generating non-random association between the alleles at the two loci. Haplotype frequencies are given in brackets.*

genotype, is 1.39 (95% C.I. 1.00–1.93). These computations can be carried out in standard statistical packages, such as SPSS or Stata.[§§]

Significance levels

Owing to the ease with which case-control series can be collected and the rapid improvements in genotyping technology, large numbers of association studies are now being conducted, principally concentrating on polymorphisms in 'candidate' genes thought to be functionally important in cancer development (e.g. genes involved in DNA repair). This has led to many apparently significant associations. The number of polymorphisms truly associated with disease will be small, however, and most associations significant at, say, the 5 per cent level are likely to be type I errors. This is confirmed by the fact that almost all reported associations cannot be replicated (e.g. Dunning *et al.*[69]).

To guard against spurious associations, the appropriate significance threshold needs to be stringent. One approach to this, by analogy with LOD score threshold for linkage searches, is to set the threshold such that the probability of a significant association by chance across all polymorphisms tested is less than, say, 5 per cent. On this basis, for candidate gene studies (in which there may ultimately be several hundred polymorphisms) a threshold of 10^{-4} might be appropriate. At this level, only a very small number of cancer susceptibility alleles been have definitively established by association. These include the associations between HLA alleles and nasopharyngeal cancer and Hodgkin's disease, and the recent association between *CHEK2* 1100delC and breast cancer (see Chapter 18).

The appropriate significance threshold for a whole genome search will depend on how many polymorphisms are required, but thresholds of 10^{-7}–10^{-8} have been suggested.[70]

Linkage disequilibrium

In allelic associations, the observed high-risk allele need not be a disease-causing mutation itself. Another possible cause of the association is *linkage disequilibrium*. Linkage disequilibrium is the non-random assortment of alleles at linked loci. When a new allele arises in a population, it will be associated with alleles at other loci that are on the same haplotype (see Figure 3.6). This association will be maintained in the population unless destroyed through recombination. Thus, an association between a disease and given polymorphism will induce an association with any other polymorphism that is in linkage disequilibrium with it. This is both an advantage and a disadvantage; it does allow associations to be detected without necessarily testing the true functional polymorphism but, on the other hand, further evaluation is required to determine which polymorphism is truly causing disease.

Disequilibrium is reduced by recombination at a rate $(1 - \theta)$ per generation, where θ is the recombination fraction.[71] Since most common polymorphisms are very old, linkage disequilibrium is typically found over very small distances. Recent evidence suggests that blocks of disequilibrium in humans are typically 5–50 kb in length, although some can be 100 kb or more.[72] Consequently, a very high density of polymorphisms would be required to be confident of mapping any disease susceptibility allele by linkage disequilibrium. Projects to define such haplotype blocks across the whole genome are currently ongoing.

The power to detect an association by linkage disequilibrium will depend on the strength of linkage disequilibrium between the tested markers. Two commonly used measures of linkage disequilibrium between single nucleotide polymorphisms (SNPs) are D' and r.[¶¶] Both take values between −1 and 1, with 0 being no linkage disequilibrium. However, they differ in that D' takes its

---

[§§] An alternative presentation of the uncertainty in the risks associated with each genotype is to use so-called *floating risks*.[68] This approach assigns a confidence interval to all three categories and avoids the arbitrary choice of a reference category. In this simple case, the floating standard errors associated with the three genotype categories are $\sqrt{(1/a + 1/b)}$, $\sqrt{(1/c + 1/d)}$ and $\sqrt{(1/e + 1/f)}$.

[¶¶] If the haplotype frequencies are given by the table:

	SNP2		
SNP1	p_{11}	p_{12}	$p_{1.}$
	p_{21}	p_{22}	$p_{2.}$
	$p_{.1}$	$p_{.2}$	

then, if $D = p_{11} - p_{1.}p_{.1}$, $r = D/\sqrt{(p_{1.}p_{2.}p_{.1}p_{.2})}$ and $D' = D/D_{max}$ if $D > 0$, $D' = D/D_{min}$ if $D < 0$ where D_{max} and D_{min} are the maximum and minimum values that D can take for any set of haplotype frequencies with the same marginal allele frequencies.

maximum absolute value whenever only three of the four possible haplotypes formed by the four SNPs are observed. This reflects the situation that occurs if there have been no recombinants between the markers since their creation. In contrast, r is 1 (or -1) only if just two of the possible haplotypes are observed, i.e. the marker genotypes are completely correlated. Thus, while D' reflects the degree of recombination between markers and is useful in defining haplotype blocks, r is more relevant to the design of the association studies. In fact, the sample size required to map a susceptibility allele by linkage disequilibrium will be greater than that required if the functional polymorphism itself is typed by a factor $1/r^2$, where r is the linkage disequilibrium coefficient between the functional polymorphism and the typed marker. This is illustrated by the polymorphisms in Figure 3.6. The disequilibrium coefficients between the two markers are $D' = 1$ and $r = 0.41$. If A is the disease-causing polymorphism, the sample size required to map it by linkage disequilibrium using marker B will be increased by approximately six times over that required using A itself, despite the fact that there are no recombinant haplotypes. This effect is particularly an issue for mapping rarer susceptibility alleles using commoner SNPs, where r is small even if $D' = 1$.*** To some extent this can be reduced by using haplotypes rather than individual SNPs, since r between the SNP and the relevant haplotype on which the disease allele resides will be greater; nevertheless, mapping of rare disease alleles by linkage disequilibrium remains problematic.

Common SNPs tend to be found in all major population groups, but the distance over which linkage disequilibrium between common SNPs is observed is somewhat shorter in African than in European or Asian populations.[72] This is likely to be a reflection of bottlenecks in the populations that founded non-African populations. Rarer SNPs (e.g. those with frequencies of 1 per cent or less) are more likely to be population specific, reflecting a more recent origin. These SNPs are expected to be in linkage disequilibrium with markers over larger regions, particularly in so-called 'founder' populations with more recent population bottlenecks (e.g. Iceland). Thus, mapping of rarer disease susceptibility alleles in founder populations may require smaller sample sizes. Such populations may also be advantageous if there is allelic heterogeneity. If the disease is associated with multiple alleles in a gene, the power to detect an association by linkage disequilibrium can be greatly reduced because several haplotypes will carry high-risk alleles. In a founder population, the number of risk alleles will typically be smaller (as observed, for example, in the case of *BRCA1* and *BRCA2* mutations).

Confounding and stratification

In addition to true 'causal' associations and those due to linkage disequilibrium, spurious associations may also be caused by confounding. In most epidemiological studies, age and sex are considered to be potential confounding factors that must be controlled for by matching or adjustment, but these are not important in genetic studies (except for sex in the case of X-linked genes) because allele frequencies do not depend strongly on them. Similarly, lifestyle risk factors will not normally be important confounding factors, except in situations where genotype may be associated with certain behaviours, for example, smoking. However, allele frequencies do vary markedly between populations, and particularly between ethnic groups, and such confounding does need to be controlled. Usually, this can be dealt with by suitably chosen matched population-based controls, or by adjusting for geographical region or ethnic group in the analysis, using stratified logistic regression. Nevertheless, choosing suitable controls for a sample of cases drawn from, say, a hospital in a large ethnically diverse city can be problematic.

A more subtle manifestation of this problem is hidden population stratification. If the population consists of multiple substrata that do not interbreed and between which the disease varies, differences in allele frequencies between strata will give rise to artefactual disease associations. One way to circumvent this problem is to make use of within-family controls. One of the simplest approaches is to use the marker alleles in the parents of an affected individual that are not transmitted to their affected offspring.[73,74] The statistical analysis of such data is extremely simple, but elegant – one simply compares the proportion of alleles of a given type that are transmitted from a heterozygous parent with its expected proportion under independent Mendelian segregation, namely 1/2. This procedure (which is identical to McNemar's test in classical statistics) is known as the transmission disequilibrium test, or TDT.[73] One can also use this design to compute relative risks of disease due to a given allele, using the methodology of matched case-control analysis. The only difficulty with this approach is that, for many common cancers, a high proportion of parents will already be deceased. However, it is possible to construct a similar test, albeit with reduced power, using unaffected siblings as controls.

In reality, marked population stratification sufficient to cause serious confounding is unlikely to be a problem in most association studies. It is possible to detect such stratification by testing for associations between unlinked markers.[75] Moreover, where such stratification does exist, methods for correcting the association tests using the association between unlinked markers (so-called 'genomic control') have been developed.[76–78]

*** If $D' = 1$, then $r = p_1.p_2/p_2.p_1$, that is, the ratio of the odds of the allele frequencies of the two polymorphisms.

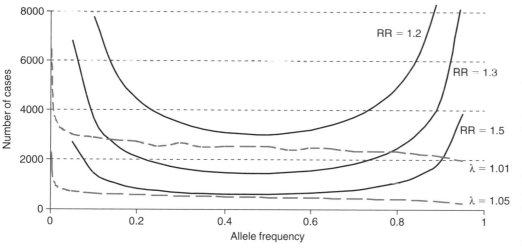

Figure 3.7 *Sample sizes required to detect association, for a dominant susceptibility allele, assuming 90 per cent power and a significance level of 0.0001. Sample sizes are given for different relative risks (RR; solid lines) and for different familial relative risks (λ; dashed lines).*

Design considerations

Figure 3.7 illustrates the sample sizes required to detect associations for different allele frequencies and relative risks. The figure assumes a dominant susceptibility allele, a significance level of 0.0001 and 90 per cent power. For a whole genome search, where a significance level of 10^{-7} or 10^{-8} would be more appropriate, the required sample sizes would be approximately doubled. The figure illustrates that 1000 cases and controls should be sufficient to detect susceptibility alleles, with frequencies of 10 per cent or more, provided that the relative risk is two or more. However, the sample size increases rapidly with reducing relative risk and is also greater for rarer alleles. The figure also illustrates power in terms of the familial relative risk (λ) to siblings of affected individuals attributable to the polymorphism. Thus, if λ = 1.05, less than 1000 cases and controls are required at most allele frequencies, whereas if λ = 1.01, over 2000 cases and controls will be required. Since for many common cancers, the overall familial risk is approximately twofold, λ = 1.01 represents 1 per cent of the overall genetic variation. Thus, a study of 2000 cases and controls will not reliably detect polymorphisms that are less than 1 per cent of the genetic variance, and hence, less than 100 disease-causing polymorphisms would be detectable by this approach.[†††] This derivation explains why prior probability of any tested polymorphism being disease associated at a detectable level is extremely small, and hence why the large majority of 'significant' associations are spurious.

As previously noted, larger sample sizes will be required if one wishes to test reliably for associations across whole regions (e.g. genes) by linkage disequilibrium, rather than just functional polymorphisms. There are, however, some possibilities for reducing the amount of genotyping required. One is to use subsets of cases where the effects of polymorphisms are likely to be stronger. Calculations have shown, for example, that use of cases with a family history will typically reduce the required sample sizes by twofold or more.[79] Use of cases diagnosed at an early age, where the familial risks are higher, may also be more efficient. Another approach is to use a two-stage design, in which polymorphisms are initially tested in a smaller number of cases and controls, and polymorphisms showing some evidence of an association (say $P < 0.05$) are then followed up in a further series.

Notwithstanding the large sample sizes required for association studies, they provide a method for detecting effects that would be undetectable by linkage studies. For example, suppose a particular allele has a population frequency of 5 per cent and causes a twofold risk of cancer. This effect could be detected with a sample size of about 190 cases and matched controls, with 50 per cent power and a significance level of 0.0001. To detect the same effect by linkage would require about 22 000 affected sibling pairs, even assuming no genetic heterogeneity!

Admixture mapping

A somewhat different approach to disease gene mapping is to utilize populations that have resulted from the recent admixture of two previously isolated populations. Such admixture has occurred, for example, in African–American and Hispanic populations. If a disease susceptibility allele has markedly different frequencies in the two populations, the disease will be associated with alleles originating in the high-risk population for markers in

---

[†††] The precise number of polymorphisms will depend not only on their effect size but also on the degree of 'interaction' between them. For example, if all polymorphisms combine additively, 100 polymorphisms each with λ = 1.01 would give rise to an overall familial relative risk of two, whereas, if they combine multiplicatively, only 70 polymorphisms would be required

the vicinity of the causative polymorphism. This association will persist across distances of several centimorgans for several generations.[80,81] Prostate cancer, which is much commoner in African–American populations, might be amenable to this approach.

DISCUSSION

Linkage analysis has proved an extremely powerful tool for mapping and hence identifying cancer susceptibility genes. With the quantity and quality of DNA polymorphisms now available for typing, any gene responsible for a substantial fraction of high-risk cancer families should be mappable by this approach. Cancer susceptibility genes identified to date explain relatively little of the observed familial aggregation of the disease and, at first sight, further linkage analysis in multiple families would appear to be an attractive strategy to map further genes. Those cancers that would appear to be most amenable to this approach include prostate cancer, breast cancer not due to BRCA1 or BRCA2 mutations (although suitable families are rather rare, as BRCA1 and BRCA2 mutations account for the majority of high risk families), and perhaps lung cancer. Linkage studies in colorectal cancer families may also still be worthwhile, if a sufficient number of informative high-risk families not due to the mismatch repair genes can be identified. It should also be feasible to map susceptibility genes for some of the rarer cancers by linkage in small families (such as relative pairs), where the familial relative risk is high, provided that one or two genes explain a high fraction of the familial effect. These include testis cancer, non-medullary thyroid cancer, laryngeal cancer, chronic lymphocytic leukaemia, non-Hodgkin's lymphoma and myeloma.[52]

After notable successes in the early 1990s, linkage studies in the common cancers have been relatively unsuccessful in identifying novel susceptibility genes. The difficulties have been particularly apparent in prostate and breast cancer, where apparently promising linkage results could not be replicated.[82–84] Such results lend weight to the theory that most of the unexplained familial aggregation is due to a large number of genes, perhaps combining in a complex fashion.

Common low-risk polymorphisms should be identifiable by association studies. Many such studies are underway, but these have met with limited success so far. Some of this may be attributable to insufficient sample size, but perhaps more important is the fact that only a very small proportion of plausible candidate genes have yet been tested in any disease. Another potential problem is that much of the important variation may be in regulatory rather than coding regions, and perhaps not in strong linkage disequilibrium with tested polymorphisms.

Fortunately, progress with genotyping technology is such that whole genome association studies to identify empirically any common polymorphisms associated with disease will soon become feasible.

Most problematic of all is the possibility that much of the variation in the disease risk is attributable to rare variants. It has been argued on theoretical grounds that selection against disease alleles may result in most such alleles being rare.[85] If this is the case, they may be undetectable until further advances in technology allow large-scale resequencing. In the near future, eludicating further susceptibility genes may depend on a broad range of strategies, including linkage analysis on a larger scale, use of associated phenotypic markers, association studies and direct analysis of candidate genes.

KEY POINTS

- Linkage analysis of the cosegregation of genetic markers with disease can be used to locate high/moderate cancer-predisposition genes in families.
- Association studies can be used to find low penetrance genes.
- Genetic heterogeneity reduces the power of linkage analysis.
- Whole genome association studies will soon be feasible and will improve prospects for detection of lower penetrance cancer-predisposition genes.

REFERENCES

1. Dausset J, Colombani J, Hors J. Major histocompatibility complex and cancer. *Cancer Surveys* 1982; **1**:120–147.
2. Simons MJ, Wee GB, Chan SH, *et al.* Probable identification of an HLA second locus antigen associated with a high risk of nasopharyngeal carcinoma. *Lancet* 1975; **i**:142–143.
3. Hoskins LC, Loux HA, Britten A, Zamcheck N. Distribution of ABO blood groups in patients with pernicious anemia, gastric carcinoma and gastric carcinoma associated with blood group A. *N Engl J Med* 1965; **273**:633–637.
4. Botstein D, White R, Skolnick MH, Davis R. Construction of a genetic linkage map in map using restriction fragment length polymorphisms. *Am J Hum Genet* 1980; **32**:314–331.
5. Bodmer WF, Bailey CJ, Bodmer J, *et al.* Localisation of the gene for familial adenomatous polyposis on chromosome 5. *Nature* 1987; **328**:614–616.
6. Mathew CGP, Chin KS, Easton DF, *et al.* A linked genetic marker for multiple endocrine neoplasia type 2A on chromosome 10. *Nature* 1987; **328**:527–528.
7. Simpson NE, Kidd KK, Goodfellow PJ, *et al.* Assignment of multiple endocrine neoplasia type 2A to chromosome 10 by linkage. *Nature* 1987; **328**:528–530.

8. Peltomaki L, Aaltonen LA, Sistonen P, *et al*. Genetic mapping of a locus predisposing to human colorectal cancer. *Science* 1993; **260**:810–812.

9. Lindblom A, Tannergard P, Werelius B, Nordenskjord M. Genetic mapping of a second locus predisposing to hereditary non-polyposis colon cancer. *Nature Genet* 1993; **5**:279.

10. Cannon-Albright LA, Goldgar DE, Meyer LJ, *et al*. Assignment of a locus for familial melanoma, *MLM*, to chromosome 9p13–p22. *Science* 1992; **258**:1148–1152.

11. Hall JM, Lee MK, Morrow J, *et al*. Linkage analysis of early onset familial breast cancer to chromosome 17q21. *Science* 1990; **250**:1684–1689.

12. Wooster R, Neuhausen S, Mangion J, *et al*. Localization of a breast cancer susceptibility gene to chromosome 13q12–q13. *Science* 1994; **265**:2088–2090.

13. Easton DF, Bishop DT, Ford D, Crockford GP, Breast Cancer Linkage Consortium. Genetic linkage analysis in familial breast and ovarian cancer: results from 214 families. *Am J Hum Genet* 1993; **52**:678–701.

14. Narod SA, Ford D, Devilee P, *et al*. An evaluation of genetic heterogeneity in 145 breast–ovarian cancer families. *Am J Hum Genet* 1995; **56**:254–264.

15. Ford D, Easton DF, Stratton M, *et al*. Genetic heterogeneity and penetrance analysis of the *BRCA1* and *BRCA2* genes in breast cancer families. *Am J Hum Genet* 1998; **62**:334–345.

16. Ott J. *Analysis of human genetic linkage*, 3rd edn. Baltimore: Johns Hopkins University Press, 1999.

17. Morton NE. Sequential tests for the detection of linkage. *Am J Hum Genet* 1955; **7**:277–318.

18. Lander ES, Schork NJ. Genetic dissection of complex traits. *Science* 1994; **265**:2037–2048.

19. Sawcer S, Jones HB, Judge D, *et al*. Empirical genomewide significance levels established by whole genome simulations. *Genet Epidemiol* 1997; **14**:223–229.

20. Skolnick MH, Thompson EA, Bishop DT, Cannon LA. Possible linkage of a breast cancer susceptibility locus to the ABO locus: sensitivity of LOD scores to a single new recombinant observation. *Genet Epidemiol* 1984; **1**:363–373.

21. Weeks DE, Ott J, Lathrop GM. SLINK: a general simulation program for linkage analysis. *Am J Hum Genet* 1990; **47**:A204.

22. Lathrop GM, Lalouel JM, Julier C, Ott J. Strategies for multilocus linkage analysis in humans. *Proc Natl Acad Sci USA* 1984; **81**:3443–3446.

23. Cottingham RW Jr, Idury RM, Schäffer AA. Faster sequential genetic linkage computations. *Am J Hum Genet* 1993; **53**:252–263.

24. O'Connell JR, Weeks DE. The VITESSE algorithm for rapid exact multilocus linkage analysis via genotype set-recoding and fuzzy inheritance. *Nature Genet* 1995; **11**:402–408.

25. Cohen BB, Porter DE, Wallace MR, *et al*. Linkage of a major breast cancer gene to chromosome 17q12–21: results from 15 Edinburgh families. *Am J Hum Genet* 1993; **52**:723–729.

26. Lander ES, Green P. Construction of multilocus genetic linkage maps in humans. *Proc Natl Acad Sci USA* 1987; **84**:2363–2367.

27. Kruglyak L, Daly MJ, Reeve-Daly MP, *et al*. Parametric and nonparametric linkage analysis: a unified multipoint approach. *Am J Hum Genet* 1996; **58**:1347–1363.

28. Kong A, Cox N, Frigge M, Irwin M. Sequential imputation and multipoint linkage analysis. *Genet Epidemiol* 1993; **10**:483–488.

29. Guo SW, Thompson EA. A monte carlo method for combined segregation and linkage analysis. *Am J Hum Genet* 1992; **51**:1111–1126.

30. Claus EB, Risch NJ, Thompson WD. Age at onset as an indicator of familial risk of breast cancer. *Am J Epidemiol* 1990; **131**:961–972.

31. Weeks DE, Sobel E, O'Connell JR, Lange K. Computer programs for multilocus haplotyping of general pedigrees. *Am J Hum Genet* 1995; **56**:1506–1507.

32. Hastbacka J, de la Chapelle A, Mahtani MM, *et al*. The diastrophic dysplasia gene encodes a novel sulfate transporter – positional cloning by fine structure linkage disequilibrium mapping. *Cell* 1994; **78**:1073–1087.

33. Southern EM. Detection of specific sequences among DNA fragments separated by gel electrophoresis. *J Mol Biol* 1975; **98**:503–517.

34. Jeffreys AJ, Wilson V, Thein SL. Hypervariable minisatellite regions in human DNA. *Nature* 1985; **314**:67–73.

35. Weber JL, May PE. Abundant class of human DNA polymorphisms which can be typed using the polymerase chain reaction. *Am J Hum Genet* 1989; **44**:388–396.

36. Eeles RA, Stamps AC. *Polymerase chain reaction (PCR): the technique and its applications*. Austin TX: RG Landes, 1993.

37. Kruglyak L. The use of a genetic map of biallelic markers in linkage analysis. *Nature Genet* 1997; **17**:121–124.

38. Smith CAB. Homogeneity test for linkage data. *Proc Second Int Congr Hum Genet* 1961; **1**:212–213.

39. Nyström-Lahti M, Parsons R, Sistonen P, *et al*. Mismatch repair genes on chromosomes 2p and 3p account for a major share of hereditary nonpolyposis colorectal cancer families evaluable by linkage. *Am J Hum Genet* 1994; **55**:659–665.

40. Leach FS, Nicolaides NC, Papadopoulos N, *et al*. Mutations of a *mutS* homolog in hereditary nonpolyposis colorectal cancer. *Cell* 1993; **75**:1215–1225.

41. Lander ES, Botstein D. Strategies for studying heterogeneous genetic traits in humans by using a linkage map of restriction fragment length polymorphisms. *Proc Natl Acad Sci USA* 1986; **83**:7353–7357.

42. Chiano MN, Yates JR. Linkage detection under heterogeneity and the mixture problem. *Ann Hum Genet* 1995; **59**:83–95.

43. Holmans P. Asymptotic properties of affected-sib-pair linkage analysis. *Am J Hum Genet* 1993; **52**:362–374.

44. Risch N. Linkage strategies for genetically complex traits. II. The power of affected relative pairs. *Am J Hum Genet* 1990; **46**:226–241.

45. Bishop DT, Williamson JA. The power of identity-by-state methods for linkage analysis. *Am J Hum Genet* 1990; **46**:254–265.

46. Weeks DE, Lange K. The affected-pedigree-member method of linkage analysis. *Am J Hum Genet* 1988; **42**:315–326.

47. Clerget-Darpoux F, Bonaiti-Pellie C, Hochez J. Effects of misspecifying genetic parameters in LOD score analysis. *Biometrics* 1985; **42**:393–399.

48. Risch N, Giuffra L. Model misspecification and multipoint linkage analysis. *Hum Hered* 1992; **42**:77–92.

49. Green P. Genetic linkage and complex diseases: a comment. *Genet Epidemiol* 1990; **7**:25–27.

50. MacClean CJ, Bishop DT, Sherman SL, Diehl SR. Distribution of LOD scores under uncertain mode of inheritance. *Am J Hum Genet* 1993; **52**:354–361.

51. Ploughman LM, Boehnke M. Estimating the power of a proposed linkage study for a complex genetic trait. *Am J Hum Genet* 1989; **44:**543–551.

52. Goldgar DE, Easton DF, Cannon-Albright LA, Skolnick MH. A systematic population based assessment of cancer risk in first-degree relatives of cancer probands. *J Natl Cancer Inst* 1994; **86:**1600–1608.

53. Goldgar DE, Easton DF. Optimal strategies for mapping complex disease loci in the presence of genetic heterogeneity. *Am J Hum Genet* 1997; **60:**1222–1232.

54. Risch N. Segregation analysis incorporating linkage markers. I. Single-locus models with an application to type 1 diabetes. *Am J Hum Genet* 1984; **36:**363–386.

55. Greenberg DA. Inferring mode of inheritance by comparison of LOD scores. *Am J Med Genet* 1989; **35:**480–486.

56. Burt RW, Cannon-Albright LA, Bishop DT, *et al.*. Familial factors in sporadic adenomas and colorectal cancer. *Problems Gen Surg* 1993; **10:**688–694.

57. Green A, Swerdlow AJ. Epidemiology of melanocytic naevi. *Epidemiol Rev* 1989; **11:**204–221.

58. Day N, Warren R. Mammographic screening and mammographic patterns. *Breast Cancer Res* 2000; **2:**247–251.

59. Boyd NF, Dite GS, Stone J, *et al.* Heritability of mammographic density, a risk factor for breast cancer. *N Engl J Med* 2002; **347:**886–894.

60. The Endogenous Hormones and Breast Cancer Collaborative Group. Endogenous sex hormones and breast cancer in postmenopausal women: reanalysis of nine prospective studies. *J Natl Cancer Inst* 2002; **94:**606–616.

61. Scott D, Jones LA, Elyan SAG, *et al.* Identification of A-T heterozygotes. In: Gatti RA, Painter RB (eds) *Ataxia-telangiectasia*. Berlin: Springer-Verlag, 1992;101–116.

62. Goldgar DE, Cannon-Albright LA, Meyer LJ, *et al.* Inheritance of nevus number and size in melanoma/DNS kindreds. *Cytogenet Cell Genet* 1992; **59:**200–202.

63. Risch N, Sherman S. Genetic Analysis Workshop 7: summary of the melanoma workshop. *Cytogenet Cell Genet* 1992; **59:**148–158.

64. Page GP, Amos CI, Boerwinkle E. The quantitative LOD score: test statistic and sample size for exclusion and linkage of quantitative traits in human sibships. *Am J Hum Genet* 1998; **62:**962–968.

65. Healey CS, Dunning AM, Teare MD, *et al.* A common variant in *BRCA2* is associated with both breast cancer risk and prenatal viability. *Nature Genet* 2000; **26:**362–364.

66. Sasieni PD. From genotypes to genes: doubling the sample size. *Biometrics* 1997; **53:**1253–1261.

67. Breslow NE, Day NE. Statistical methods in cancer research Vol I. The design and analysis of case-control studies. IARC scientific publication no. 32. Lyon: IARC, 1980.

68. Easton DF, Peto J, Babiker A. Floating absolute risks – an alternative to choosing an arbitrary reference group in survival analysis and case-control studies. *Statistics Med* 1991;**10:**1025–1035.

69. Dunning AM, Healey CS, Pharoah PDP, *et al.* A systematic review of genetic polymorphisms and breast cancer risk. *Cancer Epidemiol Biomarkers Prev* 1999; **8:**843–854.

70. Risch N, Merikangas KR. The future of genetic studies of complex human diseases. *Science* 1996; **273:**1516–1517.

71. Weir BS. *Genetic data analysis: methods for discrete population genetic data.* Sunderland, MA: Sinauer, 1990.

72. Gabriel SB, Schaffner SF, Nguyan H, *et al.* The structure of haplotypes in the human genome. *Science* 2002; **296:**2225–2229.

73. Spielman RS, McGinnis RE, Ewens WJ. Transmission disequilibrium test for linkage disequilibrium: the insulin gene region and insulin-dependent diabetes mellitus (IDDM). *Am J Hum Genet* 1993; **52:**506–516.

74. Self S, Longton G, Kopecky K, Liang K-Y. On estimating HLA/disease association ith application to a study of aplastic anaemia. *Biometrics* 1991; **47:**53–61.

75. Goode EL, Dunning AM, Healey CS, *et al.* Assessment of population stratification in a large population-based cohort. *Genet Epidemiol* 2002; **21:**A126.

76. Devlin B, Roeder K. Genomic control for association studies. *Biometrics* 1999; **55:**997–1004.

77. Pritchard JK, Rosenberg NA. Use of unlinked genetic markers to detect population stratification in association studies. *Am J Hum Genet* 1999; **65:**220–228.

78. Reich DE, Goldstein DB. Detecting association in a case-control study while correcting for population stratification. *Genet Epidemiol* 2001; **20:**4–16.

79. Antoniou A, Easton DF. Polygenic inheritance of breast cancer: implications for design of association studies. *Genet Epidemiol* 2003; Nov **25**(3):190–202.

80. Stephens JC, Briscoe D, O'Brien SJ. Mapping by admixture linkage disequilibrium in human populations: limits and guidelines. *Am J Hum Genet* 1994; **55:**603–624.

81. McKeigue PM. Mapping genes underlying ethnic differences in disease risk by linkage disequilibrium in recently admixed populations. *Am J Hum Genet* 1997; **60:**188–196.

82. Kainu T, Juo SH, Desper R, *et al.* Somatic deletions in hereditary breast cancers implicate 13q21 as a putatitve novel breast cancer susceptibility locus. *Proc Natl Acad Sci USA* 2000; **97:**9603–9608.

83. Thompson D, Szabo CI, Mangion J, *et al.* Evaluation of linkage of breast cancer to the putative *BRCA3* locus on chromosome 13q21 in 128 multiple case families from the Breast Cancer Linkage Consortium. *Proc Natl Acad Sci USA* 2002; **99:**827–831.

84. Ostrander EA, Stanford JL. Genetics of prostate cancer: too many loci, too few genes. *Am J Hum Genet* 2000; **67:**1367–1375.

85. Pritchard JK. Are rare variants responsible for susceptibility to complex diseases? *Am J Hum Genet* 2001; **69:**124–137.

4

From chromosomes to genes: how to isolate cancer-predisposition genes

RICHARD WOOSTER

INTRODUCTION

A central aim of cancer research over the last 20 years has been the identification of genes involved in the development and behaviour of cancer. These genes have formed a foundation for understanding the biological abnormalities within neoplastic cells, have provided information on the function of gene products and shed light on more complex questions, such as the relationships between genes and biochemical pathways. As our understanding of the underlying biology of cancer has grown, the strategies for the development of new therapeutic and preventive agents in cancer have become increasingly dependent upon modulation of critical molecular targets. A number of avenues of investigation have revealed:

- new cancer genes;
- the use of biological assays for transforming activity;
- primary localization to a small part of the genome (e.g. by genetic linkage analysis or loss of heterozygosity analysis) followed by mutational analysis of the genes within the restricted region;
- the mutational analysis of candidate genes that recommend themselves on the basis of predicted or proven functions.

All of these approaches may yield new therapeutic targets and tools for cancer classification. However, genetic linkage analysis has the added value of discovering genes that predispose individuals to cancer. Knowledge of these genes can provide information before the onset of disease and has proved influential in the management of high-risk cancer families. While many cancer predisposition genes have been cloned, there are a number that have been elusive to date, for example, those involved in prostate cancer[1] and testicular cancer.[2] The methods employed to search for the chromosomal location of highly penetrant predisposition genes have changed little over the past 10 years with genetic linkage analysis still forming the backbone of this science. However, the approaches available for the final identification of the genes have changed dramatically with the availability of the human genome sequence. This chapter will provide a historical view of gene identification before the genome sequence, a present-day approach with the available mass of sequence data and will conclude with predictions for the future.

FINE MAPPING

One of the underlying goals during the genetic mapping of genes is to place the gene in the smallest possible segment of the genome. To this end, there is a balance between mapping the gene to a large interval of perhaps 5 cM and reducing the map interval to a fraction of a centimorgan. The balance is dictated on the one hand by the ease of reducing the size of the interval by further rounds of fine mapping and on the other hand by the information available for the region in terms of DNA sequence, gene content and physical mapping data. A number of approaches are available to either provide direct genetic mapping information to reduce the size of a critical region or provide supporting evidence of the genes location.

Genetic markers

A reasonable scan of the genome would use perhaps 400 polymorphic markers, such as the Genethon CA/GT set, spread evenly across the genome.[3] At this density, approximately one marker every 10 cM, there is plenty of scope to develop a denser set of genetic markers and refine the location of critical recombinants. There are at least 5000 published CA/GT markers spread throughout the genome.[3] The bulk of these were isolated in a random fashion and were genetically mapped using the CEPH families. Closer inspection of the exact physical location of the markers suggests discrepancies between the genetic and physical maps. However, they provide a very good starting point to refine recombinants.

The sequence of the human genome allows the original CA/GT markers to be placed on an accurate physical metric. This makes it possible not only to use existing CA/GT markers but also to search the DNA sequence for new markers. Previous experience suggests that longer runs of CA dinucleotides are more polymorphic than shorter runs with repeats of more than 15 CAs, i.e. $(CA)_n$, where $n = 15$, being almost always polymorphic. A simple search of the entire 35 Mb of chromosome 22 shows there is on average one CA/GT repeat (where n is >11) every 53 kb with a minimum gap of a few bases between adjacent repeats and a maximum of 400 kb. If this is true for the rest of the genome, there will be in excess of 60 000 $(CA)_{11}$ repeats across the genome. For the more determined mapper, there will undoubtedly be a higher density of single nucleotide polymorphisms (SNPs) across the genome. With estimates suggesting there is one SNP every 500 bp, it will be possible to map recombinants to a very small interval.[4] Indeed, nearly 1.5 million SNPs have been identified across the genome[5] giving an estimated average density of one SNP per 1.9 kb of sequence. Even at this density it is possible to analyse inheritance patterns, for example, map regions of the genome that show low levels of recombination.[6] However, the time expended mapping to this resolution could be better spent looking for mutations to identify the gene.

Other mapping information

It is possible that a cancer predisposition gene might reveal itself by leaving other clues in the genome either of normal or tumour cells. There is a wide selection of associated techniques that can assist cancer predisposition gene

mapping. It could be argued that few of these additional methods have borne fruit; however, they can, in theory, provide a very rapid shortcut to the cancer predisposition gene.

Loss of heterozygosity (LOH) mapping has commonly been used as a mapping tool in its own right.[7] This approach assumes the gene is a tumour suppressor where one copy is inactivated in the tumour by a small intragenic mutation and the other by a larger deletion. The larger deletions can be detected with a low resolution map of perhaps one polymorphic marker every 500 kb with the aim of providing additional breakpoints to define the minimal region. Unfortunately, many tumours are characterized by tumour cells in close proximity to normal cells and extracting DNA from this mixed population does not provide conclusive evidence of LOH. Furthermore, other allelic imbalances might appear as LOH, whereas, in fact, they are a duplication of one chromosome. Finally, the deletions are often large, encompassing many tens of megabases, if not whole chromosome arms or whole chromosomes, and provide little useful data.[8]

An extension of LOH mapping is to search for homozygous deletions. If both alleles are deleted and the distance between the markers is less than the size of the smaller deletion, there is a chance of finding a homozygous loss. Homozygous deletions can be very small, perhaps due to flanking genes that are critical to the survival of the cell, and can reduce a critical region very quickly. Indeed, homozygous deletion mapping has been far more successful than LOH mapping.[9]

New families

In addition to new genetic markers and other mapping techniques, new families can provide fresh recombinants that may reduce the critical interval. Therefore, there is always pressure to ascertain new families in the hope that they will reduce the size of the critical region and hence the number of candidate genes that need to be screened. Even if new families do not provide recombinant information, they are always a valuable source of material for mutation screening and their contribution should not be underestimated.

A general trawl for new families segregating the same disease is one way to collect new data. However, selective collections can provide added value. For example, specific phenotype characteristics may enhance the chance of finding further linked kindreds, e.g. X-linked families with testicular cancer.[2] The use of founder-effect populations can give what at first sight appear to be many small nuclear families that are in fact descended from a common ancestor.[10,11] If the density of polymorphic markers across the critical interval is dense enough, it is possible to calculate the frequency of the haplotype in the various families. This might suggest the haplotype is so rare that the families are likely to be derived from a founder in the population.

FROM GENETIC TO PHYSICAL MAPS

The translation of a genetic map to a physical map has changed dramatically over the past year with the availability of large amounts of the human genome sequence. In the near future, it will be unnecessary to build and analyse a new physical map for any part of the human genome. However, an understanding of the process is still relevant and can assist in the analysis of the genome sequence (see Figure 4.1).

The markers that are routinely used to map predisposition genes, be they RFLPs, microsatellite markers or SNPs, are usually located on genetic maps. In the absence of the genome sequence, genes can be placed on the same genetic maps so long as the genes contain suitable polymorphisms that can be typed through the appropriate families. This is time consuming and requires a prior knowledge of the gene and its sequence. More often, there will be anecdotal evidence, perhaps from cytogenetic data or previous mapping experiments that will place a number of genes either in the candidate region or nearby. In order to build a complete physical map, it is necessary to take the existing data and build a set of overlapping large insert genomic clones to cover the region of interest, a physical map of clones. The conventional route to construct the physical map is to hybridize known DNA sequences to genomic libraries to identify clones for the interval. The known DNA sequences can be the polymorphic markers that fall in the region, cDNAs that represent genes in the region and any other cloned DNA thought to be from the critical region. For example, a cDNA that represents a gene in the interval is labelled with ^{32}P. Clones from a P1 artificial chromosome (PAC) are screened with the labelled cDNA and positive clones isolated for further investigation. The relationship of the PAC clones to one another can be determined by short tag sequence (STS) content mapping or through one of many fingerprinting methods. PACs contain an average insert size of 100 kb and screening a library with a series of genes or markers, etc. spread at 50 kb intervals can produce a complete clone contig. If the clone contig is not complete, it is necessary to walk from the ends of each clone contig to fill the gaps. This can be achieved by either randomly creating new probes from the PACs towards the ends of the existing contigs, or by isolating sequence or probes from the ends of the appropriate clones. This walking process can be cycled until the gaps are closed and the physical map is complete.

It can take 6 months to a year to build a clone contig covering 3 megabases of genome. However, this just represents the time to obtain the clones without any additional knowledge of the genes or features in the clones, let alone the sequence of the clones. The process of sequencing a set of PAC clones covering 3 megabases could only be attempted by larger labs and was generally avoided. By contrast, the human genome sequence provides a direct route from genetic makers to the sequence of the interval.

Having identified the makers that define the minimal interval for the gene of interest, modern scientists will turn to their computers and the internet in preference to their laboratories and chemicals. There are many websites that will provide access and tools to interrogate the human genome sequence. Many of the genome centres responsible for generating the genome sequence have web tools to browse and query the sequence from their part of the genome (e.g. www.sanger.ac.uk/HGP and genome. wustl.edu/gsc/), while other national and international repositories and informatics institutes have extensive websites (e.g. www.ensembl.org and www.ncbi.nlm.nih. gov). These portals to the human genome sequence can provide the raw DNA sequence for the critical region and a list of genomic clones that were used to derive the sequence. Through this route, in a sense reverse mapping, it is possible to order the genomic clones from the critical interval and wait for your physical map to arrive in the post (www.chori.org/bacpac/orderingframe.htm). The clones themselves can be important tools in the quest for genes in the critical interval. However, the sequence itself and the existing analysis of these data can be searched for genes and other features that are relevant for the isolation of the predisposition gene.

ANALYSING THE HUMAN GENOME SEQUENCE

Computer-based approaches: the dry laboratory

There are many tools that can be used to analyse genome sequence. For the purposes of this text, the tools will concentrate on those designed to find genes.

The best approach to finding genes in the sequence of your candidate region is to look for known genes that have been confirmed by wet laboratory experiments. These can be found by BLASTing your genome sequence against public databases, such as EMBL (www.ebi.ac.uk) and GenBank (www.ncbi.nlm.nih.gov) through various web pages. This will give you all of the sequences that are similar to your sequence. As the size of the public databases has expanded, the number of hits one can expect to record has also increased. This is now at a stage where a 3-megabase interval will return many thousands of hits to both human and other sequences. The amount of data

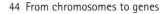

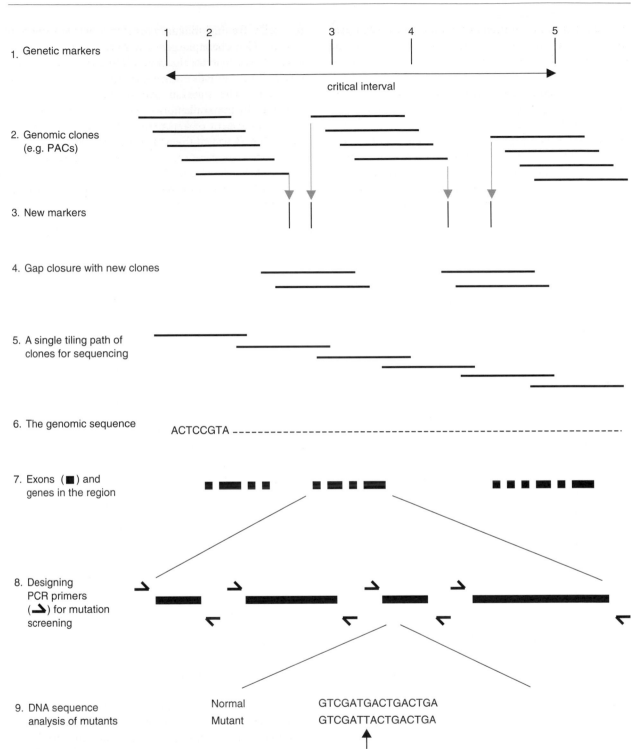

Figure 4.1 *From disease to mutation. The process of genetic mapping, sequencing, gene discovery and mutation detection has been very successful. Genetic markers (1) used to define the critical region can also be used to identify genomic clones for the region (2). The genomic clones can be used to identify new genetic markers (3) that extend the clone set (4) leading to a minimum set of overlapping clones that encompass the region of interest (5). The sequence of the clones (6) can be used to discover the genes in the interval (7). In most cases disease-causing mutations fall within the gene sequence and this is targeted for mutation screening (8). The final product is sequence from the samples with the disease showing the exact location of the mutation (9). The human genome sequence removes the need to work through steps 2–6, and enables step 1 and the final stages of the process.*

is so large that this approach should only be attempted once easier routes have been exhausted, and this method repeats work that has already been done by other genome annotators.

A comprehensive and dynamic analysis of the human genome can be viewed at www.ensembl.org and www.ncbi.nlm.nih.gov/genome/guide with a list of other sites at www.ensembl.org/genome/central. Both of these sites will let you access information about your region of interest in conjunction with various BLAST hits from known genes. In addition, they will display predicted genes and other features that may be useful. There are a number of features present in genes that, in theory, make it possible to locate genes in genomic sequence without the aid of any laboratory data. Examples of the features include splice sites, a contiguous open reading frame in the spliced form of the gene and perhaps a CpG island towards the start or 5′ end of the gene. In practice, the programs that search for genes are far from perfect. Many of the gene features can vary around a consensus, ideal, sequence. Setting strict search criteria minimizes the number of false positives in the results, but also misses many true, known, genes. Conversely, relaxing the search criteria finds most of the known genes, but introduces so many false positives that a sea of artefacts swamps the true data. Therefore, the use of prediction tools, such as Grail or Genescan, should be used as a final search mechanism. Furthermore, any data from prediction software should be confirmed by wet laboratory experiments before proceeding to mutation screening.

Although the human genome is nearing completion, the analysis of the sequence is in a state of flux and the websites and tools are likely to change. However, many of the core centres listed above will undoubtedly continue as the initial portals to these data and they should be reviewed on a regular basis.

Finding genes in the wet laboratory

The human genome offers a reference sequence that can be used in many experiments. It does not automatically identify all the genes. Many genes have already been identified in the wet laboratory; however, there is still the possibility that one will screen all the known genes in a critical interval and find no mutations that implicate the genes in your disease. Either the location of the disease is wrong or the mutation does not conform to the previous dogma, or there are unknown genes lurking in the sequence. Computer programs may indicate some potential new genes and wet laboratory experiments can either confirm these observations or identify genes that have not been predicted. Methods such as exon trapping[12] and solution hybrid capture[13] use genomic clones to either look for coding region based on its ability to be spliced by

the cell's transcriptional machinery or by using the Watson–Crick base pairing of complementary strands to select cDNAs that have sequence similarity to the genomic clones. Both methods make few assumptions in their trawl for genes. The solution hybrid capture approach is restricted by the availability of the correct cDNAs. If the gene is not expressed in the tissue that was used to create the cDNA, it will not be discovered through this route. Therefore, a number of tissues should be used as the source of the cDNA pool.

Wet laboratory experiments can be useful in confirming computer-predicted data. For example, a series of consecutive exons that are predicted to form a single mRNA can be confirmed by reverse transcription polymerase chain reaction (RT-PCR). PCR primers are designed in each exon (in the appropriate orientation) and used in an attempt to amplify the sequence from cDNA. Again, successful results are dependent on the expression of the gene in the cDNA pool and, assuming a product is made during the RT-PCR, it is worthwhile confirming the identity of the product by sequencing. A similar approach can be used to extend partial genes, for example, where ESTs (expressed sequence tags) are located in the critical region. ESTs are usually neither full length (containing the complete coding region of the gene) or completely sequenced (see www.ncbi.nlm.nih.gov/UniGene). Hence some wet work is essential to confirm the extent and exact nature of partial genes.

Even before defining the whole coding region of a gene, it is possible to pass known coding fragments for mutation screening. Early evidence of disease-causing mutations can focus work and remove the need to identify the other genes in the minimal interval.

MUTATION SCREENING

Many techniques have been developed for the identification of DNA sequence changes. The ultimate test is a comparison of the DNA sequence itself. This is, however, often time consuming and rapid screening methods offer a fast route to identify those DNA fragments or exons that potentially contain interesting sequence changes. Automated sequencing machines have improved over the past decade; however, throughput is still an order of magnitude lower compared to rapid mutation detection techniques. DNA microarrays offer an alternative approach where a whole gene can be resequenced on one array (see Hacia and Collins[14] and references therein). However, this technology is currently inflexible, does not cover every gene in the genome and is relatively expensive. Therefore, there is still extensive reliance upon rapid screening techniques that can quickly identify a subset of samples that appear to have novel sequence changes.

Examples of such screening techniques include:

- the protein truncation test – PTT;[15]
- denaturing gradient gel electrophoresis – DGGE;[16]
- chemical cleavage of mismatches – CMC;[17]
- single-strand conformation polymorphism – SSCP;[18]
- conformation-sensitive gel electrophoresis – CSGE.[19]

These are discussed further in Chapter 5. To be useful, these techniques should have a very high sensitivity (ideally as high as determining the DNA sequencing itself) and a higher throughput than determination of the DNA sequence.

The existing techniques have many advantages and disadvantages. Some rapid screening techniques are costly for a small number of samples (e.g. the GC clamps required for DGGE), while others are not amenable to high throughput (again DGGE and PTT). Most of these methods have their limitations. For example, PTT, as its name implies, can only detect changes that introduce a premature stop codon in coding sequences, while SSCP has limited sensitivity. CSGE or heteroduplex analysis can detect most types of sequence changes within certain parameters, for example, PCR primers are designed at least 50 bp either side of the region of interest with limits on the length of the PCR product. Recent developments of CSGE have included the use of fluorescent labels and automated DNA sequencers to resolve the normal homoduplex bands and aberrant heteroduplex products,[20,21] and transfer of the technique to automated capillary-based platforms.[22] The move to automated platforms has enabled projects that were untenable only a few years ago. The Cancer Genome Project at the Wellcome Trust Sanger Institute is screening 50 genes a day in 50 tumour samples to identify somatic mutations. At this pace it will take approximately 4 years to trawl the whole genome and corroborate any discoveries. The utility of this approach is exemplified by the discovery of mutations in the B-RAF gene in four out of five malignant melanomas.[23]

In most mutation screening methods, PCR primers are designed to amplify the region of interest, for example, an exon. Some of the methods have a limit in the amount of sequence they can analyse and multiple overlapping PCR products must be designed to encompass larger exons. If a rapid screening method is used, it will reveal PCR fragments that contain putative mutations or sequence variants. These must be analysed further by DNA sequencing. The discovery of disease-causing mutations usually requires a comparison between DNA from an affected individual with DNA from a normal, control sample. This is true for both the rapid approaches and the final DNA sequence analysis. Some sequence variants or mutations can have a serious impact on gene translation, and function of the protein product, or change a critical amino acid in the protein sequence. These changes are usually sufficient to implicate the gene in the development of the disease, especially if there are multiple independent examples of different mutations. If the sequence variant has a more subtle effect on the coding region, it may not implicate the gene as the disease gene. Segregation with the disease phenotype may be due to linkage disequilibrium and functional experiments may be required to ascertain functional significance of the sequence variation in this case.

THE FUTURE

The arrival of the human genome sequence has changed the approach used to identify predisposition genes. Genes that took decades to clone at the end of the twentieth century can be identified in a matter of months. Many common predisposition genes that have a high penetrance have been mapped and cloned. The evidence for other cancer predisposition genes is compelling; however, without the human genome sequence, it would be difficult to justify the time required to isolate these genes. In the future it will be possible to tackle larger and larger projects. This is partly due to increased levels of automation in the mapping of genes, but also because of a reduction in the time it takes to identify the gene in a critical region. The human genome sequence continues to be a tool that few have used. Anyone who begins to use it will soon realize it is not the perfect tool and has its defects. However, the identification of predisposition genes completely *in silico* has never been closer.

KEY POINTS

- The human genome sequence is revolutionizing cancer genetics with the potential to discover cancer genes at an ever increasing pace.
- In the next few years it is likely that most cancer genes will be identified.
- On the horizon is the possibility of large-scale genomic sequencing of individuals and their tumours to determine the somatic alterations that have occurred.
- To make the best use of this information we need the appropriate health care strategies to benefit patients.

REFERENCES

1. Smith JR, Freije D, Carpten JD, et al. Major susceptibility locus for prostate cancer on chromosome 1 suggested by a genome-wide search. *Science* 1996; **274**:1371–1374.

2. Rapley EA, Crockford GP, Teare D, *et al*. Localization to Xq27 of a susceptibility gene for testicular germ-cell tumours. *Nature Genet* 2000; **24**:197–200.

3. Dib C, Faure S, Fizames C, *et al*. A comprehensive genetic map of the human genome based on 5,264 microsatellites. *Nature* 1996; **380**:152–154.

4. Wang DG, Fan J, Siao C, *et al*. Large-scale identification, mapping, and genotyping of single-nucleotide polymorphisms in the human genome. *Science* 1998; **280**:1077–1082.

5. Sachidanandam R, Weissman D, Schmidt SC, *et al*. A map of human genome sequence variation containing 1.42 million single nucleotide polymorphisms. *Nature* 2001; **409**:928–933.

6. Gabriel SB, Schaffner SF, Nguyen H,*et al*. The structure of haplotype blocks in the human genome. *Science* 2002; **296**:2225–2229.

7. Munn KE, Walker RA, Varley JM. Frequent alterations of chromosome 1 in ductal carcinoma *in situ* of the breast. *Oncogene* 1995; **10**:1653–1657.

8. Collins N, McManus R, Wooster R, *et al*. Consistent loss of the wild type allele in breast cancers from a family linked to the *BRCA2* gene on chromosome 13q12–13. *Oncogene* 1995; **10**:1673–1675.

9. Versteege I, Sevenet N, Lange J, *et al*. Truncating mutations of *hSNF5/INI1* in aggressive paediatric cancer. *Nature* 1998; **394**:203–206.

10. Friedman LS, Szabo CI, Ostermeyer EA, *et al*. Novel inherited mutations and variable expressivity of *BRCA1* alleles, including the founder mutation 185delAG in Ashkenazi Jewish families. *Am J Hum Genet* 1995; **57**:1284–1297.

11. Neuhausen S, Gilewski T, Norton L, *et al*. Recurrent *BRCA2* 6174delT mutations in Ashkenazi Jewish women affected by breast cancer. *Nature Genet* 1996; **13**:126–128.

12. Duyk GM, Kim SW, Myers RM, Cox DR. Exon trapping: a genetic screen to identify candidate transcribed sequences in cloned mammalian genomic DNA. *Proc Natl Acad Sci USA* 1990; **87**:8995–8999.

13. Futreal PA, Cochran C, Rosenthal J, *et al*. Isolation of a diverged homeobox gene, *MOX1*, from the *BRCA1* region on 17q21 by solution hybrid capture. *Hum Mol Genet* 1994; **3**:1359–1364.

14. Hacia JG, Collins FS. Mutational analysis using oligonucleotide microarrays. *J Med Genet* 1999; **36**:730–736.

15. Roest PA, Roberts RG, van der Tuijn AC, *et al*. Protein truncation test (PTT) to rapidly screen the *DMD* gene for translation terminating mutations. *Neuromuscul Disord* 1993; **3**:391–394.

16. Fischer SG, Lerman LS. DNA fragments differing by single base-pair substitutions are separated in denaturing gradient gels: correspondence with melting theory. *Proc Natl Acad Sci USA* 1983; **80**:1579–1583.

17. Cotton RG, Rodrigues NR, Campbell RD. Reactivity of cytosine and thymine in single-base-pair mismatches with hydroxylamine and osmium tetroxide and its application to the study of mutations. *Proc Natl Acad Sci USA* 1988; **85**:4397–4401.

18. Orita M, Iwahana H, Kanazawa H, *et al*. Detection of polymorphisms of human DNA by gel electrophoresis as single-strand conformation polymorphisms. *Proc Natl Acad Sci USA* 1989; **86**:2766–2770.

19. Ganguly A, Rock MJ, Prockop DJ. Conformation-sensitive gel electrophoresis for rapid detection of single-base differences in double-stranded PCR products and DNA fragments: evidence for solvent-induced bends in DNA heteroduplexes. *Proc Natl Acad Sci USA* 1993; **90**:10325–13029.

20. Ganguly T, Dhulipala R, Godmilow L, Ganguly A. High throughput fluorescence-based conformation-sensitive gel electrophoresis (F-CSGE) identifies six unique *BRCA2* mutations and an overall low incidence of *BRCA2* mutations in high-risk *BRCA1*-negative breast cancer families. *Hum Genet* 1998; **102**:549–556.

21. Spitzer E, Abbaszadegan MR, Schmidt F, *et al*. Detection of *BRCA1* and *BRCA2* mutations in breast cancer families by a comprehensive two-stage screening procedure. *Int J Cancer* 2000; **85**:474–481.

22. Rozycka M, Collins N, Stratton MR, Wooster R. Rapid detection of DNA sequence variants by conformation-sensitive capillary electrophoresis. *Genomics* 2000; **70**:34–40.

23. Davies H, Bignell GR, Cox C, *et al*. Mutations of the *B-RAF* gene in human cancer. *Nature* 2002; **417**:949–954.

5

Screening for mutations in cancer-predisposition genes

JAN VIJG AND YOUSIN SUH

INTRODUCTION

With the publication of the results of the Human Genome Project, near-complete sequence information has become available theoretically to permit presymptomatic screening of all genes identified as relevant to cancer risk for the presence of heritable variation. This would include not only high-penetrance mutations but also polymorphic variants influencing cancer risk to a lesser degree. However, before genetic screening on such a large scale becomes a serious option, several issues remain to be addressed. The predominant issue in this respect is the clinical utility of genetic screening as standard practice. That is, does it reduce cancer morbidity and mortality through interventions that decrease cancer risk? Although genetic screening does exactly that in some isolated cases, at this stage it is fair to say that for many cancers the clinical validity and utility of such testing is debatable and more data are needed.[1] While these issues are dealt with elsewhere in this book, the central question in this chapter is whether the state of current mutation analysis technology is actually capable of meeting the potential demand for large-scale genetic screening (for earlier reviews of the subject, see Mathew,[2] and Eng and Vijg[3]). Here, we will address the issue by first discussing the various criteria for an optimal genetic screening test in relation to its application. We will then present an overview of current and experimental methods for the detection of point mutations and small insertions, and deletions in clinical diagnostics. Finally, the future technological prospects in this field will be discussed.

CRITERIA FOR A GENETIC SCREENING TEST

Some major criteria for a genetic test are listed in Table 5.1. The most obvious criterion is a high accuracy, as determined by a high sensitivity and specificity. Indeed, without a high sensitivity (i.e. the ability of the test to identify correctly those samples with a mutation), individuals at high genetic risk would go undetected. Likewise, a low specificity (i.e. a low ability of the test to identify samples without a mutation correctly) would lead to false positives. Other criteria are less straightforward and their importance relates to other issues; for example, health economic

Table 5.1 *Requirements of a genetic screening test*

- High accuracy
  - High sensitivity
  - High specificity
- Low cost
- Robust and easy
- High sample throughput
- Small DNA usage requirements
- Short hands-on time

considerations. It also depends on the number and size of the gene(s) and the number of mutations that need to be detected. On the assumption that, ultimately, genetic screening tests will be applied to large groups of people, cost becomes a major issue and should be ranked immediately after accuracy.

A third important criterion is the reliability of a test. This is basically determined by its reproducibility, which in turn is likely to be higher when the test is robust and easy to perform. A final criterion of major importance is throughput. Throughput is basically defined as the amount of DNA sequence analysed per assay time. To some extent this is related to the cost, since throughput can be increased, simply by increasing the number of technicians, instruments, etc. However, in some cases, time can be an issue, as well as laboratory space, which make it opportune for a test to be rapid. Another criterion is the amount of sample DNA available, which is of high relevance when many genes need to be analysed and sample quantity is limited. Finally, automation of a test to reduce hands-on time can be expected to reduce human error as a major factor in determining accuracy.

TYPES OF GENETIC SCREENING TESTS

Genetic screening tests differ with respect to the type of biological material that is needed. Indeed, genetic screening tests have been described that detect the presence or absence of a particular gene function, for example, microsatellite instability in tumors of hereditary non-polyposis colon cancer (HNPCC) patients,[4] alterations at the protein or mRNA level or alterations at the genomic DNA level. In general, genetic screening tests should be applicable to DNA alterations at the genomic DNA level. This is necessary, since gene functional changes and/or changes at protein or mRNA level cannot always be readily detected in a blood or mouth wash sample, but only in the target tissue(s) or the tumour. Moreover, a number of cases have been described in which the wild-type allele is preferentially or exclusively transcribed, which leads to false negative reporting for heterozygous mutations. Hence, the best genetic screening tests at present are those that are readily applicable to genomic DNA. Targeting genomic DNA is technologically complicated by the fact that, for virtually all genes, the coding region is scattered over multiple exons amidst many sometimes very large introns (Figure 5.1).

A second criterion by which to distinguish genetic screening tests involves their relative capacity actually to scan the target gene(s) for all possible mutations. Most tests advocated for their high throughput at low cost are actually mutational screening tests. That is, they screen samples for the presence of one or multiple previously identified and well-characterized mutations. Since, thus

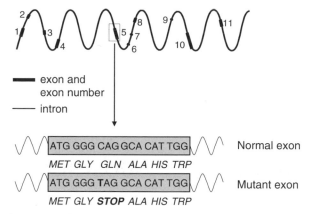

Figure 5.1 *Schematic representation of the genomic organization of a human gene. The use of genomic DNA as the starting material for mutation scanning requires enough intronic sequence information to allow amplification of each of the sometimes many exons of a cancer predisposition gene. (Courtesy of Dr Nathalie van Orsouw.)*

far, there are few instances where only one or very few mutations occur in a gene, such screening methods are only useful when they are capable of detecting all the mutations one can expect to find in a particular gene. For many genes, e.g. *BRCA1*, hundreds of different mutations have been discovered. Exhaustive screening in the majority of these cases renders most mutational screening tests uneconomical, even when they can operate at high throughput. Moreover, the distribution of mutations is not uniform among ethnic groups and complete mutational spectra in this respect are not presently available for any gene. Finally, new mutations continue to be generated *de novo*. Solely for this latter reason, mutational screening tests will never provide reliable pre-screening utility. Once a positive diagnosis of an individual case of hereditary cancer has been made, however, it is then economical to analyse family members for the same mutation, which then greatly reduces the cost. Below we will critically evaluate some of the major mutational scanning and screening methods.

CURRENT AND EXPERIMENTAL METHODS FOR MUTATION DETECTION

Basic principles

In the application of methods for mutation detection, four stages can be distinguished:

1 sample preparation and preparation of the target sequence;
2 mutation detection;
3 readout;
4 interpretation of the results.

In stage 1, DNA extraction is of critical importance for obtaining interpretable and reproducible results. For routine testing, a number of high-quality DNA extraction systems are commercially available and, in our experience, are worth the marginal additions to cost that accompany their use. The main reason high-quality DNA is needed to obtain optimal template DNA is for polymerase chain reaction (PCR) amplification, which is by far the most frequently used method for target sequence preparation. Optimal DNA quality is especially important for multiplex PCR or long-distance PCR. PCR amplification can be a major determinant of the cost of an assay. Indeed, a large cancer susceptibility gene, such as *BRCA1*, may require as many as 30–40 PCR amplicons to generate all the coding sequences for mutation analysis. The reagent costs alone for this number of PCR amplifications can easily amount to US $20–30, depending on the type of enzyme used and the reaction volumes. Therefore, co-amplification of multiple fragments in the same tube (multiplex PCR) can greatly reduce the costs as well as the labour required for detecting mutations in large or multiple genes. DNA extraction and PCR set-up can be automated. This has several advantages, the most important being a reduction of the costs (less labour and sometimes also fewer reagents) and a lower risk of human error. Liquid handlers for DNA extraction and PCR set-up are available from numerous companies.

The second stage, the actual mutation detection stage, defines the type of method used and basically determines the physical limits of its accuracy. There are a great variety of different mutation detection principles currently available (discussed below), most of which can be used in combination with PCR and various readout systems. Virtually all of these methods have been designed to detect point mutations, and small deletions or insertions. While on the one hand this represents a positive step because it is this type of mutation that has been previously difficult to detect with conventional methods (i.e. Southern hybridization) the disadvantage is that large mutations, deleting entire exons or the entire gene often go undetected. In such cases, PCR amplification generates target sequence only from the wild-type allele, which limits the sensitivity of the test. This is true for almost all mutation detection tests, including sequencing.

To visualize the result of the actual mutation detection stage, a readout system is required. This usually involves a separation step (e.g. electrophoresis). More recently, alternatives have been developed, such as hybridization or mass spectrometry. Sometimes, but not always, the readout system itself is part of the mutation detection principle (see later). When talking about throughput, this step is usually considered the most important, but it should be realized that much of the time involved in a genetic screening test is the actual sample preparation,

DNA extraction and PCR amplification. Indeed, while it can be argued that the actual readout of mass spectrometry is only milliseconds, such an advantage is not very useful when the entire test still takes many hours owing to the need for sample preparation, DNA extraction, PCR amplification, mutation detection and result interpretation.

Finally, the interpretation of the results of a genetic screening test, whether in the form of a band pattern after electrophoresis or a hybridization pattern, can be automated by image analysis. This not only serves to reduce the overall time involved in a given assay, but also helps minimize human error and allows the results to be automatically logged into a database. Many, if not most, of the currently available genetic screening tests lack suitable image analysis and database systems.

Below, we discuss a number of mutational scanning and screening methods with the focus on scanning methods, since we believe those to be the most relevant to future screening for mutations in cancer susceptibility genes. All methods have been distinguished on the basis of their mutation detection principle. For mutational scanning assays, we have indicated their accuracy and cost in comparison to nucleotide sequencing, which is generally considered the gold standard, although mutations can even escape detection by sequencing (see later). Since most of these methods can be carried out in different formats, such a comparison is necessarily arbitrary. In this respect, we have made the assumption that each method is carried out only once under a given set of conditions and we have decided to ignore human error. For mutational screening methods, the costs are expressed per mutation/sample analysed, while their accuracy is assumed to be close to 100 per cent.

MUTATIONAL SCANNING METHODS

DNA sequencing

The most familiar of the mutational scanning methods listed in Table 5.2 and generally considered to be the gold standard is DNA sequencing. Virtually all DNA sequencing protocols are now based on dideoxy chain termination, as originally developed by Sanger *et al.*[5] This technique depends on 2′,3′-dideoxyribonucleotide triphosphates (ddNTPs) being incorporated into an extending copy of a template DNA from a primer, which then leads to chain termination due to lack of the 3′-OH group required for phosphodiester bond formation. With multiplex fluorescence labels in the form of either primer or terminator to identify the A, C, G and T extensions, four sequencing reactions can be performed simultaneously in one tube and all four reaction products can be fractionated

Table 5.2 *Mutation scanning methods*

Method[a]	Accuracy[b]	Cost[c]	Genes[d]	References
Sequencing	High	High	BRCA1/BRCA2	63, 68
Conformation based				
SSCP	Low	Medium	BRCA1/BRCA2, ATM	9, 69, 77
CFLP	Medium	Medium	BRCA1, TP53	70, 71
CSGE	Low	Medium	BRCA1, MSH6	72, 73
Melting based				
DGGE	High	Medium	BRCA1/BRCA2, PTEN	74, 75
TDGS	High	Low	BRCA1, TP53	21, 76
DHPLC	Medium	Medium	BRCA1/BRCA2	29, 77
Mismatch scanning				
CCM	High	Medium	ATM, TP53	78, 79
EMC	Medium	Medium	TP53	80
Protein truncation testing	Low	Medium	BRCA1/BRCA2	81, 82
DNA array	Medium	High	BRCA1,TP53, ATM	47–49

[a] Categories of methods, modifications are discussed in main text.
[b] Assuming one set of conditions, no human error and a 100 per cent accuracy of sequencing as the arbitrary standard.
High = 100%; medium = 90–99%; low = 60–89%.
[c] Cost/bp: high = 10–20 US cents/base, medium = 5–9 US cents/base, low = <5 US cents/base.
[d] Examples of cancer predisposition gene(s) exhaustively analysed by the method.
CCM, chemical cleavage of mismatches; CFLP, cleavage fragment length polymorphism; CSGE, conformation-sensitive gel electrophoresis; DGGE, denaturing gradient gel electrophoresis; DHPLC, denaturing high-performance liquid chromatography; EMC, enzymatic mismatch cleavage; SSCP, single-strand conformation polymorphism; TDGS, two-dimensional gene scanning.

by size through electrophoresis in a slab gel, capillary gel or microchip in a single lane.[6]

Despite some obvious advantages of DNA sequencing (e.g. high level of automation, commercial availability of dedicated equipment and reagents, and ability to provide complete information about the location and nature of the sequence variants), DNA sequencing is still labour intensive. In addition, it is sometimes difficult to accurately identify heterozygous mutations because of background noise, suggesting mutations where there are none,[7] owing to software errors. This is illustrated in Plate 1, where a real mutation was detected and confirmed by sequencing in two directions. However, the overlapping peaks in Plate 1 reflect an apparent artefact because they could not be reproduced by reversed sequencing or by using an alternative method (e.g. DGGE, see later). This illustrates the importance of sequencing in two directions when confirming the presence of a mutation. Although adopted as the gold standard, sequencing can miss mutations and, therefore, does not have 100 per cent accuracy.

The high overall cost of sequencing essentially constrains routine use of the technique for genetic screening in most laboratories. A hierarchical approach with stepwise use of a combination of methods, first employing an accurate prescreening method to scan mutations in an entire gene of interest prior to direct sequencing of only the mutation-containing fragment, will dramatically reduce labour and cost. In Table 5.2 we have compared accuracy between different mutation scanning methods, assuming sequencing to be the arbitrary standard of 100 per cent accuracy, under one set of conditions excluding human error. The mutational scanning methods have been broadly categorized according to their principles of mutation detection. They all use PCR to obtain the target sequence. The principle of each mutation scanning method is discussed with special reference to modifications adopted to improve assay sensitivity as well as throughput, although this is at the sacrifice of cost since it adds complexity.

SSCP

Single-strand conformation polymorphism (SSCP) analysis, first described by Orita et al.,[8] is based on the fact that under non-denaturing conditions a single-stranded DNA molecule will adopt a conformation that is uniquely dependent on its sequence context, owing to the formation of intrastrand base pairing. Such conformations are often different enough to distinguish a single base change by an alteration in electrophoretic mobility. Conventional SSCP analysis requires denaturation of the double-stranded PCR product by heating, immediate chilling on ice, followed by gel electrophoresis under non-denaturing conditions. Traditionally, slab gel electrophoresis and autoradiography of the radiolabelled fragments are employed for the readout. However, as with other mutation scanning methods based on electrophoresis, increased convenience, improved safety and greater efficiency of detection, as well as increased speed, can be obtained by the application of a fluorescent label in combination with high-speed separation. The latter may vary from minigels and capillary gels to microchip-based analysis.[9] However, in most cases, this requires expensive equipment.

Although SSCP is one of the most popular and widely used methods for its simplicity, its disadvantages are the requirement to perform analysis under more than one electrophoretic condition to detect all possible conformational changes. Even under multiple conditions, its sensitivity is between 60 per cent and 95 per cent, depending on the gene and fragment size, and the assay is unreliable with fragments greater than about 200 bp. This is understandable because not all point mutational differences necessarily lead to differences in secondary structure. The use of restriction digestion (REF-SSCP; restriction endonuclease fingerprinting[10]) or a combination of SSCP and direct sequencing (DDF-SSCP; dideoxy fingerprinting[11]) have been adopted to increase accuracy, but at the expense of added complexity and cost.

CFLP

Cleavage fragment length polymorphism (CFLP) is based upon the same principle as SSCP, that is, the fact that single-stranded DNAs form reproducible hairpin duplexes during self-annealing. In CFLP, rather than relying on mutation-dependent differences in secondary structure, the hairpins are cleaved by endonuclease cleavage I (Cleavase 1), a structure-specific endonuclease, at the 5′ side of the junctions between the single stranded and the duplex region.[12] The cleavage products reveal sequence-specific patterns of bands on a gel, which can be distinguished by the appearance, disappearance, increase or decrease in the signal intensity of one or more bands, and the patterns often reflect the locations of the sequence differences. Compared with SSCP, CFLP is more rapid, more accurate and permits the analysis of larger DNA fragments.[13] However, to generate a reproducible fragment pattern, assay time and temperature have to be optimized for each type of DNA fragment to be analysed to stabilize characteristic intrastrand hairpin duplexes. A recently introduced 'ramping' protocol eliminates the need for optimizations by enabling all DNA fragments to be analysed under identical reaction conditions.[14]

A different approach to exploit the variation in DNA secondary structure for mutation scanning is conformation-sensitive gel electrophoresis (CSGE), which is based on differences in conformation between homoduplex and heteroduplex double-stranded DNA fragments.[15] Heteroduplexes are generated by heat denaturation and reannealing of a mixture of wild-type and mutant DNA molecules. The resulting homoduplexes and heteroduplexes exhibit either distinct electrophoretic mobility or

distinct cleavage patterns under appropriate conditions. Only when combined with SSCP can the mutation detection rate of CSGE approach 100 per cent.

DGGE

Denaturing gradient gel electrophoresis (DGGE), first described by Fischer and Lerman,[16] is based on the physical property of DNA to denature in distinctive domains and not all at once, resulting in a branched structure. Since the stability of each domain is dependent upon base composition, single nucleotide differences are sufficient to alter melting behavior. When a DNA fragment reaches a denaturant concentration or temperature equivalent to the melting temperature of its lowest melting domain, partial strand separation, branching and reduction in electrophoretic mobility occurs in a gradient gel of increasing denaturant concentration (DGGE) or increasing temperature (TGGE; temperature gradient gel electrophoresis;[17]). The sensitivity of DGGE has been improved to virtually 100 per cent by:

1 the attachment of a GC-rich sequence (known as a GC-clamp) to serve as the highest melting domain;[18]
2 the use of a computer program to predict optimal melting profiles for the sequence to be scanned;[19]
3 applying heteroduplexing.

Figure 5.2 shows two applications of DGGE. In Figure 5.2a a heterozygous polymorphism in exon 8 of the DNA mismatch repair gene, *MLH1*, is revealed by 4 bands, that is, the two homoduplex fragments and the two heteroduplex fragments, as compared to the homozygous state in the control fragment in the left lane. The same polymorphism can be detected as part of a comprehensive display of all *MLH1* exons separated in two dimensions on the basis of both size and melting temperature, using two-dimensional gene scanning (Figure 5.2b). Two-dimensional gene scanning (TDGS) is based on DGGE in a two-dimensional (2D) format enabling analysis of an entire gene for all possible mutations in one gel under one set of conditions.[20,21] A simple automated 2D instrument has been developed allowing the entire 2D electrophoresis process to be completed well within 3 hours, using ultrathin gels and high voltage.[22,23] Because the 2D format permits the analysis of many fragments in parallel, TDGS is one of a few techniques known to allow extensive multiplex PCR, that is, up to 26 fragments in one single reaction, resulting in a significant cost reduction.[24]

DHPLC

Denaturing high-performance liquid chromatography (DHPLC), first described by Oefner and Underhill[25] and Oefner *et al.*[26] has rapidly gained popularity.[26–29] DHPLC uses ion-pair reverse phase liquid chromatography to

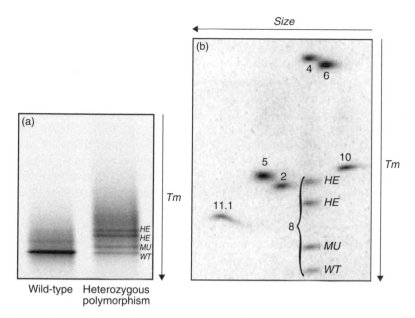

Figure 5.2 *Example of the use of denaturing gradient gel electrophoresis (DGGE) or its derivative, two-dimensional gene scanning (TDGS), to scan the hereditary non-polyposis colorectal cancer (HNPCC) susceptibility gene MLH1. (a) Two lanes of a DGGE gel. Electrophoresis of the polymerase chain reaction (PCR)-amplified exon 8 results in one band for the homozygous control sample, while the polymorphic heterozygote state results in four bands: two homoduplex variants (wild-type/wild-type; WT, or mutant hybridized to mutant; MU) and two heteroduplex (wild-type/mutant strands; HE) variants. (b) Detail of a TDGS gel. In TDGS, all PCR-amplified exons are first separated by size in the top part of a DGGE gel. The same polymorphism in exon 8 is detected, while the other six exon fragments visible are homozygous. (Courtesy of Dr Nathalie van Orsouw.)*

detect DNA heteroduplexes. Under partially denaturing conditions within a linear acetonitrile gradient, heteroduplexes denature more readily and display reduced column reten- tion time relative to their fully complementary homoduplex counterparts, which are detected as new chromatographic peaks at a lower retention time (Figure 5.3). DHPLC offers the major advantage of being an automated hands-free alternative to gel-based techniques, requiring no post-PCR sample processing. Moreover, the ion-pairing agent (i.e. triethylammonium acetate) compresses the melting range of the amplicons, reducing the need for GC-clamped PCR primers, unlike other melting-based methods. However, in order to detect a heteroduplex molecule, the system's operating temperature must be optimized for each amplicon tested, which is facilitated by an algorithm available at the Stanford University website (http://insertion.standford.edu/melt. html). For some fragments, however, it is only when tried empirically with ±1°C changes from the theoretically optimal temperature that a sequence variant becomes obvious from the chromatogram as multiple peaks instead of one.[30] Therefore, sensitivity of DHPLC is given as below 100 per cent under one set of conditions in Table 5.2. Analysis time is rapid, ranging from 6 to 10 minutes per sample for fragment sizes from 200 up to 700 bp. However, with present instruments, only one sample can be analysed at a time and parallel analysis is not (yet) possible. In view of this low throughput, DHPLC is not very

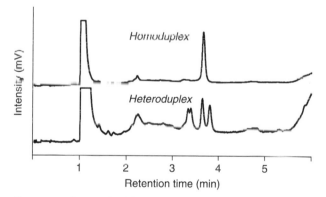

Figure 5.3 *Denaturing high-performance liquid chromatography (DHPLC) separation patterns of a homozygous (top) normal and heterozygous mutated DNA fragment. The first, very large peak in the chromatogram is the injection peak, representing primers, deoxyribonucleotide triphosphates (dNTPs) and salts. The peak around 2 minutes represents the primer dimer. The four-peak pattern in the lower chromatogram represents a heterozygous mutation, with the early eluting peaks being the heteroduplexes. As in denaturing gradient gel electrophoresis, heterozygous mutations or polymorphisms can be detected by the appearance of more than one peak, as compared to the single peak for the homozygous situation. (Courtesy of Varian Inc.)*

suitable for large-scale testing. It is, however, used in several clinical diagnostic laboratories with a moderate sample throughput load.

CCM

Chemical cleavage of mismatch (CCM) is based on the susceptibility of mismatched bases in a heteroduplex to modification by chemicals.[31] Initially, hydroxylamine or osmium tetroxide were used for modification of mismatched cytosine or thymine residues, respectively, which are then cleaved with piperidine for analysis of cleavage products on gel. If both sense and antisense strands are analysed, all point mutations can be detected with an accuracy approaching 100 per cent, because mutations of adenine and guanine will also be detected as a mismatched T or C on the other strand.[32] Moreover, CCM can localize the sites of the mismatch, reducing the need for extensive DNA sequencing to characterize a mutation. Recent protocols replace the toxic osmium tetroxide with potassium permanganate.[33] Moreover, modifications, such as fluorescent multiplexing and solid phase reactions, open the way to complete automation for high throughput analysis.[34] Compared to other mutation scanning methods, CCM has the ability to scan large PCR fragments up to 2 kb with a high sensitivity of detection. The usefulness of being able to scan large fragments in most cases of cancer predisposition screening, however, is doubtful since the average exon size is not much higher than 200 bp and cDNA is not the optimal target for genetic screening (see earlier).

EMC

Enzymatic mismatch cleavage (EMC) uses specific enzymes to cleave at the site of the heteroduplex. The enzymes used for this purpose range from the classical RNase and S1 nuclease to a relatively new class of enzymes, the bacteriophage resolvases, all of which are able to recognize and cleave DNA containing unpaired bases *in vitro*.[35,36] Despite the capability of resolvases to cleave at all possible mispairings, relative cleavage efficiencies vary considerably for individual mismatches and may escape detection if located in an unfavourable surrounding sequence.[37] Moreover, non-specific cleavage between different batches of enzyme and difficulties in interpreting results by the inexperienced user preclude the routine use of this method in the clinical setting.

PTT

The protein truncation test (PTT) is a method to detect premature translation-terminating mutations due to stop codons created by point mutations or as a consequence of frameshift mutations. PTT protocols have not been greatly improved from the method originally described.[38] After reverse transcription of RNA, PCR-amplified cDNA is used for *in vitro* transcription-translation to generate peptide fragments, which are then analysed on a sodium dodecyl sulphate–polyacrylamide gel electrophoresis (SDS-PAGE) gel for identification of shortened (truncated) proteins, that is, translation-terminating mutations. The important feature of PTT is a specially designed tailed sense primer enabling the transcription and translation of PCR products. The primer contains an RNA polymerase promotor (T7, SP6 or T3), a eukaryotic translation initiation sequence (consensus Kozak sequence) and an ATG start codon in-frame with the target gene sequence.[39] Recently, a PTT primer containing an N-terminal myc-tag has been used for antibody detection of correctly initiated translation product.[40] Because PTT targets a gene-coding region of RNA, large segments (up to 2–4 kb) can be screened in a single assay. In some cases, PTT can be used to scan a large portion of a gene for truncating point mutations using genomic DNA as a template.[41,42]

Because almost all translation-termination mutations have been proven to be disease related, PTT pinpoints clinically relevant mutations only. This method is, therefore, useful for scanning genes in which translation-terminating mutations are known to dominate, such as the *APC*, *BRCA1* and *BRCA2* tumour suppressor genes, in which most mutations result in truncated proteins. However, missense mutations yielding amino acid substitutions, which have been shown to account for a significant fraction of the mutations in many cancer genes, cannot be detected by PTT. Moreover, in common with other RNA-based mutation detection methods, mutated transcripts are often under-represented due to the instability of transcripts carrying truncating mutations compared with the transcripts derived from the wild-type allele; this is termed nonsense-mediated mRNA decay,[43,44] leading to false negatives. In addition, mutations near the extreme N- or C-terminus of the protein or tissue-specific splicing variants will lead to false negatives or false positives, respectively.

DNA arrays

DNA microarrays on glass or so-called 'DNA chips' offer one of the most promising solutions for cost-effective, accurate, high-throughput mutational scanning. DNA chip-based technology allows large numbers of hybridization experiments in parallel using high-density, 2D arrays of oligonucleotide probes.[45] The currently used oligonucleotide arrays consist of short oligonucleotides (up to 25 nt) synthesized directly on a solid support using sequentially masked photolabile nucleotide chemistry developed by Affymetrix.[46] This allows for approximately 300 000 polydeoxynucleotides to be synthesized on a small glass surface of 1.28 cm². To scan a sequence of interest for all possible changes, four 25-mer sequencing probes are designed to interrogate the identity of each target nucleotide. One probe is designed to be perfectly complementary to a target sequence, whereas the other three are identical to the first, except at the interrogation position where one of the other three bases is substituted in the central position. By analysing hybridization patterns, nucleotide identities are assigned. Therefore, in theory, sequence information for virtually any sequence could be obtained when an oligonucleotide array is designed to interrogate sense and antisense strand sequence, because all possible complementary sequences are present in the array. However, the system is not well suited for detection of large deletions and insertions. Key to the approach is the use of probe redundancy, which improves signal-to-noise ratio, which in turn increases assay sensitivity and specificity by compensating for non-specific signals.[47] Oligonucleotide arrays for a number of cancer genes have been developed and their use for mutation scanning demonstrated. Examples are *TP53* with 65 000 different oligonucleotide probes of about 18 bases in length,[48] *ATM* with >90 000 oligonucleotide probes of 25 bases in length[47] and *BRCA1* with >97 000 oligonucleotide probes of 25 bases in length.[49] Only the *TP53* chip is presently commercially available and appears to function at high accuracy.[48] However, its high cost effectively constrains application on a large scale (see also later).

The DNA array principle of simultaneously analysing an entire gene-coding sequence as one set of automatically interpreted hybridization signals makes it a powerful and effective tool for high-throughput mutational analysis. It is also one of the few methods that can be used in combination with PCR multiplexing. However, for the moment, at least for most genes, the accuracy of the system is well below 100 per cent because it is very difficult to create one set of conditions to fulfil all hybridization requirements of so many different sequences. Current protocols are suitable under conditions where a modest false-negative error rate (5–10 per cent) is permitted and to reduce the false-negative rate is the greatest challenge in hybridization-based mutational analysis.[45] Modifications adapted to increase sensitivity and specificity of hybridization include the use of modified triphosphates[49] and peptide nucleic acid arrays.[50]

MUTATIONAL SCREENING METHODS

It goes without saying that all of the mutational scanning methods described above can be used to screen multiple samples for known, previously identified mutations. However, once a recurrent mutation has been identified, it becomes infinitely easier and less expensive to detect its presence in a DNA fragment by using one of the available mutational screening tests. Table 5.3 lists a number of mutational screening principles. What all these methods have in common is a very low cost per assay/mutation (around one dollar or less per assay/mutation), a high throughput and a high accuracy.

Table 5.3 *Mutation screening methods*

Method	References
Restriction analysis	
Minisequencing	
Pyrosequencing	51
Mass spectrometry	53
Allele-specific oligonucleotide hybridization	55, 56
Allele-specific amplification	
ARMS	57
Oligonucleotide-specific ligation	58, 59
Invasive cleavage	60
Rolling circle amplification	61

ARMS, amplification refractory mutation system.

Restriction analysis

The most simple method to detect known point mutations, which is still widely used, is restriction analysis. By selecting a restriction enzyme that cuts at the site of the mutation, it is possible to differentiate between the mutant and wild-type allele as obtained, for example, by PCR amplification, on the basis of the appearance of one or two fragments. The readout system can be a simple gel or more advanced systems of fragment size separation, such as mass spectrometry. The potential disadvantages of this method can be the lack of suitable restriction enzymes and incomplete digestion. (Of note, in the case of a deletion or insertion, the size of the PCR fragment itself can be analysed without restriction digestion.)

Minisequencing

Although sequencing *per se* can obviously be used to detect known mutations, its general format does not lend itself for an economic mutational screening test. However, minisequencing is a cost-effective alternative. Pyrosequencing, for example, is a new method for real-time minisequencing, typically of up to 20 nucleotides, simultaneously on 96 different templates.[51] First, sequencing primers are chosen close to the specific mutation. Then the target locus is PCR-amplified, using one biotinylated and one standard PCR primer. Single-stranded template is obtained by magnetic strand separation on streptavidin-coated beads and, finally, several bases, including the site of the mutation, are sequenced on the bead-bound template. Incorporation is detected in real time by pyrophosphate detection. Both instrumentation and reagent kits are commercially available.

Another fast minisequencing method to detect a known mutation in multiple samples is based on mass spectrometry. Using matrix-assisted laser desorption/ionization time of flight (MALDI-TOF) mass spectrometry, one or a few base differences can be distinguished very rapidly, i.e. in milliseconds.[52] After PCR amplification of the target fragment, a primer is annealed to the template adjacent to the region containing the mutation. For example, when one needs to distinguish a one-base difference, a mixture of one dideoxynucleotide triphosphate and the three other deoxy-NTPs will allow the primer to be extended by one or more bases. The resulting two different products are differentiated by mass spectrometry. By using such a primer extension assay it has been demonstrated that it is possible to analyse up to 12 loci together in one single tube.[53] It is also possible actually to sequence by using mass spectrometry in combination with the dideoxy Sanger sequencing principle, but not more than up to 35 bases.[54] Also for this minisequencing/primer extension principle, equipment and reagent kits are commercially available.

Allele-specific oligonucleotide hybridization

An accepted way of detecting known mutations is by allele-specific oligonucleotide (ASO) hybridization. In such assays, an oligonucleotide is synthesized specific for the wild-type or mutant allele and immobilized (e.g. on membrane or glass supports). Subsequent hybridization with PCR-amplified labelled target sequence allows discrimination between the mutant and wild-type allele by differential hybridization signals.[55] Alternatively, it is possible to immobilize the target sequence, which is then interrogated using labelled oligonucleotides specific for the mutant or wild-type sequence. ASO can be used in so-called homogeneous assays in which the actual mutation detection step is combined with PCR target amplification. For example, TaqMan or Molecular Beacon technology allow the distinction in real time between PCR-amplified mutant and wild-type alleles.[56] These assays are based on PCR amplification of the target sequence in the presence of the two allele-specific probes labelled with different fluorophores. Only perfect hybridization provides for fluorescence emission, which is monitored in real time. The changes in fluorescence during cycling reflect the different genotypes.

Allele-specific amplification

A variant of ASO is allele-specific amplification in which primers are designed with mismatches at their terminal 3′ nucleotide with the wild-type refractory to PCR of the mutant allele and vice versa. The best known example is the ARMS (amplification refractory mutation system) test.[57]

Oligonucleotide ligation assay

Another system to detect known mutations or polymorphisms is the oligonucleotide ligation assay (OLA). In this assay, PCR-amplified target sequence is used as template for two oligonucleotide probes, one for a common sequence and the other for either the mutant or the wild-type sequence immediately adjacent to the common sequence. Using thermostable DNA ligase, only the perfectly complementary pair of oligonucleotides is joined. Various ways, including electrophoresis and DNA microarrays, have been described as readouts for this system.[58,59]

Invasive cleavage

An example of a method that combines the mutation detection step with an amplification step (homogeneous assay) is based on the use of flap endonucleases (FENs) isolated from archaea.[12] Originally used for the development of a signal amplification system, these enzymes are capable of cleaving overlapping pairs of oligonucleotide probes, that is, an invasive and a signal probe, complementary to a predetermined region of target DNA.[60] Cleavage is highly specific, in the sense that mismatches between the signal probe and the target at the nucleotide immediately upstream of the intended cleavage site preclude the creation of the overlap. This enables discrimination of point mutations. Elevated temperature and an excess of one of the probes enable multiple probes to be cleaved for each target sequence present without temperature cycling. These cleaved probes then direct cleavage of another labelled probe, which is quenched by an internal dye. Upon cleavage, the fluorescein-labelled product can be detected using a standard fluorescence plate reader. Hence, this assay is not dependent on PCR, but includes its own signal amplification step. The same cleavase enzymes can also be used in a variant of this method (i.e. CFLP), which is capable of scanning a DNA fragment for all possible mutations (see earlier).

Rolling circle amplification

A second option for diagnostic mutation analysis in the absence of PCR amplification is rolling circle amplification. In this method, circularizable, so-called padlock probes are used to bind the target DNA, leaving a small gap of 8 bp. Addition of allele-specific eight-base oligonucleotides permit subsequent ligation and rolling circle amplification, providing for an isothermal signal amplification step.[61]

CONCLUSIONS AND FUTURE PROSPECTS

The last 10 years have witnessed the metamorphosis of molecular genetics from primarily individual-driven research to a highly automated, computerized factory science. In this respect, it is highly appropriate that, with the virtual completion of the human genome project, a landmark in the history of science, essentially all human genes have become accessible for research. It is reasonable to expect that this will greatly accelerate the pace at which novel cancer-related genes are identified and characterized. This, however, should only be considered as the foundation of further exploratory endeavours into the realm of human variability. Indeed, one of the most challenging prospects in this respect is the possibility that has now emerged to screen human populations genetically for all possible gene variants conferring increased risk for various cancers. In spite of all this progress, many challenges still lie ahead, both in testing procedures and in the interpretation of test results, before genetic screening becomes daily routine. In this chapter we have critically evaluated the situation with respect to present and future procedures to screen large numbers of individuals for mutations and polymorphic variants in multiple genes, based on their identification as cancer susceptibility genes and the availability of full sequence information.

While a number of methods can now be identified that are capable of accurately detecting a given known mutation, the real challenge in this field is to find a 100 per cent effective method for scanning entire genes for all possible mutations, including as yet unidentified ones. Some significant progress in this respect has now been made; there are now a few mutational scanning methods that have virtually a 100 per cent accuracy to detect previously unknown small mutations in a cancer susceptibility gene correctly. Unfortunately, this does not mean that we now have methods that are 100 per cent accurate in correctly identifying genetic changes that predispose to cancer. First of all, none of the PCR-based methods described has the capacity to detect large deletions. Hence, it will remain necessary to include cytogenetic, loss of heterozygosity or deletion detection methods to rule out such mutations. Second, mutations can occur in the promoter regions as well as in non-coding regions, which are usually not subjected to analysis in standard genetic tests. Finally, the possibility of additional genes can never be ruled out.

Of the other criteria mentioned in Table 5.1, almost none are universally met by any system currently available. Most importantly, no methods are as yet cost-effective enough to allow large-scale genetic screening, that is, involving multiple genes and pathways. Sequencing, which is still considered as the gold standard of genetic screening, is also the most expensive, which is illustrated by the cost of a commercial BRCA1 and BRCA2 sequence analysis of over US $2600. (Myriad is now licensing the sequencing service to National Institutes of Health scientists for less for research purposes.[62]) Recent developments in the form of increased electrophoresis speed and throughput have made improvements, but almost completely automated, computerized platforms for mutation detection in large cancer genes, such as the Myriad company's platform for BRCA1 and BRCA2 sequencing,[63] are relatively rare. New sequencing principles, such as sequencing by hybridisation,[64] are still far away from practical application. Hence, sequencing is unlikely to be the near-future technology platform of choice for large-scale genetic predisposition testing.

There is very little information available about the performance of any of the alternative prescreening methods, such as SSCP or DGGE, as automated platforms in a routine, clinical environment. Nevertheless, some of these methods are clearly an order of magnitude less expensive than sequencing at the same or higher accuracy. Most of them also lend themselves well to similar automation and computerization as sequencing. Therefore, it is reasonable to expect that particularly the multiplex PCR-based methods will be able to compete very well with sequencing now that novel readout systems, such as capillary electrophoresis, high-performance liquid chromatography (HPLC), 2D electrophoresis, and electrophoresis in microplates or on glass chips have become available. Indeed, based upon the rapid progress in the development and improvement of alternative prescreening methods for mutational scanning, it seems realistic to predict that, several years from now, one or more of these systems will be capable of offering tests at a cost well below US $100 per average gene of 15 exons, including labour and overheads.

Somewhat surprisingly, the microarray-based DNA chip methods, heralded as the potentially least expensive gene mutational scanning method with the highest throughput, are as yet among the most expensive and not as accurate as, for example, DGGE-based methods. The only chip for gene mutational scanning that is presently commercially available is the TP53 array,[48] a relatively small gene, which costs about US $500 for five disposable arrays, excluding reagents and PCR primers. Although it is realistic to assume that mass production will lower the price, thus far it has proved costly to make such DNA arrays by photolithography. Novel, more cost-effective technology might become available over the next few years, which would improve cost efficiency.[65] A major strength of the DNA array method is its ability to scan multiple fragments, up to entire genes or multiple genes in parallel in a relatively short time (i.e. about 4.5 hours from purified DNA to data analysis[48]). In this respect, however, it is no longer unique. Other parallel methods based on extensive PCR multiplexing are available to scan entire genes in hours,[24] while increased efficiency of multicapillary electrophoresis or HPLC systems permit parallel analysis of hundreds of PCR amplicons simultaneously.[66] That would leave the DNA-array approach with its single advantage of being able to identify the mutation immediately without further sequencing.

More recent advances in this field include anchored multiplex amplification using SDA (strand displacement amplification), an isothermal amplification method. This amplification procedure can be carried out directly on microelectronic chip arrays and allows target amplification (in large multiplex groups) and mutation detection to be performed on the same platform.[67]

Where does this leave the mutational screening methods? Such methods are especially useful in rapid and cost-effective screening of a limited number of mutations or polymorphisms. Since even more modern mutational scanning methods cannot attain 100 per cent sensitivity, it can be argued that to test for only a limited number of mutations should be acceptable in many cases. On the somewhat longer term, however, it is likely that even the most inexpensive mutational screening methods will be superseded by equally inexpensive scanning methods.

ACKNOWLEDGEMENTS

We thank Dr Nathalie van Orsouw and Mr David Rines for critically reading the manuscript of this chapter and the many useful suggestions. We are grateful to Nathalie van Orsouw for Figures 5.1, 5.2 and 5.3. We thank Mr Eric Gerber of Varian Inc. for providing us with Figure 5.4 and some of the information he provided on DHPLC. The authors of the chapter have a commercial interest in one of the mutational scanning methods discussed: two-dimensional gene scanning (TDGS).

KEY POINTS

- Screening for genetic mutations is becoming highly automated and computerized.
- The human genome project will enable all human genes to become accessible for research, which will accelerate the pace at which novel cancer-related genes are identified and characterized.
- There are still many challenges, both in testing procedures and in the interpretation of test results before genetic screening becomes daily routine.
- While a number of methods can detect a known mutation, the real challenge in this field is to find a 100 per cent effective method for scanning entire genes for all possible mutations, including as yet unidentified ones.
- It is likely that even the most inexpensive mutational screening methods will be superseded by equally inexpensive scanning methods.

REFERENCES

1. Eng C. From bench to bedside ... but when? *Genome Res* 1997; **7**:669–672.
2. Mathew CG. Screening for mutations in cancer predisposition genes. In: Eeles RA, Ponder BAJ, Easton DF, Horwich A (eds) *Genetic predisposition to cancer.* London: Chapman & Hall, 1996:372–382.
3. Eng C, Vijg J. Genetic testing: the problems and the promise. *Nature Biotechnol* 1997, **15**:422–426.
4. Liu B, Parsons R, Papadopoulos N, *et al.* Analysis of mismatch repair genes in hereditary non-polyposis colorectal cancer patients. *Nature Med* 1996; **2**:169–173.
5. Sanger F, Nicklen S, Coulson AR. DNA sequencing with chain-terminating inhibitors. *Proc Natl Acad Sci USA* 1977; **74**:5463–5467.
6. Schmalzing D, Koutny L, Salas-Solano O, *et al.* Recent developments in DNA sequencing by capillary and microdevice electrophoresis. *Electrophoresis* 1999; **20**:3066–3077.
7. Phelps RS, Chadwick RB, Conrad MP, *et al.* Efficient, automatic detection of heterozygous bases during large-scale DNA sequence screening. *BioTechniques* 1995; **19**:984–989.
8. Orita M, Iwahana H, Kanazawa H, *et al.* Detection of polymorphisms of human DNA by gel electrophoresis as single-strand conformation polymorphisms. *Proc Natl Acad Sci USA* 1989; **86**:2766–2770.
9. Tian H, Jaquins-Gerst A, Munro N, *et al.* Single-strand conformation polymorphism analysis by capillary and microchip electrophoresis: a fast, simple method for detection of common mutations in *BRCA1* and *BRCA2. Genomics* 2000; **63**:25–34.
10. Liu Q, Sommer SS. Restriction endonuclease fingerprinting (REF): a sensitive method for screening mutations in long, contiguous segments of DNA. *Biotechniques* 1995; **18**:470–477.
11. Lancaster JM, Berchuck A, Futreal PA, *et al.* Dideoxy fingerprinting assay for *BRCA1* mutation analysis. *Mol Carcinogen* 1997; **19**:176–179.
12. Lyamichev V, Brow MA, Dahlberg JE. Structure-specific endonucleolytic cleavage of nucleic acids by eubacterial DNA polymerases. *Science* 1993; **260**:778–783.
13. Rossetti S, Englisch S, Bresin E, *et al.* Detection of mutations in human genes by a new rapid method: cleavage fragment length polymorphism analysis (CFLPA). *Mol Cell Probes* 1997; **1**:155–160.
14. Oldenburg MC, Siebert M. New cleavase fragment length polymorphism method improves the mutation detection assay. *Biotechniques* 2000; **28**(2):351–357.
15. Ganguly A, Rock MJ, Prockop DJ. Conformation-sensitive gel electrophoresis for rapid detection of single-base differences in double-stranded PCR products and DNA fragments: evidence for solvent-induced bends in DNA heteroduplexes. *Proc Natl Acad Sci USA* 1993; **90**(21):10325–10329.
16. Fischer SG, Lerman LS. DNA fragments differing by single base-pair substitutions are separated in denaturing gradient gels: correspondence with melting theory. *Proc Natl Acad Sci USA* 1983; **80**:1579–1583.
17. Riesner D, Steger G, Zimmat R, *et al.* Temperature-gradient gel electrophoresis of nucleic acids: analysis of conformational

transitions, sequence variations, and protein-nucleic acid interactions. *Electrophoresis* 1989; **10**:377–389.

18. Sheffield VC, Cox DR, Lerman LS, *et al.* Attachment of a 40-base-pair G + C-rich sequence (GC-clamp) to genomic DNA fragments by the polymerase chain reaction results in improved detection of single-base changes. *Proc Natl Acad Sci USA* 1989; **86**:232–236.

19. Lerman LS, Silverstein K. Computational simulation of DNA melting and its application to denaturing gradient gel electrophoresis. *Methods of Enzymology* 1987; **155**:482–501.

20. Vijg J, van Orsouw NJ. Two-dimensional gene scanning: exploring human genetic variability. *Electrophoresis* 1999; **20**:1239–1249.

21. van Orsouw NJ, Dhanda RK, Elhaji Y. A highly accurate, low cost test for *BRCA1* mutations. *J Med Genet* 1999; **36**:747–753.

22. Dhanda RK, Smith W, Scott CB, *et al.* A simple system for automated two-dimensional electrophoresis: applications to genetic testing. *Genet Testing* 1998; **2**:67–70.

23. McGrath SB, Bounpheng M, Torres L, *et al.* High-speed, multicolor fluorescent two-dimensional gene scanning. *Genomics* 2001; **78**:83–90.

24. van Orsouw NJ, Li D, van der Vlies P, *et al.* Mutational scanning of large genes by extensive PCR multiplexing and two-dimensional electrophoresis: application to the *RB1* gene. *Hum Mol Genet* 1996; **5**:755–761.

25. Oefner PJ, Underhill PA. Comparative DNA sequencing by denaturing high-performance liquid chromatography (DHPLC). *Am J Hum Genet* 1995; **57S**:A266.

26. Underhill PA, Jin L, Lin AA, *et al.* Detection of numerous Y chromosome biallelic polymorphisms by denaturing high performance liquid chromatography. *Genome Res* 1997, **7**:996–1005.

27. Liu W, Smith DI, Rechtzigel KJ, *et al.* Denaturing high performance liquid chromatography (DHPLC) used in the detection of germline and somatic mutations. *Nucl Acids Res* 1998; **26**:1396–1400.

28. O'Donovan MC, Oefner PJ, Roberts SC, *et al.* Blind analysis of denaturing high-performance liquid chromatography as a tool for mutation detection. *Genomics* 1998; **52**:44–49.

29. Wagner T, Stoppa-Lyonnet D, Fleischmann E, *et al.* Denaturing high-performance liquid chromatography detects reliably *BRCA1* and *BRCA2* mutations. *Genomics* 1999; **62**:369–376.

30. Arnold N, Gross E, Schwarz-Boeger U, *et al.* A highly sensitive, fast, and economical technique for mutation analysis in hereditary breast and ovarian cancers. *Hum Mutat* 1999; **14**:333–339.

31. Ellis TP, Humphrey KE, Smith MJ, *et al.* Chemical cleavage of mismatch: a new look at an established method. *Hum Mutat* 1998; **11**:345–353.

32. Condie A, Feles R, Borresen AL, *et al.* Detection of point mutations in the *p53* gene: comparison of single-strand conformation polymorphism, constant denaturant gel electrophoresis, and hydroxylamine and osmium tetroxide techniques. *Hum Mutat* 1993; **2**:58–66.

33. Lambrinakos A, Humphrey KE, Babon JJ, *et al.* Reactivity of potassium permanganate and tetraethylammonium chloride with mismatched bases and a simple mutation detection protocol. *Nucl Acids Res* 1999; **27**:1866–1874.

34. Rowley G, Saad S, Giannelli F, *et al.* Ultrarapid mutation detection by multiplex, solid-phase chemical cleavage. *Genomics* 1995; **30**:574–582.

35. Youil R, Kemper BW, Cotton RG. Screening for mutations by enzyme mismatch cleavage with T4 endonuclease VII. *Proc Natl Acad Sci USA* 1995; **92**:87–91.

36. Mashal RD, Koontz J, Sklar J. Detection of mutations by cleavage of DNA heteroduplexes with bacteriophage resolvases. *Nature Genet* 1995; **9**:177–183.

37. Youil R, Kemper B, Cotton G. Detection of 81 of 81 known mouse beta-globin promoter mutations with T4 endonuclease VII-the EMC method. *Genomics* 1996; **32**:431–435.

38. Roest PA, Roberts RG, Sugino S, *et al.* Protein truncation test (PTT) for rapid detection of translation-terminating mutations. *Hum Mol Genet* 1993; **2**:1719–1721.

39. Den Dunnen JT, Van Ommen GJ. The protein truncation test: a review. *Hum Mutat* 1999; **14**:95–102.

40. Rowan AJ, Bodmer WF. Introduction of a myc reporter tag to improve the quality of mutation detection using the protein truncation test. *Hum Mutat* 1997; **9**:172–176.

41. Groden J, Thliveris A, Samowitz W, *et al.* Identification and characterization of the familial adenomatous polyposis coli gene. *Cell* 1991; **66**:589–600.

42. Miki Y, Swensen J, Shattuck-Eidens D, *et al.* A strong candidate for the breast and ovarian cancer susceptibility gene, *BRCA1*. *Science* 1994; **266**:66–71.

43. Hentze MW, Kulozik AE. A perfect message: RNA surveillance and nonsense-mediated decay. *Cell* 1999; **96**:307–310.

44. Culbertson MR. RNA surveillance. Unforeseen consequences for gene expression, inherited genetic disorders and cancer. *Trends Genet* 1999; **15**:74–80.

45. Hacia JG. Resequencing and mutational analysis using oligonucleotide microarrays. *Nature Genet* 1999; **21**(1 Suppl): 42–47.

46. Lipshutz RJ, Fodor SP, Gingeras TR, *et al.* High density synthetic oligonucleotide arrays. *Nature Genet* 1999; **21**(1 Suppl):20–24.

47. Hacia J.G, Sun B, Hunt N, *et al.* Strategies for mutational analysis of the large multiexon *ATM* gene using high-density oligonucleotide arrays. *Genome Res* 1998; **8**:1245–1258.

48. Wen WH, Bernstein L, Lescallett J, *et al.* Comparison of *TP53* mutations identified by oligonucleotide microarray and conventional DNA sequence analysis. *Cancer Res* 2000; **60**:2716–2722.

49. Hacia JG, Woski SA, Fidanza J, *et al.* Enhanced high density oligonucleotide array-based sequence analysis using modified nucleoside triphosphates. *Nucl Acids Res* 1998; **26**:4975–4982.

50. Weiler J, Gausepohl H, Hauser N, *et al.* Hybridisation based DNA screening on peptide nucleic acid (PNA) oligomer arrays. *Nucl Acids Res* 1997; **25**:2792–2799.

51. Ahmadian A, Gharizadeh B, Gustafsson AC, *et al.* Single-nucleotide polymorphism analysis by pyrosequencing. *Analyt Biochem* 2000; **280**:103–110.

52. Little DP, Braun A, Darnhofer-Demar B, *et al.* Detection of *RET* proto-oncogene codon 634 mutations using mass spectrometry. *J Mol Med* 1997; **75**:745–750.

53. Ross F, Hall L, Smirnov I, *et al.* High level multiplex genotyping by MALDI-TOF mass spectrometry. *Nature Biotech* 1998; **16**:1347–1351.

54. Fu D-J, Tang K, Braun A, *et al.* Sequencing exons 5 to 8 of the *p53* gene by MALDI-TOF mass spectrometry. *Nature Biotechnol* 1998; **16**:381.

55. Shuber AP, Michalowsky LA, Nass GS, *et al.* High throughput parallel analysis of hundreds of patient samples for more than 100 mutations in multiple disease genes. *Hum Mol Genet* 1997; **6**:337–347.

56. Täpp I, Malmberg L, Rennel E, *et al.* Homogeneous scoring of single-nucleotide polymorphisms: Comparison of the 5'-nuclease TaqMan assay and molecular beacon probes. *BioTechniques* 2000; **28**:732–738.

57. Newton CR, Graham A, Heptinstall LE. Analysis of any point mutation in DNA. The amplification refractory mutation system (ARMS). *Nucl Acids Res* 1989; **17**:2503–2516.

58. Brinson EC, Adriano T, Bloch W, *et al.* Introduction to PCR/OLA/SCS, a multiplex DNA test, and its application to cystic fibrosis. *Genet Test* 1997; **1**:61–68.

59. Favis R, Day JP, Gerry NP, *et al.* Universal DNA array detection of small insertions and deletions in *BRCA1* and *BRCA2*. *Nature Biotechnol* 2000; **18**:561–564.

60. Lyamichev V, Mast AL, Hall JF, *et al.* Polymorphism identification and quantitative detection of genomic DNA by invasive cleavage of oligonucleotide probes. *Nature Biotechnol* 1999; **17**:292–296.

61. Lizardi PM, Huang X, Zhu A, *et al.* Mutation detection and single-molecule counting using isothermal rolling-circle amplification. *Nature Genet* 1998; **19**:225–232.

62. Hollon T. NIH researchers receive cut-price *BRCA* test. *Nature Med* 2000; **6**:610.

63. Tavtigian SV, Oliphant A, Shattuck-Eidens D, *et al.* Genomic organization, functional analysis, and mutation screening of *BRCA1* and *BRCA2*. In: Fortner JG, Sharp PA (eds) *General Motors Cancer Research Foundation accomplishments in cancer research.* Philadelphia: Lippincott–Raven, 1996:189–204.

64. Southern EM. DNA chips: analysing sequence by hybridization to oligonucleotides on a large scale. *Trends in Genetics* 1996; **12**:110–115.

65. Blanchard AP, Friend SH. Cheap DNA arrays – it's not all smoke and mirrors. *Nature Biotechnol* 1999; **17**:953.

66. Gao Q, Yeung ES. High-throughput detection of unknown mutations by using multiplexed capillary electrophoresis with poly(vinylpyrrolidone) solution. *Analyt Chem* 2000; **72**:2499–2506.

67. Westin L, Xu X, Miller C, *et al.* Anchored multiplex amplification on a microelectronic chip array. *Nature Biotechnol* 2000; **18**:199–204.

68. Spitzer E, Abbaszadegan MR, Schmidt F, *et al.* Detection of *BRCA1* and *BRCA2* mutations in breast cancer families by a comprehensive two stage screening procedure. *Int J Cancer* 2000; **85**:474–481.

69. Castellvi-Bel S, Sheikhavandi S, Telatar M, *et al.* New mutations, polymorphisms, and rare variants in the *ATM* gene detected by a novel SSCP strategy. *Hum Mutat* 1999; **14**:156–162.

70. Eisinger F, Jacquemeier J, Charpin C, *et al.* Mutations at *BRCA1*: the medullary breast carcinoma revisited. *Cancer Res* 1998; **58**:1588–1592.

71. Okamoto Y, Nakano H. Detection of *p53* gene mutations in its full translational sequence by cleavase fragment length polymorphism analysis. *Ann Clin Biochem* 1999; **36**:511–513.

72. Blesa JR, Hernandez-Yago J. Adaptation of conformation-sensitive gel electrophoresis to an ALFexpress DNA sequencer to screen *BRCA1* mutations. *Biotechniques* 2000; **28**:1019–1025.

73. Parc YR, Halling KC, Wang L, *et al.* *hMSH6* alterations in patients with microsatellite instability-low colorectal cancer. *Cancer Res* 2000; **60**:2225–2231.

74. Sibille-Hoang C, de ter Beerst J, Froment O, *et al.* *BRCA1* and *BRCA2* mutations in Belgian families with a history of breast and/or ovarian cancer. *Eur J Cancer Prev* 1998; **7**(Suppl. 1):S3–S5.

75. Marsh DJ, Dabia PL, Kum CS, *et al.* Germline *PTEN* mutations in Cowden syndrome-like families. *J Med Genet* 1998; **35**:881–885.

76. Rines RD, van Orsouw NJ, Sigalas I, *et al.* Comprehensive mutational scanning of the *p53* coding region by two-dimensional gene scanning. *Carcinogenesis* 1998; **19**:979–984.

77. Gross E, Arnold N, Goette J, *et al.* A comparison of *BRCA1* mutation analysis by direct sequencing, SSCP and DHPLC. *Hum Genet* 1999; **105**:72–78.

78. Izatt L, Vessey C, Hodgson SV, *et al.* Rapid and efficient *ATM* mutation detection by fluorescent chemical cleavage of mismatch: identification of four novel mutations. *Eur J Hum Genet* 1999; **7**:310–320.

79. Sheridan E, Hancock BW, Goyns MH. High incidence of mutations of the *p53* gene detected in ovarian tumours by the use of chemical mismatch cleavage. *Cancer Lett* 1993; **68**:83–89.

80. Giunta C, Youil R, Venter D, *et al.* Rapid diagnosis of germline *p53* mutation using the enzyme mismatch cleavage method. *Diagn Mol Pathol* 1996; **5**:265–270.

81. Hogervorst FB, Cornelis RS, Bout M, *et al.* Rapid detection of *BRCA1* mutations by the protein truncation test. *Nature Genet* 1995; **10**:208–212.

82. Friedman LS, Gayther SA, Kurosaki T, *et al.* Mutation analysis of *BRCA1* and *BRCA2* in a male breast cancer population. *Am J Hum Genet* 1997; **60**:313–319.

PART 2

Inherited cancer syndromes

6

Retinoblastoma: the paradigm for a genetically inherited cancer syndrome

CHRISTOPHER MITCHELL

INTRODUCTION

Genetic analysis of human hereditary cancer has identified the chromosomal location of genes that predispose to tumorigenesis. In the majority of cases, it has been shown that loss of function of both alleles of these genes is required for tumour initiation. Such genes have collectively been called 'tumour-suppresser genes' because at least one functional copy of the gene product is required to prevent tumour initiation. Since their normal function is to ensure that differentiation and signal transduction occurs in the appropriate cell type, tumorigenesis cannot be initiated so long as one functional allele is present. The first tumour suppresser gene to be isolated was the retinoblastoma gene (*RB*), the inheritance of which predisposes to the children's eye cancer, retinoblastoma (Rb). The study of this gene has established many of the precedents for the analysis and the cloning of other tumour suppresser genes.

RETINOBLASTOMA (RB) GENETICS

As the name implies, Rb is a tumour of retinal cells. With only rare exceptions, it affects children under the age of 5 years, the majority of tumours occurring before 2 years of age. Individuals can present with Rb at birth, which suggests that the tumours have been growing since early fetal life. This view is supported by the histopathology of the tumour, which shows a relatively undifferentiated, embryonic-like organization, implying arrest in the development of a retinal precursor cell. Thus, clones of cells are arrested in a state in which further genetic changes can occur, thus giving rise to the full tumour phenotype. The exact identity of these precursor cells, however, remains unknown.

Approximately 10 per cent of patients will have a family history, while the remaining cases are apparently sporadic. Since the new mutation rate is relatively high,[1] many of these apparently sporadic cases will carry new germline mutations. In the familial form, the tumour phenotype segregates as an autosomal dominant trait, implying that predisposition is due to inheritance of a single mutation. In fact, pedigree analysis shows that, in 10 per cent of cases, individuals who inherit the mutant gene do not develop a tumour – so-called 'incomplete penetrance' – so, clearly, it is only a predisposition to tumorigenesis that is inherited, and other genetic events or mutations, must also occur.

To estimate how many additional mutations are required, Knudson[2] analysed the incidence of tumours by age and devised the 'two-hits' hypothesis. In hereditary cases, the first mutation is present in all cells of the body. Only one additional mutation is required for tumour development. This event mainly affects the developing retina, which suggests a highly tissue-specific and developmental stage-specific role for this gene. Since only one additional mutation is required for tumour formation and the chances of this event are high, hereditary Rb is characterized by the presence of multiple tumours in both eyes. For this reason, all bilaterally affected individuals must be considered to be carriers of an *RB1* gene mutation. This group accounts for 40–50 per cent of all patients. In truly sporadic cases, both mutations must occur, one in each allele of the *RB* gene, in the same cell during an early stage of development. The possibility of these events occurring by chance is very small. Sporadic cases, therefore, are generally characterized by the presence of unilateral unifocal tumours. We know empirically, however, that approximately 10–15 per cent of families have unilaterally affected individuals. Therefore, some unilaterally affected sporadic cases will carry a predisposing mutation, although it is difficult to identify which ones, but this group probably represents less than 5 per cent of cases. In some families, apparently unaffected individuals have been seen to have retinal scars, which resemble successfully treated tumours (Figure 6.1). These lesions have been described as benign tumours.[3] Occasionally, several affected children can be born to unaffected parents with no prior family history. One possibility in such cases is that an unusual insertional translocation is segregating in the affected family and individuals should certainly be referred for cytogenetic analysis. It is also possible, however, that one of the parents is a mosaic carrying the mutation in the germ cells, but not in their own retinal cells.

If tumours are detected early they are usually smaller, and hence more easily treated than those presenting late. The location of the tumour within the eye is also important. Treatment of small tumours usually involves cryosurgery, photocoagulation or radiation therapy, whereas larger tumours usually require enucleation. Tumours left to develop in the eye will eventually spread locally, often down the optic nerve, or metastasize. The prognosis in these cases is very poor indeed. Since early diagnosis offers a better prognosis, all 'at-risk' patients are screened regularly during the first years of life. In practice, screening involves all first-degree relatives of Rb patients, since the possibility of incomplete penetrance means that lack of family history is not always an indication of the absence of heritable disease. Tumour formation is, for most patients, the only unequivocal clinical means of identifying mutant gene carriers. Clearly a system to identify those patients with germline mutations would make the clinical management of this disease more efficient (see later).

DEFINING THE *RB* LOCUS

The first clues to the location of the *RB1* gene came from the cytogenetic analysis of rare Rb patients with mental retardation and other developmental abnormalities. These patients invariably had constitutional deletions of chromosome 13, the commonly deleted region being 13q 14.3.[1,4] Only 3 per cent of Rb patients harbour cytogenetic deletions, but in most cases, the deletion also includes the adjacent esterase-D gene (*ESD*). The gene responsible for the familial form of Rb was shown to lie in 13q14 because of close genetic linkage between the disease locus and the *ESD* locus.[5] Subsequently, sporadic tumours from individuals who were constitutionally heterozygous for polymorphic *ESD* alleles were shown to be homozygous at this locus.[6] This 'loss of heterozygosity' (LOH) was confirmed using polymorphic DNA probes.[7] The interpretation of these observations was that the

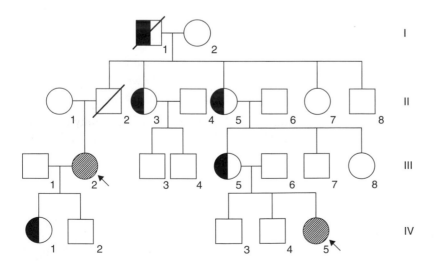

Figure 6.1 *Example of family pedigree segregating a 'mild' form of the disease. Individuals who have developed tumours are only unilaterally affected and two patients (arrows) have regressed tumours. (Half shading indicates unilateral tumours and ⊘ regressed tumours.)*

chromosome 13 homologue bearing the *RB1* mutation in retinal precursor cells was duplicated at some stage and the normal chromosome 13 homologue was then lost. In this way, the cell becomes homozygous for the initial *RB1* mutation, which presumably leads to failure to produce a functional protein. Cavenee *et al.* confirmed this hypothesis[8] by showing that, in a tumour from a patient with hereditary Rb, the allele that was retained was the one contributed by the affected parent. The mechanism by which LOH occurs most frequently is non-disjunction of chromosome 13, although, in some cases, mitotic recombination, hitherto a mechanism that was considered very infrequent in mammalian cells, was the mechanism responsible. It appears that 70 per cent of tumours arise as a result of LOH; presumably the other 30 per cent are due to two independent mutations within the two copies of the *RB1* gene itself (see later).

Similar molecular analyses allowed the parental origin of the *RB1* mutation to be determined.[9] In new heritable cases, the mutation arose on the paternally derived chromosome. In sporadic cases, however, there was no differential susceptibility to somatic mutation between the homologous copies of the gene. These findings argue against genomic imprinting as an explanation for the parental origin, and new mutations point to new mutational events arising predominantly during spermatogenesis. There does not, however, seem to be a paternal age effect.[10]

ISOLATION OF THE *RB1* GENE

Following the random isolation of only 12 DNA probes from a flow sorted chromosome 13-specific DNA library, one – H3-8 – was shown to lie within the smallest of the constitutional deletions identified in Rb patients. A chromosome 'walk' from this locus generated adjacent probes, which showed homozygous deletions in some tumours and which recognized a region of DNA highly conserved between species, suggesting it was within a gene. Using this probe, Friend *et al.*[11] soon identified a cDNA, 4.7 kb long, which detected structurally abnormal mRNAs in Rb tumours. Constitutional reciprocal translocations pre-disposing to Rb were shown to interrupt the *RB1* gene, confirming its authenticity.[12,13] The tissue distribution of expression of *RB1*, however, was surprising. Since the hypothesis was that this gene controls important aspects of the developing fetal retina, the finding of expression at high levels in all tissues examined was unexpected.[11] The *RB1* gene spans approximately 200 kb of genomic DNA and consists of 27 exons encoding 928 amino acids. There are no distinctive motifs in the gene structure or its promoter that clearly identify its function.

MUTATIONS IN THE *RB1* GENE

Only 20 per cent of tumours showed structural abnormalities of *RB1*, so clearly the majority of mutations were more subtle. The nature of these mutations in tumours was demonstrated in a variety of ways. Dunn and colleagues[14] analysed RNA from tumour cells and identified a variety of different mutations in tumours and cell lines. Demonstrating constitutional mutations in the *RB1* gene in Rb patients, however, would provide the formal proof of the role of *RB1* in predisposition to Rb. Following the cloning of *RB1*, the exon structure of the gene was established and sequence surrounding the 27 exons determined.[15] There then followed an exon-by-exon survey of the gene, using polymerase chain reaction (PCR) amplification of the individual exons and flanking intron regions followed by sequencing.[16] The efficiency of this procedure was improved by screening the amplified exons before sequencing to identify those exons most likely to carry mutations.[17] In a survey of tumours and constitutional cells from bilaterally affected patients, it was clear that mutations were resulting in a non-functional protein. It was also possible in some tumours to show homozygous mutations, confirming predictions suggested by LOH. In other tumours, two independent mutations were found in the two alleles of *RB1*, thus confirming the two-hit theory.[18]

Mutations could be divided into three broad classes: those affecting correct splicing of the gene (presumably resulting in exon deletions); small deletions and insertions (which invariably generate premature stop codons downstream); and point mutations, which generate stop codons directly.[18] The most common type of point mutation was a C to T transition, 70 per cent of which converted CGA-arginine codons or splice sites to TGA-stop codons. With few exceptions, patients heterozygous for this type of mutation develop bilateral Rb.[19]

Dryja *et al.*[9] had previously presented evidence that the majority of new mutations arise in the male germline. Since these cells are rapidly dividing, and go through many generations, these mutations could be due to carcinogens or replication errors. Replication errors were responsible for the majority of mutations reported by Hogg *et al.*[18] Deletions and insertions occurred between direct repeat sequences, the intervening bases being lost, and point mutations occurred in the vicinity of quasi-repeats. If base pairing slipped during replication, the quasi-repeat sequence would be copied instead of the normal one (Figure 6.2).

Missense mutations, simply substituting one amino acid for another, appear to be less common, as are in-frame deletions. A missense mutation in exon 20 was found in a hereditary Rb patient, which was associated with a 'low-penetrance' phenotype.[20] This finding raises

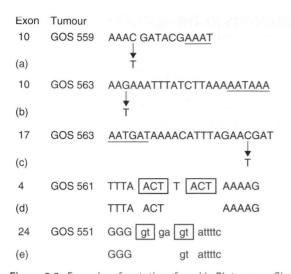

Exon	Tumour	
10	GOS 559	AAAC GATACGAAAT
(a)		↓
		T
10	GOS 563	AAGAAATTTATCTTAAAAATAAA
(b)		↓
		T
17	GOS 563	AATGATAAAACATTTAGAACGAT
(c)		↓
		T
4	GOS 561	TTTA [ACT] T [ACT] AAAAG
(d)		TTTA ACT AAAAG
24	GOS 551	GGG [gt] ga [gt] attttc
(e)		GGG gt attttc

Figure 6.2 *Examples of mutations found in Rb tumours. Single base-pair mutations (a, b, c) induce stop codons directly but the mutated sequence is usually an identical copy of the same sequence (underlined) either upstream (c) or downstream (a, b), suggesting they may arise as a result of replication errors. Small deletions (d, e) occur between perfect repeats (boxed). Again, slipped mispairing during replication results in one of the repeats, and the intervening sequence, being excised.*

the possibility that the substitution of a single amino acid only compromises the function of the protein. Unless the second mutation in the tumour precursor cell causes complete loss of *RB1* function, duplication of the 'weak' mutation would allow sufficiently functional RB protein to be produced, so inhibiting tumorigenesis. This suggestion is consistent with the observation that in this particular family many of the mutant gene carriers were either unaffected or have regressed tumours. Sakai *et al.*[21] also investigated low-penetrance families and found mutations in recognition sequences for different transcription factors in the *RB1* promoter region. Again the suggestion is that, as a result of this type of mutation, a quantitative decrease in transcription occurs, rather than complete inactivity. Sufficient RB protein is produced, however, so that any phenotypic consequences are mild. Whether single amino acid changes will generally be found in patients with mild phenotypes remains to be determined.

Although there have still been too few mutations reported in Rb patients, there do not appear to be any 'hot spots' within *RB1*.

CLINICAL APPLICATIONS IN THE IDENTIFICATION OF *RB1*

The autosomal dominant mode of inheritance of Rb predisposition makes genetic linkage analysis relatively straightforward, although there is some heterogeneity in

the phenotype. In the majority of families, affected individuals have bilateral multifocal tumour with early-age onset and, since there is a family history of Rb, early detection is guaranteed because newborns are screened regularly and tumours treated as they arise. Genetic linkage studies in these families have identified, unequivocally, which individuals are at risk of tumour development and which are not.[22] In the majority of cases, it is sufficient to use one or two very highly polymorphic probes, e.g. RS 2.0 or RB 1.20.[22] Using these tests, over 95 per cent of families are informative, meaning that mutant gene carriers can be identified; just as importantly, so too can those individuals who do not carry the mutant allele because they and their children will not have to undergo repeated ophthalmological examination. This type of linkage analysis has also proved useful in families where incomplete penetrance is observed.[20] In these families, unaffected mutant gene carriers can be identified and their children screened. It has also been possible to offer prenatal screening using chorionic villus sampling[23] and, so far, this screening programme has proved to be very successful. Only 10–12 per cent of Rb cases, however, have a prior family history of the disease. Of the remaining 85 per cent, approximately half will be bilaterally affected[24] and so, presumably, carry a germline mutation as a result of a new mutation. To offer these individuals screening for their firstborn, it is necessary to identify the causative mutation. Since the majority of patients have their tumours successfully treated, this identification has to be carried out on constitutional cells where the mutation will be heterozygous. A number of techniques have been developed for this purpose, but perhaps the most commonly used is single-strand conformation polymorphism (SSCP). This method depends on the alteration in mobility in polyacrylamide gels caused by single basepair changes in single-stranded DNA molecules (Figure 6.3). This procedure screens the *RB1* exons quickly and likely mutations can be identified and then confirmed by sequencing (Figure 6.4). This approach has been successfully applied to the *RB1* gene[17] and it is now theoretically possible that the mutations in all individuals could be identified. It is still not clear, however, whether in individuals where a mutation is not identified, it has been missed, or the gene is normal. The fact that several exons can be analysed simultaneously makes the procedure less labour intensive. PCR analysis can also be carried out on formalin-fixed, paraffin-embedded tissue sections,[25] which means archival material can also be used to identify causative mutations.

THE FUNCTION OF THE *RB1* GENE

The undifferentiated appearance of Rb tumours and the restriction of the Rb phenotype suggest that the retinal

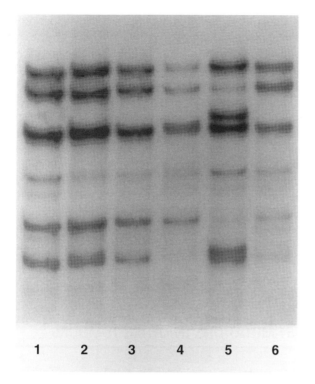

Figure 6.3 *Single-strand conformation polymorphism (SSCP) gel showing DNA samples from exon 18 from six different patients. The only aberrant banding pattern is seen in lane 5, where two novel bands appear that are not present in the other samples. For details of the technique used, see Chapter 5.*

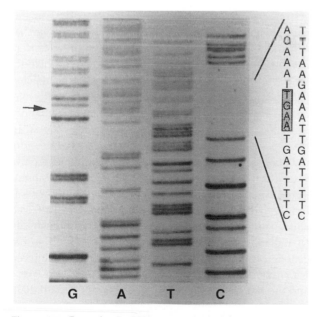

Figure 6.4 *Example of a DNA sequencing gel from exon 4 from an Rb patient showing a four-basepair deletion (boxed). Because this mutation is heterozygous, the normal and the mutant sequence are superimposed from the point of the deletion (arrow), whereafter two bands are present at each position on the gel.*

precursor cell has been arrested at an early stage of its the development. The implication of this suggestion is that *RB1* somehow controls the progression of the immature precursor into a photoreceptor. The finding, however of widespread RB expression, implied a more fundamental role in control of cell differentiation and development. Analysis of the gene sequence did not reveal any motifs that typified a known class of gene; *RB1* is now recognized as the prototype of the 'pocket protein' family. Its function is to connect the cell-cycle clock with the cell's transcriptional machinery. In this role, RB allows the clock to control the expression of genes that serve to advance the cell through its growth cycle, and exerts its influence in the first two-thirds of G1. Cells entering G1 from mitosis are serum dependent, a state reflecting their requirement for mitogens present in serum. This serum-dependent state is maintained continuously in G1 until a few hours before the onset of S-phase, when the cells become serum independent. The passage from serum dependence to independence has been termed the R (for restriction) point.[26] Once the cell has passed the R point, it is, excluding extreme disturbance such as DNA damage, irrevocably committed to progress through the remainder of the cell cycle. There is now considerable evidence that the retinoblastoma protein (RB) is the factor controlling progression through the R point.

The first clue to the function of RB came from the demonstration that it could bind to proteins from certain dominantly transforming DNA tumour viruses. After entry into a cell, DNA tumour viruses produce an 'early' set of proteins that trigger division of in a normally quiescent cell. This process is essential for successful virus replication. The transforming viral proteins, E1A from adenovirus, large-T antigen (LT) from SV40 and E7 from human papilloma virus, all share conserved regions that are necessary for the transforming functions, and form complexes with RB protein.[27] Mutations within the conserved regions not only negate their transforming potential but also prevent binding to RB protein. The RB protein itself can be phosphorylated at a number of sites. In an early G1 cell it is unphosphorylated, but as the cell moves into the later stages of G2, and subsequently into S phase, RB becomes phosphorylated and remains so until the end of mitosis, when it becomes dephosphorylated again.[28] This finding led to the notion that the unphosphorylated form of RB protein promotes cell quiescence. LT binds specifically to the unphosphorylated form of RB protein and LT–RB complexes are found only in G0/G1 when the unphosphorylated form of RB is present. Thus, by sequestering RB during G0/G1, the viral-transforming proteins permit progress of the cell through the R point into S-phase. The E1A viral protein is thought to transform cells by altering the activity of cellular transcription factors. One such protein is E2F, which has been shown to be a transcriptional regulator of several cellular genes.[29] Ordinarily, E2F forms a complex with specific cellular proteins, which effectively suppress its function. E1A, however, can dissociate E2F from its protein complexes, releasing free E2F. To exert its transcriptional regulation, E2F must form a stable complex with other proteins so as to bind specific DNA sequences in the promoter regions of the genes it controls. The conserved regions of E1A facilitate E2F binding and the same regions are also responsible for binding RB. It is not surprising, therefore, to find that RB protein also forms complexes with E2F and that E1A can dissociate them. The E2F–RB protein complex ordinarily dissociates as the cell approaches the G1–S boundary, thus releasing free E2F. Another protein, p107, which is highly homologous to RB, recaptures E2F after it has exerted its effect on transcription, to again inactivate it.[30] The association of the viral early proteins with the RB protein is almost certainly an *in vitro* phenomenon, since it is unlikely that fetal retinal cells have been infected with these viruses. Rather, this model system points to associations of RB protein with other naturally occurring proteins.

A further link of RB with the cell cycle is the interaction between the calcium/calmodulin kinase (CamK) and the retinoblastoma protein/SP1 pathway. CamK II and IV activate c-*fos* transcription through a short promoter region, which contains the retinoblastoma control element (RCE), and a cAMP response element (CRE). Deletion analysis showed that the RCE is responsive to CamK, and is sufficient to transfer CamK and calcium regulation to a minimal promoter. CamK-dependent transcription is regulated by the RB protein and the p107Rb-related protein. The stimulatory effects of RB and CamK on c-*fos*, however, are blocked by overexpression of both proteins, effects that are directly mediated by SP1.[31]

Other evidence that phosphorylation of RB is an underlying mechanism in cell-cycle control is that the unphosphorylated form of RB appears to bind and hence control the effects of a number of other cellular proteins, a property which the phosphorylated form loses. In addition, conditions that favour phosphorylation of the RB favour cell proliferation.[32]

These data led to the development of a model in which a cell advances through the cell cycle to the R point, where further progress is checked by the presence of dephosphorylated RB. If conditions are appropriate for continued advance, RB becomes phosphorylated and the cycle proceeds. If a cell lacks RB function, it will proceed through the cycle unchecked by RB or those factors that influence RB phosphorylation status.[33]

The RB protein can be phosphorylated at a number of serine and threonine residues, each of which seems to have a distinct effect on the ability of RB to interact with its various partner proteins. Thus, phosphorylation at S780 abolishes binding to E2F, while at S807 and S811 it abolishes binding to c-abl, and at T821 or T826 to SV40 large T. The amino-acid sequences surrounding the phosphorylation sites are typical of sites modified by cyclin-dependent kinases (CDKs). Cyclins of the D group are induced in resting cells exposed to mitogens and are expressed throughout G1, and Cyclin E expression is induced in mid-G1, at a time when RB is becoming phosphorylated. It now appears that D-type cyclins, acting with *CDk* 4/6 partly phosphorylate RB, and the process is then completed by cyclin E-*CDK*2. Once RB is fully phosphorylated, it is no longer capable of binding the transcription factor E2F, which is then liberated to initiate transcription of a further cascade of genes whose products are also participants in the cell-cycle programme.[34,35]

RB1 MUTATIONS IN OTHER TUMOURS

Patients carrying a constitutional *RB1* gene mutation are also at significantly higher risk of developing second, non-ocular tumours later in life.[24] In childhood and early adulthood these are usually osteosarcomas and soft-tissue sarcomas. Both of these tumours have been shown to lose heterozygosity for markers on chromosome 13. The same classes of tumour also show frequent structural and transcriptional abnormalities of *RB1*, suggesting it plays a role in the development of the malignant phenotype in these cells. There is also evidence that *RB1* mutation confers an increased risk of other cancers later in life, such as small-cell lung cancer and bladder cancer. Recent work has also shown that the unaffected parents of children with the hereditary form of Rb may be more sensitive than normal to cell killing by radiation, as well as to enhanced radiation-induced G1 arrest. In five families studied, at least one parent was as or more radiation-sensitive than the probands. In four of the five cases, the *RB1* mutation found in the proband was absent in the parental cells. In one case, an affected father was found to harbour the same mutation as his affected child. This apparently increased parental cell sensitivity to radiation suggests that some as yet unrecognized genetic event occurs in one or both parents of children with retinoblastoma, although the nature of the event and the mechanism by which it exerts its effects remain conjectural.[36]

Structural abnormalities in *RB1* are also found in breast cancer[37] and small-cell lung carcinoma tumour DNA.[38] Horowitz *et al.* presented data on a series of other tumours showing less frequent involvement of *RB1*.[39] It is likely, however, that *RB1* mutations in these other tissues only contribute to tumour progression because, in many cases, the frequency of tumours with mutations is still relatively low.

SUPPRESSION OF THE MALIGNANT PHENOTYPE

Loss of function of the *RB1* gene is clearly vital for the development of tumours. It would be predicted, therefore, that the introduction of a normal *RB1* gene into cells with no RB function would reverse the malignant phenotype. Results from this type of experiment, however, have been difficult to interpret. Depending on the vector used, the nature of the recipient cell line, and the *in vivo* system being used to monitor the effects on tumorigenicity, different laboratories report different results.[40] In some cases, transfected cells continued to grow in culture but did not produce tumours in nude mice. In other systems, malignancy was apparently suppressed but, when the inoculation was intraocular, the same cells produced tumours, albeit at a slower rate than normal. All of these experiments, however, used an *RB1* gene that was not under the control of its own promoter, which was technically a more complicated procedure. However, when the *RB1* gene is in its normal chromosomal environment, it can suppress the malignant phenotype, because introduction of an intact chromosome 13 into cell lines lacking a functional *RB1* gene causes the cells to cease proliferation. It appears, therefore, that *RB1* expression promotes arrest in G0. The same kinds of experiments have shown that reconstituting *RB1* (deficient) cell lines derived from bladder, prostate and lung cancers with *RB1* will also suppress malignancy in these cell types. This finding was unexpected, since multiple genetic events appear to be responsible for the development of the malignant phenotype in these tumours. However, it has been shown in other tumours that malignancy can be suppressed by correcting any one of the defects in the multistep chain leading to malignancy with the introduction of the relevant wild-type gene.[41]

TRANSGENIC MOUSE STUDIES

If the *RB1* gene is responsible for tumour initiation in retinal precursor cells, it might be expected that disrupting this gene in mouse embryos would predispose them to Rb. Whether this would prove to be a realistic animal model was questionable because, for unknown reasons, mice do not naturally develop Rb. Using homologous recombination, one copy of the *rb1* gene was 'knocked out' in mouse embryonic stem cells, which were then used to create chimeric mice, leading eventually to the production of mice heterozygous for the inactivated *rb1*

gene.[42,43] In contradiction to Knudson's prediction, none of these mice developed tumours. A random mutational event in the homologous normal gene should have initiated tumorigenesis. When the heterozygous mice were interbred, however, fetuses, which were *rb1*−/*rb1*− developed apparently normally up to 11 days but then died *in utero* after 13–14 days of gestation. These mice did not have Rb or retinal defects but, instead, showed abnormal development of the midbrain and haematopoietic system. Neuronal cell death was most obvious in the spinal cord and hindbrain. Aberrant haematopoiesis was characterized by the deficiency of mature red cells, which reflected an abnormal proliferation of immature erythrocytes in the liver. Clearly the *rb1* gene is very important for normal development of mice, but loss of *rb1* function does not appear to predispose to Rb. Remarkably, *rb1* does not appear to be important for normal early development and is not crucial for normal cell division during this period in mice. When heterozygous mice were followed for longer periods, they were shown to develop adenocarcinoma of the pituitary, which is not one of the tumours often seen in hereditary cases of Rb in humans. These tumours showed loss of the normal *rb1* allele.[43] The reason why *rb1* mutation should predispose to pituitary tumours in mice, but retinal tumours in humans, is still not understood.

APPLICATION OF MOLECULAR BIOLOGY TO THERAPY

Although the prognosis for life of Rb patients is excellent, that for vision is often less good, particularly when the tumours are large or adjacent to the ophthalmic nerve. In addition, in patients carrying the Rb predisposition, the risk of second tumours is greatly enhanced by the use of radiotherapy. Smaller tumours, though, can be managed conservatively by laser or cryotherapy. Some success has been enjoyed using chemotherapy, but an alternative method that is now being explored is gene therapy. The Y79 retinoblastoma cell line can be killed *in vitro* when transduced with an adenoviral vector containing the herpes simplex thymidine kinase gene (*AdV-TK*) followed by treatment with the prodrug ganciclovir. Y79 cells can be injected into the vitreous humour of immunodeficient mice to produce an aggressive murine model of retinoblastoma. If these tumours are transduced *in vivo* with *AdV-TK* and the animals treated with ganciclovir, there is complete ablation of the tumour in 70 per cent of the animals with significant prolongation of the progression free survival compared to control animals.[44] This work suggests that it may be possible, in due course, to develop an effective alternative to enucleation.

Table 6.1 *Screening of siblings of proband. All siblings and both parents should have fundi examined at time of proband's diagnosis. Subsequent screening requirements can be based on the presence or absence of an identifiable mutation within the* RB1 *gene*

All new siblings
- Dilated fundus examination within 1 week of birth

Proband has unilateral disease but no mutation identified
- Examination every 2 months to 12 months
- then examination every 4 months to 2 years
- then examination every 6 months to 5 years

Proband has bilateral disease but no mutation identified
- Examination every 2 months to 2 years
- then examination every 4 months to 3 years
- then examination every 6 months to 5 years

Mutation identified in proband, regardless of unilateral/bilateral status
- If new sibling is negative for mutation no further examinations are necessary
- or if positive for mutation, fundus examinations every 4 weeks and treatment as necessary.

CLINICAL FOLLOW-UP

The identification of predisposing lesions within the *RB1* gene of affected children should permit the restriction of frequent ophthalmological examination to those patients who are predisposed to bilateral or multifocal tumours, and their predisposed siblings. It has been proven that genetic testing improves clinical management by avoiding unnecessary anaesthesia in non-carriers in families with proven mutations.[45] Families with low-penetrance mutations would still be identified as being at risk, albeit reduced, of tumour and could be enrolled in an appropriate screening programme.[46] Typical intervals for ophthalmological examination of predisposed siblings are shown in Table 6.1.

Screening for second tumours, such as osteosarcoma, is difficult because of the multiplicity of tumours and the different sites at which they might arise. It is difficult to envisage a sensible and effective screening programme for second tumours that might have any useful effect on treatment or long-term outcome beyond regular clinical contact between an educated patient or parent, and a knowledgeable clinician.

SUMMARY

The *RB1* gene has proved to be the model tumour suppressor gene. Inactivation of this gene alone leads to the development of a highly specific type of cancer and its less frequent involvement in other tumours explains the increased risk that mutant gene carriers have to these malignancies. Reintroduction of a wild-type gene into cells deficient for its function apparently reverses the malignant phenotype. At present, it seems that variations in phenotypic expression seen in different families are due to subtle differences in mutations in the *RB1* gene. Hereditary cases carry inactivating mutations, and their tumours either become homozygous for these initial mutations or sustain different inactivating mutations in the homologous gene. Molecular analysis of *RB1* allows prenatal identification of mutant gene carriers and makes risk assessment for hereditary cases straightforward. *RB1* appears to control the developmental process in immature retinal cells through interaction with cell-specific proteins, which remain to be discovered. The interaction with dominant transforming genes was unexpected but allowed the integration of RB into the control of the cell cycle, and hence has allowed a better understanding and development of many difficult but related areas of cancer research.

KEY POINTS

- Retinoblastoma (Rb) usually affects children at <5 years (most are <2 years).
- Hereditary Rb is caused by mutations in a gene, *RB*, on chromosome 13q14.3.
- There is a high new mutation rate.
- Bilateral Rb cases should all be considered to be *RB* mutation carriers.
- Ten per cent of Rb cases have a family history of the disease.
- Tumour development follows the 'two-hit' hypothesis.
- A lot of mutations are small genetic deletions.
- Genetic testing improves quality of life by avoiding unnecessary screening in non-carriers.

REFERENCES

1. Vogel F. Genetics of retinoblastoma. *Hum Genet* 1979; **52**:1–54.
2. Knudson AG. Mutation and cancer: statistical study of retinoblastoma. *Proc Natl Acad Sci USA* 1971; **68**:820–823.

3. Gallie BL, Ellsworth RM, Abramson DH, Phillips RA. Retinoma: spontaneous regression of retinoblastoma or benign manifestation of the mutation? *Br J Cancer* 1982; **45:**513–521.

4. Cowell JK, Hungerford J, Rutland P, Jay M. A chromosomal breakpoint which separates the esterase D and retinoblastoma predisposition loci in a patient with del(13) (q14–q31). *Cytogenet Cell Genet* 1987; **27:**27–31.

5. Sparkes RS, Murphree AL, Lingua RW, *et al.* Gene for hereditary retinoblastoma assigned to human chromosome 13 by linkage to esterase-D. *Science* 1983; **219:**971–973.

6. Godbout R, Dryja TP, Squire J, *et al.* Somatic inactivation of genes on chromosome 13 is a common event in retinoblastoma. *Nature* 1983; **304:**451–453.

7. Cavenee WK, Dryja TP, Phillips RA, *et al.* Expression of recessive alleles by chromosomal mechanisms in retinoblastoma. *Nature* 1983; **305:**779–784.

8. Cavenee WK, Hansen MF, Nordenskjold M, *et al.* Genetic origin of mutations predisposing to retinoblastoma. *Science* 1985; **228:**501–503.

9. Dryja TP, Mukai S, Petersen R, *et al.* Parental origin of mutations of the retinoblastoma gene. *Nature* 1989; **339:**556–558.

10. Matsunaga E, Minoda K, Sasaki MS. Parental age and seasonal variation in the births of children with sporadic retinoblastoma: a mutation–epidemiological study. *Hum Genet* 1990; **84:**155–158.

11. Friend SH, Bernards R, Rogelj S, *et al.* A human DNA segment with properties of the gene that predisposes to retinoblastoma and osteosarcoma. *Nature* 1986; **323:**643–646.

12. Goddard AD, Balakier H, Canton M. *et al.* Infrequent genomic rearrangement and normal expression of the putative *RB1* gene in retinoblastoma tumours. *Mol Cell Biol* 1988; 8:2082–2088.

13. Mitchell CD, Cowell JK. Predisposition to retinoblastoma due to a translocation within the 4./R locus. *Oncogene* 1989; 4:263–267.

14. Dunn JM, Phillips RA, Zhu X, *et al.* Mutations in the *RB1* gene and their effects on transcription. *Mol. Cell. Biol.* 1989; 9:4596–4604.

15. McGee TL, Yandell DW, Dryja TP. Structure and partial genomic sequence of the human retinoblastoma susceptibility gene. *Gene* 1989; **80:**119–128.

16. Yandell DW, Campbell TA, Dayton SH, *et al.* Oncogenic point mutations in the human retinoblastoma gene: their application to genetic counselling. *N Engl J Med.* 1989; 321:1689–1695.

17. Hogg A, Onadim Z, Baird PN, Cowell JK. Detection of heterozygous mutations in the *RB1* gene in retinoblastoma patients using single-strand conformation polymorphism analysis and polymerase chain reaction sequencing. *Oncogene* 1992; 7:1445–1451.

18. Hogg A, Bia B, Onadim Z, Cowell JK. Molecular mechanisms of oncogenetic mutations in tumours from patients with bilateral and unilateral retinoblastoma. *Proc Natl Acad Sci USA* 1993; **90:**7351–7355.

19. Lohman DR. *RB1* mutations in retinoblastoma. *Hum Mutat* 1999; **14:**283–288.

20. Onadim Z, Hogg A, Baird PN, Cowell JK. Oncogenic point mutations in exon 20 of the *RB1* gene in families showing incomplete penetrance and mild expression of the retinoblastoma phenotype. *Proc Natl Acad Sci USA* 1992; **89:**6177–6181.

21. Sakai T, Ohtani N, McGee TL, *et al.* Oncogenic germline mutations in Ap1 and ATF sites in the human retinoblastoma gene. *Nature* 1991; **353:**83–86.

22. Onadim ZO, Mitchell CD, Rutland PC, *et al.* Application of intragenic DNA probes in prenatal screening for retinoblastoma gene carriers in the United Kingdom. *Arch Dis Child* 1990; **65:**651–656.

23. Onadim Z, Hungerford J, Cowell JK. Follow-up of retinoblastoma patients having prenatal and perinatal predications for mutant gene carrier status using intragenic polymorphic probes from the *RB1* gene. *Br J Cancer* 1992; **65:**711–716.

24. Draper GJ, Sanders BM, Brownbill P-A, Hawkins MM. Patterns of risk of hereditary retinoblastoma and applications to genetic counselling. *Br J Cancer* 1992; **66:**211–219.

25. Onadim Z, Cowell JK. Application of PCR amplification from paraffin embedded tissue sections to linkage analysis in familial retinoblastoma. *J Med Genet* 1991; **28:**312–316.

26. Pardee AB. G1 events and regulation of the cell cycle. *Science* 1989; **246:**603–608.

27. Weinberg RA. Tumour suppresser genes. *Science* 1991; **254:**1138–1146.

28. Mihara K, Cao XR, Yen A, *et al.* Cell cycle-dependent regulation of phosphorylation of the human retinoblastoma gene product. *Science* 1989; **246:**1300–1303.

29. Nevins JR. Transcriptional activation by viral regulatory proteins. *Trends Biochem Sci* 1991; **16:**435–439.

30. Horowitz JM. Regulation of transcription by the retinoblastoma protein. *Genes Chromosomes Cancer* 1993; **6:**124–131.

31. Sohm F, Gaiddon C, Antoine M, *et al.* The retinoblastoma susceptibility gene product/SP1-signalling pathway is modulated by Ca^{2+}/calmodulin kinases II and IV activity. *Oncogene* 1999, **18:**2762–2769.

32. Cobrinik D, Whyte P, Peeper DS, *et al.* Cell cycle specific association of E2F with the p130 E1A-binding protein. *Genes Dev* 1992; **7:**2392–2404.

33. Weinberg RA. The retinoblastoma protein and cell cycle control. *Cell*, 1995; **81:**323–330.

34. Herrera RA, Sah VP, Williams BO, *et al.* (1996). Altered cell cycle kinetics, gene expression and G$_1$ restriction point regulation in Rb-deficient fibroblasts. *Molec Cell Biol* 1996; **16:**2402–2407.

35. Lundberg AS, Weinberg RA. Functional inactivation of the retinoblastoma protein requires sequential modification by at least two distinct cyclin–cdk complexes. *Molec Cell Biol* 1998; **18:**753–761.

36. Fitzek MM, Dahlberg WK, Nagasawa H, *et al.* Unexpected sensitivity to radiation of fibroblasts from unaffected parents of children with hereditary retinoblastoma. *Int J Cancer* 2002; **99:**764–768.

37. T'Ang A, Varley JM, Chakraborty S, *et al.* Structural rearrangement of the retinoblastoma gene in human breast carcinoma. *Science* 1988; **242:**263–266.

38. Harbour JW, Lai S-L, Whang-Peng J, *et al.* Abnormalities in structure and expression of the human retinoblastoma gene in SCLC. *Science* 1988; **241:**353–357.

39. Horowitz JM, Park S-H, Bogenmann E, *et al.* Frequent inactivation of the retinoblastoma anti-oncogene is restricted

to a subset of human tumour cells. *Proc Natl Acad Sci USA* 1990; **87:**2775–2779.

40. Xu HJ, Sumegi J, Hu SX, *et al.* Intraocular tumor formation of RB reconstituted retinoblastoma cells. *Cancer Res* 1991; **51**(16):4481–4485.

41. Stanbridge, E.J. Functional evidence for human tumour suppresser genes: chromosome and molecular genetic studies. *Cancer Surv* 1992; **12:**5–24.

42. Jacks T, Fazeli A, Schmitt EM, *et al.* Effects of an *rb1* mutation in the mouse. *Nature* 1992; **359:**295–300.

43. Lee EY-HP, Chang C-Y, Hu N, *et al.* Mice deficient for *rb1* are nonviable and show defects in neurogenesis and haematopoiesis. *Nature* 1992; **359:**288–294.

44. Hurwitz MY, Marcus KT, Chevez-Barrios P, *et al.* Suicide gene therapy for treatment of a retinoblastoma model. *Hum Gene Ther* 1999; **10:**441–448.

45. Raizis A, Clemett R, Corbett R, *et al.* Improved clinical management of retinoblastoma through genetic testing. *N Z Med J* 2002; **115:**231–234.

46. Cowell JK, Gallie BL. Which retinoblastoma patients should be screened? *Eur J Cancer* 1998; **34:**1825–1826.

7

Neurofibromatosis types 1 and 2

SUSAN M. HUSON AND AURELIA NORTON

INTRODUCTION

In contrast to the majority of other genetic cancer syndromes reviewed in this book, neurofibromatosis 1 (NF1) and neurofibromatosis 2 (NF2) do not result in cancer developing in the majority of affected individuals. In NF1, the tumours that develop in the majority of patients are benign cutaneous neurofibromas. People with NF1 have a small but significant risk of specific cancers developing; these include malignant peripheral nerve tumours (MPNST), rhabdomyosarcomas, atypical forms of childhood leukaemia and astrocytomas. In NF2, the tumours are nearly always histologically benign and include vestibular Schwannomas (also called acoustic neuromas), meningiomas, Schwannomas and spinal ependymomas. Although these tumours are not malignant, curative surgery is often difficult, and NF2 is associated with significant disease-related morbidity and mortality.

Both the *NF1* and *NF2* genes have been cloned and function as tumour suppressors. Clinically, NF2 fits well into the Knudson model.[1] In NF1 there are many non tumorous manifestations, the cause of which is the focus of intense study.

Historical perspective

Although the earliest reports of NF1[2] and NF2[3] appear to describe quite distinct diseases, following von Recklinghausen's report, patients with NF2 were recognized that had cutaneous features similar to those in NF1 and, in many reports in the first half of this century, NF1 and NF2 were not clearly distinguished and were combined together under the umbrella term 'von Recklinghausen's

disease'. As the inheritance of both NF1 and NF2 is autosomal dominant, this did not help to distinguish the different forms of neurofibromatosis. Gardiner and Frazier, in reporting a large family in 1930, did point out that the uniform expression of 'acoustic neurofibromas' in their family, with limited cutaneous involvement, was unusual for von Recklinghausen's disease.[4] Despite this, cases of NF1 and NF2 continued to be considered together until the early 1970s. In 1970, Young *et al.* reported a follow-up of the Gardiner and Frazier family.[5] Their report resulted in NF2 becoming established as a distinct entity. They emphasized that the major disease feature in the family was bilateral vestibular Schwannomas and that the cutaneous features, present in a few of the family, were much less prominent than in NF1. Other NF1 complications were notably absent.

Until the 1970s, although there are many case reports in the literature of one or more patients with particular disease features, there was little in the way of systematic clinical or laboratory research. Since the 1970s, there has been an escalation of activities specific to neurofibromatosis, stimulated by the developments in genetic research and the formation of organizations for patients and their families (e.g. the National Neurofibromatosis Foundation (NNFF) in the USA, formed in 1978, and the UK Neurofibromatosis Association, formed in 1981). From a clinical perspective, work has concentrated on clearly delineating the different forms of neurofibromatosis and studying the natural history of NF1 and NF2. 'Splitting' of the various forms of the disease from the all-embracing umbrella of von Recklinghausens disease may seem at first an academic exercise. It was vital for genetic linkage studies but, in addition, the clinical importance cannot be overstated: the management and genetic advice for patients with variant forms is quite different. The most significant advances in neurofibromatosis research in the last two decades have been in molecular genetics and cell biology. The gene for NF1 was cloned in 1990[6–8] and for NF2 in 1993.[9,10]

Nosology and classification

As discussed above, in many of the early reports, NF1 and NF2 are reported under the umbrella term of von Recklinghausen's disease. Later authors, aware of the different forms of the disease, used a number of terms, which have now been superseded by the numerical classification recommended by the National Institutes of Health (NIH) Consensus Conference on Neurofibromatosis.[11] Prior to this conference, NF1 was most commonly called von Recklinghausen's, multiple or peripheral neurofibromatosis, and NF2 bilateral acoustic or central neurofibromatosis. These eponyms told us nothing about the nature of the underlying disease; the concept of peripheral and central disease seemed superficially sound but confusion was created in those cases of NF1 with central nervous system (CNS) involvement. Bilateral acoustic neurofibromatosis now seems unsatisfactory because the acoustic neuromas actually arise from the vestibular rather than the acoustic part of the eighth cranial nerve and are Schwannomas histologically. Throughout this chapter acoustic neuromas are referred to as vestibular Schwannomas, as recommended by the NIH Consensus Conference on Acoustic Neuroma in 1992.[12]

In addition to NF1 and NF2, there are other rarer forms of neurofibromatosis. In 1982, Riccardi[13] proposed a classification that included seven different types of neurofibromatosis and an eighth category for cases 'not otherwise specified'. Definition of the different forms depended on variations of the occurrence, number and distribution of the major defining features and associated complications, particularly tumours of the nervous system. Riccardi's classification has not come into widespread use, particularly because several of the forms are not defined sufficiently to permit their general use. At the 1988 NIH Consensus Conference, the panel concluded that, although other forms did exist, they could not be precisely classified at that time. To review all the other forms of neurofibromatosis is beyond the scope of this chapter. Readers should, however, be aware that they do exist and that, when they see patients that do not seem clearly to fit into either NF1 or NF2, an opinion from someone with a particular interest in neurofibromatosis may be of value. Viskochil and Carey more recently proposed an approach to classification,[14] which has the attraction that it takes a combined molecular and clinical approach. The best defined of the other forms is segmental neurofibromatosis, where patients present with the cutaneous features of NF1 limited to one or more body segments.[15] Another recently recognized, related phenotype of significance to oncologists is patients homozygous for mismatch repair gene mutations. These conditions are discussed in the sections on differential diagnosis and malignancy in NFI respectively.

NEUROFIBROMATOSIS 1

NF1 is one of the commonest single-gene disorders in humans. It is by far the most frequent form of neurofibromatosis. It has an estimated birth incidence of 1 in 2500 to 1 in 3300.[16,17] Population-based studies have found the prevalence of NF1 to be between 1 in 4000 and 1 in 5000.[18]

Clinically, the disease features are usefully divided into major defining features (café au lait spots, peripheral neurofibromas and Lisch nodules), minor disease features (short stature and macrocephaly) and disease complications. The morbidity and mortality caused by NF1 are largely dictated by the occurrence of complications; these are numerous and can involve any of the body systems. Their development is not predictable even within families. The diagnosis is a clinical one based on the criteria shown in Table 7.1.[11] These have stood the test of time remarkably well.[19] The only proviso is that patients with segmental NF1 may have >6 café au lait spots and neurofibromas or freckling, thus satisfying the diagnostic criteria.[15] However, the features are limited to one body segment. It is important these patients are distinguished – they have a very low risk of disease complications and of transmitting the disease to their children.

Pathogenesis

NF1 is virtually 100 per cent penetrant by 5 years of age.[18] Approximately 50 per cent of cases represent new

Table 7.1 *National Institutes of Health consensus statement, 1988:[11] diagnostic criteria for neurofibromatosis 1 (NF1)*

The diagnostic criteria for NF1 are met in an individual if two or more of the following are found:

- Six or more café au lait macules of over 5 mm in greatest diameter in prepubertal individuals and over 15 mm in greatest diameter in postpubertal individuals
- Two or more neurofibromas of any type or one plexiform neurofibroma
- Freckling in the axillary or inguinal regions
- Optic glioma
- Two or more Lisch nodules (iris hamartomas)
- A distinctive osseous lesion such as sphenoid dysplasia or thinning of the long bone cortex with or without pseudarthrosis
- A first-degree relative (parent, sibling, or offspring) with NF1 by the above criteria

mutations and the NF1 mutation rate is one of the highest in man. The reason for this is not understood.

The cloning of the *NF1* gene in 1990[6–8] represented the first major step towards an eventual understanding of disease pathogenesis. Studies before those involving molecular genetics were relatively few and arose from clinical observations. Bolande proposed that NF1 results from an abnormal migration, growth or cytodifferentiation of primitive neural crest cells at various stages of development.[20] The majority of NF1 manifestations arise in tissue of neural crest origin but others, such as the orthopaedic problems (scoliosis, pseudarthrosis – mesodermal origin) and learning difficulties (neural tube origin) probably do not. Riccardi, based on clinical and pathological observations, proposed that mast cells may contribute to the origin and growth of neurofibromas.[21] They form a major component of neurofibromas and NF1 patients often complain of intense itching at the site of neurofibroma development. Riccardi also suggested that trauma may have a role in the origin and/or progression of neurofibromas.[22] As will be seen later in the text, recent data from animal models support these observations.

Clinical studies have given rise to a number of questions that may give clues to disease pathogenesis. The timing and rate of progression of different lesions in NF1 is striking. For example, why do café au lait spots appear during childhood, but then remain static or even disappear in adults?

THE *NF1* GENE AND ITS PROTEIN PRODUCT NEUROFIBROMIN

As there was no information available on the structure and function of the *NF1* gene before the late 1980s, the only feasible approach available to identify the gene was positional cloning, which was achieved in 1990.[6–8] A large number of publications have followed providing information regarding the action and distribution of the protein, the nature of mutations and studies of animal models. In this chapter it is only possible to provide a brief overview of these exciting developments and interested readers are referred to recent reviews.[23–26]

The gene spans over 350 kb of genomic DNA, has 60 exons and encodes mRNA of 11–13 kb. Its protein product, 'neurofibromin', contains 2818 amino-acid residues and has an estimated molecular mass of 220 kDa. Neurofibromin is expressed ubiquitously, although expression is highest in the nervous system (in neurones, oligodendrocytes and Schwann cells). In the brain, it is expressed in neuronal dendrites and axons, and might be associated with the neuronal cytoskeleton.

Several alternatively spliced transcript isoforms of *NF1* have been identified. They result from the variable inclusion of three alternatively spliced exons (9a, 23a and 48a). Exon 23a appears to be widely expressed. The 48a form seems to be found in muscle tissues alone and the 9a isoform in forebrain neurones, where it appears to be developmentally regulated.[23]

The only region of the protein whose biological function is known is a 360-amino-acid region, which shows homology to the catalytic domain of the mammalian guanosine triphosphate-activating protein (GAP). Neurofibromin is a GAP protein for members of the p21 ras-protein family. Loss of neurofibromin function leads to downstream cell growth activation because neurofibromin negatively regulates ras output by accelerating the conversion of active ras-GTP to inactive ras-GDP. In this function at least, therefore, neurofibromin is acting as a tumour suppressor, with inactivation of neurofibromin resulting in higher levels of active ras and, therefore, cell proliferation.

There is one other intriguing aspect of the *NF1* gene. Within one large intron are nested three genes that are transcribed in the opposite direction. The genes are the human homologues of the murine leukaemia genes *Evi2a* and *Evi2b*, and the oligodendrocyte myelin glycoprotein (OMGP) gene. The significance of this genomic organ-ization is not known but OMGP has been reported to function as a negative growth regulator for Schwann cells.[27]

MUTATION ANALYSIS

The large size of the *NF1* gene and lack of a major mutational hotspot within it has made NF1 mutation analysis relatively laborious.[28] Recent developments in detection techniques promise to improve this situation.[29,30] A wide variety of gene mutations has been identified in NF1 patients. Exhaustive analysis of the *NF1* gene, using a variety of techniques, allowed Messiaen et al. [31] to identify 95 per cent of mutations in a cohort of 67 unrelated patients. They identified one translocation through the gene, one deletion of the entire gene, 25 nonsense mutations, 12 frameshift mutations, 19 splicing-site mutations, and 6 missense mutations or small in-frame deletions. Exons 10a–10c and 37 were particularly rich in mutations, accounting for 30 per cent of the mutations in their cohort.

GENOTYPE–PHENOTYPE ANALYSIS

The studies published to date have failed to identify any genotype–phenotype correlation,[28,31] except in those cases where the whole of one copy of the *NF1* gene and several surrounding genes are deleted.[32–34] Most of the NF1 microdeletions have a size of around 1.5 Mb and arise because of unequal meiotic crossovers, mediated by misalignment of flanking paralagous sequences.[34] These patients have a more severe phenotype with dysmorphic facies, high trapezius insertion (giving a webbed neck appearance), and an increased frequency of particular disease features. They have early onset of large numbers of neurofibromas, a higher frequency of learning problems and MPNST. In our series of 15 patients, two have died from MPNST, and three have had cervical root neurofibromas removed.

RNA processing may be one factor contributing to the clinical variability in NF1. Ars *et al.*[35] in a series of 80 unrelated NF1 patients, found that 50 per cent of the mutations identified in their series resulted in splicing alterations. They hypothesized that variations in the RNA splicing mechanism may lead to differential expression of the splicing mutation, and hence to different levels of the aberrantly spliced mRNA. Skuse and Cappioni argued that variations in normal NF1 RNA processing at a number of levels may be involved.[36] The evidence they cite to support their argument included:

- the difference seen in the relative ratios of different splice variants in NF1 tumours compared with non-tumour tissue;
- the unequal expression of mutant and normal NF1 alleles in cultured cells derived from NF1 patients;
- the existence of NF1 tumours, which display NF1 mRNA editing levels that are greater than seen in non-NF1 tumours;
- finally, tissue-specific and developmental stage-specific expression of particular alternative NF1 transcripts.

Other evidence points to the role of modifying genes in the variable expression of NF1. Easton and colleagues, in order to distinguish between genetic influences on the one hand, and environmental and/or chance influences on the other, examined a series of monozygotic twins concordant for NF1 and compared them with affected relatives of different degrees of relationship.[37] There was a significant correlation in the number of café au lait spots and neurofibromas between identical twins with a lower but significant correlation in first-degree relatives, and almost no correlation between distant relatives. This suggests that these features are controlled by other genetic influences but that the specific mutation in the *NF1* gene itself plays a minor role. Of the complications seen in the twin pairs, optic glioma, scoliosis, epilepsy and learning disability were concordant, but plexiform neurofibromas were not. All of these complications, with the exception of plexiform neurofibromas, showed a decreasing concordance with an increasing degree of relationship. There was no evidence of any association between the different traits in affected individuals. The study concluded that the phenotypic expression of NF1 is to a large extent determined by the genotype of other modifying loci, and that these modifying genes are trait specific. The identification of these modifying genes is the focus of active research at the present time. Further support for the role of modifying genes comes from work with animal models. The tumour phenotype in both *Nf1* heterozygote mice[38] and mice with mutations in both *Nf1* and *Tp93*[39] shows strain-specific effects.

ANIMAL MODELS OF NF1

In the absence of naturally occurring animal models, much focus has been placed on the development of animal models using recombinant technology. Human neurofibromin shows 98 per cent and 60 per cent sequence homology with its mouse and *Drosophila* equivalent, respectively. Although both mouse and *Drosophila* models have been developed, it is those in the mouse that have provided the most insight into tumour development.[24]

The first mouse models were created using homologous recombination.[40,41] *Nf1* homozygous mice (*Nf1*[-/-]) died *in utero* with severe cardiac defects (double-outlet right ventricle). The heterozygous mice are viable and, although they show none of the major disease features, do have cognitive problems[42] and die at around 15 months of age from specific tumours also seen in humans with NF1: phaeochromocytomas and myeloid leukaemia. Models that replicate the human disease more closely, in terms of neurofibroma formation, have come from the study of chimeras,[43] mice with mutations in both *Nf1* and *p53*,[39] and models using tissue-specific *Nf1* gene activation.[44,45]

In summary, animal models that develop one or more of the disease features are now available. These have already significantly advanced our understanding of the mechanism of tumorigenesis, and are beginning to act as a resource for testing potential therapies.[24,26] Our current understanding of the pathogenesis of the different NF1-related tumours is discussed individually. As predicted by the Knudson model, a second mutation is found in the majority of tumours. However, there is increasing evidence that haploinsufficiency of NF1 is also essential for some disease features to develop.[44,46]

The major disease features

Café au lait spots are the first major disease feature to appear, and may be present at birth. They are present in virtually all patients by the age of 2. In some patients, they are associated with freckling in specific sites. The next disease feature to develop during childhood is Lisch nodules. The peripheral neurofibromas develop from early adolescence onward in the majority of patients.

CAFÉ AU LAIT SPOTS AND FRECKLING

Café au lait spots are not unique to NF1 sufferers. A number of studies have shown that between 10 and 25 per cent of the general population have 1–3 of these lesions.[18] Clinically, there are no differences between the café au lait spots in NF1 patients and those in the general population; it is the increased number that is significant. The presence of six or more café au lait spots of a significant diameter should lead to the presumptive diagnosis of NF1 in the absence of a family history. Some patients with NF1 have only four or five café au lait spots; these are usually older people with other disease features, the number of café au lait spots decreases with age.[47,48] There are some rare families with <6 café au lait spots from childhood, but with typical other features and proven NF1 mutations[49] (and personal observation).

Café au lait spots may be present at birth, they increase in number throughout childhood and appear to stop developing or even disappear in adulthood. Though varying in diameter from 0.5 to 50 cm or more, the majority are less than 10 cm (Figure 7.1). They usually have smooth contours, although some larger lesions may have irregular outlines. The intensity of their colour depends on the background skin pigmentation. In some children with very pale complexions, the spots can be

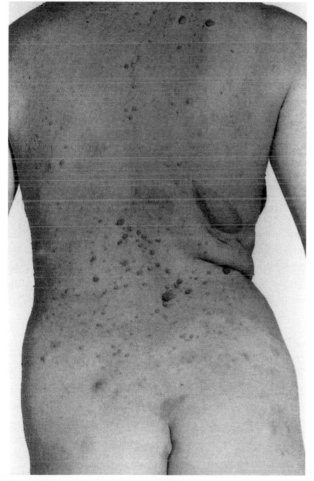

Figure 7.1 *Typical appearance of café au lait spots and cutaneous neurofibromas in an adult with neurofibromatosis type 1 (NF1). In childhood, only the café au lait spots would have been present, making the skin appearance less obvious. The significance of multiple café au lait spots in childhood is often not appreciated unless other disease features are present.*

difficult to recognize with the naked eye and are best assessed with an ultraviolet lamp.

The other characteristic form of skin pigmentation, which appears to be unique to NF1, is freckling in the axilla, around the base of the neck, in the groins and in the submammary regions in women. In obese people with NF1, freckles can often be seen between skin folds. In some patients, there seems to be no demarcation in the zones of freckling and the patients have small freckles all over the trunk and proximal extremities. The freckles resemble café au lait spots and are 1–3 mm in diameter. Freckling tends to appear after the café au lait spots, from around 3 years of age.[47] The pigmentation in NF1 is asymptomatic and is not associated with a predisposition to malignant change.

The pathogenesis of the pigmentary anomalies in NF1 remains to be elucidated. It is the one feature not observed in animal models to date and no evidence has been found for loss of heterozygosity (LOH) in cultured café au lait melanocytes.[50]

PERIPHERAL NEUROFIBROMAS

Clinically, one can distinguish dermal and nodular peripheral neurofibromas.[47,51] Dermal neurofibromas lie within the dermis and epidermis and move passively with the skin (Figure 7.1). Most adults with NF1 have dermal neurofibromas. The majority appear as discrete nodules with a violatious colour; they feel soft, almost gelatinous on palpation and vary from 0.1 cm to several centimetres in diameter. In older patients and in those with many lesions, some of the dermal neurofibromas become papillomatous and grow larger. Dermal neurofibromas develop principally on the trunk. They are only present in large numbers on the face and other exposed areas of the body in more severe cases. They usually begin to appear around the onset of adolescence and the number of lesions increases linearly with age, but this is very variable even within families. There is no way to predict the number of neurofibromas that will develop. A small number of patients just have pigmentary changes even in adult life.

Although the majority of patients, once they understand the nature of the disease, come to accept the appearance of the dermal neurofibromas, some patients are continually distressed by their appearance and require the support of a sympathetic plastic or dermatological surgeon. It is unrealistic to have all the neurofibromas that will develop removed, but patients often appreciate surgery for the largest lesions, particularly in exposed areas. Dermal neurofibromas only occasionally cause symptoms, the commonest being pruritis over the lesions particularly as they first develop. They are rarely painful. Women with NF1 often comment that their neurofibromas increase in size and number during pregnancy, often with a partial regression after delivery. These lesions rarely, if ever, undergo sarcomatous change. However, haemorrhage into them may cause sudden painful enlargement.

The other form of peripheral neurofibroma is the nodular neurofibroma. These arise on the major peripheral nerve trunks, have a much firmer consistency and more defined margins than dermal neurofibromas. As they are on major nerve trunks, they often give rise to neurological symptoms, which rarely occur with true dermal lesions. Removal of the nodular lesions is more difficult than for dermal neurofibromas because of major nerve trunk involvement, and requires the expertise of a surgeon experienced in peripheral nerve surgery. No one has recorded systematically how many NF1 patients develop nodular neurofibromas; we would estimate that it is in the region of 5 per cent. It is this kind of neurofibroma, particularly when lying in deeper tissues, that can undergo malignant change, although the risk of this in any one lesion is small.

Histologically, neurofibromas are heterogeneous tumours containing four cell types: Schwann cells, neurones, fibroblasts, and perineurial cells. One of the unanswered questions until recently has been which was the primary cell type in these tumours. Although evidence pointed to the Schwann cell (reviewed in Zhu and Parada[24]), this has only recently been confirmed. Rutkowski et al. found no NF1 mRNA in neurofibroma-derived Schwann cells, but reduced levels (consistent with haploinsufficiency) in the fibroblasts.[52] Sherman et al. found increased ras-GTP levels in Schwann cells from neurofibromas, but normal levels in neurofibroma-derived fibroblasts.[53] Serra et al. added molecular proof, finding loss of both NF1 alleles in a subset of neurofibroma-derived Schwann cells, but not in fibroblasts.[54] Through use of a conditional (Cre/Lox) allele, Zhu et al. confirmed the loss of both copies of NF1 in Schwann cells as the primary event in neurofibroma formation.[44] Furthermore, they showed that this event alone was insufficient for tumour formation. They only saw tumours in mice with mast cells haploinsufficient for NF1. It is known that mast cells from NF1 heterozygote mice have enhanced proliferative properties.[46] Zhu et al. speculate that sensitized heterozygote mast cells homing to nullizygous Schwann cells in peripheral nerves create a cytokine-rich microenvironment permissive for tumour growth.[44] This model could have major clinical implications. It may be possible to prevent or delay tumour formation in NF1 by designing therapies to neutralize the effects of the mast cells, a concept originally proposed by Riccardi based on clinical and pathological observations.[22]

LISCH NODULES

Lisch nodules are asymptomatic, harmless iris hamartomas. Although they can occasionally be seen by the naked eye, slit-lamp examination is advisable to distinguish them from the more common iris nevus.[55] Using the slit lamp, they appear as smooth domed lesions, which are usually brown in colour but can be much paler, particularly on dark irides. As they develop in childhood after the café au lait spots but before peripheral neurofibromas, they are useful for confirming the diagnosis in children with no family history and only multiple café au lait spots. They are also useful in distinguishing NF1 and NF2, as they only occur in the former. Over 90 per cent of adults with NF1 have Lisch nodules.[47]

Minor disease features

These are features that occur in quite a high proportion of NF1 patients that are not specific to the disease. The main ones are macrocephaly and short stature,[47,56] neither of which is associated with significant morbidity. In a Welsh study, after excluding patients with complications of the disease, such as scoliosis and known unrelated causes of short stature, 31.5 per cent of patients were at or below the third centile for height.[47,56] When compared with the height of their normal siblings, the reduced height of NF1 patients was highly significant. Affected males are 8 cm under expected height and females 7.6 cm under. No cause for this short stature has been found in those patients who have had full endocrinological work-ups. One must be aware, however, that very occasionally patients with pituitary/hypothalamic involvement from an optic chiasm tumour may have growth disturbance as one of the complications of this lesion.

Macrocephaly, or large heads, are a well-recognized feature of NF1. In the Welsh population study, 45 per cent of patients had head circumferences at or above the 97 centile. Again, the reason for this is unknown. In clinical practice, if children have large heads that are growing parallel to the 97 centile, we would not necessarily investigate the cause for the large head. Cranial neuroimaging studies should be reserved for patients with other symptoms and signs, or an increasing head circumference.

Differential diagnosis

The clinical diagnosis of NF1 is usually straightforward. The most common misdiagnosis relates to other forms of neurofibromatosis not being distinguished. Patients with NF1 are rarely misdiagnosed as having another form, but patients with NF2 or one of the rarer forms have often been originally diagnosed as NF1. If a patient is being assessed who has some of the features of NF1 but who does not satisfy the diagnostic criteria given in Table 7.1, it is important to consider an alternative form of neurofibromatosis.

Segmental or mosaic localized NF1 are the terms used to describe patients with features of NF1 limited to one or more body segments.[15] It has long been assumed that patients with segmental NF1 represented somatic mosaics of the *NF1* gene and this has now been proven at the molecular level.[57] Within a segment there may be sufficient disease features to satisfy the diagnostic criteria for generalized NF1. The importance of distinguishing this form is the different natural history, as disease complications are uncommon and unlikely to occur in areas outwith the skin changes. Patients with segmental NF1 have a small but definite risk of having a child with classic NF1. It is assumed that they represent gonosomal mosaics for the *NF1* gene (i.e. they have both somatic and gonadal involvement). It is important to realize that, even though the skin segment is distant from the gonads, there can still be gonadal involvement.

Numerous genetic syndromes are reported as having café au lait spots as a disease feature; we feel this simply reflects the fact that 10–15 per cent of the general population have one or two café au lait spots. There are a few very rare conditions where six or more café au lait spots can occur, distinguishable from those seen in NF1. These include the various ring chromosome syndromes[58] and Schimke immuno-osseous dysplasia.[59] In both of these conditions, other syndrome features are so striking (particularly the short stature) that the diagnosis of NF1 is soon discarded as a possibility. The only condition that usually presents with multiple café au lait spots, and no other major physical features, is the newly recognized phenotype caused by homozygosity for mismatch repair gene mutations. This is discussed in the section on NF1 and malignancy.

The other conditions that tend to be confused with NF1 either have abnormal skin pigmentation, which is confused with the café au lait spots, or some form of cutaneous tumour. In the former group, we have seen patients with McCune–Albright syndrome, Leopard syndrome and urticaria pigmentosa misdiagnosed as NF1. With regard to conditions with cutaneous/subcutaneous swellings, the commonest condition misdiagnosed as NF1 is multiple lipomatosis. Other, much rarer conditions in this group are the Proteus syndrome, Cowden syndrome and congenital generalized fibromatosis. One of the most famous patients originally diagnosed as having NF1 was Joseph Merrick, the 'Elephant Man'. It has now been realized that he had the much rarer Proteus syndrome; some of the swellings in this condition can be misdiagnosed initially as plexiform neurofibromas.

Complications

We define a complication of NF1 as any condition that occurs at an increased frequency in patients with the disease compared with the general population. Many of the complications are also seen as isolated problems in the general population (e.g. scoliosis and the malignancies which occur). Others are relatively specific to NF1, such as sphenoid wing dysplasia. Table 7.2 shows the frequency of

NF1 complications in the Welsh population along with their age and presentation where this is known.[47] Other problems that we feel are definitely associated with NF1 but were not seen in the study population are also listed; their presumed frequency is $\leqslant 1$ per cent. Some may argue that some of the disease complications listed are actually disease associations (e.g. juvenile xanthogranulomas), but this further distinction seems unnecessary.

It is the complications that make NF1 a disease with significant morbidity and mortality. They only occur in a proportion of affected individuals and their occurrence cannot be predicted, even within families. This makes management of NF1 extremely difficult in terms of achieving the balance between appropriate disease monitoring and creating unnecessary anxiety for the patient. For patients and their families, learning to deal with NF1 involves coming to terms with continuing uncertainty. Giving families detailed information about the frequency and age of presentation of the different NF1 complications is compounded by our lack of detailed knowledge about the natural history of NF1. Many of the complications of NF1 were initially identified through case reports of one or more patients, which gave little sense of a denominator to permit quantification of risk. A more complete picture comes from cross-sectional studies of large series of NF1 patients,[16,47,60] even then methods of case ascertainment tend to identify patients preferentially with more severe disease. The ideal study would be to follow a cohort of children with NF1 from birth in a defined geographical population; this has not been done.

For discussion about presentation and management of the majority of complications of NF1, the interested reader is referred to one of the texts concentrating purely on neurofibromatosis.[51,61] Before moving on to the specific malignancies associated with NF1, it is worth briefly mentioning the two most frequent complications: learning difficulties and plexiform neurofibromas.

LEARNING DIFFICULTIES

Learning difficulties affect at least one-third of children with NF1. They are usually not severe and may be associated with a tendency for the child to be generally clumsy. Because they are mild, in a classroom setting, the child may appear to have good verbal skills and be labelled as being lazy when they fail to perform in their numerical or written work. For this reason, it is important that children with NF1 are assessed with a view to learning difficulties around the time they enter school. There is also a high incidence of Attention-Deficit-Hyperactivity-Disorder in NF1.[62]

PLEXIFORM NEUROFIBROMAS

Plexiform neurofibromas were found in 30 per cent of the Welsh NF1 population.[47] They are quite distinct both clinically and pathologically from dermal neurofibromas[63,64]

Table 7.2 *Frequency of neurofibromatosis 1(NF1) complications in the Welsh study. The age range at which these can present is also given unless it is obvious. (Data derived from Huson et al.[47])*

Complication	Frequency (%)	Age range (years) of presentation
Plexiform neurofibromas		
All lesions	30.0	0–18
Large lesions of head and neck	1.2	0–1
Limbs/trunk lesions associated with significant skin/bone hypertrophy	5.8	0–5
Intellectual handicap		
Severe	0.8	
Moderate	2.4	
Minimal/learning difficulties	29.8	
Epilepsy		
No known cause	4.4	
Secondary to disease complications	2.2	Lifelong[a]
Hypsarrhythmia	1.5	0–5
Central nervous system (CNS) tumours		
Optic glioma	1.5	0–20
Other CNS tumours	1.5	Lifelong
Spinal neurofibromas	1.5	Lifelong
Aqueduct stenosis	1.5	Lifelong
Malignancy		
Peripheral nerve sarcoma	1.5	Lifelong
Pelvic rhabdomyosarcoma	1.5	0–5
Orthopaedic complications		
Scoliosis – requiring surgery	4.4	0–18
Scoliosis – less severe	5.2	
Pseudarthrosis of tibia and fibula	3.7	0–5
Gastrointestinal neurofibromas	2.2	Lifelong
Renal artery stenosis	1.5	Lifelong
Phaeochromocytoma	0.7	From 10 years
Duodenal carcinoid	1.5	onwards
Congenital glaucoma	0.7	0–1
Juvenile xanthogranuloma	0.7	0–5
Complications not seen in Welsh study but definitely associated with NF1		
Sphenoid wing dysplasia		Congenital
Lateral thoracic meningocoele	Presumed frequency ≤1%	Lifelong
Atypical forms of childhood leukaemia		0–18
Cerebrovascular disease		Usually in childhood

[a] 'Lifelong' indicates cases have been reported presenting in all age groups.

and can be divided into two types: the more common diffuse plexiform neurofibroma, and nodular plexiform neurofibromas.

Diffuse plexiform neurofibromas present as large subcutaneous swellings, they have ill-defined margins and vary from a few centimetres in diameter to those that involve a whole area of the body (Figure 7.2). They have a soft consistency, although sometimes hypertrophied nerve trunks can be palpated within the mass. The skin over the lesions is abnormal in about 50 per cent of cases,

owing to a combination of hypertrophy, café au lait pigmentation or hypertrichosis. When these lesions occur on the trunk, they are often asymptomatic but those occurring on the face or on the limbs (particularly when they are associated with underlying bone hypertrophy) are a cause of significant cosmetic burden. Diffuse plexiform neurofibromas develop much earlier than other neurofibromas in NF1. The largest lesions are all probably obvious on careful clinical examination within the first year or two of life.

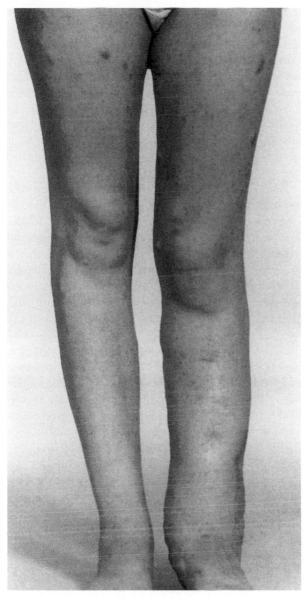

Figure 7.2 *Plexiform neurofibroma of the left leg in a 39-year-old patient with NF1. This resulted in overgrowth of the left leg in childhood. Several operations were performed to control this but the normal limb then outgrew the affected limb, leaving the patient with the disproportion seen above.*

A less common form of plexiform neurofibroma is the nodular form. The skin and other tissue surrounding the nerve trunks appear normal, but the nerve trunks themselves develop multiple nodular neurofibromas, which seem to run into one another. The distribution of age of onset of these lesions is not known precisely, although patients tend to become symptomatic in their teens. They are much less frequent than the diffuse plexiform neurofibroma: in the Welsh study, none of the patients had a nodular lesion.[47]

In terms of malignancy, plexiform neurofibromas are important, as it is they, rather than dermal neurofibromas,

that harbour the potential for malignant change. Increasingly, clinicians working with the NF1 patients feel the risk of malignant change is greatest in deep-seated nodular tumours.

The management of plexiform neurofibromas is complex because their size and impingement on surrounding structures often precludes total removal. Furthermore, they are very vascular, complicating life for the surgeon even further. In addition, there is a risk of bleeding into superficial lesions after trauma. There are no published natural history studies of plexiform neurofibromas. An international study addressing this problem using clinical assessment and volumetric magnetic resonance imaging is ongoing.[63] Clinical trials have also begun. A randomized placebo control trial is currently assessing an oral farnesyl-transferase inhibitor, the hypothesis being that this would inhibit neurofibroma growth by impeding the ability of ras to reach the membrane where it is activated.[63] The antifibrotic agent pirfenidone, which inhibits cytokines such as platelet-derived growth factor and fibroblasts and epidermal growth factors, and reduces proliferation and collagen matrix synthesis in human fibroblasts, is being evaluated in clinical trials with adults who have progressive plexiform and spinal neurofibromas.[63]

NF1 and malignancy

Cancer is a frequently cited and much feared complication of NF1. The association of specific tumour types, often occurring at a younger age than usual, was first recognized through case reports. Reliable estimates for the frequencies of the different tumour types are limited because of the paucity of formal epidemiological studies. The frequency of a particular malignancy in some published series of NF1 patients is vastly overestimated because of ascertainment bias. Another compounding factor in some earlier studies is that NF1 and NF2 are not clearly distinguished. In the present authors' opinion there is no clear evidence any longer for stating that there is an increased frequency of meningiomas or Schwannomas either of the eighth nerve or elsewhere in the nervous system in NF1. Overall, cancer only occurs slightly more frequently in NF1 patients than in the general population. The relative risk of some specific tumour types is high:[65] the majority of these are so rare in the general population, however, that the absolute risk of a patient with NF1 developing a particular tumour is usually small. For the purpose of this section, we have defined malignancy as a malignant neoplasm or benign CNS tumour; deep or cutaneous neurofibromas are excluded.

As stated in the section on NF1 complications, the ideal epidemiological study would be to follow a cohort of NF1 children in a defined population from birth; this has not been done. Two cohorts have been retrospectively followed up. Sorenson *et al.* followed up a Danish cohort identified 39 years previously.[66] Seventy (33 per cent) of the original cohort of 212 individuals had developed a malignancy (defined as a malignant neoplasm or benign CNS tumour). The numbers of expected cancers were calculated by applying the age-, year- and sex-specific incidence of total cancer to the corresponding numbers of years of risk in the cohort. For the total cohort, the point estimate of relative risk of malignancy was 2.5 (95 per cent confidence interval (CI) 1.9–3.3) with 53 observed cases vs. 20.8 expected. The excess was largely in the probands, whose relative risk was 4 (CI 2.8–5.6). The relative risk was higher in female cases. The cancers observed were very different from the general population, 47 per cent of all malignant tumours in the cohort occurred in the nervous system, whereas in the general population lung, prostate and large bowel in men, and breast, large bowel and uterus in women account for over 50 per cent of all cancers. Finally, in the general population, a second cancer develops in 4 per cent of persons with a first cancer, whereas 15 out of 70 NF1 patients (21 per cent) with a first malignancy developed a second malignancy. A Swedish follow-up study of a cohort of 70 adult patients[67] estimated that the relative risk was four (CI 2.1–7.6) during an 11-year follow-up period (1978–89).

At present, patients with NF1 who develop particular tumours are usually treated in the same way as individuals with the same kind of tumour but who do not have NF1, and this seems appropriate. There are very few data reviewing the natural history of the different kinds of tumours in NF1 and when they occur in NF1 compared within the general population. The notable exception to this is the optic glioma, which appears to follow a more benign course in NF1.[68]

CNS TUMOURS

As mentioned above, when reviewing the early literature about CNS tumours and NF1, the reader must be alert as to whether the particular article combines NF1 and NF2 or clearly distinguishes between the two conditions. As will be seen later in the chapter, CNS tumours are the hallmark of NF2 but occur relatively infrequently in NF1.

Optic nerve gliomas
Approximately 15 per cent of children with NF1 display thickening of the optic nerve by computed tomography or magnetic resonance imaging (MRI).[69–71] However, only 2–5 per cent of these became symptomatic.[47,68,69] Although biopsy is rarely done, this is attributed to optic glioma. Where pathology is available, it is typically a pyelocytic astrocytoma. The tumour may involve the orbital portion of the optic nerve, the retroorbital portion, the chiasm or any combination of these. Orbital tumours can produce proptosis, interference with extraocular movement and loss of visual acuity or visual fields. Visual loss can also occur from retro-orbital or chiasmatic tumours, and the latter may involve the hypothalamus, usually presenting as precocious puberty.[72] Spontaneous plateau of tumour growth is common and regression has even been seen in untreated patients.[73,74]

When optic gliomas are diagnosed incidentally by MRI, asymptomatic children should be followed clinically with repeated ophthalmological assessment and MRI. Treatment is not indicated unless visual impairment occurs.[68] Growth by MRI in the absence of visual signs is not an indication for treatment because spontaneous cessation of growth or even recession can occur. In the past, symptomatic optic gliomas were treated with radiation, but cranial radiation in young children results in a high frequency of cognitive, endocrine and vascular complications. Chemotherapy is more commonly used now, particularly Vincristine and Carboplatin.[75,76] Surgery is rarely indicated because the diagnosis does not require biopsy and there is a high likelihood of visual impairment after surgery. Surgical treatment is reserved for orbital tumours that are causing pain or proptosis.

Other CNS tumours
These are principally astrocytomas, which can occur anywhere in the nervous system, particularly in the cerebral and cerebellar hemispheres and brain stem. Reviewing the literature, Hughes concluded that, as neurological series of NF1 patients only identify 2–3 per cent of patients with primary CNS tumours, the incidence of glioma in NF1 is at most four times greater than the general population in which 0.7 per cent of deaths are caused by primary malignant brain tumours.[77] In the Welsh population,[47] none of the living patients had CNS tumours other than optic gliomas, although one deceased affected family member had died from a frontal astrocytoma and another (where the diagnosis of NF1 was uncertain) died of a cerebellar astrocytoma, giving an overall frequency of 0.7–1.5 per cent in the cohort used for this part of the study, depending on whether the case with an uncertain NF1 diagnosis is included.

MALIGNANT PERIPHERAL NERVE SHEATH TUMOURS

In the past, MPNSTs were described as 'neurofibrosarcomas' or 'malignant Schwannomas'. The diagnostic term 'malignant peripheral nerve sheath tumour' was introduced for both under the World Health Organization classification of nervous system tumours.[78]

The frequency of these tumours has been greatly overestimated in some series. Brasfield and Das Gupta found a frequency of 29 per cent (32 out of 110);[79] this was a hospital-based series and one of the hospitals was a cancer centre. Subsequent hospital studies have shown a much lower frequency: based on his large experience, Riccardi gives a lifetime risk of 5 per cent.[80] In the Welsh population-based study, the frequency was 1.5 per cent (2 out of 138).[47] The low risk in the Welsh study may be an underestimate because of the limitations of a cross-sectional study. In their longitudinal, population-based study, Evans et al. estimate that the lifetime risk may be as high as 8–13 per cent.[81] The mean age of diagnosis in patients with NF1 (28.7 years) is younger than for non-NF1 patients (34.0 years) with a 5-year survival of 16 per cent in NF1 patients, compared with 53 per cent for non-NF1 patients. This prognosis correlated with tumour size and extent of resection, but not with radiotherapy or chemotherapy.[82–84] Therefore, patients with NF1 need to be aware of the importance of reporting growths that suddenly become large, or painful, to their doctor. Peripheral nerve malignancies in NF1 usually arise through malignant change in an existing plexiform neurofibroma, less commonly de novo. Cutaneous neurofibromas probably do not harbour the potential for malignant change. Mutation of both copies of the NF1 gene has been demonstrated in both MPNST and benign neurofibromas. This differs from the usual 'two-hits' model in which the second hit involves loss of heterozygosity. Other hypotheses have been postulated, including microsatellite instability, promotor methylation, RNA editing and the possibility of a second functional domain in the NF1 gene.[35,36,85,86] It is also likely that additional genetic and molecular changes contribute to malignant change, such as the presence of modifier genes, loss of p53 and abnormal expression of EGFR.[87–90]

RHABDOMYOSARCOMAS

Several series of rhabdomyosarcoma cases have shown a higher than expected number of patients with NF1. In a US series of 84 consecutive patients with rhabdomyosarcoma seen at the Children's Hospital of Philadelphia, and the National Cancer Institute, five had NF1 (0.03 were expected by chance).[91] Hartley et al. found a similar excess in a UK series of childhood sarcomas.[92] They drew attention to the fact that the tumours in their series all arose in the pelvis, and had presented between 7 and 13 months of age, compared with a median age at diagnosis for all cases in the series of 48 months. In retrospect, seven of the ten children who presented at 5 years or under in the US series[91] had a rhabdomyosarcoma originating in the pelvis. In the Welsh population study, the estimated frequency of rhabdomyosarcoma was 1.5 per cent, both of which arose in the pelvis, one of

which presented at 6 months of age and the other at 2 years.[47]

ENDOCRINE TUMOURS

The association of phaeochromocytoma with NF1 is well established: again, despite a very large relative risk, the absolute risk to an NF1 patient of developing a phaeochromocytoma is small. Seven of 72 patients (9.7 per cent) in one series of patients with phaeochromocytoma had NF1.[93] In the Welsh study, 1 out of 135 (0.7 per cent) had a phaeochromocytoma.[47]

Duodenal carcinoid is known to be associated with NF1.[94] In the Welsh study, 2 out of 135 patients had NF1, one of these was the patient who also had a phaeochromocytoma, and the duodenal carcinoid was an incidental finding at operation, the surgeon being aware of the possible association. There is now a small but significant literature on the association of phaeochromocytoma and duodenal carcinoid occurring together in NF1. The practical outcome of this is that, whenever a patient is diagnosed as having one of these tumours with NF1, then a search must be made for the presence of the other.

HAEMATOLOGICAL MALIGNANCY

Like gliomas and sarcomas, it is well known that there is an elevated risk of leukaemia, particularly of chronic myeloid leukaemia, in children with NF1. Again the absolute risk to an NF1 patient of developing this complication is small, but the relative risk is quite large. In the series of Stiller et al. there was a 200-fold risk of chronic myelomonocytic leukaemia (CMML) in children with NF1, but no evidence for an increased risk of adult Philadelphia chromosome positive chronic myeloid or acute non-lymphocytic leukaemia. For acute lymphoblastic leukaemia (ALL) and non-Hodgkins lymphoma the results were consistent with a 5–10-fold risk in association with NF1.[95] However, neither of the authors, who have a personal experience of some 1500 NF1 patients, has seen an NF1 patient with either leukaemia or lymphoma and so, although it is a real association, it is an extremely rare occurrence. Bader and Miller, in a US series, found the usual ratio of ALL to non-lymphoblastic leukaemia in childhood of 4 to 1 to be reversed among NF1 patients to 9 to 20, with the rare subtypes CMML and acute myelomonocytic leukaemia comprising 13 out of 18 cases.[96] The medical literature draws our attention to the association of xanthogranuloma with NF1 and leukaemia.[97] Xanthogranuloma are benign cutaneous lesions, which develop in early childhood and resolve with age; they are usually multiple when seen in NF1. They are reported to occur in NF1 both with and without leukaemia. We believe there is a real association of NF1 and xanthogranuloma (seen in approximately 1 per cent of children in our clinic), but that the triple association reflects reporting bias. In practice, we do not perform any kind of monitoring of haematological indices in children presenting with NF1 and xanthogranuloma.

NF1, HAEMATOLOGICAL MALIGNANCY AND HOMOZYGOSITY FOR MISMATCH REPAIR GENE MUTATIONS

There have now been four families published[98-101] where one or more offspring with NF1 were homozygote for mismatch repair gene mutations (in three *MLH1* and in one *MSH2*). Of the seven children reported, all but one have had a haematological malignancy (two NHL, one AML, one atypical CML, one 'acute leukaemia' and one T cell ALL). The seventh child died from a haemorrhage into an asymptomatic glioma. Six of the seven had definite features of NF1, which were generalized in five, but limited to half of the body in the sixth. Wang *et al.* suggest that there may be further cases described in the older literature.[98,102]

These cases suggest that the *NF1* gene may be a particular target for mismatch repair (MMR) mutogenesis. Two studies have further explored this *in vitro*. Wang *et al.*[103] identified *NF1* mutations in 5/10 tumour cell lines with microsatellite instability (MSI) compared with 0/5 MMR proficient lines. They also identified *NF1* mutations in two primary tumours that exhibited MSI. Finally they found a mosaic *NF1* mutation in embryonic fibroblasts derived from *mlh* −/− mice. However, no constitutional *MLH1* or *MSH2* alterations were found in 20 patients with *de novo NF1* mutations. Therefore, this mechanism is not a common cause of *de novo* NF1 in families. Gutmann *et al.*[104] showed an acceleration of myeloid leukaemogenesis in *mlh* −/−; *Nf1* +/− mice. These mice all died by day 260 compared with none of the mice that were just heterozygous for *Nf1*. Furthermore, 50 per cent of the *mlh* −/−; *Nf1* +/− mice had died by 150 days compared with 252 days for *mlh* −/− mice.

This MMR deficient phenotype is important to recognize for two reasons, the much higher risk of early malignancy in the patient, and the risk of hereditary non-polyposis colon cancer (HNPCC) related malignancy in the heterozygote parents. None of the parents in the reports have shown any features of NF1. All but one of the reported children have been born into known HNPCC families; in two of the four families the parents were first cousins.

OTHER MALIGNANCIES

Hope and Mulvihill[105] and, subsequently, Mulvihill[106] have provided overviews of malignancy in NF1. Although in the earlier review a possible association with neuroblastoma and Wilms' tumour was thought possible, by

1994, Mulvihill did not think that any further evidence for this had emerged and we would agree. Given the abnormal pigmentation found in NF1, it is perhaps surprising that there is no clear evidence from the literature of an increased frequency of malignant melanoma. However, interestingly desmoplastic neurotrophic melanoma, an uncommon subtype of melanoma but one that is similar morphologically to nerve sheath tumours, has in one series shown LOH in intron 38 of the *NF1* gene in 10 out of 15 tumours.[107]

Although the frequency of NF1 in cohorts of children with cancer has been studied,[65] similar studies of adult cancer patients have not been performed. The NF1 cross-sectional and the Danish retrospective cohort study (reviewed by Mulvihill[106]) do not suggest this, but the individual studies are probably too small to definitively address the question.

Natural history

Because the morbidity and mortality of NF1 are largely dictated by the occurrence of its complications, all the limitations of our knowledge regarding frequency of those discussed above apply to our understanding of the natural history of NF1. The one consistent feature in all the large studies of NF1 populations has been the extreme variation of the disease, even within families, with neither the expression of the major defining features nor the occurrence of complications showing tight intrafamilial correlation except in monozygotic twins.[37] The only long-term follow-up of NF1 patients available at this time is that from the Danish NF1 cohort study.[66] Mortality rates to June 1983 of patients who were alive on 1 January, 1944 were higher than those in the general population. Mortality was increased among probands, especially females, compared with affected relatives; female relatives had a mortality rate slightly higher than that of the general population. The probands had been originally identified through hospital in-patient records and the authors concluded that patients requiring admission to hospital had a poor prognosis, whereas incidentally diagnosed relatives had a considerably better outcome. In the Welsh study, we assessed the contribution of NF1 to mortality in two ways.[47] First, we looked at disease prevalence with age and found a decrease in prevalence from the second decade onwards, which could not be accounted for solely by underascertainment. Mortality attributable to NF1 was also assessed by looking at the cause of death in 25 deceased affected relatives. Death was definitely attributable to NF1 in six cases (24 per cent). Causes of death were rhabdomyosarcomas in two children; a frontal astrocytoma in a 32-year-old; neurofibrosarcoma in a 24-year-old; obstructive hydrocephalus following the removal of a neurofibroma at C1–2 in a

51-year-old; and acute left ventricular failure and haemorrhage into an undiagnosed phaeochromocytoma in a 54-year-old.

The largest study looking at mortality in NF1 was done by analysis of death certificates in the US.[108] Rasmussen *et al.* used multi-cause mortality files compiled from death certificates by the National Centre for Health Statistics for the period 1983–1987. They identified 3770 cases of presumed NF1 amongst 32 722 122.00 deaths. This gave a frequency of NF1 of 1 per 8700 which is a lower prevalence than found in cross population based studies, the majority of which have given a prevalence in the region of 1 per 4–5000. This under ascertainment could be the cause of bias if NF1 is more likely to be listed on the death certificates of persons who had severe disease. Patients with NF1 had a reduced life expectancy with a mean of 54.4 years and median of 59 years, compared with 70.1 and 74 years in the general population. This 15 year reduction is similar to that found in the Swedish follow up study.[67] There is a suggestion in the data that survival of females with NF1 is more affected than males. Previous studies[66,67] have suggested this, and it is an area that requires further study. When the ages at death were studied for the group that had survived to the age of 40, the mean and median ages were decreased by 9 years when compared with overall American population. Therefore NF1 affects mortality at all ages, although more so in the younger age group.

Proportionate mortality ratio (PMR) analyses showed that people with NF1 were 34 times more likely to have a malignant collective or other soft tissues neoplasm listed on their death certificates than were the general population (PMR = 34.3, 95 per cent CI 30.8–38). This is the group of neoplasms in which MPNSTs fall. The PMR for this group was raised at all ages, but was particularly high in the group aged 10–29 years. An increased risk of brain tumours was found at all ages, but for myeloid leukaemia only in those under 10 years of age. The other major cause of premature death was related to vascular disease, but this was only the case for people under the age of 29 years. A similar pattern was seen when cerebrovascular disease was considered alone, but for hypertensive disease the PMR was increased only amongst subjects who died at 20–29 years of age.

Management

Because of its extreme variability and large number of complications, NF1 is an extremely difficult disease to manage. As so many different specialties may be involved in the care of any one patient, the coordination of medical care presents a significant challenge. Yet many NF1 patients will not develop major disease complications, and so the health professional is continually performing

a difficult 'balancing act' between providing adequate information and follow-up, but not creating unnecessary anxiety. Until the last 10–15 years, the majority of NF1 patients did not receive any special form of health care and were independently managed by each specialty as complications arose. Although most patients were told the name of the disease, few received adequate information about NF1 and its genetic implications.

In the Welsh study, 94 out of 135 cases had had at least one hospital consultation for NF1 before their assessment for the study.[47] Only 30 out of 135 were being regularly followed up in a hospital clinic and, in half of these, it was to monitor a specific disease complication. Medical histories of many of the patients demonstrated that regular follow-up with more awareness of the disease would have avoided delay in diagnosis of complications and distress caused by uncertainty. Only nine individuals from seven families had received genetic counselling and in four cases this was after they had completed their families.

Fortunately, over the last two decades, the approach to health care for NF1 patients has gradually changed, largely due to pressure from lay groups and the example of pioneering health professionals in the field, such as Riccardi.[13,109] It is now recommended that individuals with NF1 attend an annual clinical review, with a general physical examination geared to monitoring for complications. As shown in Table 7.2, the age at which particular complications may develop varies. For example, if a child reaches 2 years without obvious pseudarthrosis or a large superficial plexiform neurofibroma, the parents can be reassured that these complications will not develop. Particular care over spinal examinations needs to be taken during childhood, particularly through the adolescent growth spurt. The blood pressure needs to be monitored at all ages, as hypertension secondary to phaeochromocytoma may not be symptomatic until a relatively advanced stage, although renal artery stenosis usually presents under the age of 20 years.

There are times when the NF1 patients and their families need more support. The time of diagnosis is particularly important, and the authors frequently offer a combination of two or three clinic and/or home visits with the clinic nurse to help families come to terms with the diagnosis and to learn about the natural history. As children enter full-time education, it is important that they are assessed from the viewpoint of learning difficulties, so that, if these are present, they can receive appropriate help from an early age. Another important time is when adolescents and young adults begin to think about their own genetic risk, and referral for genetic counselling at an appropriate point is helpful.

The coordination of care of NF1 patients varies from country to country. In the USA, Riccardi and others developed the concept of the multidisciplinary NF clinic.[109]

This involves one or two clinical coordinators, who are usually clinical geneticists, paediatricians or neurologists who liaise closely with identified colleagues in other specialties pertinent to NF1 complications (e.g. ophthalmologists, plastic surgeons, etc.). It is not considered that all NF1 patients need to attend a specialist NF clinic on a regular basis. Although each country needs a number of specialist clinics to be available for diagnostic assessment of unusual cases, to assess cases with particular severe manifestations and to coordinate research programmes, most NF1 patients should be cared for in a 'local' setting, whether by a hospital consultant or a family physician.

The question of which specialist should follow-up NF1 patients then arises. Because many NF1 complications present in childhood, an annual follow-up by a consultant paediatrician is recommended during this period. In adults, the family physician or any one of a number of specialists (e.g. clinical geneticists, neurologists or dermatologists) are equally appropriate. In addition to medical care, many families find it helpful to be in touch with a lay organization. All the lay groups provide written literature and many now have their own website. The British Neurofibromatosis Patients' Association employs family support workers who act as a source of information and support for families.

Some people feel that annual clinical examination of NF1 patients should be supplemented by screening investigations for particular disease complications. Riccardi argued that because of the high frequency of asymptomatic optic gliomas, NF1 patients should have cranial neuroimaging at least on their initial assessment.[109] Evidence from using this approach does not support this,[19,110] because so few of these lesions become symptomatic and treatment is only offered for progressive, symptomatic lesions.

There are no specific treatments for NF1, or any drug therapy that prevents growth or development of neurofibromas themselves. Patients with troublesome neurofibromas are helped by being in touch with sympathetic plastic surgeons for removal of particularly unsightly or troublesome lesions. The treatment of specific complications is beyond the scope of this chapter and is reviewed in detail elsewhere.

Genetic counselling

The risk of a child inheriting the mutation from an affected parent is 50 per cent and the gene is 100 per cent penetrant. However, the risk of developing complications is more difficult to predict, as these do not breed true, even within families. This is particularly important to mention if the affected parent has a disease complication, as they often think children will have the same presentation of NF1. Rather than go through the risks of each disease complication separately, the authors find it useful to group the complications together as to how they will affect the patient, using data derived from the Welsh population study.[48] The frequency of complications that fall into a particular group were totalled and then halved (and rounded to the nearest 0.5 per cent) to give the risk to offspring of an affected parent. The groups are as follows:

1 intellectual handicap, 16.5 per cent (moderate/severe retardation, 1.5 per cent; minimal retardation/learning difficulties, 15 per cent);
2 complications developing in childhood and causing lifelong morbidity (severe plexiform neurofibromas of the head and neck, severe orthopaedic complications), 4.5 per cent;
3 treatable complications (aqueduct stenosis, epilepsy, internal neurofibromas, endocrine tumours, renal artery stenosis) that can develop at any age, 8 per cent;
4 malignant or CNS tumours, 2.3 per cent.

For some couples, this approach is too complex, at which point it is important to try to identify those complications the couples would find a particular problem should they occur in the child, and talk about them. If it is assumed that these include moderate to severe retardation, the different complications that develop in childhood and cause lifelong morbidity, and the risk of developing a CNS or malignant tumour, then the combined risk to the offspring of an affected parent is 8 per cent. The majority of people with NF1 choose to have children without prenatal testing. Many couples say they would have testing if it predicted disease severity rather than just disease status. At-risk children need to be monitored for signs of the disease. The majority of affected individuals have developed multiple café au lait spots by the end of the second year of life. In practice, if at-risk children reach the end of the second year of life with no café au lait spots, we are reassuring to the parents but perform one final examination at the age of 5 years.

As 50 per cent of patients represented are the first case in their family (new mutations), the most common question in clinical practice is 'what is the risk of recurrence?' It is not possible to answer this without a careful examination of the skin and irides of the parents. This is because occasionally one finds a parent who is so mildly affected that they are not aware of having the disease. Also there are a few individuals with segmental neurofibromatosis that have been reported[15] who have children with full-blown NF1. It is presumed that these represent gonosomal mosaics for the *NF1* gene; in other words, a mutation in the *NF1* gene happened in early development that involved both the segment involved with NF1 features and gonadal tissue. If the examination of the parents is entirely normal, then the chance of recurrence is barely increased above the background population risk of another new mutation. Certainly the large clinical studies of NF1 have not shown gonadal mosaicism to occur at the very high frequency and there are only a handful of families in the literature where two affected siblings are born to unaffected parents.

Molecular genetic diagnosis

The large size of the gene and absence of a particular mutation hotspot delayed widespread introduction of molecular genetic diagnosis for NF1 into service laboratories. Recent developments in mutation detection[29–31] are changing this. For prenatal and pre-symptomatic diagnosis in familial cases, intragenic and closely linked DNA markers have been available for some years. However, uptake of their use has been limited. With regard to pre-symptomatic diagnosis, as the café au lait spots develop within the first two years of life, most parents accept this time period and do not want to know as soon as possible after birth. With regard to prenatal diagnosis, the majority of couples decline testing. Many say that they would only use a prenatal test if it could predict disease severity.

The diagnosis of NF1 is usually straightforward clinically and so, again, confirmation at a molecular genetic level is usually not necessary. Even in cases where the diagnosis is not certain, clinical examination by a neurofibromatosis expert is probably preferable until the time that mutation detection is routinely diagnosing more than 99 per cent of cases. The only cases that we routinely ask for mutation analysis on are those patients in whom we suspect hold gene deletion – they are initially screened using fluorescent *in situ* hybridization (FISH). The reason for testing is the higher frequency of disease complications in this group.

Future prospects

The last decade has seen major advances in our understanding of the pathogenesis of NF1. In particular, the work on neurofibroma formation[44] raises several possible approaches to developing treatment that would prevent neurofibroma formation. With good animal models in place in which to test potential treatments, there is now realistic hope that specific therapies for NF1 may one day be possible.

NEUROFIBROMATOSIS 2

Neurofibromatosis 2 is much less common than NF1, the only study of disease prevalence finding only 1 in 210 000 individuals to be affected.[111] The same study estimated the birth incidence to be between 1 in 33 000–40 000. The large difference between prevalence and incidence

is explained by the late mean age of diagnosis of NF2 (usually in the late 20s) and the fact that many affected patients die from their disease at a relatively young age.

The original NIH diagnostic criteria proved too narrow for routine clinical use.[11,12] As a result of their large clinical study of NF2 in the United Kingdom,[112] Evans *et al.* suggested a further revision of criteria. Finally a group of experts convened by the NNFF in the US proposed a further set of criteria in 1997.[19] The latter criteria are shown in Table 7.3. They are probably the most used at the present time, but all of them have been shown to have limitations.[113] The NNFF have recently convened an international working party to develop a single revised set of diagnostic criteria. The main limitation of the present criteria is that they do not allow for the fact that, when the severe form of NF2 presents early in childhood, vestibular Schwannomas are rarely the presenting feature. The disease features are summarized in Table 7.4.

Pathogenesis

From a clinical viewpoint, NF2 fits well into the pattern of other hereditary cancers that have been shown to be caused by tumour suppressor genes. In the general population, unilateral vestibular Schwannomas develop in middle or old age. In NF2, vestibular Schwannomas occur bilaterally and are often associated with other neoplasms,

Table 7.3 *The NF2 diagnostic criteria proposed by Gutmann et al.*[19]

Definite NF2
Bilateral vestibular Schwannomas (VS)
or
Family history of NF2 (first degree relative)
Plus
1 Unilateral VS < 30 years or
2 Any two of the following:
  (a) meningioma
  (b) glioma
  (c) schwannoma
  (d) juvenile posterior subcapsular lenticular opacities

Presumptive of probable NF2
Unilateral VS < 30 years plus at least one of the following:
  (a) meningioma
  (b) glioma
  (c) schwannoma
  (d) juvenile posterior subcapsular lenticular opacities
or
Multiple meningiomas (two or more) plus unilateral VS < 30 years or one of the following:
  (a) glioma
  (b) schwannoma
  (c) juvenile posterior subcapsular lenticular opacities

Table 7.4 *Neurofibromatosis 2 (NF2): clinical features in the 120 patients studied by Evans et al.[112]*

Feature	Frequency
Tumours of the nervous system	
Bilateral VS	85
Unilateral VS	6
Meningiomas	45
Spinal tumours (meningiomas, Schwannomas)	26
Astrocytomas[a]	4
Ependymomas[a]	3
Café au lait spots (*n* = 100)	
1–4	42
6	1
Skin tumours	
Overall	68
>10 (maximum number: 27)	10
Cataracts and lens opacities (*n* = 55)[b]	60
Peripheral neuropathy	3

VS = vestibular Schwannoma.
[a] All located in brainstem and/or upper cervical cord.
[b] Only 55 individuals had slit-lamp examination.

all of which develop at a relatively young age. Before the molecular genetic era, cytogenetic analysis of meningiomas had shown loss of the whole or part of chromosome 22 in 10–30 per cent of tumours.[114,115] With the development of molecular genetic techniques, this led Seizinger and colleagues[116] to focus on chromosome 22 in their molecular genetic analysis of isolated vestibular Schwannomas. Their hypothesis proved correct and preferential loss of chromosome 22 was found in unilateral vestibular Schwannomas, in the general population. The studies were then extended to vestibular Schwannomas from patients with NF2 who showed a similar loss of chromosome 22.[117] This gave strong evidence that the most likely localization for the *NF2* gene was on chromosome 22, which was confirmed by study of the segregation of chromosome 22 markers in a large NF2 kindred.[118] Subsequent studies in other families has given no suggestion of genetic heterogeneity in NF2.[119]

THE *NF2* GENE: MERLIN/SCHWANNOMIN

The *NF2* gene was isolated in 1993 by positional cloning techniques which were facilitated by the identification of a number of patients with germline deletions.[9,10] Since that time, significant advances in our understanding as to how the NF2 protein acts as a tumour suppressor have been made.[120–122] The *NF2* gene spans 100 kb, and has 17 exons (16 constitutive and 1 alternatively spliced). Alternative splicing of exon 16 gives rise to 2 isoforms. The NF2 sequence shows strong homology to the protein 4.1 super family, particularly the ERM sub-group. It encodes

for a 595 amino acid protein that has been named Merlin (for Moesin, Ezrin and Radixin like protein[10]), although others prefer the name Schwannomin.[9] The primary role of the protein 4.1 family appears to be in communicating between the extra cellular matrix and cytoskeleton.[123]

Merlin is expressed at high levels in large numbers of tissues during embryonic development. In adult tissue, significant expression is detected in Schwann cells, meningeal cells, the lens and nerves compatible in the development of the major disease features in these tissues. Within the cell, Merlin appears to localize in cell membranes at sites involved in cell/cell contact and motility. The protein interactions and exact mechanism that underly Merlin's role as a tumour suppressor are gradually being elucidated.[120]

MOUSE MODELS FOR NF2

There are no naturally occurring animal models for the disease. Mice with targeted NF2 deficiency have now been created. Inactivation of both copies of the gene leads to early embryonic death.[124] The heterozygotes develop metastatic osteosarcomas and other tumours at increased frequency, but not tumours typical of NF2.[125] Improved mouse models have come from conditional inactivation of the gene in specific cell types.[126] When NF2 is inactivated specifically in Schwann cells it results in Schwann cell hyperplasia and then Schwannoma formation. Likewise, inactivation in the leptomeninges gives rise to hyperplasia and meningiomas. MRI scanning has detected Schwannoma development in the animal model, and the infectibility of the tumours with vectors that could be used for therapeutic gene delivery has been demonstrated.[127]

Nervous system tumours occurring in NF2

VESTIBULAR SCHWANNOMAS (ACOUSTIC NEUROMAS)

These are the most consistent disease features and were the cause of the initial symptom in the majority of cases in both of the largest clinical studies.[112,128] Early symptoms included hearing loss with tinnitus or vertigo resulting from pressure on the cochlear nerve. Compared with their unilateral counterparts, vestibular Schwannomas in NF2 present at a younger age (median age of onset 27 years compared with over 50 years in non-NF2 cases usually). They also tend to have grown to a larger size before causing symptoms, which presents difficulties in management[129] (Figure 7.3).

SCHWANNOMAS

In addition to the eighth nerve, Schwannomas can develop in any of the other cranial nerves (except 1 and 2), on the

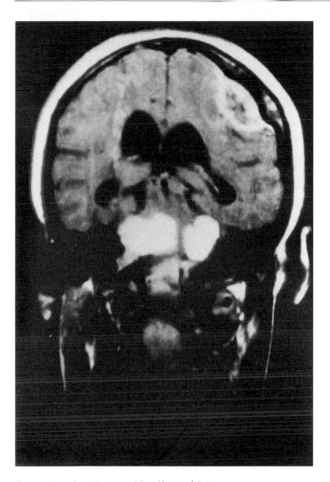

Figure 7.3 An 18-year-old patient with severe neurofibromatosis type 2 (NF2). The cranial T1-weighted gadolinium-enhanced magnetic resonance image demonstrates bilateral enhancing vestibular schwannomas dramatically compressing the brain stem. The brain stem and upper cervical cord are also expanded by an enhancing mass consistent with a brain stem glioma. There is also a left convexity meningioma.

dorsal nerve roots of the spinal cord and on the major peripheral nerves. There may be multiple nerve involvement. The presenting features of the tumours are related to their anatomical localization.

The peripheral nerve Schwannomas in NF2 appear clinically very like the nodular fibromas in NF1 and, if they are the initial presentation of NF2, this often results in initial misdiagnosis as NF1 until other disease features develop.

MENINGIOMAS

Meningiomas were present in 45 per cent of the patients in a large UK study.[112] There is no site where they are particularly prone to occur, but symptoms are related to location. Meningioangiomatosis is a distinctive lesion with a meningiothelial and vascular component that can

be associated with NF2. Although the lesions have been reported adjacent to meningiomas, it is thought that they present a dysplastic hamartomatous lesion rather than a neoplastic process.

GLIAL TUMOURS

Glial tumours are much less common in NF2 than Schwannomas or meningiomas. They include pilocytic astrocytomas of the brain and spinal cord, cerebral and spinal ependymomas. Optic nerve gliomas do not occur with increased frequency in NF2. In the UK study,[112] 4 per cent of patients had an astrocytoma and 2.5 per cent ependymomas; they were low-grade tumours and affected the lower brain stem or upper cervical cord. Syringomyelia can develop in association with intramedullary tumours.

CUTANEOUS TUMOURS

These occur less consistently and in much smaller numbers than in NF1. The most common kind, occurring in 48 per cent of patients in the UK study,[112] are sometimes referred to as NF2 plaques and have a distinctive appearance. They are discrete, well-circumscribed, slightly raised cutaneous lesions, usually <2 cm in diameter. Their surface may be slightly pigmented, roughened and often contain excess hair. Less commonly, NF2 patients have cutaneous tumours indistinguishable from the dermal lesions seen in NF1. They occurred in 27 per cent of patients seen in the UK study but were much fewer in number than would be normally seen in an adult with NF1. Histologically the cutaneous tumours in NF2 are usually Schwannomas.

Other disease features

CAFÉ AU LAIT SPOTS

Some 43 per cent of the patients in the UK study[112] had café au lait spots. Of these, 24 patients had one, 11 had two, four had three and three had four spots. Only one patient had six café au lait spots. Hence, although café au lait spots occur more frequently in NF2 than in the general population, they are much less frequent in number than in NF1. Axillary and groin freckling are not seen in NF2.

OPHTHALMOLOGICAL FEATURES

Lisch nodules do not occur in NF2. Characteristic eye findings are posterior subcapsular lens opacities and sometimes cataracts. Kaiser-Kupfer et al. found these changes in 18 of 22 affected individuals (82 per cent).[130] In the UK study, opacities were found in 60 per cent of the patients who had slit-lamp examinations. Fifteen had been identified as having cataracts in childhood, of which four had minimal vision in the affected eye, probably from birth.

The other eye findings in NF2 are retinal astrocytic hamartomas, found by Ragge et al.[131] in eight of 21 patients.

Because the eye changes are present from infancy, individuals at risk of NF2 should be screened for their presence from that time. If these eye changes are found in otherwise asymptomatic individuals with no family history, then the diagnosis of NF2 should be considered as a possible underlying cause.

OTHER FEATURES

Peripheral neuropathy is seen in patients with severe NF2. This can take the form of a mixed peripheral motor and sensory neuropathy or isolated mononeuropathy.[132,133] Histology of the nerves shows the axonopathy to be caused, not only by tumour growth, but also by multiple tumourlets and proliferation of Schwann and perineural cells[134,135] – it is interesting to note the similarities in the nerve pathology seen in mouse models.

Intracranial calcifications on cranial neuroimaging not due to tumour and somewhat similar to those in tuberous sclerosis have been reported in a number of patients. However, their frequency in a large series of patients has not been studied, nor is the pathological nature of the lesions known.

Differential diagnosis

The most common misdiagnosis in the authors' experience is that patients with NF2 and marked cutaneous features are labelled as having NF1. The possibility of NF2 must be borne in mind when assessing young adults referred as having NF1 who subsequently have enough café au lait spots to satisfy diagnostic criteria or who have atypical cutaneous tumours.

Another problem in misdiagnosis is that the possibility of NF2 is not considered when young people present with single vestibular Schwannomas, meningiomas or spinal Schwannomas. It is important that other signs of NF2 are sought in such patients and that they are offered long-term follow-up.

Bilateral vestibular Schwannomas appear to be unique to NF2. However, there are rare families in which multiple meningiomas segregate as an autosomal trait, and others where spinal Schwannomas with or without peripheral nerve Schwannomas segregate without other NF2 features.[129,136,137]

Natural history

In the UK study, the mean age at first symptom was 21.6 (range 2–52) years and at diagnosis 27.6 (range 5–66) years.[112] Eleven patients (10 per cent) presented before the age of 10 years. The mean age at onset of deafness was 24.3 (range 4–50) years in 87 patients. The natural history of NF2 is affected by the rate of growth of the vestibular Schwannomas and the number of other tumours the individual may develop. The natural history is also affected by the surgical management. Inappropriate operations on large vestibular Schwannomas can hasten the course of the disease. In the large family followed up by Young et al.,[5] the 20 deceased members who did not undergo surgery had a mean survival from onset of symptoms of 18.5 (range 4–44) years. The nine deceased members who had surgery had a mean survival of 9.2 (range 3–19) years. In the UK study, the mean age at death in 40 cases was 36.3 years.[112] The mean actuarial survival from diagnosis was 15 years, which gave a mean age at death of 42–6 years, if mean age at diagnosis was used. Overall, the mean actuarial survival from birth for 150 cases was 62 years; however, over 40 per cent would be expected to have died by 50 years and all cases by 70 years.

Baser et al.[138] looked at predictors of mortality in NF2 in 368 patients from 261 families in the UK NF2 registry. Relative risk of mortality increased the younger the age of diagnosis and with the presence of meningiomas. Conversely those patients treated in NF2 speciality centres had a significantly lower mortality than those treated in non-speciality centres.

Some studies have suggested a deleterious effect of pregnancy on the natural history of NF2. The UK study, however, did not find evidence that pregnancy or indeed gender were associated with natural history.[108]

Genetics

NF2 is an autosomal dominant condition with almost complete penetrance by the age of 60 years.[112] Approximately half the cases of NF2 are the first in their family and are presumed to be the result of new gene mutation. The mutation rate has been calculated to be 6.5×10^{-6} per allele per generation.

In contrast to NF1, all studies of NF2 have shown strong intrafamilial correlation in disease course but marked interfamilial variation. Families fall into two main groups (two references) as follows:

1 Mild (Gardener type) – these families are characterized by a relatively late onset after the age of 20 years. Bilateral vestibular Schwannomas with only minimal skin manifestations and occasional other CNS tumours are the clinical features.
2 Severe (Wishart) – these patients present before the age of 20 and have multiple meningiomas and spinal tumours in addition to their bilateral vestibular Schwannomas. It is in this category one sees

intra-medullary spinal tumours. They are also the patients that have problems with peripheral neuropathy and have the most florid ophthalmological manifestations, particularly retinal hamatomas.

In clinical practice, defining these sub-types is clinically useful in counselling families. However, a cautious approach is warranted as there are families which do not fall easily into either group. As will be seen below, missense mutations have been associated with intrafamilial variability. Likewise, many of the milder cases, who are the first person in their family to be diagnosed with NF2, actually represent somatic mosaics.

Early studies[139] showing younger age of onset in maternally inherited cases have not been supported by more recent data.[140,141]

MOSAICISM IN NF2

As molecular analysis in NF2 patients became available it was realized that a significant number of de novo cases actually had somatic mutations, despite satisfying the diagnostic criteria.[142,143] The importance of this clinically is that these patients have a lower offspring risk (only 1 of 9 affected children were born to 3 mosaic patients in the Evans et al. series[142]). However, the disease may be more severe as they will be non-mosaic.[144] It is estimated that approximately 20 per cent of de novo cases may be somatic mosaics. This fact means that it is unsafe to use DNA marker studies for presymptomatic testing in the children of the first case in a family, where a mutation cannot be detected, as they may well be mosaics.[145]

Mosaic patients where the features of NF2 are limited to a specific part of the nervous system are very common, although they are more easily recognized in clinical practice as scanning techniques have developed.[15]

GENOTYPE–PHENOTYPE CORRELATION

Since the cloning of the gene in 1993, there have been numerous studies of genotype phenotype correlation that have recently been reviewed by Baser et al.[120] and MacCollin and Gusella.[146] The correlations are strong but not complete and caution must be used in interpreting them clinically. In general, people with constitutional nonsense and frameshift mutations have severe disease, and those with missense mutations in-frame or large deletions have mild disease. Those with splice-site mutations have variable disease severity. The latter group of mutations are the only ones where variable disease severity may be associated with the location of the mutation.[147] In the study of Baser et al. looking at predictors of mortality in NF2, missense mutations were found to have a lower risk of mortality than other types of mutation.[138]

MOLECULAR GENETIC DIAGNOSIS

In contrast with NF1, molecular genetic diagnosis in NF2 is of enormous value clinically. Both DNA marker studies and mutation analysis are available. As discussed in the section on mosaicism, caution must be used in terms of the family structure where DNA marker studies are undertaken. The percentage of patients where mutations are detected is gradually improving.[120,148] The detection rate in de novo cases is much lower than in second generation familial cases; this is due to the presence of mosaicism in such a high proportion of de novo cases. When a mutation is not identified in the lymphocyte DNA of de novo cases, mutation analysis in tumours can be undertaken. The addition of techniques that enable the detection of deletions, which account for approximately 30 per cent of mutations in NF2 patients, will increase mutation detection in non-mosaic patients.[148]

Management

In contrast to NF1, the authors recommend that all patients with NF2 and at-risk family members are followed in centres with experience of management of the condition.[138] This is because the successful management of NF2 patients involves coordination between several different specialties, principally neurosurgeons, otolaryngologists, ophthalmologists and geneticists. All patients with the condition, because of the high frequency of vestibular Schwannomas and other serious nervous system tumours, need this multidisciplinary follow up. Patients also need ongoing support from other health professionals, such as teachers of communication to the deaf, and social workers. Several studies have shown improved surgical outcome when vestibular Schwannoma surgery in NF2 is performed in centres specializing in this kind of surgery.[12,138] The study of Evans et al. also showed that very few families had any understanding of the natural history or genetic nature of their condition.[112,139] Only 44 of 120 patients had received genetic counselling and many people were unaware that NF2 could be inherited.[139]

MANAGEMENT OF AFFECTED INDIVIDUALS

Once an individual has been diagnosed as having NF2, they need lifelong follow-up because monitoring for the early diagnosis of developing tumours is essential. Even if patients only present with symptomatic vestibular Schwannomas, they should always have a spinal MRI scan to exclude spinal tumours before any surgery is undertaken. The rate of growth of the tumours in NF2 is very variable and, with the advent of MRI imaging, many asymptomatic tumours are being found in individuals with NF2, which, when followed for a number of years, either remain the same size or take several years before they become large enough to cause symptoms.

Surgery is geared toward the treatment of symptomatic lesions. For meningiomas and spinal tumours occurring in NF2, the surgical approach is the same as when these lesions arise in the general population. The management of the vestibular Schwannomas in NF2 is still the subject of debate. The long-term goal is to develop a treatment for small tumours that leads to preservation of hearing. Neither early proactive surgery[149] or stereotactic radio surgery[150] can guarantee this. Furthermore, there are concerns that long-term follow-up of patients with stereotactic radio surgery will see more cases of malignant change in the residual tumour being reported.[120] In the Oxford NF2 clinic, we follow a relatively conservative approach in the management of NF2. The patients have regular audiological examinations and neuroimaging studies (4–6 six monthly initially and annually in tumours that are not growing or growing very slowly). In patients with no symptoms or mild stable symptoms and where MRI shows no increase in tumour size, conservative observation is indicated. For symptomatic or growing tumours, the different treatment options are discussed in detail with the patients.

The significant development in NF2 management in recent years has been the development of brain stem implants to provide some restoration of hearing in patients with bilateral deafness.[151,152] Where the cochlear nerve is left intact after surgery, use of cochlear implants offers even better restoration of hearing.[153]

GENETIC COUNSELLING AND THE MANAGEMENT OF AT-RISK INDIVIDUALS

In families with established NF2, children of affected individuals have a 50 per cent risk of inheriting the condition. Approximately half of NF2 patients will have no obvious family history, even after a detailed family tree has been drawn up. If a mutation is identified in the patient, then we offer mutation testing to their parents (unless they are asymptomatic and over the age of 60) and first degree relatives (the latter is done because of the possibility a parent could be a mosaic). In families where no mutation is identified we offer to screen the relevant relatives with clinical and ophthalmological examination and neuroaxis MRI scans.

With regard to children at risk, we follow them annually from birth. In the early years we offer an annual review of symptoms with ophthalmological screening for cataracts and retinal changes. The timing of molecular genetic diagnosis in at risk children is discussed with the parents from birth. Our preferred option is to delay it until around the age of 10 years of age when we would be considering the initial neuroimaging of those with the gene. This allows the child to be involved in discussion with regard to testing. Some children and their parents prefer to continue with imaging rather than have a definitive answer from mutation testing.

Once a child is found to have the gene mutation then their follow-up is as for affected individuals from around the age of 10 years. In families where mutation analysis is not available, depending on the age of onset of disease in the family we offer annual examinations with audiological and clinical assessments, and MRI of the cerebellopontine angle. The frequency with which full neuroaxis scanning should be done in this group is still being determined. In our own practice we perform it in the early teens and five yearly thereafter until around the age of 30 years. In the majority of families, if screening is negative at this point, it will mean that the child has not inherited the gene. However, in families with a later onset of disease, screening should be continued as appropriate.

In our experience prenatal testing is requested more frequently by NF2 patients than those with NF1. Preimplantation genetic diagnosis is also possible.[154]

FUTURE PROSPECTS

With increasing understanding of tumour pathogenesis and reliable animal models, the prospect of development of a medical treatment for the tumours in NF2 is now a realistic goal for the next decade.

KEY POINTS

Neurofibromatosis type 1 (NF1)

- There are diagnostic criteria (see Table 7.1).
- The prevalence is 1 in 4000–5000.
- The majority of features are benign.
- The condition is due to mutations in a large gene, *NF1*, and 50 per cent are new mutations and there is therefore no family history.
- The lifetime risk of disease related cancers is around 5–10%.

Neurofibromatosis type 2 (NF2)

- There are diagnostic criteria (see Table 7.3); the most characteristic is acoustic neuroma.
- It is less common than NF1 (1 in 210 000).
- Fifty per cent are due to new mutations in the *NF2* gene on chromosome 22.
- The most common malignancies are in the CNS.

REFERENCES

1. Knudson AG Jr. Mutation and cancer: statistical study of retinoblastoma. *Proc Natl Acad Sci USA* 1971; **68**:820–823.
2. von Recklinghausen FD. *Üeber die multiplen Fibrome der Haut und ihre Beziehung zu den multiplen Neuromen.* Berlin: Hirschwald, 1882.

3. Wishart J. Cases of tumors in the skull, dura mater and brain. *Edin Clin Surg J* 1822; **18**:393–397.

4. Gardiner WT, Frazier CH. Bilateral acoustic neurofibromas: a clinical study and field survey of a family of five generations with bilateral deafness in 38 members. *Arch Neurol Psychiat* 1930; **23**:266–300.

5. Young DF, Eldridge R, Gardner WJ. Bilateral acoustic neuromas in a large kindred. *J Am Clin Assoc* 1970; **214**:347–353.

6. Cawthon RM, Weiss R, Xu G, *et al*. A major segment of the neurofibromatosis type 1 gene: CDNA sequence, genomic structure and point mutations. *Cell* 1990; **62**:193–201.

7. Viskochil D, Buchberg AM, Xu G. *et al*. Deletions and a translocation interrupt a cloned gene at the neurofibromatosis type 1 locus. *Cell* 1990; **62**:187–192.

8. Wallace MR, Marchuk DA, Anderson LB, *et al*. Type 1 neurofibromatosis gene: identification of a large transcript disrupted in three NF1 patients. *Science* 1990; **249**:181–186.

9. Rouleau GA, Merel P, Lutchman M, *et al*. Alteration in a new gene encoding a putative membrane organizing protein causes neurofibromatosis type 2. *Nature* 1993; **363**:515–521.

10. Trofatter JA, MacCollin MM, Rutter JL, *et al*. A novel moesin, ezrin, radixin-like gene is a candidate for the neurofibromatosis 2 tumour suppressor. *Cell* 1993; **72**:791–800.

11. NIH Consensus Development Conference. Neurofibromatosis conference statement. *Arch Neurol* 1988; **45**:575–578.

12. NIH Consensus Development Conference. Conference statement: acoustic neuroma. *Neurofibromatosis Res Newslett* 1992; **8**:1–7.

13. Riccardi VM. Neurofibromatosis: clinical heterogeneity. *Curr Probl Cancer* 1982; **VII** (2):1–34.

14. Viskochil D, Carey JC. Nosological considerations of the neurofibromatoses. *J Dermatol* 1992; **19**:873–880.

15. Ruggieri M, Huson SM. The clinical and diagnostic implications of mosaicism in the neurofibromatoses. *Neurology* 2001; **56**:1433–1443.

16. Crowe FW, Schull WJ, Neel JV. *A clinical, pathological and genetic study of multiple neurofibromatosis*. Springfield, IL: Charles C Thomas, 1956.

17. Huson SM, Clark P, Compston DAS, Harper PS. A genetic study of von Recklinghausen's neurofibromatosis in South East Wales I: prevalence, fitness, mutation rate and effect of parental transmission on severity. *J Med Genet* 1989; **26**:704–711.

18. Huson SM. Neurofibromatosis I: a clinical and genetic overview. In: Huson SM, Hughes RAC (eds) *The neurofibromatoses: a pathogenetic and clinical overview*. London: Chapman and Hall, 1994:160–203.

19. Gutman DH, Aylsworth A, Carey JC, *et al*. The diagnostic evaluation and multidisciplinary management of Neurofibromatosis 1 and Neurofibromatosis 2. *JAMA* 1997; **278**:91–97.

20. Bolande RP. Neurofibromatosis – the quintessential neurocristopathy: pathogenetic concepts and relationships. *Adv Neurol* 1981; **29**:67–75.

21. Riccardi VM. Cutaneous manifestations of neurofibromatosis: cellular interaction, pigmentation, and mast cells. *Birth Defects Orig Article Ser* 1981; **17**:129–149.

22. Riccardi VM. The potential role of trauma and mast cells in the pathogenesis of neurofibromas. In: Ishibashi Y, Hori Y (eds) *Tuberous sclerosis and neurofibromatosis: epidemiology, pathophysiology, biology and management*. Amsterdam: Elsevier, 1990;167–190.

23. Reed N, Gutman DH. Tumorigenesis in neurofibromatosis: new insights and potential therapies. *Trends Mol Med* 2001; **7**:157–162.

24. Zhu Y, Parada LF. Neurofibromin, a tumour suppressor in the nervous system. *Exp Cell Res* 2001; **264**:19–28.

25. Ferner RE, O'Doherty MJ. Neurofibroma and schwannoma. *Curr Opin Neurol* 2002; **15**:679–684.

26. Das Gupta B, Gutmann DH. Neurofibromatosis 1: closing the gap between mice and men. *Curr Opin Genet Dev* 2003; **13**:20–27.

27. Habib AA, Gulcher JR, Hognason T, *et al*. The *Omgp* gene, a second growth suppressor within the *NF1* gene. *Oncogenesis* 1998; **16**:1525–1531.

28. Upadhyaya M, Cooper DN. The mutational spectrum in neurofibromatosis 1 and its underlying mechanisms. In: Upadhyaya M, Cooper DN (eds) *Neurofibromatosis type 1 from genotype to phenotype*. Oxford: 1998:65–88.

29. Luc AD, Buccino A, Gianni D, *et al*. *NF1* gene analysis based on DHDLC. *Hum Mutat* 2003; **21**:171–172.

30. Gite S, Lim M, Carlson R, *et al*. A high throughput nonisotopic protein truncation test. *Nature Biotechnol* 2003; **21**:194–197.

31. Messiaen LM, Callens T, Mortier G, *et al*. Exhaustive mutation analysis of the *NF1* gene allows identification of 95 per cent of mutations and reveals a high frequency of unusual splicing defects. *Hum Mutat* 2000; **19**:941–999.

32. Kayes LM, Burke W, Riccardi VM, *et al*. Deletions spanning the neurofibromatosis 1 gene: identification and phenotype of five patients. *Am J Hum Genet* 1994; **54**:424–436.

33. Wu B-L, Austin MA, Schneider GH, *et al*. Deletion of the entire *NF1* gene detected by FISH: four deletion patients associated with severe manifestations. *Am J Med Genet* 1995; **59**:528–539.

34. Lopez Correa C, Brems H, Lazaro C, *et al*. Unequal meiotic crossover: a frequent cause of *NF1* microdeletions. *Am J Human Genet* 2000; **66**:1969–1974.

35. Ars E, Serra E, Garcia J, *et al*. Mutations affecting mRNA splicing are the most common molecular defects in patients with neurofibromatosis type 1. *Hum Mol Genet* 2000; **9**:237–247.

36. Skuse G, Cappione AJ. RNA processing and clinical variability in neurofibromatosis type 1 (NF1). *Hum Mol Genet* 1997; **6**:1707–1712.

37. Easton DF, Ponder MA, Huson SM, Ponder BAJ. An analysis of variation in expression of *NF1*: evidence for modifying genes. *Am J Hum Genet* 1993; **53**:305–313.

38. Tischler A, Shih T, Williams B, Jacks T. Characterisation of phaeochromocytomas in a mouse strain with a targeted disruptive mutation of the neurofibromatosis gene *NF1*. *Endocrine Pathol*. 1995; **6**:323–335.

39. Reilly KM, Loisel DA, Bronson RJ, *et al*. Nf1: Trp53 mutant mice develop glioblastoma with evidence of strain-specific effects. *Nature Genet* 2000; **26**, 109–113.

40. Brannan CI, Perkins AS, Vogel KS, *et al*. Targeted disruption of the neurofibromatosis type 1 gene leads to developmental abnormalities in heart and various neural crest-derived tissues. *Genes Dev* 1994; **8**:1019–1029.

41. Jacks T, Shaneshih T, Schmitt EM, *et al*. Tumour predisposition in mice heterozygous for a targeted mutation in *Nf1*. *Nature Genet* 1994; **7**:353–361.

42. Silva AJ, Frankland PW, Marowitz Z, *et al*. A mouse model for the learning and memory deficits associated with neurofibromatosis type 1. *Nature Genet* 1997; **15**:281–284.

43. Cichowski K, Shih TS, Schmitt E, *et al.* Mouse tumour model for neurofibromatosis type 1. *Science* 1999; **286:**2172–2176.

44. Zhu Y, Ghosh P, Charnay P, *et al.* Neurofibromas in NF1: Schwann cell origin and role of tumour environment. *Science* 2002; **296:**920–922.

45. Gitler AD, Zhu Y, Ismat FA, *et al.* NF1 has an essential role in endothelial cells. *Nature Genet* 2003; **33:**75–79.

46. Ingram DA, Yang F-C, Travers JB, *et al.* Genetic and biochemical evidence that haploinsufficiency of the *NF1* tumor suppressor gene modulates melanocyte and mast cell fates *in vivo. J Exp Med* 2000; **191:**181–187.

47. Huson SM, Harper PS, Compston DAS. von Recklinghausen neurofibromatosis: a clinical and population study in South East Wales. *Brain* 1998; **III:**1355–1381.

48. Huson SM, Compston DAS, Harper PS. (1989) A genetic study of von Recklinghausen neurofibromatosis in Sough East Wales II (guidelines for genetic counseling). *J Med Genet* 1989; **26:**712–721.

49. Faravelli F, Upadhyaya M, Osborn M, *et al.* Unusual clustering of brain tumours in a family with NF1 and variable expression of cutaneous features. *J Med Genet* 1999; **36:**893–896.

50. Eisenbarth I, Assum G, Kaufmann D, Krong W. Evidence for the presence of the second allele of the neurofibromatosis type 1 gene in cultivated melanocytes from patients with neurofibromatosis 1. *Arch Dermatol Res* 1997; **287:**413–416.

51. Friedman JC, Gutmann DH, MacCollin M, Riccardi VM. *Neurofibromatosis: phenotype, natural history and pathogenesis,* 3rd edn. Baltimore, MD: Johns Hopkins University Press, 1999.

52. Rutkowski JL, Wu K, Gutmann DH, Boyer PJ, Legius E. Genetic and cellular defects contributing to benign tumour formation in neurofibromatosis type 1. *Hum Mol Genet* 2000; **9:**1059–1066.

53. Sherman LS, Atit R, Rosenbaum T, *et al.* Single cell ras-GTP analysis reveals altered ras activity in a single population of neurofibroma schwann cells but not fibroblasts. *J Biol Chem* 2000; **275:**30740–30745.

54. Serra E, Rosenbaum T, Winner U, *et al.* Schwann cells harbor the somatic *NF1* mutation in neurofibromas: evidence of two different schwann cell subpopulations. *Hum Mol Genet* 2000; **9:**3055–3064.

55. Ragge NK, Falk RE, Cohen WE, Murphree AL. (1993) Images of Lisch nodules across the spectrum. *Eye* 1993; **7:**95–101.

56. Cnossen MH, Moons KGM, Garssen MPJ, *et al.* Minor disease features in neurofibromatosis type 1 (NF1) and their possible value in diagnosis of NF1 in children ≤6 years and clinically suspected of having NF1. *J Med Genet* 1998; **35:**624–627.

57. Tinschert S, Naumann I, Stegmann E, *et al.* Segmental neurofibromatosis is caused by somatic mutation of the neurofibromatosis type 1 (*NF1*) gene. *Eur J Hum Genet* 2000; **8:**455–459.

58. Gardner RJM, Sutherland GR. *Chromosome Abnormalities and Genetics Counselling.* Oxford: Oxford University Press, 1996.

59. Ludman MD, Cole DEC, Crocker JFS, Cohen MM. Schimke immuno-osseus dysplasia: case report and review. *Am J Med Genet* 1993; **47:**793–796.

60. Friedman JM, Birch PH. Type 1 neurofibromatosis: a descriptive analysis of the disorder in 1728 patients. *Am J Med Genet* 1997; **70:**138–143.

61. Huson SM, Hughes RAC (eds) *The neurofibromatoses: a clinical and pathogenetic overview.* London: Chapman & Hall, 1994.

62. Mautner VF, Kluwe L, Thakker SD, Leark RA. Treatment of ADHD in neurofibromatosis type 1. *Dev Med Child Neurol* 2002; **44:**164–170.

63. Packer RJ, Gutmann DH, Rubenstein A, *et al.* Plexiform neurofibromas in NF1. *Neurology* 2002; **58:**1461–1470.

64. Huson SM. Neurofibromatosis 1: a clinical and genetic overview. In: Huson SM, Hughes RAC (eds) *The neurofibromatoses: a pathogenetic and clinical overview.* London: Chapman & Hall, 1994.

65. Narod SA, Stiller C, Lenoir GM. An estimate of the heritable fraction of childhood cancer. *Br J Cancer* 1991; **63:**993–999.

66. Sorenson SA, Mulvihill JJ, Nielsen A. (1986) Long-term follow up of von Recklinghausen neurofibromatosis: survival and malignant neoplasms. *N Engl J Med* 1986; **314:** 1010–1015.

67. Zoller MET, Rembeck B, Oden A, *et al.* Malignant and benign tumours in patients with neurofibromatosis type 1 in a defined Swedish population. *Cancer* 1997; **79:**2125–2131.

68. Listernick R, Charrow J, Greenwald MJ, Mets M. Natural history of optic pathway tumours in children with neurofibromatosis type 1: a longitudinal study. *J Pediatr* 1994; **125:**63–66.

69. Lewis RA, Gerson LP, Axelson KA, *et al.* von Recklinghausen neurofibromatosis II. Incidence of optic gliomata. *Ophthalmology* 1984; **91:**929–935.

70. Listernick R, Lovis DN, Packer RJ, Gutmann DH. Optic pathway glioma in children with neurofibromatosis type 1: consensus statement from the Optic Pathway Glioma Task Force. *Ann Neurol* 1997; **41:**143–149.

71. Kuenzle C, Weissert M, Roulet E, *et al.* Follow-up of optic pathway gliomas in children with neurofibromatosis type 1. *Neuropaediatrics* 1994; **25:**295–300.

72. Cnossen MH, Stam EN, Cooiman CMG, *et al.* Endocrinologic disorders and optic pathway gliomas in children with neurofibromatosis type 1. *Pediatrics* 1997; **100:**667–670.

73. Brzowski AE, Bazan C, Mumma JV, Ryan SG. Spontaneous regression of optic glioma in a patient with neurofibromatosis. *Neurology* 1992; **42:**679–681.

74. Perilongo G, Moras P, Carollo C, *et al.* Spontaneous partial regression of low-grade glioma in children with neurofibromatosis-1: a real possibility. *J Child Neurol* 1999; **14:**352–356.

75. Packer RJ, Sutton LN, Bilaniuk LT, *et al.* Treament of chiasmatic/hypothalamic gliomas of childhood with chemotherapy: an update. *Ann Neurol* 1988; **23:**79–85.

76. Listernick R, Charrow J, Tomita T, Goldman S. Carboplatin therapy for optic pathway tumours in children with neurofibromatosis type-1. *J Neurooncol* 1999; **45:**185–190.

77. Hughes RAC. Neurological complications of neurofibromatosis 1. In: Huson SM, Hughes RAC (eds) *The neurofibromatoses: a clinical and pathogenetic overview.* London: Chapman & Hall, 1994:204–232.

78. Kleihus P, Burger PC, Scheithauer BW. *Histological typing of tumours of the central nervous system,* 2nd edn. Berlin: Springer Verlag, 1993.

79. Brasfield RD, Das Gupta TK. Von Recklinghausen's disease: a clinicopathological study. *Ann Surg* 1972; **175:**86–104.

80. Riccardi VM. *Neurofibromatosis: phenotype, natural history and pathogenesis,* 2nd edn. Baltimore, MD: Johns Hopkins University Press, 1992.

81. Evans DGR, Baser ME, McGaughran J, et al. Malignant peripheral nerve sheath tumour in neurofibromatosis. J Med Genet 2002; **39**:311–314.

82. Ramanathan RC, Thomas JM. Malignant peripheral nerve sheath tumours associated with Von Recklinghausen's neurofibromatosis. Eur J Surg Oncol 1999; **25**:190–193.

83. Korf BR. Malignancy in neurofibromatosis type 1. Oncologist 2000; **5**:477–485.

84. King AA, Debaun MR, Riccardi VM, Gutmann DH. (2000). Malignant peripheral nerve sheath tumors in neuro-fibromatosis type 1. Am J Med Genet 2000; **93**:388–392.

85. Horan MP, Cooper DN, Upadhyaya M. Hypermethylation of the neurofibromatosis type 1 gene promoter is not a common event in the inactivation of the NF1 gene in NF1 specific tumours. Hum Genet 2000; **107**:33–39.

86. Chester A, Scott J, Anant S, Navaratnam N. RNA editing: cytidne to uridine conversion in apolipoprotein B mRNA. Biochim Biophys Acta 2000; **1494**:1–13.

87. Mechtershiemer G, Otano-Joos M, Ohl S, et al. Analysis of chromosomal imbalances in sporadic and NF1-associated peripheral nerve sheath tumours by comparative genomic hybridisation. Genes Chromosomes Cancer 1999; **25**:362–369.

88. Schmidt H, Taubert H, Meye A, et al. Gains in chromosome 7, 8q, 15q and 17q are characteristic changes in malignant but not benign peripheral nerve sheath tumors from patients with Recklinghausen disease. Cancer Lett 2000; **155**:181–190.

89. Weijzen S, Velders MP, Kast WM. Modulation of the immune response and tumour growth by activated Ras. Leukaemia 1999; **13**:502–513.

90. Feldkamp MM, Angelov L, Guha A. Neurofibromatosis type 1 peripheral nerve tumors: aberrant activation of the Ras pathway. Surg Neurol 1999; **51**:211–218.

91. McKeen EA, Bodurtha J, Meadows AT, et al. (1978) Rhabdomyosarcoma complicating multiple neurofibromatosis. J Paediatr 1978; **93**:992–993.

92. Hartley AL, Birch JM, Marsden HB, et al. Neurofibromatosis in children with soft tissue sarcoma. Pediatr Hematol Oncol 1988; **5**:7–16.

93. Modlin IM, Farndon JR, Shepherd A, et al. Phaeochromocytoma in 72 patients: clinical and diagnostic features, treatment and long-term results. Br J Surg 1979; **66**:456–465.

94. Griffiths DFR, Williams GT, Williams ED. (1987) Duodenal carcinoid, phaeochromocytoma and neurofibromatosis: islet cell tumor, phaeochromocytoma and the von Hippel Lindau complex: two distinctive neuroendocrine syndromes. Q J Med 1987; **64**:69–82.

95. Stiller CA, Chessells JM, Fitchett M. Neurofibromatosis and childhood leukaemia/lymphoma: a population-based UKCCSG study. Br J Cancer 1994; **70**:969–972.

96. Bader JL, Miller RW. Neurofibromatosis and childhood leukaemia. J Paediatr 1978; **92**:925–929.

97. Morier P, Merot Y, Paccaud D, et al. Juvenile chronic granulocytic leukaemia, juvenile xanthogranulomas and neurofibromatosis. Case report and review of the literature. J Am Acad Dermatol 1990; **22**:962–965.

98. Wang Q, Lasset C, Desseigne F, et al. Neurofibromatosis and early onset of cancers in MLH1-deficient children. Cancer Research 1999; **59**:294–297.

99. Ricciardone MD, Ozcelik T, Cevher B, et al. Human MLH1 deficiency predisposes to haematological malignancy and neurofibromatosis type 1. Cancer Research 1999; **59**:290–293.

100. Vilkki S, Tsao J-L, Loukola A, et al. Extensive somatic microsatellite mutations in normal human tissue. Cancer Research 2001; **61**:4541–4544.

101. Whiteside D, McLeod R, Graham G, et al. A homozygous germ-line mutation in the human MSH2 gene predisposes to hematological malignancy and multiple café au lait spots. Cancer Research 2002; **62**:359–362.

102. Pratt CB, Parham DM, Rao BN, et al. Multiple colorectal carcinomas, polyposis coli, and neurofibromatosis. J Natl Cancer Inst 1988; **80**:1170–1172.

103. Wang Q, Montmain G, Ruano E, et al. Neurofibromatosis type 1 gene as a mutational target in a mismatch repair-deficient cell type. Hum Genet 2003; **112**:117–123.

104. Gutmann DH, Winkeler E, Kabbarah O, et al. Mlh1 deficiency accelerates myeloid leukemogenesis in neurofibromatosis 1 (Nf1) heterozygous mice. Oncogene 2003; **22**(29):4581–4585.

105. Hope DG, Mulvihill JJ. Malignancy in neurofibromatosis. Adv Neurol 1981; **29**:33–35.

106. Mulvihill JJ. (1994) Malignancy: epidemiologically associated cancers. In: Huson SM, Huughes RAC (eds) The neuro-fibromatoses: a clinical and pathogenetic overview. London: Chapman & Hall, 1994:305–315.

107. Gutzmer R, Herbst RA, Mommert S, et al. Allelic loss at the neurofibromatosis type 1 (nf1) gene locus is frequent in desmoplastic neurotropic melamona. Hum Genet 2000; **107**:357–361.

108. Rasmussen S, Yang Q, Friedman JM Mortality in Neuro-fibromatosis 1: An Analysis using U.S. Death Certificates. Am J Hum Genet 2001; **68**:1110–1118.

109. Riccardi VM. von Recklinghausen neurofibromatosis. N Engl J Med 1981; **309**:1617–1627.

110. Listernick R, Charrow J, Greenwald M. (1992) Emergence of optic pathway gliomas in children with neurofibromatosis-1 following normal neuroimaging studies. J Paediatr 1992; **121**:1584–1587.

111. Evans DGR, Huson SM, Donnai D, et al. A genetic study of type 2 neurofibromatosis in the United Kingdom: I. Prevalence, mutation rate, fitness and confirmation of maternal transmission effect on severity. J Med Genet 1992; **29**:841–846.

112. Evans DGR, Huson SM, Neary W, et al. A clinical study of type 2 neurofibromatosis. Q J Med 1992; **304**:603–618.

113. Baser ME, Friedman JM, Wallace AJ, et al. Evaluation of clinical diagnostic criteria for neurofibromatosis 2. Neurology 2002; **59**:1759–1765.

114. Zang KD, Singer H. Chromosomal constitution of meningiomas. Nature 1967; **216**:84–85.

115. Zang KD. Cytological and cytogenetical studies on human meningioma. Cancer Genet Cytogenet 1982; **6**:249–274.

116. Seizinger BR, Martuza RL, Gusella JF. Loss of genes on chromosome 22 in tumorigenesis of human acoustic neuroma. Nature 1986; **322**:644–647.

117. Seizinger BR, Rouleau G, Ozelius L, et al. A common patho-genetic mechanism for three different tumour types in bilateral acoustic neurofibromatosis. Science 1987; **236**:317–319.

118. Rouleau G, Wertelecki W, Haings JL, et al. Genetic linkage analysis of bilateral acoustic neurofibromatosis to a DNA marker on chromosome 22. Nature 1987; **329**:246–248.

119. Narod SA, Parry DM, Parboosingh J, et al. Neurofibromatosis type 2 appears to be a genetically homogeneous disease. Am J Hum Genet 1992; **51**:486–496.

120. Baser ME, Evans DGR, Gutmann DH. Neurofibromatosis 2. *Curr Opin Neurol* 2003; **16**:27–33.

121. Uhlmann EJ, Gutmann DH. Tumour Suppressor Gene Regulation of Cell Growth: recent insights into Neurofibromatosis 1 and 2 gene function. *Cell Biochemistry and Biophysics* 2001; **34**:61–71.

122. Sun C-X, Robb VA, Gutmann DH. Protein 4.1 tumor suppressors: getting a FERM grip on growth regulation. *J Cell Science* 2002; **115**:3991–4000.

123. Tsukita S, Yonemura S, Tsukita S. ERM Family: from cytoskeleton to signal transduction. *Curr Opin Cell Biol* 1997; **9**:70–75.

124. McClatchey AI, Saotome I, Ramesh V, *et al.* The *NF2* tumour suppressor gene product is essential for extraembryonic development immediately prior to gastrulation. *Genes Dev* 1997; **11**:1253–1265.

125. McClatchey AI, Saotome I, Mercer K, *et al.* Mice heterozygous for a mutation at the NF2 tumour suppressor locus develop a range of highly metastatic tumours. *Genes Dev* 1998; **12**:1121–1133.

126. Giovannini M, Robanus-Maandag E, Niwa-Kawakita M, *et al.* Schwann cell hyperplasia and tumours in transgenic mice expressing a naturally occurring mutant NF2 protein. *Genes Dev* 1999; **13**:978–986.

127. Messerli SM, Tang Y, Giovanni M, *et al.* Detection of spontaneous schwannomas by MRI in a transgenic murine model of neurofibromatosis type 2. *Neoplasia* 2002; **4**(6):501–509.

128. Parry DM, Eldridge R, Kaiser-Kupfer MI, *et al.* Neurofibromatosis 2 (NF2); clinical characteristics of 63 affected individuals and clinical evidence of heterogeneity. *Am J Med Genet* 1994; **52**:450–461.

129. MacCollin M. Neurofibromatosis 2 (Clinical aspects and associated tumours). In Friedman J, Gutmann DH, MacCollin M, Riccardi VM (eds) *Neurofibromatosis: phenotype, natural history and pathogenesis* 3rd edition. Baltimore MA: Johns Hopkins University Press, 1999:299–250.

130. Kaiser-Kupfer MI, Friedlin V, Datiles MB, *et al.* The association of posterior capsular lens opacities with bilateral acoustic neuromas in patients with *neurofibromatosis* type 2. *Arch Ophthalmol* 1989; **107**:541–544.

131. Ragge NK, Baser M, Falk RE, *et al.* Presymptomatic diagnosis of NF2: ocular expression. *Am J Hum Genet* 1992; **51** (suppl.) A51:113 (abstract).

132. Gijtenbeek JM, Gabreels-Festen AA, Lammens M, *et al.* Mononeuropathy multiplex as the initial manifestation of neurofibromatosis type 2. *Neurology* 2001; **56**:1766–1768.

133. Trivedi R, Byrne J, Huson SM, Donaghy M. Focal amyotrophy in neurofibromatosis 2. *J Neurol Neurosurg Psychiatry* 2000; **69**:257–261.

134. Sperfeld AD, Hein C, Schroder JM, *et al.* Occurrence and characterization of peripheral nerve involvement in neurofibromatosis type 2. *Brain* 2002; **125**:996–1004.

135. Hagel C, Lindenau M, Lamszus K, *et al.* Polyneuropathy in neurofibromatosis 2: clinical findings, molecular genetics and neuropathological alterations in sural nerve biopsy specimens. *Acta Neuropathol (Berl)* 2002; **104**:179–187.

136. Pulst SM, Rouleau G, Marineau C, *et al.* Familial meningioma is not allelic to neurofibromatosis 2. *Neurology* 1993; **43**:2096–2098.

137. MacCollin M, Willett C, Heinrich B, *et al.* Familial schwannomatosis: Exclusion of the NF2 locus as the germline event. *Neurology* 2003; **60**(12):1968–1974.

138. Baser ME, Friedman JM, Aeschliman D, *et al.* Predictors of the risk of mortality in neurofibromatosis 2. *Am J Hum Genet* 2002; **71**:715–723.

139. Kanter WR, Eldridge T, Fabricant R, *et al.* Central neurofibromatosis with bilateral acoustic neuroma: genetic, clinical and biochemical distinctions from peripheral neurofibromatosis. *Neurology* 1980; **30**:851–859.

140. Evans DGR, Huson SM, Neary W, *et al.* A genetic study of type 2 neurofibromatosis: II guidelines for genetic counselling. *J Med Genet* 1992; **29**:847–852.

141. Baser M, Friedman JM, Evans GDR. Maternal gene effect in Neurofibromatosis 2: fact or artefact? *J Med Genet*; **38**:783–784.

142. Evans DGR, Wallace AJ, Wu CL, *et al.* Somatic Mosaicism: A common cause of classic disease in tumour-prone syndromes? Lessons from type 2 Neurofibromatosis. *Am J Hum Genet* 1998; **63**:727–736.

143. Kluwe L, Mautner VF. Mosaicism in sporadic neurofibromatosis 2 patients. *Hum Mol Genet* 1998; **7**(13):2051–2055.

144. Bourn D, Carter SA, Evans DGR, *et al.* A mutation in the neurofibromatosis type 2 tumour suppressor gene, giving rise to widely different clinical phenotypes in two unrelated individuals. *Am J Hum Genet* 1994; **55**:69–73.

145. Moyhuddin A, Baser ME, Watson C, *et al.* Somatic mosaicism in neurofibromatosis 2: prevalence and risk of disease transmission to offspring. *J Med Genet* 2003; **40**:459–463.

146. MacCollin M, Gusella JF. Molecular Biology of NF2. In: Friedman JM, Gutmann DH, MacCollin M, Riccardi VM (eds) *Neurofibromatosis: phenotype, natural history and pathogenesis*. 3rd edition. Baltimore MA: Johns Hopkins University Press, 1999; 351–362.

147. Kluwe L, Friedrich RE, Tatagiba M, Mautner V. Presymptomatic diagnosis for children of sporadic neurofibromatosis 2 patients: a method based on tumour analysis. *Genet Med* 2002; **4**:27–30.

148. Mantripragada KK, Buckley PG, Jarbo C, *et al.* Development of NF2 gene specific, strictly sequence defined diagnostic microarray for deletion detection. *J Mol Med* 2003; **81**(7):443–451.

149. Brackmann DE, Fayad JN, Slattery WH, *et al.* Early proactive management of vestibular Schwannomas in neurofibromatosis type 2. *Neurosurgery* 2001; **49**(2):274–283.

150. Rowe JG, Radatz MWR, Walton L, *et al.* Clinical experience with gamma knife stereotactic radiosurgery in the management of vestibular schwannomas secondary to type 2 neurofibromatosis. *J Neurol Neurosurg Psychiatry* 2003; **74**:1–7.

151. Nevison B, Laszig R, Sollmann W-O, *et al.* Results from a European Clinical Investigation of the Nucleus Multichannel Auditory Brainstem Implant. *Ear & Hearing* 2002; **23**:170–183.

152. Bance M, Ramsden RT. Management of neurofibromatosis type 2. *Ear, Nose & Throat Journal* 1999; **78**(2):91–96.

153. Graham J, Lynch C, Weber B, *et al.* The magnetless Clarion® cochlear implant in a patient with neurofibromatosis 2. *J Laryngology & Otology* 1999; **113**:458–463.

154. Verlinsky J, Zverina E, Betka J, *et al.* Preimplantation diagnosis for neurofibromatosis. *Reprod Biomed Online* 2002; **4**:218–212.

Multiple endocrine neoplasia type 1

TERESA RUDKIN AND WILLIAM D. FOULKES

INTRODUCTION

The clinical entity now known as multiple endocrine neoplasia type 1 (MEN 1, OMIM# 131100) was identified as a distinct genetic syndrome in 1954 by P. Werner when he reported a family in which the father and four of nine siblings were affected by adenomas of the parathyroids, anterior pituitary, and the pancreatic islets.[1] MEN 1 is now recognized as the most common multiglandular syndrome. Although the majority of known families are of Caucasian origin, in which the estimated prevalence is 0.02–0.2/1000, MEN 1 occurs in families from other ethnic backgrounds.

MEN 1 is an autosomal dominant inherited endocrine disease with high penetrance. The clinical manifestations of this disease are diverse, even within families. The glandular organs which are most susceptible to tumour development in those with germline *MEN 1* mutations are the parathyroid glands, the anterior pituitary, and the enteropancreatic glands. More rarely, patients also develop thymic, bronchial, and gastrointestinal carcinoid tumours, lipomas, angiofibromas, and adrenocortical tumours (Table 8a.1).

The morbidity related to being a carrier of an *MEN 1* mutation can be significant. In one retrospective study of 34 MEN 1 kindreds, 46 per cent of mutation carriers

Table 8a.1 *Endocrine and non-endocrine manifestations of MEN 1*

Endocrine tumours	Non-endocrine tumours
Parathyroid adenomas/hyperplasia	Lipomas (subcutaneous, visceral)
Enteropancreatic tumours	Collagenomas, facial angiofibromas
Non-functioning (including polypeptide secreting)	Leimyomeiomas (oesophagus, lung, uterus)
Gastrinomas	Meningiomas, Ependymomas, Schwannomas
Insulinomas	
VIP-omas, Somatostatinomas	
Anterior pituitary adenomas	
Prolactinomas	
Somatostatinomas	
Other	
Carcinoids	
Thymus, Bronchus, Gastrointestinal tract	
Adrenocortical tumours	
Thyroid	

Adapted from Chandrasekharappa SC and Teh BT. 2003, **253**.007.[7]

died of MEN 1-related causes at a median age of 47 years.[2] (It is worth noting, however, that poor outcome was restricted to a subset of mutation carriers and that, overall, carrier status for an *MEN 1* mutation did not affect survival.) The screening required to detect occult neoplasms in suspected carriers is extensive. Unfortunately, in up to 20 per cent of clinically diagnosed MEN 1 patients, the mutation is not found with clinically available mutation analysis. In these kindreds, if linkage is not feasible, there will inevitably be family members who needlessly undergo inconvenient and laborious biochemical and radiological investigations.

In this chapter, we review the tremendous progress that has been made towards understanding the molecular basis of this disease since the gene was first identified in 1997. We also review the diverse clinical presentation of the disease and some relevant issues with respect to its diagnosis and management.

MOLECULAR ASPECTS

In 1988, Larsson *et al.*,[3] were able to map the *MEN 1* gene to chromosome 11q13. It was finally cloned in 1997.[4,5] The *MEN 1* gene (GenBank accession no. U93237) comprises 10 exons extending across 7.2 kb and expresses a 2.8 kb transcript. It codes for a 610-amino acid protein called menin. Recent data suggest that the expression of the *MEN 1* gene is regulated by feedback from its product.[6] The protein sequence of menin is highly conserved across species: menin from mouse, rat, and zebrafish share 96.7 per cent, 97.2 per cent, and 67 per cent homology with the human menin protein respectively.[7] This protein, however, shares no similarity to any other known protein and does not contain recognizable functional motifs.

Recently, a mouse MEN 1 knockout model was generated.[8] Homozygotic *men[1]* null mice die early *in utero*. Heterozygotes develop tumours of the endocrine pancreas, parathyroid, and pituitary. These tumours are associated with loss of heterozygosity of the wild-type *men[1]* allele.[9] Because these mouse models appear to mimic the human MEN 1 phenotype, *men[1]* mutant mice are likely to prove to be a useful model for this disease.

The functions of MEN 1 and its role in tumourigenesis are not entirely clear. Kim *et al.* illustrated the tumour suppressing function of menin by demonstrating that overexpression of menin in ras-transformed NIH 3T3 cells results in growth and tumour suppression.[10] Tumour development is consistent with Knudson's two-hits model in which tumours require somatic loss of the wild type allele in those patients who have inherited a germline mutation of the other allele. Although menin is expressed in most organ tissues and is expressed in all stages of

development, loss of menin leads primarily to tumours affecting endocrine organs.

Menin is localized mainly to the nucleus,[11] and it is likely that it exerts its function of growth suppression via interactions with specific transcription factors. For a thorough review of the studies that have contributed to the knowledge amassed about the structure and function of MEN 1 and its protein menin, readers are encouraged to consult a recent report by Chandrasekharappa and Teh.[7] To briefly summarize, thus far, menin has been found to interact with various nuclear proteins including JunD, NF-κB, Smad3, Pem, Nm23, glial fibrillary acidic protein (GFAP), vimentin, and replication protein A (RPA2).[6,7] Menin probably acts as a growth suppressor protein through interactions with the AP-1 and TGF-β pathways. It is involved with the AP-1 pathway through a direct interaction with JunD. JunD is a member of the AP-1 transcription factor that is composed of c-Jun, JunB, and JunD and the Fos system of proteins. In contrast to other AP-1 components, JunD has been shown to inhibit cell proliferation. JunD can be manipulated to act as a growth promoter when its binding to menin is prevented either by a *MEN 1* null genetic background or by a JunD mutant incapable of binding to menin.[12] Menin appears to have an inhibitory effect upon JunD transcriptional activity, possibly via recruitment of an mSin3A-histone deacetylase complex.[10] An additional mechanism by which menin is thought to suppress cell proliferation is via the TGF-β system through its interaction with Smad3. The TGF-β signaling pathway ultimately causes inhibition of most epithelial, endothelial, fibroblast, neuronal, lymphoid, and hematopoietic cells. The Smad family of proteins is a critical effector of the TGF-β pathway. When Smad2 and Smad3 are phosphorylated, they associate with Smad4. These complexes then activate transcription of specific genes. Inactivation of menin antagonizes TGF-β growth inhibition. When menin is inactivated, Smad3 is unable to associate with Smad4 and inhibits the Smad complex from binding to specific transcriptional regulatory sites.[13]

Approximately 10 per cent of germline mutations are *de novo*. These account for so-called 'sporadic' cases of MEN 1. To date, more than 350 different germline and somatic mutations of the *MEN 1* gene have been described. These include frameshift, nonsense, missense, and in-frame deletion and insertion mutations. Approximately two thirds of the mutations identified thus far are nonsense frame-shift and splice sequence mutations causing truncation of menin. The remaining one third are missense and in-frame deletions that result in normal levels of a structurally abnormal protein product. These mutations are equally distributed throughout the length of the coding sequence. Many of these involve domains in which menin interacts with JunD, Smad3, and NF-κB.[14] However, there are no identified mutational hot-spots and no single mutation accounts for more than 2 per cent of mutations thus far identified. For this reason, genetic testing must be performed by complete sequence analysis.

GENOTYPE/PHENOTYPE ASSOCIATIONS

Despite many large studies, no genotype–phenotype correlations have been found. The time of onset and the clinical manifestations differ substantially, even within families. In addition, unrelated families with the same mutation do not consistently share the same clinical features. Some studies have suggested that a so-called Burin-MEN 1 variant exists. This variant is composed of the clinical association of hyperparathyroidism, prolactinoma, and carcinoids, and is apparently restricted to those originating from the Burin peninsula of Newfoundland, Canada. All such affected individuals carry R460X mutation occurring on the same haplotype.[15]

In general, information of the particular gene defect involved in an individual patient is useful for confirming the diagnosis of MEN1, and in predictive testing. It does not yet play a role in predicting prognosis or in directing subsequent clinical management.

CLINICAL ASPECTS

It is generally accepted that the clinical diagnosis of MEN 1 is based upon the following: 1) two major lesions involving the parathyroid, endocrine pancreas, and/or anterior pituitary in the proband either present synchronously or in a metachronous fashion, *or* 2) one major MEN 1-related lesion occurring in a first degree relative of a person previously diagnosed with MEN 1. Accurate clinical diagnosis of MEN 1 in a given patient, however, may be complicated by at least two considerations. First, it is unclear how frequently sporadic endocrine neoplasias are falsely attributed to MEN 1. This is known as an 'MEN 1

phenocopy', the frequency of which is uncertain but which in some studies has approached 10 per cent.[16] In general, endocrine disease in MEN 1 patients occurs earlier than sporadic endocrine disease, although this appears not to be the case for pituitary lesions (Table 8a.2). It has been previously reported that 95 per cent of carriers of *MEN 1* mutations exhibit clinical manifestations by age 40. A recent study, however, estimated that the age specific penetrance of *MEN 1* mutations was 45 per cent at 30 years, 82 per cent at 50 years, and 96 per cent at 70 years of age. Two patients in this study were diagnosed after the age of 70.[17]

A relatively common clinical scenario is one in which the clinical diagnosis of MEN 1 is strictly fulfilled, but the disease is not MEN1. For example, an elderly patient may be found to have the combination of an anterior pituitary adenoma detected incidentally following brain imaging for an unrelated symptom (sometimes facetiously called an 'incidentaloma') and asymptomatic primary hyperparathyroidism based on the finding of hypercalcemia following routine bloodwork. Disentangling these cases from 'true' cases of MEN 1 is complicated by the observation that the causal mutation is never found in up to 20 per cent of patients with clinically probable MEN 1.

Other clinical entities that might be mistaken for MEN 1 include familial isolated hyperparathyroidism (OMIM 145000; *HRPT1* gene) and some familial pituitary adenomas, including isolated familial somatotropinomas (OMIM 102200; *GNAS* gene), MEN 2 (OMIM 171400; *RET* oncogene), and rarely with Carney complex (OMIM 160980; *CNC1* gene) – an autosomal dominant multiple neoplasia syndrome associated with endocrine (thyroid, pituitary, adrenocortical, and gonadal), non-endocrine (myxomas, nevi, and other cutaneous pigmented lesions), and neural lesions (schwannomas).

Primary hyperparathyroidism

The most common manifestation of MEN 1 is primary hyperparathyroidism involving the parathyroid chief cells. The age-specific penetrance by age 50 years is 73–95 per

Table 8a.2 *Comparison of sporadic and MEN 1 associated neoplasms*

Affected organ	Sporadic	MEN 1 associated
Parathyroid		
Average age of onset:	55–60 years	25–30 years
Tumour characteristics	Most commonly single	Most commonly multifocal, asymmetric
Entero-pancreatic	Lesions usually solitary	Often multicentric
Anterior pituitary		
Average age of onset	38 years	38 years
Tumour characteristics	Non-functional most common. At time of diagnosis, most likely to be microadenoma, non-invasive	Prolactinomas most common. At time of diagnosis, more likely to be macroadenoma, invasive. Hypersecretion less likely to normalize following treatment

cent. Approximately 65 per cent of patients with MEN 1 have this as their presenting feature.[17] The neoplasms are either adenomas or hyperplasias. Parathyroid carcinomas are rarely, if ever, a manifestation of MEN 1.

The prevalence of sporadic primary hyperparathyroidism in the general population increased significantly in the early 1970s following the introduction of widespread measurement of serum calcium levels in asymptomatic individuals. The prevalence has subsequently declined such that the most recent epidemiologic data estimate a prevalence of 3–4.3/1000 in Europe[18] and an annual incidence of 20/100 000 in Minnesota.[19] The fraction of these attributable to MEN 1 has been estimated at between 2 and 5 per cent[20] although some report up to 15 per cent of patients under 50 years of age.[17,21] The hyperparathyroidism of MEN 1 tends to occur earlier than sporadic hyperparathyroidism (Table 8a.2). The average age of onset in MEN1 is during the third decade, whilst sporadic disease tends to manifest in the fourth to sixth decades. Another differentiating feature in MEN 1 is that the parathyroid tumours tend to be multiple and asymmetric in size.[22]

There are certain therapeutic considerations in those patients with hyperparathyroidism and known MEN 1. First, since multiple parathyroid tumours are frequently present in MEN 1 and not all tumours are detected preoperatively by Tc-99m-sestamibi scanning and ultrasound, intraoperative rapid PTH (parathyroid hormone) assay may be helpful to ensure that no hyperfunctioning tissue remains. Second, all patients undergoing surgical parathyroidectomy should have concomitant transcervical thymectomy in order to prevent thymic carcinoma. More controversial management issues include prophylactic parathyroidectomy in patients with gastrinomas, since it is known that hyperparathyroidism exacerbates gastrin secretion. However, since proton pump inhibitors effectively decrease gastrin secretion, most advocate that concomitant gastrinoma is an insufficient indication for parathyroid surgery.[22] The success of elective subtotal parathyroidectomy varies. Persistent hyperparathyroidism occurs in 10–15 per cent and half of initially successful cases recur in 8–12 years.[22] When synthetic PTH becomes available, total parathyroidectomy could become a reasonable option for patients with MEN 1.

Screening for hyperparathyroidism includes yearly ionized calcium and PTH starting at age 8 years (Table 8a.3); imaging is not yet recommended for periodic surveillance.[23]

Entero-pancreatic glands

Pancreatic or duodenal endocrine tumours are the second most frequent manifestation of MEN 1 with approximately 30–80 per cent of patients with MEN 1 affected. Although subject to ascertainment bias, it has been estimated that 30 per cent of patients with pancreatic endocrine neoplasms are found to have MEN 1.[21]

Pancreatic endocrine tumours are the most likely cause of death in MEN 1 patients. In a retrospective study of 34 MEN 1 kindreds with 1838 members, 46 per cent (27/59) of MEN 1 patients died of MEN1-related causes. The most frequent cause of death in this series was pancreatic islet cell tumours and ulcer disease.[2] Clinical symptoms vary according to the specific tissue type involved and typically occur in the fourth or fifth decade. However, biochemical abnormalities can precede symptoms by 10–15 years.[24]

NON-FUNCTIONAL NEOPLASMS

In most series, the most common pancreatic tumours overall are non-functional neuroendocrine tumours, of

Table 8a.3 *Screening recommendations for known or suspected carriers of MEN 1 mutations*

Tumour	Age to begin (yr)	Biochemical analyses	Radiological analyses
Parathyroid	8	Annual serum PTH, ionised calcium	None
Entero-pancreatic			
Gastrinoma	20	Annual serum fasting gastrin. If elevated: gastrin output, secretin stimulated gastrin level	None
Insulinomas	5	Annual fasting serum glucose, insulin, proinsulin	
Other	20	Fasting and meal stimulated Pancreatic Polypeptide, Fasting VIP, Glucagon	SRS/CT scan of thorax and abdomen every 2–3 years EUS if biochemical evidence of disease and normal SRS/CT
Anterior pituitary	5	Annual serum prolactin, IGF-1	Brain imaging (preferably MRI) every 3 years
Foregut carcinoids	20	None	CT scan every 3 years

Adapted from Brandi *et al. J Clin Endo* 2001; **86**(12): 5560.[23]
VIP, vaso-intestinal peptide; SRS, somatostatin receptor scintigraphy; EUS, endoscopic ultrasound; IGF-1, insulin growth factor-1; PTH, parathyroid hormone.

which three quarters secrete pancreatic polypeptide. These tumours are clinically silent and may be large at presentation. Many of these are malignant at time of diagnosis.

GASTRINOMAS

The most common functional neuroendocrine neoplasms are gastrinomas resulting in autonomous hypersecretion of gastrin. These occur in up to 54 per cent of patients with MEN 1. The majority of these occur in the duodenum or the head of the pancreas. It can present symptomatically as part of Zollinger Ellison (ZE) syndrome with elevated gastrin secretion and peptic ulcer disease. The diagnosis of Zollinger Ellison syndrome can be made if the fasting serum gastrin level is >1000 pg/mL and gastric pH 3.0. Most patients have a basal acid output of over 15 meq/hr. In patients with a lower gastrin level, a secretin stimulation test must be performed. Intravenous secretin (2 units/kg) produces a rise in serum gastrin of over 200 pg/mL with 2–30 minutes in 85 per cent of patients with a gastrinoma. Approximately 25 per cent of cases of ZE are associated with MEN 1. These tend to be muticentric and are, therefore, typically more difficult to resect than sporadic gastrinomas. Management generally involves the use of proton pump inhibitors. Patients with ZE syndrome due to MEN 1 have a better prognosis than do patients with sporadic ZE. The 5-, 10-, and 20-year survival rates with MEN 1 are 94 per cent, 75 per cent, and 58 per cent respectively, compared to 62 per cent, 50 per cent and 31 per cent of those with sporadic disease.[25]

INSULINOMA (B CELL ADENOMA)

Less than 10 per cent of patients with MEN 1 have insulinomas and less than 10 per cent of patients with insulinomas have MEN 1.[26] Patients usually present with Whipple's triad of: 1) a history of hypoglycemic symptoms, 2) an associated fasting glucose of <2.0 mmol/L, 3) immediate recovery following administration of glucose. A diagnosis of inappropriate insulin secretion is made with an insulin level of 6 µU/mL or more in the presence of blood glucose <2.0 mmol/L. An elevated circulating proinsulin level (>0.2 ng/mL) in the presence of fasting hypoglycemia differentiates between an insulinoma and factitious insulinaemia secondary to insulin use.

GLUCAGONOMAS

Glucagonomas occur in 3 per cent of all MEN 1 patients. Symptoms can include hyperglycemia, migratory necrolytic erythema, weight loss, and other symptoms. These are often large at presentation (5–10 cm) and are frequently malignant with liver metastases often present at diagnosis. The diagnosis can be made by a glucagon level >1000 pg/mL.

Other more rare pancreatic-duodenal tumours include those that secrete growth hormone releasing factor (GRF), vasoactive intestinal protein (VIP), and somatostatin. Endocrine tumours that secrete growth hormone releasing factor (GRF) are a rare cause of acromegaly. (A more common cause of acromegaly in patients with MEN 1 is growth hormone secreting pituitary adenomas.) It is estimated that 30 per cent of GRF-omas and 1 per cent of VIP-omas are associated with MEN 1. The diagnosis is made by a GRF level exceeding 300 pg/mL, VIP level >170 pg/mL, and increased serum somatostatin. All of these tumour types are often multiple, large, and metastatic at time of diagnosis.[26]

Screening for pancreatic-duodenal neoplasms for MEN 1 carriers should include baseline levels of insulin, proinsulin, glucagon, pancreatic polypeptide, and gastrin. As mentioned earlier, biochemical abnormalities can precede symptomatic disease by 15–20 years (by the third decade). A combination of CT scan and somatostatin receptor scintigraphy (SRS) of the abdomen and thorax every 2–3 years, even with normal biochemistry, has been advocated in order to detect non-functional lesions. A SRS has the advantage of identifying tumours based upon the size of the mass and the concentration of somatostatin receptors. What it lacks in anatomical specificity is supplemented by the concomitant use of CT imaging.[27] SRS can also detect intrathoracic disease from either metastatic disease or carcinoid and thymic tumours. In patients with biochemical evidence of tumours but negative imaging, an endoscopic ultrasound screen is the most sensitive imaging modality for small pancreatic endocrine tumours confined to the pancreatic parenchyma and peri-pancreatic lymph nodes. Many of the issues related to entero-pancreatic manifestations of MEN 1 are well described in a recent review by Doherty and Thompson, 2000.[26] Prospective trials will be necessary to determine whether aggressive screening prolongs survival in these patients.

Anterior pituitary

Anterior pituitary adenomas occur in 20–50 per cent of patients with MEN 1. These lesions are also common in the general population. Computed tomography or magnetic resonance imaging of normal subjects has demonstrated microadenomas in 10 per cent of subjects. Eleven per cent of pituitaries are found to have adenomas at autopsy.[28] Approximately 1–3 per cent of pituitary adenomas are attributable to MEN 1. When compared to sporadic pituitary adenomas, those associated with MEN 1 are more likely to be functional – most commonly hypersecreting growth hormone (somatotropinomas) or prolactin. Two thirds of MEN 1-related pituitary tumours are prolactinomas. The remaining pituitary tumours are non-secretory, GH-secreting, and ACTH secreting. Like non-MEN 1 patients, there is a slightly increased female to male ratio observed (F:M ratio; 1.5:1) as is observed in sporadic pituitary adenomas. Age of onset does not appear to occur earlier than non-MEN 1-related adenomas (mean age 38 years).[29] However, the earliest reported age of onset for a pituitary adenoma in a patient with MEN 1 is 5 years.[30]

In the past, pituitary lesions associated with MEN 1 have been considered to be a relatively benign manifestation of the syndrome. However, since 1996, there have been several reports that suggest that MEN 1 associated lesions tend to be larger than sporadic cases.[29,31,32] In one series, 85 per cent of MEN 1 related lesions were macroadenomas versus 42 per cent in non-MEN 1 patients, $p < 0.001$.[29] The lesions were more often associated with headache and visual defects. Unlike sporadic cases, 32 per cent of lesions were invasive, and hormone hypersecretion only normalized in 42 per cent of patients (versus 90 per cent of sporadic cases). These imply that MEN 1 is associated with pituitary lesions that are more aggressive and less responsive to treatment. There are no special considerations for treatment of MEN 1 associated pituitary lesions. Prospective studies are needed to determine whether earlier and more aggressive treatment would result in improved outcome.

Since smaller, less advanced lesions are generally easier to treat, there would seem to be a role for presymptomatic screening beginning in childhood. Annual prolactin and IGF-1 levels are recommended annually starting at age 5 years and imaging, preferably magnetic resonance imaging, every three years.[23]

Carcinoid tumours

Most carcinoids are found in the hind-gut. In MEN 1 syndrome, however, they are usually found in the fore-gut (the thymus, the bronchus or the stomach). They are usually non-functioning and can develop malignancy at a late stage. Up to 25 per cent of thymic carcinoids are MEN 1-related. It has a male predominance, usually presenting in the fourth and fifth decades.[33] There is no effective treatment and the mortality rate is high. It is for this reason that it is recommended that prophylactic thymectomy be considered during parathyroidectomy on MEN 1 patients.

Adrenal tumours

Adrenocortical tumours are seen in up to 35 per cent of patients with MEN 1. Interestingly, they do not show loss of heterozygosity (LOH) at the MEN 1 locus. They are rarely part of the initial presentation. Adrenal tumours are often small, do not cause symptoms and can be managed by close surveillance. Although most lesions are asymptomatic, adrenocortical tumours can cause Cushing syndrome. It is Cushing syndrome, and not glucagonomas,

that is the commonest cause of MEN 1-related hyperglycemia. Phaeochromocytomas are rare in MEN 1 (in contrast to MEN 2), and are nearly always unilateral and benign. Some adrenal tumours have significant malignant potential and surgical resection should be considered when they are 3 cm or larger.[34]

Thyroid tumours

Although thyroid neoplasms can occur in MEN 1, but unlike MEN 2, medullary thyroid cancer is never a feature. A rare association of MEN 1 and papillary thyroid cancer has been described.[35] The relationship between the thyroid lesions seen and the malfunction of menin is not clear. In one report, genetic analysis of the thyroid lesion showed that there was no associated LOH.[35]

Other tumours

Intra-dermal lesions such as facial angiofibromas are very common in MEN 1. In fact, at least one such lesion is present in ~90 per cent of those with MEN 1, and 50 per cent have five or more.[36] These lesions show LOH at chromosome 11q13. Notably, unlike those seen in tuberous sclerosis, they are usually small and located near the upper lip. Identifying these lesions in the child of a person with MEN 1 could be useful, particularly if no mutation has been identified by complete sequencing. Leiomyomata involving the oesophagus, lung, and uterus have also been seen, albeit rarely, in MEN 1.[37]

GENETIC TESTING

The diagnosis of relatives of affected individuals has traditionally relied upon radiological and biochemical screening. Since MEN 1 is an autosomal dominant disorder, 50 per cent of children of affected parents will inherit the predisposition to developing MEN 1-related tumours. Up to 10 per cent of cases of MEN 1 are new mutations, implying that, in these cases, siblings of the proband are not at increased risk. If the proband's mutation can be identified, it is possible to test relatives and thereby determine whether intensive biochemical and radiological screening is necessary.

As mentioned earlier, molecular diagnosis of MEN 1 is complex. There are over 350 mutations identified thus far, there are no hot-spots, and no obvious genotype-phenotype correlations. Genetic testing for MEN 1 requires complete gene sequencing which is both labour-intensive and costly. Indications for mutation analysis have been proposed.[38] These include: 1) MEN 1 typical neoplasia at age <40 years and/or multifocal tumour; 2) MEN 1 typical neoplasia and positive family history regardless of age of onset; 3) two or more MEN 1 typical neoplasias; 4) recurrent MEN 1 typical neoplasia (occurring within three months of initial tumour).

Using the sequence analysis that is routinely available, no mutation is found within the coding region or splice junctions in approximately 5–30 per cent of families with a strong clinical history consistent with MEN 1.[36,38,39] It is not clear how frequently the diagnosis of MEN 1 is incorrectly attributed to sporadic endocrine neoplasias. Interestingly, in a recent retrospective analysis of members of a large MEN 1 family, up to 10 per cent of patients diagnosed with MEN 1 based upon clinical criteria had genetically negative disease and were essentially phenocopies.[17] Four of these cases were primary hyperparathyroidism, two were non-secretory pituitary adenomas, and one was a case of coincident prolactinoma and hyperparathyroidism.

Even when future developments in mutation analysis result in almost 100 per cent of mutations being correctly identified, there will still be a need for a fast, simple, cost effective screening tool. Conformation sensitive gel electrophoresis (CSGE)[40] and the combination of heteroduplex mutation assay (HMA) with mutation detection gel analysis (MDGA)[41] have been proposed as effective methods of screening the gene.

The long interval between the identification of the locus for MEN 1 and its ultimate identification has been matched by the time taken to understand the gene and its products. Nevertheless, the existence of a mouse model that quite closely mimics the human disease is likely to prove crucial in further advances in knowledge of this polyendocrinopathy syndrome.

KEY POINTS

- MEN 1 is a multiple endocrinopathy syndrome.
- There is no genotype/phenotype correlation, unlike MEN 2.

REFERENCES

1. Werner P. Genetic aspects of adenomatosis of endocrine glands. *Am J Med* 1954; **16**:363–371.
2. Doherty GM, Olson JA, Frisella MM, *et al*. Lethality of multiple endocrine neoplasia type 1. *World J Surg* 1998; **22**(6): 581–561.
3. Larsson C, Skogseid B, Oberg K, *et al*. Multiple endocrine neoplasia type 1 gene maps to chromosome 11 and is lost in insulinoma. *Nature* 1988; **332**:85–87.
4. Chandrasekharappa SC, Guru SC, Manickamp P, *et al*. Positional cloning of the gene for multiple endocrine neoplasia-type 1. *Science* 1997; **276**:404–407.

5. The European Consortium on MEN1. Identification of the multiple endocrine neoplasia type 1 (*MEN1*) gene. *Hum Mol Genet* 1997; **6**:1177–1183.
6. Zablewska B, Bylund L, Mandic SA, *et al*. Transcription regulation of the multiple endocrine neoplasia *type 1* gene in human and mouse. *J Clin Endo Metab* 2003; **88**(8):3845–3851.
7. Chandrasekharappa SC, Teh BT. Functional studies of the *MEN 1* gene. *J Int Med* 2003; **253**:606–615.
8. Crabtree JS, Scacheri PC, Ward JM, *et al*. A mouse model of multiple endocrine neoplasia, type 1, develops multiple endocrine tumors. *Proc Natl Acad Sci USA* 2001; **98**:1119–1123.
9. Bertolino P, Tong WM, Galendo D, *et al*. Heterozygous *men¹* mutant mice develop a range of tumors mimicking multiple endocrine neoplasia type 1. *Mol Endo* 2003; **17**(9):1880–1892.
10. Kim H, Lee JE, Cho EJ, *et al*. Menin, a tumor suppressor, represses JunD-mediated transcriptional activity by association with an mSin3A-histone deacetylase complex. *Cancer Res* 2003; **63**(19):6135–6139.
11. Guru SC, Goldsmith PK, Burns AL, *et al*. Menin, the product of the *MEN 1* gene, is a nuclear protein. *Proc Natl Acad Sci USA* 1998; **95**(4):1639–1634.
12. Agarwal SK, Novotny EA, Crabtree JS, *et al*. Transcription factor JunD, deprived of menin, switches from growth suppressor to growth promoter. *Proc Natl Acad Sci USA* 2003; **100**(19):10770–10775.
13. Kaji H, Canaff L, Lebrun JJ. Inactivation of menin, a Smad3-interacting protein, blocks transforming growth factor type β signaling. *Proc Natl Acad Sci USA* 2001; **98**(7):2837–3842.
14. Wautot V, Vercherat C, Lespinasse J, *et al*. Germline mutation profile of MEN 1 in multiple endocrine neoplasia type 1; search for correlation between phenotype and the functional domains of the *MEN 1* protein. *Hum Mut* 2002; **20**:35–47.
15. Olufemi SE, Green JS, Manickam P, *et al*. Common ancestral mutation in the *MEN 1* gene is likely reponsible for the prolactinoma variant of *MEN 1* (*MEN 1* Burin) in four kindreds from Newfoundland *Hum Mut* 1998; **11**(4):264–269.
16. Burgess JR, Nord B, David R, *et al*. Phenotype and phenocopy: relationship between genotype and clinical phenotype in a single large family with multiple endocrine neoplasia type 1 (MEN 1). *Clin End* 2000; **53**:205–211.
17. Glascock JM, Carty S. Multiple endocrine neoplasia type 1: fresh perspective on clinical features and penetrance. *Surg Oncol* 2002; **11**:143–150.
18. Adami S, Marcocci, Gatti D. Epidemiology of primary hyperparathyroidism in Europe. *J Bone Mineral Res* 2002; **17**(Suppl2):N18–N23.
19. Melton LJ 3rd. The epidemiology of primary hyperparathyroidism in North America. *J Bone Mineral Res* 2002; **17**(Suppl 2):N12–N17.
20. Uchino S, Noguchi S, Sato M, *et al*. Screening for *MEN 1* gene and discovery of germ-line and somatic mutations in apparently sporadic parathyroid tumours. *Can Res* 2001; **60**:5553–5557.
21. Calender A, Girard S, Porchet N, *et al*. Clinicogenetic study of MEN 1: recent physiopathological data and clinical applications. Study Group of Multiple Endocrine Neoplasia (GENFM). *Annales d'Endocrinologie* 1998; **59**(6):444–451.
22. Marx SJ, Simonds WF, Agarwal SK, *et al*. Hyperparathyroidism in hereditary syndromes: special expressions and special

managements. *J Bone Mineral Res* 2002; **17**(Suppl 2): N37–N43.

23. Brandi ML, Gagel RF, Angeli A, *et al.* Guidelines for diagnosis and therapy of multiple endocrine neoplasia type 1 and type 2. *J Clin Endocrinol Metab* 2001; **86**:5658–5671.

24. Skogseid B, Doherty GM. Multiple endocrine neoplasia type 1: a 10 year prospective screening study in four kindreds. *J Clin Endocrinol Metab* 1991; **73**:281–287.

25. Berger AC, Gibril F, Venzon DJ, *et al.* Prognostic value of initial fasting serum gastrin levels in patients with Zollinger Ellison syndrome. *J Clin Oncol* 2001; **19**(12):3051–3057.

26. Doherty GM and Thompson NW. Multiple endocrine neoplasia type 1: duodenopancreatic tumors. *J Intern Med* 2003; **253**:590–598.

27. Yim JH, Siegel BA, DeBenedetti MK, *et al.* Prospective study of the utility of somatostatin receptor scintigraphy in the evaluation of patients with multiple endocrine neoplasia type 1. *Surgery* 1998; **124**:1037–1042.

28. Clayton RN. Sporadic pituitary tumours: from epidemiology to use of databases. *Bailliere's Clin Endocrinol Metab* 1999; **13**(3):451–460.

29. Verges B, Boureille F, Goudet P, *et al.* Pituitary disease in MEN type 1: Data from the France-Belgium MEN1 Multicenter Study. *J Clin Endocrin Metab* 2002; **87**:457–465.

30. Stratakis CA, Schussheim DH, Freedman SM *et al.* Pituitary adenoma in a 5-year old: an early expression of multiple endocrine neoplasia type 1. *J Clin Endocrinol Metab* 2000; **85**(12):4776–4780.

31. Burgess JR, Shepherd JJ, Parameswaran V *et al.* Prolactinomas in a large kindred with multiple endocrine neoplasia, type 1: clinical features and inheritance pattern. *J Clin Endocrinol Metab* 1996; **81**:1841–1845.

32. Beckers A, Betea D, Valdes Socin H, *et al.* The treatment of sporadic versus MEN 1 related pituitary adenomas. *J Intern Med* 2003; **253**:599–605.

33. Teh BT. Thymic carcinoids in multiple endocrine neoplasia type 1. *J Intern Med* 1998; **243**:501–505.

34. Langer P, Cupisti K, Bartsch DK, *et al.* Adrenal involvement in multiple endocrine neoplasia type 1. *World J Surg* 2002; **26**(8):891–896.

35. Desai D, McPherson LA, Higgins JP, Weigel RJ. Genetic analysis of a papillary thyroid carcinoma in a patient with MEN 1. *Ann Surg Onc* 2001; **8**(4):342–346.

36. Schussheim DH, Skarulis MC, Agarwal SK, *et al.* Multiple endocrine neoplasia type 1: new clinical and basic findings. *Trends Endocrinol Metab* 2001; **12**:173–177.

37. McKeeby JL, Li X, Vortmeyer AO, *et al.* Multiple leiomyomas of the esophagus, lung, and uterus in multiple endocrine neoplasia type 1. *Am J Pathol* 2001; **159**:1121–1127.

38. Karges W, Schaaf L, Dralle H, Boehm BO. Clinical and molecular diagnosis of multiple endocrine neoplasia type 1. *Langenbeck's Arch Surg* 2002; **386**:547–552.

39. Thakker RV. Multiple endocrine neoplasia – syndrome of the twentieth century. *J Clin Endocrinol Metabol* 1998; **83**:2617–2620.

40. Arancha C, Ruiz-Llorente S, Cascon, A, *et al.* A rapid and easy method for multiple endocrine neoplasia type 1 mutation detection using conformation-sensitive gel electrophoresis. *J Hum Gen* 2002; **47**(4):190–195.

41. Crepin M, Escande F, Pigny P, *et al.* Efficient mutation detection in *MEN 1* gene using a combination of single strand conformation polymorphism and heteroduplex analysis. *Electrophoresis* 2003; **24**(1–2):26–33.

Multiple endocrine neoplasia type 2

CHARIS ENG AND BRUCE A.J. PONDER

INTRODUCTION

Genetic testing and the consequent clinical management in multiple endocrine neoplasia type 2 (MEN 2) represent an important paradigm for the practice of molecular oncology. MEN 2 is a relatively rare autosomal dominant inherited neoplasia syndrome characterized by medullary thyroid carcinoma (MTC), phaeochromocytoma (PC) and hyperparathyroidism (HPT) (reviewed in Ponder[1] and Eng[2]). Germline mutations in only one susceptibility gene, *RET* localized to 10q11.2, are responsible for ≥95 per cent of all MEN 2.[3] Because of the single susceptibility gene, the limited number of mutations involved and the high frequency of mutations in MEN 2, sensitivity, the specificity and cost effectiveness of *RET* mutation analysis are high. The accuracy of the test and the ability of such results to alter medical management have made *RET* mutation testing part of the routine clinical care of patients with known MEN 2, suspected MEN 2 and, in some countries, all isolated presentations of MTC.

CLINICAL ASPECTS

Incidence

Approximately 1 per cent of all individuals develop some form of thyroid cancer in their lifetime. Of these, 10–20 per cent are MTC, and it is believed that 25 per cent of all MTC are hereditary, i.e. MEN 2. The incidence of MEN 2 is estimated to be 1 in 500 000 live births.[4] The great majority of MEN 2 is familial. The exception is the clinical subtype known as MEN 2B (see later), where up to 40 per cent occur as isolated cases, the result of *de novo* mutations.

Diagnosis and clinical presentation

MEN 2 is divided into three clinical subtypes depending on the combination of tissues involved. MEN 2A, which is the most common subtype, is characterized by the triad of MTC in virtually all cases, PC in 50 per cent and HPT in 15–30 per cent.[5–7] MEN 2B is similar to MEN 2A except that the age of tumour onset is an average 10 years younger than that in MEN 2A, often occurring before 10 years of age,[8] and specific physical stigmata, such as mucosal neuromas, intestinal ganglioneuromatosis and marfanoid habitus, are present. Clinically apparent HPT has never been described in MEN 2B. Familial MTC (FMTC) is characterized by MTC as the only phenotype in the family, with objective evidence against the presence of PC and HPT.[9]

MEN 2 can present at any time from shortly after birth (MEN 2B) to over 70 years of age.[10,11] MTC is almost always the first tumour to present in MEN 2. Both sporadic and hereditary MTC can present clinically with a change of the thyroid contour, possibly palpable during physical examination, but almost never causing any functional disorder of the thyroid. The majority of patients

(50–80 per cent) with sporadic MTC and also those with hereditary MTC who are not diagnosed by surveillance procedures usually have lymph node metastases at the time of diagnosis. Thus, cervical lymph node metastases may be the initial symptom of MTC. In MEN 2A, lymph node metastases can be diagnosed as early as the age of 5 years and 11 months, and, in MEN 2B, even at the age of 3 years.[12] Thus, the most common presentation of MTC is a neck mass. In advanced stages, symptoms may arise from effects caused by extensive production of calcitonin, especially diarrhoea. Local symptoms caused by distant metastases are rarely the initial symptom of MTC.

Phaeochromocytoma, which may be present in up to 50 per cent of individuals in both MEN 2A and MEN 2B, can be present at the time the diagnosis of MTC is made, but often occurs subsequent to MTC diagnosis. Very rarely, symptoms caused by a PC (palpitation, nervousness, hypertension either paroxysmal or sustained), precede MTC. Of interest, not all patients with PC are hypertensive. Instead, patients with adrenalin-secreting tumours may have orthostatic hypotension. The PC seen in MEN 2 is often multifocal and bilateral. Fewer than 10 per cent are malignant. Rarely, sudden death occurs as a result of hypertensive crisis; this is a particular hazard if an MEN 2 carrier enters into pregnancy and childbirth without proper surveillance. Up to one-third of patients who undergo unilateral adrenalectomy will eventually develop a contralateral PC.

As many as 20–30 per cent of patients with MEN 2A will develop primary HPT. The absence of parathyroid abnormalities in cases of sporadic MTC with grossly elevated calcitonin levels suggests that the association of parathyroid disease with MEN 2A is a consequence of germline *RET* mutation (i.e. it is genetically determined) and not a response to elevated calcitonin levels. All four parathyroid glands can be involved. Up to 20 per cent of all MEN 2A patients have a fifth intrathymic parathyroid gland. Primary hyperparathyroidism is most often diagnosed during follow-up of patients operated on for MTC, and the clinical course of primary HPT in MEN 2A seems to be milder than in its sporadic counterpart. In MEN 2B, the occurrence of clinically apparent primary HPT is not increased over that of the general population.

Histopathology

Like many inherited cancer syndromes, the component neoplasias in MEN 2 are generally characterized by multifocal disease and bilateral involvement in paired organs (Table 8b.1). The hallmark component tumour MTC derives from the parafollicular C-cells of the thyroid. C-cells produce calcitonin (hence the name), a protein consisting of 32 amino acids with a variety of physiological effects, which include the inhibition of osteoclastic and osteocytic

Table 8b.1 *Recognition of potentially hereditary cancer*

- Clustering of cases in family
- Early age of onset
- Multiple primary tumours
- Bilateral disease in paired organs
- Different tumour types in single individual

bone resorption, as well as calciuric, saluretic and uricosuric effects on the kidneys. Since MTC does not derive from follicular cells, it does not take up radioiodine. In MEN 2, C-cell hyperplasia is believed to be the precursor (i.e. a preneoplastic lesion) of MTC. Before the discovery of the MEN 2 gene, C-cell hyperplasia was considered pathognomonic for MEN 2. However, while C-cell hyperplasia is still considered an important hallmark of MEN 2, false positives and false negatives do occur.[13–15]

The actual macroscopic and microscopic appearance of all three component tumours, MTC, PC and HPT, are no different from their sporadic counterparts. Nonetheless, multifocal tumours and/or bilateral disease should alert the pathologist that heredity should be considered (Table 8b.1).

GENETICS

The *RET* proto-oncogene

RET (*re*arranged during *t*ransfection) is the susceptibility gene for MEN 2 (reviewed in Eng[2]). This gene, located on chromosomal sub-band 10q11.2, has 21 exons, and encodes a receptor tyrosine kinase expressed in neural and neuroendocrine organs and tumours.[16–19] The extracellular domain is encoded by exons 1–10 and part of exon 11, the transmembrane domain by part of exon 11, and the remaining exons encode the cytoplasmic domain. The intracytoplasmic portion of *RET* contains tyrosine kinase domains (Figure 8b.1).

RET is an unusual receptor tyrosine kinase because it requires both ligand and co-receptor for transactivation to occur.[20] At least four related ligands belonging to the glial cell line-derived neurotrophic factor (GDNF) family have been identified: GDNF, neurturin (NTN), persephin (PSP) and artemin (ART).[20–28] Each binds differentially to one of four related co-receptors, GFRα-1, GFRα-2, GFRα-3 and GFRα-4.[20,27,29–31] Not all the natural downstream targets of *RET* activation are known, despite much knowledge gained in this regard in the last two decades. As of 2001, it appears that *RET* action can effect growth, survival or differentiative signals, depending on the specific downstream pathways used and the cell type and developmental stage. It is known that *RET* signals down the MAPK/Ras/Raf pathway as well as the PI3K/Akt pathway (reviewed by Mulligan[32]).

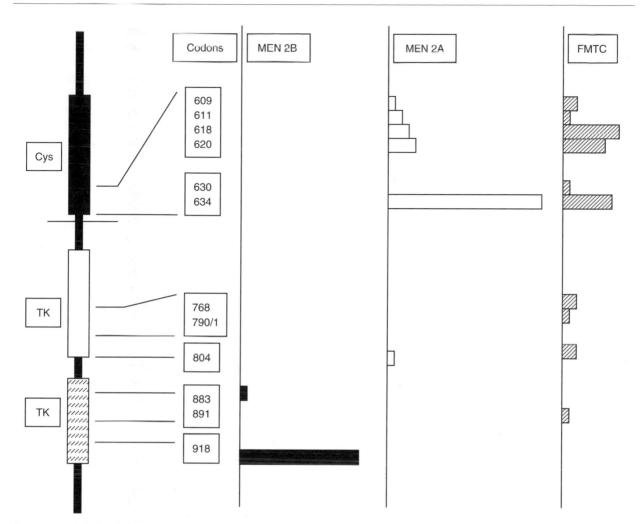

Figure 8b.1 *Relative frequency and distribution of germline* RET *mutations in MEN 2A, MEN 2B and FMTC. Cys, cysteine-rich domain; FMTC, familial medullary thyroid carcinoma; TK, tyrosine kinase domain.*

Germline *RET* mutations cause MEN 2

Germline *RET* mutations are associated with all three subtypes of MEN 2.[3,33–37] Mutations have been found in both the extracellular and the cytoplasmic domains. Germline missense mutations in the extracellular domain are always located in the juxtamembrane cysteine-rich region (Figure 8b.1). In the great majority of cases, one of five particular cysteine codons – in exon 10 (C609, C611, C618 and C620) or in exon 11 (C634) – is affected. Mutations of these codons have been found in 98 per cent of MEN 2A cases and are also found in approximately 85 per cent of FMTC families.[3] While FMTC mutations are roughly evenly distributed among codons 618, 620 and 634, mutations at codon 634 occur in at least 85 per cent of MEN 2A families (Figure 8b.1).[3] Intracellular mutations associated with MEN 2 always affect non-cysteine amino acids. Mutations have been identified in exon 13 (E768D) and exon 14 (V804L; V804M) in FMTC cases.[3,38–40] One family with a V804L mutation, and with MTC and unilateral

phaeochromocytomas in two affected members has also been reported.[41] The only two mutations associated with MEN 2B to date are both located in the intracellular tyrosine kinase domain: M918T in exon 16 (>95 per cent of cases);[3] and A883F in exon 15.[42,43]

In addition to the common mutations described above, a few rare mutations have been reported as well. In the extracellular domain, point mutations at codons 630, a cysteine codon, a 12 bp duplication, which results in an insertion of four amino acids between cysteine 634 and residue 635, and a 9 bp duplication in the cysteine-rich domain have been described in FMTC and MEN 2A families.[3,44,45] In the cytoplasmic domain, mutations at codons 790, 791 and 891 have been reported.[44,46,47] The codon 891 germline mutation has been described only twice, each occurring in an FMTC family.[44,47] Codons 790 and 791 have been reported as 'novel hot spots' for mutation resulting in FMTC and MEN 2A.[46] Interestingly, however, the codon 790 and 791 mutations have never been reported outside Germany despite many academic centres and commercial laboratories performing *RET* mutation analysis around the world. Since codons 790 and 791 lie in the same exon as codon 768, a mutation that has been commonly tested for since 1995,[38] it is difficult to imagine that the lack of reports of codon 790 and 791 mutations outside Germany is due entirely to lack of examination of those codons. This is reinforced by the fact that there are no families reported with these two novel mutations in The Netherlands, and the lack of reports emanating from neighbouring Austria and France. Perhaps the codon 790 and 791 mutations result from a founder effect peculiar only to Germany. If codon 790 and 791 mutations are discovered in individuals outside Germany, then it would be interesting to determine if these individuals were of German descent and whether a founder effect is pertinent.

Association of *RET* genotype with disease features in MEN 2

The International *RET* Mutation Consortium analysis of 477 unrelated MEN 2 families showed that specific mutations of *RET* can be associated with the development of organ-specific component tumours.[3,48] Of these 477 MEN 2 families, 42.6 per cent were classic MEN 2A, 16.6 per cent MEN 2B and 7.1 per cent FMTC.[3] The remainder were operationally classified into an 'other' category comprising 'small' FMTC ($\leq$3 affected members) and incompletely documented families. Over 98 per cent of the MEN 2A families, 95 per cent MEN 2B and 85 per cent FMTC have been found to have germline *RET* mutations.[3] There is a statistically significant association between the presence of any mutation at codon 634 (exon 11) and the presence of PC and/or primary HPT (i.e. mutation at codon 634 appears to be associated with MEN 2A). In fact, 85 per cent of the MEN 2A families were found to harbour a codon 634 mutation (Figure 8b.1). Among various codon 634 mutations, the C634R mutation, changing a cysteine to an arginine, was the most common. Whether the specific mutation, C634R, is correlated with the specific development of HPT remains open to debate.[3,49–52] From a clinical point of view, however, the C634R-HPT correlation issue is not germane: the presence of any codon 634 mutation should alert the clinician to the risk of both PC and HPT.

Mutations associated with MEN 2A can also be found in FMTC. However, it would appear that the distribution of mutations among the cysteine codons is more evenly distributed in FMTC (Figure 8b.1). For example, while 85 per cent of MEN 2A have a codon 634 mutation, only 30 per cent of FMTC families had a codon 634 mutation. Among this relatively small group of FMTC families, no C634R mutations were noted. Clinicians should, therefore, be alerted if they find an apparent FMTC family with a C634R mutation: they should rigorously pursue PC and HPT screening in all affected or mutation-positive members. Prior to the observation of a FMTC family with V804L who developed PC,[41] it was hoped that mutations at codons 768 and 804 were FMTC-specific. At present, it may be wise not to assume that particular mutations reliably predict no risk for PC.

Germline mutations at codon 918 and codon 883 are associated with MEN 2B only.[3,42,43] These two specific mutations have not been reported in patients with MEN 2A or FMTC, and, if found, may be considered diagnostic of MEN 2B. Although the number of MEN 2B cases with codon 883 mutations are limited, there does not appear to be any clinical difference between patients with M918T and those with A883F.

The above data establish clearly that different specific mutations of *RET* are associated with different patterns of MEN 2 phenotype. However, even within the same family, the occurrence and time of onset of component tumours can vary greatly, This implies that other chance environmental or genetic events are likely to have a role. Although these modifying factors have not yet been identified, there are at least preliminary data to suggest that polymorphic sequence variants within *RET* itself or perhaps with the co-receptors can modulate risk.[53,54]

Cryptic MEN 2

Determining the frequency of cryptic (occult or *de novo*) MEN 2 amongst presentations of apparently sporadic (isolated, non-familial) MTC, PC or HPT is important for clinical management. Clinical epidemiologic data suggest that 25 per cent of all MTC are hereditary, thus 75 per cent are sporadic. At least five series have examined the frequency of germline *RET* mutations in apparently sporadic MTC presentations. Four of these five studies ascertained such patients by relatively stringent criteria, including no associated features suggestive of MEN 2 in a potential subject, no known family history of MEN 2, and no family history suggestive of MEN 2 (family histories were taken to at least second-degree relatives). Data from these three series suggest that between 1.5 per cent and 10 per cent of apparently sporadic MTC cases will carry occult or *de novo* germline *RET* mutations.[7,55,56] A recent study undertaken in Poland confirmed these figures.[57] Note should be made that, because each of these projects spanned several years, the total number of known MEN 2-associated mutations examined increased as time went on. For example, the 1995 study only looked at the known hotspots within exons 10, 11, 13 and 16,[55] while the 2001 one was able to look for mutations in exons 10, 11, 13, 14, 15 and 16.[57] Because of the putative low penetrance of mutations at codon 804 (exon 14), it is conceivable that many of the so-called isolated MTC cases will carry these mutations.[11,40] A fifth series essentially took 'all comers' with MTC and found a germline *RET* mutation rate of 25 per cent,[58] which agrees with the figures obtained in prior clinical epidemiologic studies. An informal survey of over 300 apparently sporadic MTC cases collected by the International *RET* Mutation Consortium revealed an occult or *de novo* germline mutation frequency of approximately 3–4 per cent (C Eng, LM Mulligan, unpublished data). Recently, a particular polymorphic variant within *RET*, S836S (c.2439C > T; exon 15), was found to be over-represented among cases with sporadic MTC compared to region-matched controls.[53] These observations have been confirmed by several studies analysing patients originating from several countries.[59–61] This conferred a relative risk (RR) of approximately 2–3-fold. Of note, approximately 90 per cent of cases with the polymorphic variant also had MTC tumours harbouring a somatic *RET* M918T mutation.[53] These findings suggest that either the variant itself or another locus in linkage disequilibrium appears to be acting as a low-penetrance allele conferring susceptibility to 'sporadic' MTC. In addition, a variant in the 5′ untranslated region/promoter of the gene encoding the RET co-receptor GFRα-1 was also found to be over-represented in cases with isolated MTC.[54] This variant lies in a region predicted to have promoter function and, thus, the hypothesized mechanism, that the presence or absence of this variant confers differential binding of a transcription factor, is plausible.[54]

In contrast to MTC, occult or *de novo* germline *RET* mutations in apparently sporadic PC presentations are uncommon, and this is especially true if careful medical and family histories have been obtained. For example, the first series that systematically examined this issue comprised 48 apparently sporadic PC patients, among which only one (2 per cent) was shown to have a germline *RET* mutation.[62] In this instance, when the referring clinician was asked to re-examine the patient, who was already a young adult, and first-degree relatives, he discovered that the patient had an MTC, and the father had a large neck mass, which was found to be MTC as well. Furthermore, a more extensive family history revealed the index case's paternal grandfather dying of 'a goitre', which turned out to be metastatic MTC.[62] Three other series revealed no occult or *de novo* germline *RET* mutations in apparently isolated PC cases.[63–65] Leading genetic differential diagnoses to consider when faced with an apparently sporadic case of PC are von Hippel–Lindau syndrome (VHL) caused by germline *VHL* mutations or familial paraganglioma syndrome caused by germline mutations in *SDHD*, encoding a subunit of mitochondrial complex II[62,66–68] (see Chapter 10). Germline mutations in another complex II subunit SDHB may also be associated with apparently sporadic PC.[69]

No *RET* mutations have been found in apparently sporadic HPT patients,[70] or in patients presenting with non-familial HPT and PC without personal or family histories of MTC (C. Eng, unpublished data).

Gain-of-function *RET* mutations in MEN 2

The great majority of germline mutations characterizing MEN 2A and FMTC are missense mutations, which change a cysteine codon to another non-sulphydryl-containing amino acid. Similar to other receptor tyrosine kinases, the cysteines of *RET* form intramolecular disulphide bonds, which presumably determine the three-dimensional shape of the extracellular domain, critical for binding of ligand. When one of the cysteines is mutated, its partner cysteine can no longer form a disulphide bond with it, and hence, a free sulphydryl group is exposed. Two mutant receptors with free sulphydryl groups can then form intermolecular disulphide bonds, mimicking ligand activation in a constitutive manner.[71–73]

While it is true that a single gain-of-function mutation in *RET* can cause transformation, at least *in vitro*,[71,72] *in vivo*, different cysteine codon mutations result in different phenotypes[3] (see Figure 8b.1). In general, MTC, PC and HPT (i.e. classic MEN 2A) result from codon 634 mutations, and it would appear that the ages of onset are, on average, younger in families with these mutations compared to those with mutations at codons 609, 611, 618 and 620, where either MEN 2A or FMTC phenotypes may result. In stable transfection studies, the C634R mutation results in more transformants on focus assay than does the C620R mutation.[71] Subsequently, it has been shown that missense mutations affecting the extracellular domain result in *RET* molecules that fail to mature and fail to reach the cell surface.[74,75] Mutations of cysteine codons closest to the transmembrane domain (e.g. C634R) result in the greatest fraction of receptors that reach the cell surface, while those in cysteine codons furthest from the transmembrane domain (e.g. C609W) result in the lowest fraction of receptors that reach the cell surface. These observations may explain, at least partially, the relative penetrance of mutations at codon 634 and those at cysteine codons away from the transmembrane domain.

The MEN 2B-specific mutation at codon 918 occurs at a residue, which lies in the substrate recognition pocket of the catalytic core of the tyrosine kinase domain.[76] This methionine residue is highly conserved among receptor tyrosine kinases as well as across species.[76] M918T changes the methionine to a threonine. At the equivalent position, cytosolic tyrosine kinases have a threonine.[76] *In vitro*, data show that substitution of the *RET* methionine for a threonine results in a change of substrate specificity towards that characteristic of cytosolic tyrosine kinases.[71,77] While M918T-RET can be constitutively active,[71] ligand stimulation (e.g. by GDNF) of M918T-RET, can increase its activity.

The signalling pathways downstream of each mutation are being investigated; as yet what precise mechanisms mediate neoplastic transformation between mutation and phenotype is still unclear. A more comprehensive review of the signalling pathways downstream of RET, as it relates to the neurocristopathies, is beyond the scope of this chapter but may be obtained elsewhere.[32]

CANCER GENETIC ASPECTS OF THE CLINICAL MANAGEMENT OF MEN 2

Management of MEN 2 and suspected MEN 2 in the pre-*RET* era

First-degree relatives (children, parents, siblings) of affected individuals are at 50 per cent risk of inheriting the mutated gene. Before DNA-based predictive testing, all unaffected individuals at 50 per cent risk were subjected to annual screening for MTC, PC and HPT from the age of 6 to the age of 35 years. This involves pentagastrin-stimulated calcitonin levels, 24-hour urinary levels for catecholamines and serum calcium and parathyroid levels. Especially in the USA, many centres advocated prophylactic thyroidectomy in individuals who are first-degree relatives of affected individuals prior to the age of 6 for two reasons: first, the youngest age at diagnosis reported for MTC in MEN 2A is around age 6 years,[12,78] and second, MTC can be lethal.

DNA–based management of an MEN 2 family

Since mutations of the *RET* proto-oncogene have been identified in ≥95 per cent of all MEN 2 families, DNA-based testing is possible. This has distinct advantages, such as not having age-dependent sensitivity, being useful as a molecular diagnostic test to confirm a clinical diagnosis of MEN 2 and, most importantly, being useful as a predictive test for clinically asymptomatic, but at-risk individuals. *RET* testing is, therefore, considered part of the routine clinical care of MEN 2 and MTC patients.[79]

In a family with clinically evident MEN 2 or suspicious for MEN 2 where a family-specific *RET* mutation is not known, DNA testing for *RET* mutations should always begin with a clinically affected member (Figure 8b.2). Such DNA testing should always be done in the setting of a cancer genetic consultation, which includes genetic counselling (see Chapter 30). Clinicians should be aware that not all diagnostics laboratories analyse the same exons of *RET*. Thus, one must ensure that exons 10, 11, 13, 14, 15 and 16 are the ones examined. The presence of a germline *RET* mutation is diagnostic for MEN 2. Not finding a germline *RET* mutation in a clinically affected individual, which could happen in 2–15 per cent of cases, is non-diagnostic (see later).

In a known MEN 2 (MEN 2A and FMTC) family with an identified family-specific mutation (Figure 8b.2), the detection of the same mutation in a clinically at-risk individual indicates that that person has MEN 2. Conversely, if a mutation is not detected, that individual does not have MEN 2. Barring administrative errors, DNA-based predictive testing is 100 per cent accurate. Because MEN 2 is inherited as an autosomal dominant trait, first-degree relatives of an affected individual or of

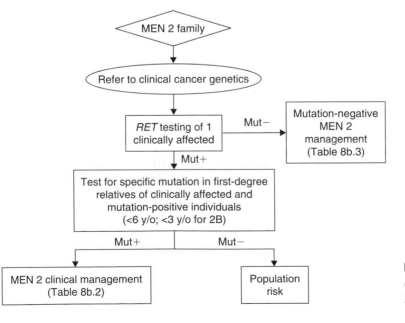

Figure 8b.2 *Algorithm for genetic management of MEN 2 family. Mut+, RET mutation positive; Mut−, RET mutation negative, y/o = years old.*

a relative with a germline *RET* mutation are at a 50 per cent likelihood of inheriting the *RET* mutation and are at-risk for MEN 2. All relatives at 50 per cent risk should undergo *RET* testing for the family-specific mutation prior to the age of 6 years (except see later for MEN 2B). Relatives found not to carry the family-specific mutation are no longer at risk for MEN 2 and can be spared unnecessary surgery, surveillance and psychological distress. Those relatives found to carry the family-specific *RET* mutation can then undergo surveillance and/or prophylactic surgery (see later for details; Table 8b.2). Because the average age of onset of MEN 2A-related MTC is in the second decade[10] and the earliest MTC has been described at age 6,[78] *RET* mutation analysis as a predictive test should be performed prior to age 6 for MEN 2A and FMTC.

Medical management for MEN 2A and FMTC *RET* mutation carriers

When a *RET* mutation carrier is identified and that person has also been shown to already have one or more of the component tumours, then the tumours need to be removed. The details of such management are noted elsewhere.[80] When a *RET* mutation carrier is identified and does not appear to have clinically apparent disease, then the mutation carrier should undergo prophylactic thyroidectomy prior to the age of 6 years[78] as well as routine surveillance for the other two component tumours (Table 8b.2). Advanced MTC is incurable and even early-stage MTC, despite appropriate surgery in the best hands, carries a relapse rate of 25 per cent (see Gimm and Eng,[80] and Eng and Ponder[81]). Once relapsed, MTC is incurable, thus, premorbid diagnosis and prophylactic treatment would be highly desirable. The evidence that early diagnosis does favourably alter outcome is highly suggestive,[13,78,82,83] although no prospective trials have been performed in this regard, nor can they be ethically performed now. The standard of care in the USA and UK, and many parts of the world, is to offer prophylactic thyroidectomy in as yet clinically unaffected *RET* mutation

carriers prior to the age of 6 years. Because of the more variable age of onset of MTC in FMTC families, the precise age to perform prophylactic thyroidectomy in mutation carriers remains controversial. Prior to thyroidectomy, PC should be ruled out. Many centres will perform prophylactic parathyroidectomy at the time of prophylactic thyroidectomy by removing three and a half glands or all four glands, with two-thirds of a gland reimplanted into an easily accessible site. After prophylactic thyroidectomy, the mutation carrier should be followed with annual serum calcitonin measurements (some advocate stimulated levels), 24-hour urine and serum catecholamines, and vanillyl mandelic acid (VMAs) as well as serum chromogranin A, and annual checks of serum ionized calcium and intact parathyroid hormone levels (Table 8b.2).

Whether both adrenal glands should be removed prophylactically in mutation carriers has recently been called into question. In the early days of gene testing for both *RET* and *VHL*, prophylactic bilateral adrenalectomies were performed in mutation-positive individuals in several centres. However, it soon became obvious that the long-term side effects from lack of adrenocortical function could be severe, possibly outweighing the benefit of PC prevention.[84] Recently, a viable alternative involving laparoscopic adrenocortical-sparing surgery has been developed.[84–86]

In the early twenty-first century, serial screening by stimulated calcitonin levels in at-risk individuals who are as yet clinically unaffected has no place in clinical care, except in special circumstances. The standard of care is to perform *RET* mutation analysis to determine molecular-based risk status. Mutation-positive individuals should undergo prophylactic thyroidectomy (see earlier). A prominent exception is if the mutation carrier does not have access to surgeons who routinely perform this operation in the paediatric age group. Then it might be safer for the young mutation-positive individual to undergo serial stimulated calcitonin screening until a rise is detected, whereupon he/she would be referred for thyroid surgery, hopefully, at a later age, where the operation would be less difficult technically. Stimulated calcitonin measurements still have a major role in detecting MTC relapses.

Table 8b.2 *Medical management of germline RET mutation-positive MEN 2*

Subtype	Prophylactic thyroidectomy	Phaeochromocytoma screen[a]	PTH and ionized calcium levels
MEN 2A	≤6 years	≥6 years	≥6 years
FMTC	≤6–10 years	>10 years	N/A
MEN 2B	<3 years	≥3 years	No

[a] Annual serum and 24-hour urine collection for catecholamines and VMA, serum chromogranin-A.
FMTC, familial medullary thyroid carcinoma; PTH, parathyroid hormone; VMA, vanillyl mandelic acid.
A single phaeochromocytoma screen should be performed prior to any surgery, e.g. before prophylactic thyroidectomy.

MEDICAL MANAGEMENT OF MEN 2A OR FMTC WITHOUT AN IDENTIFIABLE MUTATION

When a clinically affected individual with MEN 2 is said not to have a germline *RET* mutation, the physician should always check to ensure that all the pertinent exons (10, 11, 13–16) have been examined. Many reference laboratories still limit their mutation analysis to exons 10, 11 and 16.

In a syndrome where over 95 per cent of cases have identified germline mutations, it can be uncomfortable when a clinician is faced with a *RET* mutation negative MEN 2 family. The mutation negative family will most likely tend to be a 'small' FMTC family. Since MTC is rare, the occurrence of even two MTC cases in a single family is unusual. So, the chances that this has occurred entirely by coincidence are low. It would, therefore, be most conservative to treat these sorts of families as we would any MEN 2 family prior to the era of DNA-based diagnosis (Table 8b.3).

DNA–based management of apparently sporadic MTC presentations

Differentiating truly sporadic from hereditary MTC is important, as it has implications for the clinical care of the individual patient as well as his or her family. Because there is a small but finite proportion of apparently sporadic MTC cases that have been consistently found to carry occult or *de novo* germline *RET* mutation (see section earlier) and because *RET* mutation analysis has a high sensitivity, it is the clinical standard of care to perform genetic testing in all individuals presenting with MTC, regardless of age at diagnosis or family history.[2,87] An algorithm to work up such a patient is presented in Figure 8b.3. Currently, this recommendation does not hold for apparently sporadic PC and HPT presentations; if careful medical and family histories are obtained, and there is no suggestion of MEN 2, occult *RET* mutations are unlikely to be found in these cases (see earlier section on cryptic MEN 2).

When an apparently sporadic case of MTC is found to have a germline *RET* mutation, that individual has MEN 2, and genetic and clinical management follows as for any individual with MEN 2 (outlined in Figure 8b.2 and Table 8b.2). However, when an isolated MTC case is not found to have a germline *RET* mutation, clinicians are faced with a dilemma. Clinical epidemiologic data suggest that 25 per cent of all presentations of MTC are hereditary (above) and molecular epidemiologic data suggest that at least 85 per cent of MEN 2 have identifiable germline *RET* mutations.[3] Given these

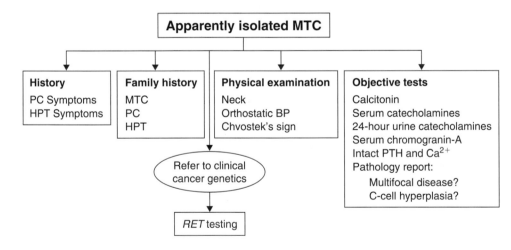

Figure 8b.3 *Algorithm for evaluation of an apparently isolated medullary thyroid carcinoma (MTC) case. BP, blood pressure; HPT, hyperparathyroidism; PC, phaeochromocytoma; PTH, parathyroid hormone.*

Table 8b.3 *Medical management of germline* RET *mutation negative MEN 2*

Consider linkage analysis
    If family is large and informative
    In the setting of clinical cancer genetics consultation only

Medical management as in pre-*RET* testing era
    Prophylactic thyroidectomy or serial stimulated serum calcitonin[a] levels for all at risk
    Annual phaeochromocytoma screen (Table 8b.2) for all at-risk individuals
    Annual serum intact PTH and ionized calcium levels for all at-risk individuals

[a] Pentagastrin is no longer available in the USA; otherwise, pentagastrin is the stimulant of choice. In the USA, it is recommended that calcium be used as the secretagogue.
PTH, parathyroid hormone.

data, a mutation-negative result in this setting would decrease the risk of an undetectable mutation to under 5 per cent (0.25 × 0.15/0.25 × 0.15 + 0.75). Each mutation-negative apparently sporadic MTC patient should be treated on a case-by-case basis. For example, if the patient were diagnosed at the age of 60 years, had unilateral disease and no C-cell hyperplasia, then in the context of no identifiable *RET* mutations it is highly likely that this person has truly sporadic disease. On the other hand, a 17-year-old diagnosed with unilateral MTC with some evidence of C-cell hyperplasia, but without a *RET* mutation, should be treated like an MEN 2 case.

Shortly after *RET* was identified as the MEN 2 gene, preliminary observations suggested that somatic *RET* M918T mutations in the MTC tumours were only found in sporadic MTC.[36,88] However, subsequent investigation has revealed that rare MEN 2-associated MTC can harbour somatic M918T as well.[89,90] Thus, although the great majority of MTC with somatic M918T are likely to be sporadic, the presence or absence of this somatic mutation in MTC should not be used to differentiate sporadic disease from MEN 2.

DNA–based management of MEN 2B

Because the age of onset of the component tumours is on average 10 years younger than in MEN 2A, genetic testing, whether for molecular diagnosis or predictive testing, should occur at birth or shortly thereafter, and certainly well before the age of 4 years, an age when metastatic disease has been found.[78,91] When MEN 2B is suspected, perhaps because of clinical features, exons 15 (codon 883) and 16 (codon 918) of *RET* should be examined. In an MEN 2B family with a known mutation, at-risk relatives should be checked only for the family-specific mutation prior to the age of 4 years. Mutation-positive individuals should then undergo a prophylactic thyroidectomy prior to the age of 4 years, after exclusion of the co-existence of PC. Thereafter, annual surveillance for PC development (Table 8b.2) should be pursued. Mutation-negative individuals who have the clinical features of MEN 2B (≤2 per cent of cases) should be treated like an MEN 2B case.

GERMLINE *RET* MUTATIONS AND HIRSCHSPRUNG DISEASE

RET and Hirschsprung disease

Hirschsprung disease (HSCR) is characterized by aganglionosis of the gut. This disorder is usually sporadic but a proportion are familial as well, although the genetics are complex.[92]

When a putative gene for HSCR was mapped to 10q11.2,[93,94] *RET*, which is expressed in the precursors of the enteric ganglia, became a prime candidate. Subsequently, loss-of-function germline *RET* mutations were found in a proportion of sporadic and familial HSCR.[95,96] Among various highly selected series, approximately 50 per cent of familial HSCR and 30 per cent of isolated cases were shown to have germline *RET* mutations scattered throughout the 21-exon gene.[16,97–100] However, an unselected, population-based HSCR series in the catchment area of Stockholm revealed a *RET* mutation frequency of 3 per cent.[101]

Whereas in the mouse, homozygous loss of Ret function was necessary to produce an HSCR phenotype, in humans, mutation of one allele may be sufficient, suggesting haploinsufficiency. The mechanism of loss-of-function can be structural, for example, whole gene deletion, nonsense mutation, frameshift mutation, or functional, such as lack of maturation of receptor to cell surface owing to missense mutations. The variable expression and penetrance of the HSCR phenotype is presumably due to the effects of modifiers on the haploinsufficient phenotype.[102,103]

Other HSCR susceptibility genes exist, including the genes encoding endothelin receptor β, its ligand endothelin-3, GDNF, NTN, and SOX10.[104–108] Interestingly, to date, germline mutations in the genes encoding three *RET* co-receptors, *GFRA1*, *GFRA2* and *GFRA3*, have not been found.[109–111] Recent data suggest that polymorphic variants within *RET* may be associated with the HSCR phenotype. Analysis of a population-based series of 64 isolated HSCR cases in Western Andalusia, Spain, revealed over-representation of polymorphic *RET* alleles in HSCR cases compared to region-matched controls.[112] One specific polymorphism at codon 45 (A45A) was highly significantly over-represented among HSCR cases compared to controls.[112] Subsequently, these data were replicated in HSCR cases from other population bases, namely, Germany, Italy and the UK.[59,60,113] Taken together, these observations suggest several hypotheses. Either the polymorphic variants themselves affect *RET* expression, for example, by introducing a cryptic splice site, or there is another locus in linkage disequilibrium with the polymorphic loci within *RET*, which predisposes to isolated HSCR in a low-penetrance manner.[112,114]

RET mutations in families with MEN 2 and HSCR

At least 14 families have been reported to segregate both MEN 2A or FMTC and HSCR. Each of these families harbours a germline *RET* mutation. The presence of both a gain-of-function and loss-of-function phenotype in the same individual appears paradoxical.[3,58,103,115–118] Most of the mutations are C618R or C620R. All of the earlier papers noted that a second, inactivating, mutation within *RET* (to explain the concurrent gain-of-function and loss-of-function phenotype in the same individual) could not be found despite complete sequencing of the gene in these families. Subsequent functional data suggest that the explanation for codon 618 and 620 mutations causing both MEN 2 and HSCR is as follows. Extracellular missense mutations, such as C618R and C620R, cause lack of maturation of mutant *RET*, and hence, lack of migration of the mutant receptors to the surface.[74,75] Thus, cysteine codon missense mutations result in functional haploinsufficiency leading to HSCR, while constitutively dimerized mutant receptors lead to the MEN 2 phenotype. These data also suggest tissue-specific sensitivity to RET signalling: for developing enteric ganglia, functional receptor number above some threshold must be important to prevent inappropriate apoptosis, while in the tissues involved in MEN 2, constitutive signalling, irrespective of numerical threshold, seems more important for development of neoplasia. However, even in MEN 2, non-634 extracellular cysteine codon mutations do result in decreased penetrance, which somehow must be related to incomplete maturation of mutant receptors.

SOMATIC *RET* MUTATIONS IN SPORADIC COUNTERPART TUMOURS

When germline mutations of a particular gene have been found to cause an inherited cancer syndrome, it is not uncommon to see somatic mutations of the same gene in sporadic component tumours as well. Somatic mutations of the *RET* proto-oncogene have been found in a subset of sporadic MTC and PC (described later), but not in the parathyroid tumours.[70] At least eight studies have been performed to analyse somatic *RET* mutations in sporadic MTC. Depending on the study and the mutation detection technology employed, the somatic mutation frequency ranges from 25 to 70 per cent in sporadic MTC.[35,36,88,119–123] Somatic M918T, the MEN 2B-associated mutation, make up the largest proportion amongst all somatic *RET* mutations. When microdissected subpopulations of MTC were examined, the somatic *RET* mutation status was found to be heterogeneous even within a single MTC and among metastases in the same individual.[90] Interestingly, there was a high concordance rate between subpopulations with *RET* mutation and *RET* expression as evidenced by immunohistochemistry.[124] Approximately 80 per cent of all MTC studies in this manner were found to harbour at least one subpopulation with somatic *RET* mutation, almost exclusively M918T.[90] These observations are likely to reflect clonal evolution within MTC, which is a relatively slow-growing

tumour and/or polyclonal origin. The latter seems to be corroborated by an independent study using X-chromosome inactivation.[125] In rare cases, somatic M918T has been detected in MTC subpopulations in MTC from MEN 2A/FMTC patients.[89,90]

Whether the presence of somatic M918T mutations is associated with prognosis for sporadic MTC remains controversial. There are three studies relating prognosis to somatic M918T status in sporadic MTC, which report varying results.[122,126,127] In the most well-controlled study, examining only the primary tumour for the presence or absence of somatic M918T, no associations with prognosis were noted. The most recent study,[127] which reports an association of M918T and poor prognosis, examined for M918T status mainly on lymph node metastases and not the primary tumours.[127] Thus, no valid conclusions can be drawn from this study.

Up to 10 per cent of sporadic PC have been found to harbour somatic *RET* mutations.[62,63,65,128] While the great majority of somatic *RET* mutations in sporadic MTC are M918T, other *RET* mutations have been reported in sporadic PC. Interestingly, the non-M918T somatic *RET* mutations in PC are not necessarily those found in the germline in patients with MEN 2.

CONCLUSIONS

Routine *RET* testing in the management of MEN 2A, MEN 2B and all presentations of MTC is the standard of clinical care. This is because such genetic testing is sensitive and specific, and the results alter medical management; it thus serves as a paradigm for the practice of molecular oncology. However, phenotypic expression, especially ages of tumour onset, are still quite variable, even within families, and this poses issues as to the timing of prophylactic surgery. This is particularly true of non-codon 634 MEN 2A and FMTC cases. The challenge for the next decade is to determine what modifies phenotypic expression and incorporate these new data into routine clinical care in addition. A second challenge lies in determining more precisely which signalling pathways lie downstream of activated *RET*, such that selective targeting of neoplastic cells may be achieved.

Note added in proof

A large population-based study accruing by symptomatic presentations of apparently sporadic phaeochromocytoma revealed that 25 per cent of all such individuals carried a germline mutation in one of four genes, VHL, SDHD, SDHB or RET.[129] These relatively high frequencies are currently being confirmed in other series. Thus, the current clinical recommendation is that all patients presenting with phaeochromocytoma or paraganglioma be offered genetic testing in a clinical cancer genetics consultation which includes genetic counseling.

KEY POINTS

- MEN 2A and MEN 2B have different phenotypic manifestations, owing to a genotype/phenotype effect in the *RET* protooncogene.
- All cases of MTC should be offered germline *RET* mutation analysis.
- Predictive testing in children can determine management.

REFERENCES

1. Ponder BAJ. Multiple endocrine neoplasia type 2. In: Vogelstein B, Kinzler KW (eds) *The genetic basis of human cancer*. New York: McGraw-Hill, 1998:475–487.

2. Eng C. *RET* proto-oncogene in the development of human cancer. *J Clin Oncol* 1999; **17**:380–393.

3. Eng C, Clayton D, Schuffenecker I, et al. The relationship between specific *RET* proto-oncogene mutations and disease phenotype in multiple endocrine neoplasia type 2: International *RET* Mutation Consortium analysis. *JAMA* 1996; **276**:1575–1579.

4. Eng C, Hampel H, de la Chapelle A. Genetic testing for cancer predisposition. *Annu Rev Med* 2001; **52**:371–400.

5. Schimke RN, Hartmann WH, Prout TW, Rimoin DL. Syndrome of bilateral pheochromoctyoma, medullary thyroid carcinoma and multiple neuromas. *N Engl J Med* 1968; **279**:1–7.

6. Schimke RN. Genetic aspects of multiple endocrine neoplasia. *Annu Rev Med* 1984; **35**:25–31.

7. Schuffenecker I, Ginet N, Goldgar D, et al. Prevalence and parental origin of de novo *RET* mutations in MEN 2A and FMTC. *Am J Hum Genet* 1997; **60**:233–237.

8. Gorlin RJ, Sedano HO, Vickers RA, Cervenka J. Multiple mucosal neuromas, phaeochromocytoma and medullary carcinoma of the thyroid – a syndrome. *Cancer* 1968; **22**:293–299.

9. Farndon JR, Leight GS, Dilley WG, et al. Familial medullary thyroid carcinoma without associated endocrinopathies: a distinct clinical entity. *Br J Surg* 1986; **73**:278–281.

10. Easton DF, Ponder MA, Cummings T, et al. The clinical and age-at-onset distribution for the MEN-2 syndrome. *Am J Hum Genet* 1989; **44**:208–215.

11. Shannon KE, Gimm O, Hinze R, Dralle H, Eng C. Germline V804M in the *RET* proto-oncogene in two apparently sporadic cases of MTC presenting in the seventh decade of life. *J Endo Genet* 1999; **1**:39–46.

12. Telander RL, Moir CR. Medullary thyroid carcinoma in children. *Sem Pediatr Surg* 1994; **3**:188–193.

13. Lips CJM, Landsvater RM, Höppener JWM, et al. Clinical screening as compared with DNA analysis in families with multiple endocrine neoplasia type 2A. *N Engl J Med* 1994; **331**:828–835.

14. Neumann HPH, Eng C, Mulligan LM, et al. Consequences of direct genetic testing for germ-line mutations in the clinical management of families with multiple endocrine neoplasia type 2. *JAMA* 1995; **274**:1149–1151.

15. Marsh DJ, McDowall D, Hyland VJ, et al. The identification of false positive responses to the pentagastrin stimulation test in *RET* mutation negative members of MEN 2A families. *Clin Endocrinol* 1996; **44**:213–220.

16. Myers SM, Eng C, Ponder BAJ, Mulligan LM. Characterization of *RET* proto-oncogene 3′ splicing variants and polyadenylation sites: a novel C-terminus for RET. *Oncogene* 1995; **11**:2039–2045.

17. Gardner E, Papi L, Easton DF, et al. Genetic linkage studies map the multiple endocrine neoplasia type 2 loci to a small interval on chromosome 10q11.2. *Hum Mol Genet* 1993; **2**:241–246.

18. Santoro M, Rosato R, Grieco M, et al. The *ret* proto-oncogene is consistently expressed in human pheochromocytomas and thyroid medullary carcinomas. *Oncogene* 1990; **5**:1595–1598.

19. Nakamura T, Ishizaka Y, Nagao M, et al. Expression of the *ret* proto-oncogene product in human normal and neoplastic tissues of neural crest origin. *J Pathol* 1994; **172**:255–260.

20. Trupp M, Raynoschek C, Belluardo N, Ibanez CF. Multiple GPI-anchored receptors control GDNF-dependent and independent activation of the c-Ret receptor tyrosine kinase. *Moll Cell Neurobiol* 1998; **11**:47–63.

21. Baloh RH, Tansey MG, Lampe PA, et al. Artemin, a novel member of the GDNF ligand family, supports peripheral and central neurons and signals through the GFRalpha-3-RET receptor complex. *Neuron* 1998; **21**:1291–1302.

22. Jing S, Wen D, Yu Y, et al. GDNF-induced activation of the Ret protein tyrosine kinase is mediated by GDNFR-a, a novel receptor for GDNF. *Cell* 1996; **85**:1113–1124.

23. Moore MW, Klein RD, Farinas I, et al. Renal and neuronal abnormalities in mice lacking GDNF. *Nature* 1996; **382**:76–79.

24. Pichel JG, Shen L, Sheng HZ, et al. Defects in enteric innervation and kidney development in mice lacking GDNF. *Nature* 1996; **382**:73–76.

25. Sanicola M, Hession C, Worley D, et al. GDNF-dependent *RET* activation can be mediated by two different cell-surface accessory proteins. *Proc Natl Acad Sci USA* 1997; **94**: 6238–6243.

26. Sánchez MP, Silos-Santiago I, Frién J, et al. Renal agenesis and the absence of enteric neurons in mice lacking GDNF. *Nature* 1996; **382**:70–73.

27. Treanor JJS, Goodman L, de Sauvage F, et al. Characterization of a multicomponent receptor for GDNF. *Nature* 1996; **382**:80–83.

28. Trupp M, Arenas E, Fainzilber M, et al. Functional receptor for GDNF encoded by the c-ret proto-oncogene. *Nature* 1996; **381**:785–789.

29. Baloh RH, Tansey MG, Golden JP, et al. TrnR2, a novel receptor that mediates neurturin and GDNF signaling through Ret. *Neuron* 1997; **18**:793–802.

30. Jing SQ, Yu YB, Fang M, et al. GFR-alpha-2 and GFR-alpha-3 are two new receptors for ligands of the GDNF family. *J Biol Chem* 1998; **272**:33111–33117.

31. Thompson J, Doxakis E, Pinon LGP, et al. GFRa-4, a new GDNF family receptor. *Mol Cell Neurosci* 1998; **11**:117–126.

32. Mulligan LM. Multiple endocrine neoplasia type 2: molecular aspects. In: Dahia PLM, Eng C (eds) *Genetic disorders of endocrine neoplasia*. Basel: Karger, 2001, 81–102.

33. Mulligan LM, Kwok JBJ, Healey CS, *et al.* Germline mutations of the *RET* proto-oncogene in multiple endocrine neoplasia type 2A. *Nature* 1993; **363**:458–460.

34. Donis-Keller H, Dou S, Chi D, *et al.* Mutations in the *RET* proto-oncogene are associated with MEN 2A and FMTC. *Hum Mol Genet* 1993; **2**:851–856.

35. Eng C, Smith DP, Mulligan LM, *et al.* Point mutation within the tyrosine kinase domain of the *RET* proto-oncogene in multiple endocrine neoplasia type 2B and related sporadic tumours. *Hum Mol Gene.* 1994; **3**:237–241.

36. Hofstra RMW, Landsvater RM, Ceccherini I, *et al.* A mutation in the *RET* proto-oncogene associated with multiple endocrine neoplasia type 2B and sporadic medullary thyroid carcinoma. *Nature* 1994; **367**:375–376.

37. Carlson KM, Dou S, Chi D, *et al.* Single missense mutation in the tyrosine kinase catalytic domain of the *RET* protooncogene is associated with multiple endocrine neoplasia type 2B. *Proc Natl Acad Sci USA* 1994; **91**:1579–1583.

38. Eng C, Smith DP, Mulligan LM, *et al.* A novel point mutation in the tyrosine kinase domain of the *RET* proto-oncogene in sporadic medullary thyroid carcinoma and in a family with FMTC. *Oncogene* 1995; **10**:509–513.

39. Bolino A, Schuffenecker I, Luo Y, *et al. RET* mutations in exons 13 and 14 of FMTC patients. *Oncogene* 1995; **10**:2415–2419.

40. Fink M, Weinäusel A, Niederle B, Haas OA. Distinction between sporadic and herditary medullary thyroid carcinoma (MTC) by mutation analysis of the *RET* proto-oncogene. *Int J Cancer* 1996; **69**:312–316.

41. Nilsson O, Tissell L-E, Jansson S, *et al.* Adrenal and extra-adrenal phaeochromocytomas in a family with germline *RET* V804L mutation. *JAMA* 1999; **281**:1587–1588.

42. Gimm O, Marsh DJ, Andrew SD, *et al.* Germline dinucleotide mutation in codon 883 of the *RET* proto-oncogene in multiple endocrine neoplasia type 2B without codon 918 mutation. *J Clin Endocrinol Metab* 1997; **82**:3902–3904.

43. Smith DP, Houghton C, Ponder BAJ. Germline mutation of *RET* codon 883 in two cases of *de novo* MEN 2B. *Oncogene* 1997; **15**:1213–1217.

44. Hofstra RMW, Fattoruso O, Quadro L, *et al.* A novel point mutation in the intracellular domain of the *RET* proto-oncogene in a family with medullary thyroid carcinoma. *J Clin Endocrinol Metab* 1997; **82**:4176–4178.

45. Höppner W, Ritter MM. A duplication of 12 bp in the critical cysteine rich domain of the *RET* proto-oncogene results in a distinct phenotype of multiple endocrine neoplasia type 2A. *Hum Mol Genet* 1997; **6**:587–590.

46. Berndt I, Reuter M, Saller B, *et al.* A new hotspot for mutations in the *RET* proto-oncogene causing familial medullary thyroid carcinoma and multiple endocrine neoplasia. *J Clin Endocrinol Metab* 1998; **83**:770–774.

47. Dang GT, Cote GJ, Schultz PN, *et al.* A codon 891 exon 15 *RET* proto-oncogene mutation in familial medullary thyroid carcinoma: a detection strategy. *Mol Cell Probes* 1999; **13**:77–79.

48. Mulligan LM, Marsh DJ, Robinson BG, *et al.* Genotype-phenotype correlation in MEN 2: Report of the International *RET* Mutation Consortium. *J Intern Med* 1995; **238**:343–346.

49. Mulligan LM, Eng C, Healey CS, *et al.* Specific mutations of the *RET* proto-oncogene are related to disease phenotype in MEN 2A and FMTC. *Nature Genet* 1994; **6**:70–74.

50. Schuffenecker I, Billaud M, Calender A, *et al. RET* proto-oncogene mutations in French MEN 2A and FMTC families. *Hum Mol Genet* 1994; **3**:1939–1943.

51. Schuffenecker I, Virally-Monod M, Broh R, *et al.* Risk and penetrance of primary hyperparathyroidism in MEN 2A families with codon 634 mutations of the *RET* proto-oncogene. *J Clin Endocrinol Metab* 1998; **83**:487–491.

52. Frank-Raue K, Höppner W, Frilling A, *et al.* Mutations of the *RET* proto-oncogene in German MEN families: relation between genotype and phenotype. *J Clin Endocrinol Metab* 1996; **81**:1780–1783.

53. Gimm O, Neuberg DS, Marsh DJ, *et al.* Over-representation of a germline *RET* sequence variant in patients with sporadic medullary thyroid carcinoma and somatic *RET* codon 918 mutation. *Oncogene* 1999; **18**:1369–1370.

54. Gimm O, Dziema H, Brown JL, *et al.* Over-representation of a germline variant in the gene encoding RET co-receptor GFRa-1 but not GFRa-2 or GFRa-3 in cases with sporadic medullary thyroid carcinoma. *Oncogene* 2001; **20**:2161–2170.

55. Eng C, Mulligan LM, Smith DP, *et al.* Low frequency of germline mutations in the *RET* proto-oncogene in patients with apparently sporadic medullary thyroid carcinoma. *Clin Endocrinol* 1995; **43**:123–127.

56. Wohlik N, Cote GJ, Bugalho MMJ, *et al.* Relevance of *RET* proto-oncogene mutations in sporadic medullary thyroid carcinoma. *J Clin Endocrinol Metab* 1996; **81**:3740–3745.

57. Wiench M, Wygoda Z, Gubala E, *et al.* Estimation of risk of inherited medullary thyroid carcinoma in apparent sporadic patients. *J Clin Oncol* 2001; **19**:1374–1380.

58. Borst MJ, van Camp JM, Peacock ML, Decker RA. Mutation analysis of multiple endocrine neoplasia type 2A associated with Hirschsprung's disease. *Surgery* 1995; **117**:386–389.

59. Ceccherini I, Griseri P, Sancandi M, *et al.* Decreased frequency of a neutral sequence variant of the RET proto-oncogene in sporadic Hirschsprung diesease. *Am J Hum Genet* 1999; **65**:A266.

60. Fitze G, Schreiber M, Kuhlisch E, *et al.* Association of the *RET* proto-oncogene codon 45 polymorphism with Hirschsprung disease. *Am J Hum Genet* 1999; **65**:1469–1473.

61. Ruiz A, Antiñolo G, Fernandez RM, *et al.* Germline sequence variant S836S in the *RET* proto-oncogene is associated with low level predisposition to sporadic medullary thyroid carcinoma in the Spanish population. *Clin. Endocrinol.* 2001; **55**:399–402.

62. Eng C, Crossey PA, Mulligan LM, *et al.* Mutations of the *RET* proto-oncogene and the von Hippel–Lindau disease tumour suppressor gene in sporadic and syndromic phaeochromocytoma. *J Med Genet* 1995; **32**:934–937.

63. Beldjord B, Desclaux-Arramond F, Raffin-Sanson M, *et al.* The *RET* proto-oncogene in sporadic pheochromocytomas: frequent MEN 2-like mutations and new molecular defects. *J Clin Endocrinol Metab* 1995; **80**:2063–2068.

64. Lindor NM, Honchel R, Khosla S, Thibodeau SN. Mutations in the *RET* protooncogene in sporadic pheochromocytomas. *J Clin Endocrinol Metab* 1995; **80**:627–629.

65. Hofstra RMW, Stelwagen T, Stulp RP, *et al.* Extensive mutation scanning of *RET* in sporadic medullary thyroid carcinoma and of *RET* and *VHL* in sporadic pheochromocytoma reveals involvement of these genes in only a minority of cases. *J Clin Endocrinol Metab* 1996; **81**:2881–2884.

66. Woodward ER, Eng C, McMahon R, *et al.* Genetic predisposition to phaeochromocytoma: analysis of candidate genes *GDNF*, *RET* and *VHL*. *Hum Mol Genet* 1997; **6**:1051–1056.

67. Gimm O, Armanios M, Dziema H, *et al.* Somatic and occult germline mutations in *SDHD*, a mitochondrial complex II gene, in non-familial pheochromocytomas. *Cancer Res* 2000; **60**:6822–6825.

68. Astuti D, Douglas F, Lennard TWJ, *et al.* Germline *SDHD* mutation in familial phaeochromocytoma. *Lancet* 2001; **357**:1181–1182.

69. Astuti D, Latif F, Dallol A, *et al.* Mutations in the mitochondrial complex II subunit SDHB cause susceptibility to familial paraganglioma and pheochromocytoma. *Am J Hum Genet* 2001; **69**:49–54.

70. Komminoth P, Roth J, Muletta-Feurer S, *et al. RET* proto-oncogene point mutations in sporadic neuroendocrine tumors. *J Clin Endocrinol Metab* 1996; **81**:2041–2046.

71. Santoro M, Carlomagno F, Romano A, *et al.* Activation of *RET* as a dominant transforming gene by germline mutations of MEN 2A and MEN 2B. *Science* 1995; **267**:381–383.

72. Borrello MG, Smith DP, Pasini B, *et al. RET* activation by germline *MEN2A* and *MEN2B* mutations. *Oncogene* 1995; **11**:2419–2427.

73. Asai N, Iwashita T, Matsuyama M, Takahashi M. Mechanism of activation of the *ret* proto-oncogene by multiple endocrine neoplasia 2A mutations. *Mol Cell Biol* 1995; **3**:1613–1619.

74. Ito S, Iwashita T, Asai N, *et al.* Biological properties of Ret with cysteine mutations correlate with multiple endocrine neoplasia type 2A, familial medullary thyroid carcinoma, and Hirschsprung's disease phenotype. *Cancer Res.* 1997; **57**:2870–2872.

75. Carlomagno F, Salvatore G, Cirafici AM, *et al.* The different *RET*-activating capability of mutations of cysteine 620 or cysteine 634 correlates with the multiple endocrine neoplasia type 2 disease phenotype. *Cancer Res.* 1997; **57**:391–395.

76. Hanks SK, Quinn AM, Hunter T. The protein kinase family: conserved features and deduced phylogeny of the catalytic domain. *Science* 1988; **241**:42–52.

77. Songyang Z, Carraway III KL, Eck MJ, *et al.* Catalytic specificity of protein-tyrosine kinases is critical for selective signalling. *Nature* 1995; **373**:536–539.

78. Wells SA, Chi DD, Toshima D, *et al.* Predictive DNA testing and prophylactic thyroidectomy in patients at risk for multiple endocrine neoplasia type 2A. *Ann Surg* 1994; **200**:237–250.

79. Offit K, Biesecker BB, Burt RW, *et al.* Statement of the American Society of Clinical Oncology – Genetic testing for cancer susceptibility. *J Clin Oncol* 1996; **14**:1730–1736.

80. Gimm O, Eng C. Medullary carcinoma of the thyroid. In: Souhami RL, Tannock I, Hohenberger P, Horiot JC (eds) *Oxford textbook of oncology.* Oxford: Oxford University Press, 2002.

81. Eng C, Ponder BAJ. Multiple endocrine neoplasia type 2 and medullary thyroid carcinoma. In: Grossman A (ed.) *Clinical endocrinology.* Oxford: Blackwell Science, 1998: 635–650.

82. Wells SA, Baylin SB, Linehan WM, *et al.* Provocative agents and the diagnosis of medullary carcinoma of the thyroid gland. *Ann Surg* 1978; **188**:139–141.

83. Telenius-Berg M, Almqvist S, Berg B, *et al.* Screening for medullary carcinoma of the thyroid in families with Sipple's syndrome: evaluation of new stimulation tests. *Eur J Clin Invest* 1977; **7**:7–16.

84. Neumann HPH, Reincke M, Bender BU, *et al.* Preserved adrenocortical function after laparoscopic bilateral adrenal sparing surgery for hereditary phaeochromocytoma. *J Clin Endocrinol Metab* 1999; **84**:1608–2610.

85. Neumann HPH, Bender BU, Reincke M, *et al.* Laparoscopic surgery for phaeochromocytoma. *Br J Surg* 1999; **84**:94–97.

86. Walther MM, Herring J, Choyke PL, Linehan WM. Laparoscopic partial adrenalectomy in patients with hereditary forms of pheochromocytoma. *J Urol* 2000; **164**:14–17.

87. Eng C. From bench to bedside ... but when? *Genome Res* 1997; **7**:669–672.

88. Eng C, Mulligan LM, Smith DP, *et al.* Mutation in the *RET* proto-oncogene in sporadic medullary thyroid carcinoma. *Genes Chrom Cancer* 1995; **12**:209–212.

89. Marsh DJ, Andrew SD, Eng C, *et al.* Germline and somatic mutations in an oncogene:*RET* mutations in inherited medullary thyroid carcinoma. *Cancer Res* 1996; **56**:1241–1243.

90. Eng C, Mulligan LM, Healey CS, *et al.* Heterogeneous mutation of the *RET* proto-oncogene in subpopulations of medullary thyroid carcinoma. *Cancer Res* 1996; **56**:2167–2170.

91. Eng C, Marsh DJ, Robinson BG, *et al.* Germline *RET* codon 918 mutation in apparently isolated intestinal ganglioneuromatosis. *J Clin Endocrinol Metab* 1998; **83**:4191–4193.

92. Badner JA, Sieber WK, Garver KL, Chakravarti A. A genetic study of Hirschsprung disease. *Am J Hum Genet* 1990; **46**:568–580.

93. Lyonnet S, Bolino A, Pelet A, *et al.* A gene for Hirschsprung disease maps to the proximal long arm of chromosome 10. *Nature Genet* 1993; **4**:346–350.

94. Angrist M, Kauffman E, Slaugenhaupt SA, *et al.* A gene for Hirschsprung disease (megacolon) in the pericentromeric region of human chromosome 10. *Nature Genet* 1993; **4**:351–356.

95. Edery P, Lyonnet S, Mulligan LM, *et al.* Mutations of the *RET* proto-oncogene in Hirschsprung's disease. *Nature* 1994; **367**:378–380.

96. Romeo G, Ronchetto P, Luo Y, *et al.* Point mutations affecting the tyrosine kinase domain of the *RET* proto-oncogene in Hirschsprung's disease. *Nature* 1994; **367**:377–378.

97. Attié T, Pelet A, Edery P, *et al.* Diversity of *RET* proto-oncogene mutations in familial and sporadic Hirschsprung disease. *Hum Mol Genet* 1995; **4**:1381–1386.

98. Attié T, Pelet A, Sarda P, *et al.* A 7 bp deletion of the RET proto-oncogene in familial Hirschsprung's disease. *Hum Mol Genet* 1994; **3**:1439–1440.

99. Luo Y, Barone V, Seri M, *et al.* Heterogeneity and low detection rate of *RET* mutations in Hirschsprung disease. *Eur J Hum Genet* 1994; **2**:272–280.

100. Angrist M, Bolk S, Thiel B, *et al.* Mutation analysis of the RET receptor tyrosine kinase in Hirschsprung disease. *Hum Mol Genet* 1995; **4**:821–830.

101. Svensson P-J, Molander J-L, Eng C, *et al.* Low frequency of *RET* mutations in Hirschsprung disease in Sweden. *Clin Genet* 1998; **54**:39–44.

102. Bolk S, Pelet A, Hofstra RMW, *et al.* A human model for multigenic inheritance: phenotypic expression in Hirschsprung disease requires both the *RET* gene and a new 9q31 locus. *Proc Natl Acad Sci USA* 1999; **97**:268–273.

103. Borrego S, Eng C, Sánchez B, et al. Molecular analysis of RET and GDNF genes in a family with multiple endocrine neoplasia type 2A and Hirschsprung disease. J Clin Endocrinol Metab 1998; **83**:3361–3364.

104. Puffenberger EG, Hosoda K, Washington SS, et al. A missense mutation of the endothelin B receptor gene in multigenic Hirschsprung's disease. Cell 1995; **79**:1257–1266.

105. Amiel J, Attè T, Jan D, et al. Heterozygous endothelin receptor B (EDNRB) mutations in isolated Hirschsprung disease. Hum Mol Genet 1996; **5**:355–357.

106. Ivanchuk SM, Myers SM, Eng C, Mulligan LM. De novo mutation of GDNF, ligand for RET/GDNFR-a receptor complex in Hirschsprung disease. Hum Mol Genet 1996; **5**:2023–2026.

107. Southard-Smith EM, Kos L, Pavan WJ. Sox10 mutation disrupts neural crest development in Dom Hirschsprung mouse model. Nature Genet 1998; **18**:60–64.

108. Doray B, Salomon R, Amiel J, et al. Mutation of the RET ligands, neurturin, supports multigenic inheritance in Hirschsprung disease. Hum Mol Genet 1998; **7**:1449–1452.

109. Myers SM, Salomon R, Gössling A, et al. Absence of germline GFRa-1 mutations in Hirschsprung disease. J Med Genet 1999; **36**:217–220.

110. Onochie CI, Korngut LM, Vanhorne JB, et al. Characterisation of the GFRalpha-3 locus and investigation of the gene in Hirschsprung disease. J Med Genet 2000; **37**:669–673.

111. Vanhorne JB, Gimm O, Myers SM, et al. Cloning and characterization of the human GFRA2 locus and investigation of the gene in Hirschsprung disease. Hum Genet 2001; **108**:409–415.

112. Borrego S, Saez ME, Ruiz A, et al. Specific polymorphisms in the RET proto-oncogene are over-represented in individuals with Hirschsprung disease and may represent loci modifying phenotypic expression. J Med Genet 1999; **36**:771–774.

113. Sancandi M, Ceccherini I, Costa M, et al. Incidence of RET mutations in patients with Hirschsprung's disease. J Pediatr Surg 2000; **35**:139–142.

114. Borrego S, Saez ME, Ruiz A, et al. RET genotypes comprising specific haplotypes of polymorphic variants predispose to isolated Hirschsprung disease. J Med Genet 2000; **37**:572–578.

115. Mulligan LM, Eng C, Attè T, et al. Diverse phenotypes associated with exon 10 mutations of the RET proto-oncogene. Hum Mol Genet 1994; **3**:2163–2167.

116. Caron P, Attè T, David D, et al. C618R mutation in exon 10 of the RET proto-oncogene in a kindred with multiple endocrine neoplasia type 2A and Hirschsprung's disease. J Clin Endocrinol Metab 1996; **81**:2731–2733.

117. Decker RA, Peacock ML. Occurrence of MEN 2a in familial Hirschsprung disease: another new indication for genetic testing of the RET proto-oncogene. J Pediatr Surg 1998; **33**:207–214.

118. Inoue K, Shimotake T, Inoue K, et al. Mutational analysis of the RET proto-oncogene in a kindred with multiple endocrine neoplasia type 2A and Hirschsprung's disease. J Pediatr Surg 1999; **34**:1552–1554.

119. Blaugrund JE, Johns MM, Eby YJ, et al. RET proto-oncogene mutations in inherited and sporadic medullary thyroid cancer. Hum Mol Genet 1994; **3**:1895–1897.

120. Zedenius J, Wallin G, Hamberger B, et al. Somatic and MEN 2A de novo mutations identified in the RET proto-oncogene by screening of sporadic MTCs. Hum Mol Genet 1994; **3**:1259–1262.

121. Komminoth P, Kunz EK, Matias-Guiu X, et al. Analysis of RET proto-oncogene point mutations distinguishes heritable from nonheritable medullary thyroid carcinomas. Cancer 1995; **76**:479–489.

122. Marsh DJ, Learoyd DL, Andrew SD, et al. Somatic mutations in the RET proto-oncogene in sporadic medullary thyroid carcinoma. Clin Endocrinol 1996; **44**:249–257.

123. Romei C, Elisei R, Pinchera A, et al. Somatic mutations of the RET proto-oncogene in sporadic medullary thyroid carcinoma are not restricted to exon 16 and are associated with tumor recurrence. J Clin Endocrinol Metab 1996; **81**:1619–1622.

124. Eng C, Thomas GA, Neuberg DS, et al. Mutation of the RET proto-oncogene is correlated with RET immunostaining in subpopulations of cells in sporadic medullary thyroid carcinoma. J Clin Endocrinol Metab 1998; **83**:4310–4313.

125. Ferraris AM, Mangerini R, Gaetani GF, et al. Polyclonal origin of medullary carcinoma of the thyroid in multiple endocrine neoplasia type 2. Hum Genet 1997; **99**:202–205.

126. Zedenius J, Larsson C, Bergholm U, et al. Mutations of codon 918 in the RET proto-oncogene correlate to poor prognosis in sporadic medullary thyroid carcinoma. J Clin Endocrinol Metab 1995; **80**:3088–3090.

127. Schilling T, Burck J, Sinn HP, et al. Prognostic value of codon 918 (ATG->ACG) RET proto-oncogene mutations in sporadic medullary thyroid carcinoma. Int J Cancer 2001; **95**:62–66.

128. Komminoth P, Kunz E, Hiort O, et al. Detection of RET proto-oncogene point mutations in paraffin-embedded pheochromocytoma specimens by nonradioactive single-strand conformation polymorphism analysis and direct sequencing. Am J Pathol 1994; **145**:922–929.

129. Neumann HPH, Brauch B, McWhinney SR, et al. Germline mutations in non-syndromic pheochromocytoma. N Engl J Med 2002; **346**:1459–1466.

9

Wilms tumour and other childhood renal tumours

KATHRYN PRITCHARD-JONES AND NORMAN BRESLOW

INTRODUCTION

Primary cancers of the kidney are rare at any age. Although only a small proportion of cases is clearly inherited, genetic predisposition is the most important aetiological factor identified in this group of tumours to date.

EPIDEMIOLOGY

Malignant kidney tumours affect about one Caucasian child in every 10 000 before 15 years of age.[1] Ninety per cent are Wilms tumour (nephroblastoma), but the histological type of tumour depends very much on the age of onset. Congenital mesoblastic nephroma, diagnosed in infancy, accounts for less than 1 per cent of the total incidence of childhood renal tumours. Rhabdoid tumour of the kidney, which presents at a median age of only 10–12 months and is associated with a high risk of independent brain tumours, accounts for another 2 per cent. The very early ages and, for rhabdoid tumour, the associated brain cancers, are suggestive of a genetic predisposition, which has recently been proven for rhabdoid tumour. Clear cell sarcoma of the kidney, which accounts for 3–4 per cent of total incidence, lacks any such feature. A few children, mostly over the age of 10, develop renal cell carcinoma similar to that seen in adults, where the incidence rises rapidly with increasing age over 40 years.

At least 90 per cent of childhood renal tumours are Wilms tumours. It is now clear that multiple genes are involved in both genetic predisposition and somatic mutations in this tumour type.[2] The median age at onset peaks at 3–4 years and the incidence declines rapidly thereafter (Figure 9.1). Wilms tumours are slightly more common in Blacks both in Africa and America, but only a third as common among Asians.[1] The age at onset distributions, and the tendency for incidence rates to vary more strongly with ethnicity than with geography or over time, suggest that genetic factors play an important role in its aetiology. It is possible that early exposure to strong environmental carcinogens, perhaps in utero or in combination with genetic factors, could also lead to tumour development. Such an intrauterine effect has been shown in the ethylnitrosourea-induced rat model of nephroblastoma.[3] A series of relatively small case-control studies of human populations have, however, failed to identify consistent environmental risk factors. Larger studies that pay greater attention to problems of measurement error and selection bias will be needed before definite conclusions about environmental effects can be drawn.

WILMS TUMOUR

Wilms tumour is one of the embryonal tumours of childhood, so-called because the growth pattern of the tumour shows a remarkable mimicry of structures seen during normal embryonic kidney development. At least

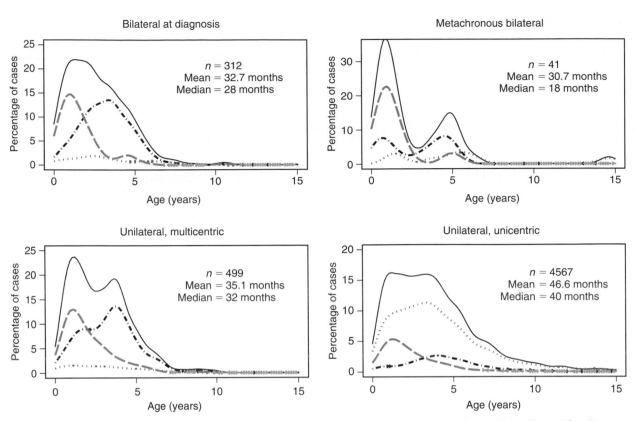

Figure 9.1 *Distributions of age-at-onset for National Wilms Tumour Study Group patients according to bilaterality and focality (centricity) of tumour. Limited to patients for whom nephrogenic rests could be evaluated. Each distribution is decomposed into three subdistributions defined by the type of rests: dashed line, intralobular nephrogenic rest (ILNR) ± perilobular nephrogenic rest (PLNR); dashed and dotted line, PLNR only; dotted line, neither.*

90 per cent of Wilms tumours occur as a sporadic event in an otherwise normal child. One to two per cent of cases have a family history of Wilms tumour and 2–3 per cent occur in children with congenital malformation syndromes that carry a greatly increased risk of Wilms tumour (Table 9.1). A further 5 per cent occur in children with an isolated malformation, either hemihypertrophy or genital abnormality in males (cryptorchidism and/or hypospadias). Wilms tumour is associated with presumed precursor lesions in the kidney, known as nephrogenic rests, which have been classified into two major types (perilobar and intralobar) according to position and morphology.[4] Intralobar nephrogenic rests (ILNRs) are thought to result from a very early, probably germline, mutation, whereas perilobar nephrogenic rests (PLNRs) are thought to represent a slightly later insult to the embryonic kidney. Overall, nephrogenic rests are found in adjacent normal kidney in up to 40 per cent of unilateral and almost 100 per cent of bilateral Wilms tumours.

Genetics of Wilms tumour and Knudson's 'two-hit' hypothesis

In 1972, Knudson proposed that his 'two-hit' mutational model, which had been formulated originally for

retinoblastoma, could also serve as a model for Wilms tumour[5,6] (see Chapter 2). Briefly, the hypothesis states that as few as two mutations are sufficient to allow tumour development and that the first of these mutations can be in the germline, in which case tumours tend to occur earlier and to be bilateral. The assumption was made that all familial and bilateral cases were carriers of a germline mutation.

Although the initial statistical analysis of small numbers of familial and bilateral cases suggested that the two-hit hypothesis should apply, the situation is now clearly more complex than for retinoblastoma. Allele loss and genetic linkage studies have provided evidence for the existence of up to 10 Wilms tumour genes, the *WT1* gene at chromosome 11p13, two or more genes involved in Beckwith–Wiedemann syndrome at 11p15, at least three familial Wilms tumour genes, *FWT1* at 17q12–21, *FWT2* at 19q, and other as yet unmapped *FWT* genes as well as genes involved in other overgrowth syndromes that have Wilms tumour as a rare component (Simpson–Golabi–Behmel syndrome, due to the *GPC3* gene; Perlman syndrome). Wilms tumour has been described in Li–Fraumeni pedigrees and the *TP53* gene is mutated somatically in anaplastic Wilms tumour. Allele loss studies have identified further loci for genes involved in

Table 9.1 *Genetics of Wilms tumour-associated syndromes*

	Wilms tumour – aniridia	Denys–Drash syndrome	Beckwith–Wiedemann syndrome (BWS)	Perlman syndrome
Prevalence among Wilms tumour cases	~1%	<1%	~0.5%[a]	Extremely rare
Risk of Wilms tumour	30–50%	High (>50%)	3–5%	High (>50%)
Genetics and mode of inheritance	*de novo* germline mutation Rarely familial (AD)	*de novo* germline mutation Rarely familial	*de novo* germline mutation Familial 15% (AD variable expressivity)	Familial (AR)
Chromosomal locus	11p13	11p13	11p15.5	Unknown
Disease gene(s)	*WT1* (and aniridia gene, *PAX6*)	*WT1*	*p57* in ~10%	Unknown
Types of mutation	Contiguous gene syndrome Complete deletion of one allele of *WT1* and *PAX6* genes	Point mutation (mainly missense) Frameshift Aberrant mRNA splicing	Polygenic disorder Alterations of *IGF2* & *H19* imprinting are common	

[a] A further 2.5% of all cases have hemihypertrophy, which may represent a 'forme fruste' of BWS.
AD, autosomal dominant; AR, autosomal recessive.

somatic mutation in Wilms tumour at 16q, 22q and 1p. In those Wilms tumours that do involve mutations in the *WT1* gene, while the majority carry mutations in both *WT1* alleles, several cases have been described where only one *WT1* allele is mutated.[7,8] Until the promoter region of the *WT1* gene has been fully examined in these tumours, one cannot be confident that they do not conform to the two-hit model, but it seems likely that other genes are interacting, particularly since several have allele loss confined to chromosome 11p15.

A further prediction of the two-hit model is the proportion of unilateral sporadic cases that represent carriers of germline predisposing mutations. For retinoblastoma, the predicted 10–12 per cent was borne out by the observed 5.5 per cent tumour rate amongst offspring. Originally, Knudson and Strong[5] calculated that 30 per cent of unilateral Wilms tumours might be prezygotically determined, based on an 8 per cent incidence of bilateral tumours and the assumption that all bilateral cases indicated a heritable mutation. The incidence of bilateral, including metachronous bilateral, disease observed in 8000 patients registered by the National Wilms Tumor Study Group (NWTSG) until 1999, is 7 per cent overall and 16 per cent among 112 confirmed familial cases. This would imply that 7 out of 16 (=44 per cent) of all Wilms tumours, and 40 per cent of unilateral cases, are hereditary (i.e. the result of a dominant germline mutation). Penetrance is believed to be variable and available estimates range from 15 per cent to as high as 63 per cent.[5,9,10] Assuming a penetrance of 20 per cent, the recurrence risk in offspring of patients with unilateral disease would be $0.40 \times 0.50 \times 0.20 = 4$ per cent. This is only slightly greater than the risk of 3 per cent estimated actuarially

from the occurrence of three Wilms tumours in 146 liveborn offspring of 78 survivors of unilateral disease in the UK.[11] The actuarial estimate is likely to be too high, however, owing to the failure to account for the statistical dependence between two of the offspring with Wilms tumour who were born to a single survivor. Two earlier series from the USA identified only one Wilms tumour among 197 liveborn offspring of 108 survivors of unilateral disease, yielding an estimated recurrence risk of 0.5 per cent.[12,13] The upper 95 per cent confidence limit for the US estimate is 2.8 per cent, however, and not all offspring had been followed beyond the period of risk for Wilms tumour. Thus, the estimate of 40 per cent for the hereditary fraction of unilateral cases, while plausible if penetrance is low, is not easily reconciled with the low recurrence risk and low percentage of familial disease.

The two-hit model predicts that patients with unilateral multifocal disease must also carry a germline mutation. Because the multiple tumours that may occur in gene carriers are assumed to be randomly distributed between the two kidneys, the model implies further that bilateral cases should outnumber unilateral multifocal cases. However, precisely the opposite has been observed in two large epidemiological studies, and the differences between the observed frequencies and those expected under the model were highly significant statistically.[14,15] It is now clear that the cases with multifocal disease are heterogeneous and it is quite possible that not all of them carry a germline mutation. Phenotypic evidence for heterogeneity comes from the bimodality of the age distributions, especially for the unilateral, multifocal and metachronous bilateral cases (Figure 9.1). The bimodality is entirely explained by the striking differences in the age distributions for the ILNR and PLNR associated cases and the fact that rest-associated tumours tend to be bilateral or multifocal.[4,14] In the NWTSG series, nephrogenic rests were found in 90 per cent of cases that were bilateral at onset, in 83 per cent of metachronous bilateral cases and in 91 per cent of the unilateral, multifocal cases. By contrast, they were found in only 30 per cent of the unilateral unifocal cases.

Wilms tumour – aniridia syndrome and the *WT1* gene

The association of aniridia (lack of iris formation) with Wilms tumour has been recognized since the 1960s. Approximately 1 per cent of children with Wilms tumour also have congenital aniridia, which is far in excess of the 1 in 50 000 population prevalence. Geneticists recognize two forms of aniridia: familial and sporadic. Only the latter group has a greatly increased risk of Wilms tumour, which affects 30–50 per cent of individuals with this phenotype. The explanation for this discrepancy is that in the familial form, the mutation is confined to the aniridia gene, whereas the sporadic form is the result of an interstitial deletion on the short arm of chromosome 11, which causes constitutional hemizygosity for both the aniridia and Wilms tumour genes as well as many other neighbouring genes. Such individuals frequently have other phenotypic abnormalities, hence the name WAGR (Wilms tumour, aniridia, genitourinary malformation and mental retardation) syndrome. Aniridia is dominant and a marker for the syndrome, whereas development of Wilms tumour is recessive at a cellular level, requiring at least a second mutation. There is a high incidence of genitourinary malformation in this syndrome, particularly amongst XY individuals, who may be phenotypically female.

High-resolution molecular mapping of the smallest regions of common overlap of chromosomal deletions from several WAGR patients has established that the aniridia gene lies about 1 Mb telomeric to the Wilms tumour gene within 11p13 and this has led to the cloning of both genes – human *PAX6* and *WT1*, respectively.[16–18] Molecular analysis of individuals with submicroscopic deletions suggests that at least some of the genitourinary abnormalities in the WAGR syndrome are due to dominant effects of mutation in the *WT1* gene rather than to deletion of neighbouring genes.[19] This has been confirmed by mutational analysis in the Denys–Drash syndrome and in two cases of familial Wilms tumour (see later).

Six out of eight WAGR patients whose Wilms tumours have been subjected to molecular analysis have a mutation in their remaining *WT1* allele, in accord with the two-hit hypothesis.[17,20–23] The two negative cases could still harbour *WT1* promoter mutations, as this region of the *WT1* gene was not examined. The nature of the second hit in the Wilms tumours developing in WAGR patients is nearly always a small deletion/insertion or point mutation, in contrast to the more usual mechanism of mitotic recombination to duplicate the mutant allele. This is because homozygous deletion of the reticulocalbin gene between *WT1* and *PAX6* is lethal to the cell.[24]

CHARACTERIZATION OF THE *WT1* GENE

The *WT1* gene encodes a 3-kb mRNA, which shows tissue-specific expression in the developing embryo, mainly in the genitourinary tract and mesothelium.[25,26] Expression continues at lower levels in the adult kidney and gonad. The predicted protein contains four zinc finger motifs and an N-terminal effector domain (Figure 9.2). *In vitro* studies have shown that the protein binds to DNA, the target sequence depending on the presence or absence of an alternative three amino acid splice (KTS) between zinc fingers 3 and 4. The effector domain appears to contain two regions, one a repressor, and the other an activator of transcription. In studies *in vitro*, the functional balance is usually in favour of repression, although the ratio of ±KTS isoforms or mutations in either the target promoter or the effector domain of *WT1* can reverse this.[27,28] The genes regulated by the WT1 protein *in vivo*

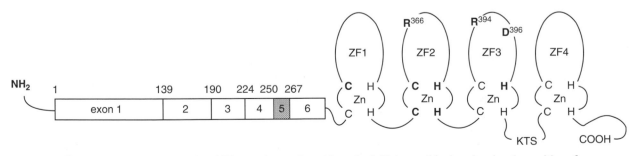

Figure 9.2 *Schematic representation of the WT1 protein, numbered from the initiator methionine, showing the position of exon boundaries. Exon 5 (shaded) and the three extra amino acids (KTS) between zinc fingers (ZF) 3 and 4 are subject to alternative splicing. Amino acids indicated in bold are sites of missense mutations in the Denys–Drash syndrome – R^{394} is by far the most common mutation, occurring in 24 out of 51 cases, with missense mutations in zinc fingers 2 or 3 accounting for a total of 41 out of 51 cases. This is in contrast to other germline intragenic WT1 mutations, where 6/7 introduce premature stop codons.*[37]

are still not fully elucidated, as all of the *in vitro* studies of WT1 transcription factor function have used single isoforms of the protein, whereas it is likely to function physiologically as a complex. However, several cell signalling or proliferative genes have been suggested, such as insulin like growth factor II, epidermal growth factor and amphireglin. WT1 is also thought to be involved in RNA metabolism, as the +KTS isoforms have been shown to co-localize with some elements of the splicing machinery in the nucleus and to bind directly to certain mRNAs. The *WT1* gene is known to be essential for formation of the metanephric kidney and gonad, as shown by the complete absence of these two organs in homozygous −wt1 null mice.[29] About 10–20 per cent of sporadic Wilms tumours have been found to have *WT1* gene mutations, most of which result in premature termination codons and presumed loss of protein function.[7,8,16,30–37] In the majority of cases, the two-hit model is followed, but several tumours have been described where only one *WT1* allele can be shown to be mutated.

Other syndromes predisposing to Wilms tumour

DENYS–DRASH SYNDROME

Denys–Drash syndrome (DDS) is a very rare, sporadic syndrome, which was described originally as a triad of male pseudohermaphroditism, early-onset protein-losing nephropathy and Wilms tumour.[38,39] The nephropathy appears to be due to a distinctive glomerular lesion, which involves the podocyte layer. It has been suggested that the syndrome should be expanded to include patients with any two of these three features and normal females with the characteristic nephropathy.[40] The risk of Wilms tumour is high, but difficult to quantify exactly as, until recently, tumour occurrence was almost a prerequisite for defining the syndrome. There is overlap with Frasier syndrome, which is characterized by later onset nephropathy and gonadal dysgenesis, with predisposition to gonadal rather than Wilms tumour. Certainly, any child with a congenital gonadal abnormality and nephropathy should be considered at greatly increased risk of Wilms and gonadal tumours.

The observation that the *WT1* gene was expressed in the three cell types showing abnormalities in DDS (i.e. metanephric blastema, podocytes, developing gonad) made it an ideal candidate gene for this syndrome.[26] This prediction was borne out when ten children with a clinical diagnosis of DDS were found to have constitutional *WT1* missense mutations in the zinc finger region.[41] Initially, it appeared that missense mutations affecting amino acids critical for the stability of DNA binding of zinc fingers 2 and 3 were responsible for the syndrome, with the genital malformation being dominant, but tumour development

requiring a second hit. Subsequently, although missense mutations of Arg[394] remain the most common group, several cases with nonsense mutations causing truncated proteins have been described (see Figure 9.2). As a unifying hypothesis, it has been suggested that the constitutionally mutant WT1 protein may behave as a dominant-negative or antimorph, somehow interfering with the function of the remaining wild-type allele.[42,43] It is also now apparent that a normal ratio of the second alternative splice in zinc finger 3 is essential for both gonadal development and podocyte function. Several patients originally diagnosed with DDS but now thought to be Frasier syndrome (gonadal tumours plus later onset nephrotic syndrome) have intronic mutations preventing formation of the +KTS splice.[44] It is perhaps debatable whether Denys–Drash and Frasier syndromes are distinct entities or form two ends of a spectrum of disorders of intersex and nephropathy.[45]

It is an interesting paradox that complete deletion of the *WT1* gene, as in the WAGR syndrome, gives a less severe genitourinary phenotype than the presence of a mutant WT1 protein. This protein must, therefore, be interfering with the function of other cellular proteins in some way. However, the final phenotypic expression of *WT1* mutations must depend on the host genetic make-up, as two children with DDS phenotype but constitutional *WT1* deletions have been described.[40,46] Conversely, the most common DDS mutation (Arg[394] → Trp) has been found in the germline of a normal female with unilateral Wilms tumour who has no evidence of nephropathy at the age of 7 years, making it unlikely that nephropathy will develop.[30] There is also a case of germline transmission of the same mutation from an unaffected father to a son with DDS.[47] Furthermore, a review of the genital phenotype of 20 children with identical Arg[394] → Trp mutations shows a wide range, from normal female to complete ambiguity.[48] This paradox is partially explained by studies in transgenic mice bearing the Arg[394] mutation.[49] Only a single heterozygote could be established, due to almost complete failure to transmit this mutant *WT1* through the germline. In both the heterozygote and chimaeras, the typical mesangial sclerosis of DDS was seen in the kidneys as well as male genital defects. In heterozygous embryonic stem cells, the mutant WT1 protein accounted for only 5 per cent of total WT1, implying that its presence has profound effects on the cellular phenotype.

BECKWITH–WIEDEMANN SYNDROME

The Beckwith–Wiedemann syndrome (BWS) is characterized by prenatal and postnatal gigantism, which may be asymmetric, leading to hemihypertrophy, as well as malformation, particularly of the heart and genitourinary system.[50] There is hyperplasia of many organs, including the tongue and intra-abdominal organs, with defects of closure of the abdominal wall (exomphalos). The kidneys often show persistent fetal characteristics and medullary dysplasia. These children have a 7.5–20.0 per cent overall risk of developing a childhood tumour, at least half of which are Wilms tumour, the remainder comprising hepatoblastoma, adrenocortical carcinoma and, occasionally, rhabdomyosarcoma and neuroblastoma.[16,50] BWS occurs in approximately 1 per cent of patients with Wilms tumour.[14] Most cases are sporadic, but familial cases have been described.

The familial cases show genetic linkage to chromosome 11p15.5 and there is an excess of maternal inheritance.[51,52] Apparently balanced 11p15 translocations occurring in BWS patients also involve the maternal allele. Several sporadic cases have been shown to have uniparental disomy or trisomy for 11p15.5, with the extra copy being of paternal origin. These findings have been interpreted as signifying involvement of genomic imprinting. Several imprinted genes within 11p15 have been identified, including the fetal mitogen, insulin-like growth factor II (IGF-II), which is normally imprinted (i.e. inactive) on the maternal allele, the H19 and KVLQT1 genes, which are paternally imprinted, and the cell cycle regulator, p57^{KIP2}, which is partially imprinted, being mainly expressed from the maternal allele.[53] Investigation of these genes in BWS show that the syndrome is genetically heterogeneous. Germline mutations of p57^{KIP2} are common in familial but rare in sporadic cases.[54] BWS-associated translocations disrupt the KVLQT1 gene (involved in long QT syndrome) and may target an antisense intronic transcript (LIT1) to cause its biallelic expression.[55] A model has been proposed whereby these genes lie within two imprinted subdomains, the more telomeric containing the IGF-2 and H19 genes, and the more centromeric including CDKN1C/p57^{KIP2}, LIT1 and KVLQT1.[55,56] Disturbances of methylation in either domain could affect imprinting and cause the BWS phenotype through biallelic expression of the growth-promoting IGF2 or silencing of the growth-suppressing CDKN1C/p57^{KIP2}. A second BWS-associated translocation cluster within 11p15 disrupts an imprinted zinc finger gene.[56] However, of these genes for which there is either direct mutational proof or suggestive evidence that they are causative for BWS none are clearly mutated in sporadic Wilms tumour.[57] This is despite allele loss data implicating the BWS locus, with one-third of sporadic Wilms tumours showing allele loss on chromosome 11p, restricted to 11p15 in a third of such cases (i.e. excludes the WT1 gene). There does, however, appear to be a common cellular phenotype of loss of imprinting (LOI) of IGFII in both BWS and sporadic Wilms tumour.[58] There is evidence that the mechanism for LOI of IGFII may involve disruption of other imprinted genes within the region. The interactions of alterations in CDKN1C/p57^{KIP2} and IGF2 have been investigated in mouse models. The cdkn1c/p57^{KIP2} knock-

out mouse has overlapping phenotypic features with BWS. By crossing these animals on to a strain with loss of imprinting of igf2, some features are shown to be igf2 independent and this may explain how BWS can arise from mutations in either gene.[59] In the future, it may be possible to predict the tumour risk in individuals with BWS by detailed molecular analysis of these two imprinted domains, but it is premature based on the current evidence to remove patients from screening programmes.[60–62]

OTHER OVERGROWTH SYNDROMES

Children with isolated hemihypertrophy, which may be of a single limb or digit, but without other stigmata of BWS, are also at increased risk of embryonal tumours, including Wilms tumour.[63] Hemihypertrophy is found in 2.5–3.3 per cent of Wilms tumour patients generally, which is about 500-fold greater than the prevalence in the general population, and in 40–45 per cent of those that occur in association with BWS.[64] It is possible that children with isolated hemihypertrophy represent a forme fruste of BWS, owing to defective imprinting and consequent overexpression of IGF-II in a mosaic fashion.[63]

Simpson–Golabi–Behmel syndrome (SGBS) is an X-linked disorder with considerable phenotypic overlap with BWS. It is associated with constitutional mutations in the glypican 3 gene, GPC3.[65] The risk of Wilms tumour in this syndrome is not well quantified, although cases do occur. However, to date, sporadic Wilms tumour does not appear to commonly involve GPC3 mutations.[66]

PERLMAN SYNDROME

Perlman syndrome is a rare congenital malformation syndrome that includes fetal gigantism, nephroblastomatosis and cryptorchidism. This syndrome has so far been reported in only ten separate families.[67–72] It shows some phenotypic overlap with BWS, but appears to be a distinct entity, with autosomal recessive inheritance, high neonatal mortality and an extremely high risk of Wilms tumour; of 18 cases reported, eight were neonatal deaths, one with a congenital Wilms tumour, and five of six survivors developed Wilms tumour at an early age, three being bilateral.

OTHER PHENOTYPES ASSOCIATED WITH WILMS TUMOUR

A retrospective study found three cases of neurofibromatosis type I among 342 children with Wilms tumour and suggested that this condition conferred a 29-fold increased risk of Wilms tumour.[73] Subsequent larger studies have failed to confirm this level of risk,[74] although anecdotal reports suggest that a link does exist.[75] Indeed, it is interesting that, in the rat, transplacental carcinogenic insults can give rise to either plexiform neurofibromas or Wilms tumour.[3]

A retrospective study of a population-based series of 176 Wilms tumour patients in Manchester suggested that up to 3 per cent of cases may occur within Li–Fraumeni syndrome families.[76] However, in one family with a *TP53* mutation affecting splicing, the child with Wilms tumour was not a mutation carrier.[77] Several other syndromes have been reported in association with Wilms tumour (e.g. trisomy 18, other overgrowth syndromes, such as Sotos–Klippel-Trelaunay), but their small numbers make the causality of these associations unknown.[78]

Familial Wilms tumour

EPIDEMIOLOGY

Familial Wilms tumour has been documented in 0.5–1.4 per cent of cases in two large series.[79,80] The rare pedigrees reported fall into two main categories: small families with an affected parent and child/children, or large pedigrees with several cases among cousins and uncles or aunts. Bilaterality and the occurrence of pulmonary metastases seem to cluster within certain families. These features have been interpreted to show autosomal dominant inheritance of the predisposition to Wilms tumour, but with variable penetrance and expressivity.[81] The age distribution of the familial cases in the large NWTSG series was similar to that of the non-familial, bilateral-at-onset cases, each having a mean of 32 months.[80] However, children with familial bilateral disease were younger still (Figure 9.3). This observation conflicts with the notion that the younger ages of the bilateral cases, whether familial or the result of a *de novo* germline mutation, are due simply to the shorter waiting time until occurrence of the second 'hit' in patients whose cells already all bear the first one.

The hereditary fraction under the two stage model (i.e. the fraction of Wilms tumour cases due to a dominant germline mutation) was originally estimated as 0.08/0.21 = 38 per cent.[5] This is quite close to the estimate of 0.07/0.16 = 44 per cent made above using recent NWTSG data. Alternatively, the hereditary fraction may be estimated as twice the concordance rate in dizygotic (DZ) twins, or as the concordance rate in monozygotic (MZ) twins, each divided by the penetrance. However, none of 31 MZ and only 1 of 35 DZ co-twins of NWTSG patients were concordant.[82] Assuming 20 per cent penetrance, the estimate of the hereditary fraction from these data on twins is only 10 per cent, but with an upper 95 per cent confidence limit of 45 per cent. Two of the MZ probands with Wilms tumour had bilateral disease. In one DZ pair, the co-twin also had hypospadias, suggesting that a shared genetic defect could manifest as either tumour or malformation. Four twin pairs had a family history of Wilms tumour in an aunt or cousin, and three were MZ pairs who remained discordant well beyond the normal risk period. Taken together, these data suggest that at least some of the Wilms tumour genes have a low penetrance or very variable expressivity. Even assuming a penetrance as low as 20 per cent, however, it is difficult to reconcile the twin data with the higher estimates of the hereditary fraction that stem from the assumption that all bilateral cases are hereditary. Additional studies of twins, and follow-up of the many children now being born to Wilms tumour survivors, will be required to resolve the issue.

GENETICS OF FAMILIAL WILMS TUMOUR

Following the cloning of *WT1*, linkage analysis of the three largest Wilms tumour pedigrees excluded both this

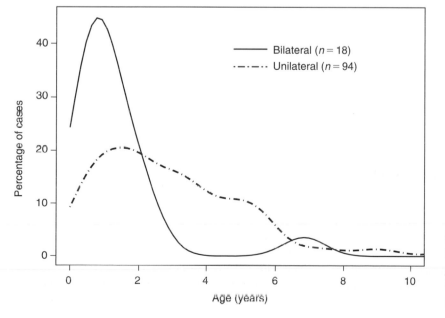

Figure 9.3 *Distributions of age at onset for National Wilms Tumour Study Group patients with familial Wilms tumour: bilateral (at onset or metachronous) vs. unilateral.*

gene, the more distal BWS locus on chromosome 11, and chromosome 16, as the site of the Wilms tumour gene in these families.[83–85] Constitutional *WT1* mutations do account for a minority of familial Wilms tumour, usually small pedigrees with parent–child transmission and genitourinary abnormalities in males.[86–88] A genomewide linkage search in a large pedigree with familial Wilms tumour localized an *FWT1* gene to 17q12–21.[89] Further analyses have confirmed linkage to this locus in an independent large pedigree, but have also shown that familial Wilms tumour is genetically heterogeneous.[90,91] The penetrance of *FWT1* has been estimated to be low, between 15 and 30 per cent.[9] Attempts to isolate this gene have been hampered by the lack of allele loss at this locus in sporadic Wilms tumour, suggesting that *FWT1* is not a tumour suppressor gene.[92] There is also linkage evidence for a further gene, *FWT2*, on 19q.[93] Both of these loci can be excluded in several small pedigrees.[91]

Identification and screening of Wilms tumour patients with genetic predispostion

The possibility of genetic predisposition should be considered in any child with Wilms tumour of early onset (<2 years) Wilms or an additional congenital abnormality, particularly of the genitourinary tract. All patients should be examined repeatedly for evidence of hemihypertrophy or neurofibromatosis, which may only become evident sometime after the diagnosis of Wilms tumour. The complete features of BWS or aniridia will usually have been diagnosed previously, and the child should be under follow-up. Wilms tumour has been observed to occur particularly in children with BWS who have persistent nephromegaly on repeated abdominal sonography, but it would be unwise at present to limit surveillance to this subgroup.[94,95] Children with bilateral and multifocal Wilms tumour should be considered to carry a germline mutation until proven otherwise. Currently, there are few survivors of bilateral disease who have gone on to reproduce, so their genetic burden is not established. Children in whom nephrogenic rests have been found, particularly when the diagnosis is made during the first year of life, should be considered at increased risk of developing another Wilms tumour in their remaining kidney.[96]

Currently all children with a presumed genetic predisposition can only be screened for *WT1* mutations or some of the genes involved in the overgrowth syndromes. Familial genes *FWT1* and *FWT2* have yet to be cloned and others remain to be discovered, while familial transmission of a mutated *WT1* is observed only rarely. Thus, the failure to identify a *WT1* mutation does not exclude a genetic predisposition. At least 90 per cent of patients, moreover, do not harbour constitutional *WT1* mutations.

An analysis of 201 unselected patients from the NWTSG revealed only eight with constitutional *WT1* mutations; seven of these were boys with genitourinary abnormalities.[97] There was no excess of *WT1* mutations among children with bilateral disease (3 out of 21), family history of Wilms tumour (1 out of 14) or presence of nephrogenic rests (2 out of 40), whereas one-quarter (7 out of 28) of boys with cryptorchidism and Wilms tumour carried a *WT1* mutation. No carrier was found among 56 patients with isolated unilateral Wilms tumour.[97]

Screening of children at known or presumed increased risk of Wilms tumour remains problematic. There are no comparative studies of ultrasound versus teaching the parents to perform regular abdominal palpation, nor of screening interval. Children with the BWS or WAGR syndromes whose tumours are detected by ultrasound screening tend to have lower stage disease.[98,99] It is suggested that the screening interval should be no greater than 3 months, at least during the period of maximum risk up to about age 5 years. Increased screening of BWS patients has apparently led to smaller Wilms tumours at nephrectomy in recent years.[100] There is no definitive evidence as yet, however, that routine radiographic screening has actually improved patient survival.

LONG-TERM FOLLOW-UP OF WILMS TUMOUR SURVIVORS IN RELATION TO GENETIC PREDISPOSITION

With the increasing number of survivors of Wilms tumour, long-term follow-up is essential in order to document the health care benefit associated with use of combination drug and radiation therapy. Patients whose disease results from a specific genetic predisposition may be at particularly high risk of late effects of treatment. Survivors of the hereditary form of retinoblastoma who received radiation therapy, for example, are prone to develop osteosarcoma in later life. The renal nephropathy associated with the DDS usually leads to end-stage renal disease either before or within a few years after the diagnosis of Wilms tumour. Children with the WAGR syndrome are also at high risk of renal failure after the onset of puberty, while those having isolated genitourinary anomalies or ILNR are at moderately increased risk (Figure 9.4).[101] It would be prudent to monitor patients in these subgroups for hypertension or other signs of incipient renal failure and to initiate appropriate intervention should this occur. These observations provide indirect evidence for a potential role of *WT1* in the aetiology of the renal pathology, but this has not been confirmed. The role of genetic factors in the occurrence of secondary malignant neoplasms and cardiomyopathies, most of which are attributed to treatment with radiation or doxorubicin, respectively, or their combination, has yet to be elucidated. However, some second primary tumours, particularly mesothelioma and

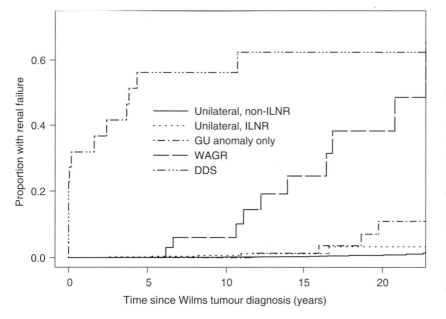

Figure 9.4 *Cumulative risk of renal failure in five subgroups of patients defined hierarchically by the presence of a specific congenital anomaly or syndrome or intralobar nephrogenic rests (ILNRs): DDS, Denys–Drash syndrome; GU anomaly only, isolated male hypospadias or cryptorchidism; unilateral ILNR, unilateral disease with ILNR but without any listed syndrome or anomaly; unilateral non ILNR, unilateral disease without ILNR and without any syndrome or anomaly; WAGR, Wilms tumour/aniridia syndrome.*

acute leukaemias, may be due to constitutional *WT1* mutation.[102–104]

OTHER RENAL TUMOURS

Malignant rhabdoid tumour of kidney (MRTK)

Rhabdoid tumour of the kidney is rare (2 per cent of childhood kidney tumours) and usually follows an aggressive course with fatal outcome, despite intensive chemotherapy. The histological appearances can be diverse, causing confusion with other renal tumours such as clear cell sarcoma and congenital mesoblastic nephroma. Approximately 10–15 per cent of cases are associated with brain tumours that are thought to be independent primaries and display a broad histological spectrum including primitive neuroectodermal tumours (PNETs) and 'atypical teratoid/rhabdoid tumour'.[105] The histogenesis of this tumour type is unknown. Cytogenetic analyses of tumours and cell lines revealed consistent translocations with breaks at 22q11. These proved to be associated with homozygous deletion of the *SNF5/INI1* gene and revealed a new class of genes involved in cancer predisposition.[106] The *INI1* gene encodes the BAF47/SNF5 subunit of an evolutionarily conserved complex involved in chromatin remodelling, which allows access of the transcriptional machinery to their targets. Germline mutations in the *INI1* gene are found in approximately half of children with MRTK, but in the one case so far examined, this was a new mutation, which was not inherited from the parents.[107,108] However, a family with multiple cases of brain tumours in infancy has been described in which there is a frameshift mutation in *INI1*.[109]

Other renal tumours

Congenital mesoblastic nephroma is generally considered benign and is the commonest renal tumour occurring in neonates. Its early age of onset would suggest a genetic predisposition that has not yet been found. The cellular subtype is more aggressive and has a greater propensity for local recurrence and, rarely, metastasis. This latter tumour has been shown to share a somatic chromosomal translocation originally diagnosed in congenital fibrosarcoma.[110] This t(12;15)(p13;q25) fuses the *TEL* (*ETV6*) gene to the *TRKC* (*NTRK3*) gene, producing a chimaeric protein tyrosine kinase with transforming properties. However, there are no reports of abnormal constitutional karyotypes in this condition.

Clear cell sarcoma of the kidney (CCSK) accounts for 4 per cent of childhood renal tumours and the age of onset is similar to sporadic Wilms tumour.[111] This is a distinct molecular entity from clear cell sarcoma of soft parts, which is associated with the somatic gene fusion *EWS-ATF1*, which rarely occurs primarily in kidney. There are no clinical indications that CCSK is due to genetic predisposition and its somatic molecular genetics are not well characterized.

Renal cell carcinoma (RCC) is rare in young children, but during the second decade of life, a primary renal tumour is as likely to be RCC as Wilms tumour.[112] RCC in children and younger adults is more likely to be of the papillary subtype.[113] Germline mutations in the *MET* oncogene have been identified in hereditary papillary RCC.[114] A subset of sporadic papillary RCC involves reciprocal somatic translocations for which the fusion genes have been identified.[115] Childhood RCC has been rarely reported in the von Hippel–Lindau syndrome.[116] (See Chapter 10 for further discussion of the genetics of RCC.)

CONCLUSION

In conclusion, the molecular basis of childhood renal cancers is beginning to be unravelled. For Wilms tumour, it is clear that multiple genes are involved in genetic predisposition. Their relative contribution to both heritable and somatic mutations must await their full identification and accurate assessment of penetrance. Studies of Wilms tumour genes, particularly *WT1*, have emphasized the intimate relationship of cancer predisposition and developmental abnormalities in childhood. In the future, it should be possible to define, at a molecular level, individuals at increased risk of childhood renal tumours, leading to a more rational approach to screening and therapy.

KEY POINTS

- There are multiple genes for Wilms tumour (WT), both for genetic predisposition and somatic mutations.
- Constitutional *WT1* mutation is rare, both in familial Wilms tumour (<10 per cent) and in sporadic cases (<5 per cent). It is usually associated with genital abnormalities and/or nephrotic syndrome, often as part of the WAGR and Denys–Drash syndromes.
- Late onset renal failure is associated with WAGR syndrome and Wilms tumours with intralobar nephrogenic rests.
- Genetic linkage studies show there are at least three familial *WT* genes: *FWT1* (17q12–21), *FWT2* (19q) and *FWT3* (locus unknown); penetrance appears to be low (15–30 per cent).
- Beckwith–Wiedemann syndrome has complex genetics involving genomic imprinting and multiple genes. It may be possible to identify subgroups at higher tumour risk but ultrasound screening is still recommended for all patients at 3-monthly intervals.
- Malignant rhabdoid tumour of kidney shares a common genetic defect (*INI1* gene mutation) with its associated second primary brain tumours.

REFERENCES

1. Stiller CA, Parkin DM. International variations in the incidence of childhood renal tumours. *Br J Cancer* 1990; **62:**1026–1030.
2. Pritchard-Jones K. Molecular genetic pathways to Wilms tumour. *Crit Rev Oncol* 1997; **8:**1–27.
3. Cardesa A, Ribalta T, Vonschilling B, *et al.* Experimental model of tumors associated with neurofibromatosis. *Cancer* 1989; **63:** 1737–1749.
4. Beckwith JB, Kiviat NB, Bonadio JF. Nephrogenic rests, nephroblastomatosis and the pathogenesis of Wilms tumour. *Pediatr Pathol* 1990; **10:**1–36.
5. Knudson AG, Strong LC. Mutation and cancer: a model for Wilms tumour of the kidney. *J Natl Cancer Inst* 1972; **48:**313–324.
6. Goodrich DW, Lee WH. The molecular genetics of retinoblastoma. *Cancer Surv* 1990; **9:**529–554.
7. Haber DA, Buckler AJ, Glaser T, *et al.* An internal deletion within an 11p13 zinc finger gene contributes to the development of Wilms tumor. *Cell* 1990; **61:**1257–1269.
8. Little MH, Prosser J, Condie A, *et al.* Zinc finger point mutations within the *WT1* gene in Wilms tumor patients. *Proc Natl Acad Sci USA* 1992; **89:**4791–4795.
9. Rahman N, Arbour L, Houlston R, *et al.* Penetrance of mutations in the familial Wilms tumor gene *FWT1. J Natl Cancer Inst* 2000; **92:**650–652.
10. Bonaiti-Pellie C, Chompret A, Tournade MF, *et al.* Genetics and epidemiology of Wilms tumor: the French Wilms tumor study. *Med Pediatr Oncol* 1992; **20:**284–291.
11. Hawkins MM, Winter D, Burton HS, Potok MHN. Heritability of Wilms tumor. *J Natl Cancer Inst* 1995; **87:**1323–1324.
12. Byrne J, Mulvihill JJ, Connelly RR, *et al.* Reproductive problems and birth defects in survivors of Wilms tumor and their relatives. *Med Pediatr Oncol* 1988; **16:**233–240.
13. Li FP, Gimbrere K, Gelber RD, *et al.* Outcome of pregnancy in survivors of Wilms tumor. *JAMA* 1987; **257:**216–219.
14. Breslow N, Olshan A, Beckwith JB, Green DM. Epidemiology of Wilms tumor. *Med Pediatr Oncol* 1993; **21:**172–181.
15. Bonaiti-Pellie C, Chompret A, Tournade MF, *et al.* Excess of multifocal tumors in nephroblastoma: implications for mechanisms of tumor development and genetic counseling. *Hum Genet* 1993; **91:**373–376.
16. Ton CC, Hirvonen H, Miwa H, *et al.* Positional cloning and characterization of a paired box- and homeobox-containing gene from the aniridia region. *Cell* 1991; **67:**1059–1074.
17. Gessler M, Konig A, Moore J, *et al.* Homozygous inactivation of *WT1* in a Wilms tumor associated with the WAGR syndrome. *Genes Chromosomes Cancer* 1993; **7:**131–136.
18. Call KM, Glaser T, Ito CY, *et al.* Isolation and characterization of a zinc finger polypeptide gene at the human chromosome 11 Wilms tumor locus. *Cell* 1990; **60:**509–520.
19. van Heyningen V, Bickmore WA, Seawright A, *et al.* Role for the Wilms tumor gene in genital development? *Proc Natl Acad Sci USA* 1990; **87:**5383–5386.
20. Baird PN, Groves N, Haber DA, *et al.* Identification of mutations in the *WT1* gene in tumours from patients with the WAGR syndrome. *Oncogene* 1992; **7:**2141–2149.
21. Brown KW, Watson JE, Poirier V, *et al.* Inactivation of the remaining allele of the *WT1* gene in a 'Wilms tumour from a WAGR patient. *Oncogene* 1992; **7:**763–768.
22. Parks S, Tomlinson G, Nisen P, Haber DA, *et al.* Altered transactivational properties of a mutated *WT1* gene product in a WAGR-associated Wilms tumor. *Cancer Res* 1993; **53:**4757–4760.

23. Santos A, Osorio-Almeida L, Baird PN, et al. Insertional inactivation of the WT1 gene in tumour cells from a patient with WAGR syndrome. Hum Genet 1993; 92:83–86.

24. Kent J, Lee M, Schedl A, et al. The reticulocalbin gene maps to the WAGR region in human and to the Small eye Harwell deletion in mouse. Genomics 1997; 42:260–267.

25. Armstrong JF, Pritchard-Jones K, Bickmore WA, et al. The expression of the Wilms tumour gene, WT1, in the developing mammalian embryo. Mech Dev 1993; 40:85–97.

26. Pritchard-Jones K, Fleming S, Davidson D, et al. The candidate Wilms tumour gene is involved in genitourinary development. Nature 1990; 346:194–197.

27. Wang ZY, Qiu QQ, Enger KT, et al. A second transcriptionally active DNA-binding site for the Wilms tumor gene product, WT1. Proc Natl Acad Sci USA 1993; 90:8896–8900.

28. Wang ZY, Qiu QQ, Deuel TF. The Wilms tumor gene product WT1 activates or suppresses transcription through separate functional domains. J Biol Chem 1993; 268: 9172–9175.

29. Kreidberg JA, Sariola H, Loring JM, et al. wt-1 is required for early kidney development. Cell 1993; 74:679–691.

30. Akasaka Y, Kikuchi H, Nagai T, et al. A point mutation found in the WT1 gene in a sporadic Wilms tumor without genitourinary abnormalities is identical with the most frequent point mutation in Denys–Drash syndrome. FEBS Lett 1993; 317:39–43.

31. Coppes MJ, Liefers GJ, Paul P, et al. Homozygous somatic WT1 point mutations in sporadic unilateral Wilms tumor. Proc Natl Acad Sci USA 1993; 90:1416–1419.

32. Huff V, Miwa H, Haber DA, et al. Evidence for WT1 as a Wilms tumor (WT) gene: intragenic germinal deletion in bilateral WT. Am J Hum Genet 1991; 48:997–1003.

33. Tadokoro K, Fujii H, Ohshima A, et al. Intragenic homozygous deletion of the WT1 gene in Wilms tumor. Oncogene 1992; 7:1215–1221.

34. Cowell JK, Wadey RB, Haber DA, et al. Structural rearrangements of the WT1 gene in Wilms tumour cells. Oncogene 1991; 6:595–599.

35. Kikuchi H, Akasaka Y, Nagai T, et al. Genomic changes in the WT-gene (WT1) in Wilms tumors and their correlation with histology. Am J Pathol 1992; 140:781–786.

36. Radice P, Pilotti S, De Benedetti V, et al. Homozygous intragenic loss of the WT1 locus in a sporadic intralobar Wilms tumor [letter]. Int J Cancer 1993; 55:174–176.

37. Little M, Wells C. A clinical overview of WT1 gene mutations. Hum Mutat 1997; 9:209–225.

38. Drash A, Sherman F, Hartmann, WH, Blizzard RM et al. A syndrome of pseudohermaphroditism, Wilms tumor, hypertension, and degenerative renal disease. J Pediatr 1970; 76:585–593.

39. Denys P, Malvaux P, Van Den Berghe H, et al. Association of an anatomo-pathological syndrome of male pseudo-hermaphroditism, Wilms tumor, parenchymatous nephropathy and XX/XY mosaicism. Arch Fr Pediatr 1967; 24:729–739.

40. Jadresic L, Leake J, Gordon I, et al. Clinicopathologic review of twelve children with nephropathy, Wilms tumor, and genital abnormalities (Drash syndrome). J Pediatr 1990; 117:717–725.

41. Pelletier J, Bruening W, Kashtan CE, et al. Germline mutations in the Wilms tumor suppressor gene are associated with abnormal urogenital development in Denys–Drash syndrome. Cell 1991; 67:437–447.

42. Little MH, Williamson KA, Mannens A, et al. Evidence that WT1 mutations in Denys–Drash syndrome patients may act in a dominant-negative fashion. Hum Mol Genet 1993; 2:259–264.

43. Hastie ND. Dominant negative mutations in the Wilms tumour (WT1) gene cause Denys–Drash syndrome – proof that a tumour-suppressor gene plays a crucial role in normal genitourinary development. Hum Mol Genet 1992; 1:293–295.

44. Klamt B, Koziell A, Poulat F, et al. Frasier syndrome is caused by defective alternative splicing of WT1 leading to an altered ratio of WT1+/−KTS splice isoforms. Hum Mol Genet 1998; 7:709–714.

45. Koziell A, Charmandari E, Hindmarsh PC, et al. Frasier syndrome, part of the Denys Drash continuum or simply a WT1 gene associated disorder of intersex and nephropathy? [see comments]. Clin Endocrinol (Oxf) 2000; 52:519–524.

46. Henry I, Hoovers J, Barichard F, et al. Pericentric intrachromosomal insertion responsible for recurrence of del(11)(p13p14) in a family. Genes Chromosomes Cancer 1993; 7:57–62.

47. Coppes MJ, Liefers GJ, Higuchi M, et al. Inherited WT1 mutation in Denys–Drash syndrome. Cancer Res 1992; 52:6125–6128.

48. Coppes MJ, Campbell CE, Williams BR. The role of WT1 in Wilms tumorigenesis. FASEB J 1993; 7:886–895.

49. Patek CE, Little MH, Fleming S, et al. A zinc finger truncation of murine wt1 results in the characteristic urogenital abnormalities of Denys–Drash syndrome. Proc Natl Acad Sci USA 1999; 96:2931–2936.

50. Pettenati MI, Haines JL, Higgins RR. Wiedemann–Beckwith syndrome: presentation of clinical and cytogenetic data on 22 new cases and review of the literature. Hum Genet 1986; 74:143–154.

51. Moutou C, Junien C, Henry I, Bonaiti-Pellie C, et al. Beckwith–Wiedemann syndrome: a demonstration of the mechanisms responsible for the excess of transmitting females [see comments]. J Med Genet 1992; 29:217–220.

52. Catchpoole D, Lam WW, Valler D, et al. Epigenetic modification and uniparental inheritance of H19 in Beckwith–Wiedemann syndrome. J Med Genet 1997; 34:353–359.

53. Feinberg AP. Imprinting of a genomic domain of 11p15 and loss of imprinting in cancer: an introduction. Cancer Res 1999; 59(7 Suppl):1743s–1746s.

54. Lam WW, Hatada I, Ohishi S, et al. Analysis of germline CDKN1C (p57KIP2) mutations in familial and sporadic Beckwith–Wiedemann syndrome (BWS) provides a novel genotype–phenotype correlation. J Med Genet 1999; 36:518–523.

55. Lee MP, DeBaun MR, Misuyaka K, et al. Loss of imprinting of a paternally expressed transcript, with antisense orientation to KVLQT1, occurs frequently in Beckwith–Wiedemann syndrome and is independent of insulin-like growth factor II imprinting. Proc Natl Acad Sci USA 1999; 96:5203–5208.

56. Alders M, Ryan A, Hodges M, et al. Disruption of a novel imprinted zinc-finger gene, ZNF215, in Beckwith–Wiedemann syndrome. Am J Hum Genet 2000; 66:1473–1484.

57. O'Keefe D, Dao D, Zhao L, *et al.* Coding mutations in *p57KIP2* are present in some cases of Beckwith–Wiedemann syndrome but are rare or absent in Wilms tumors. *Am J Hum Genet* 1997; **61**:295–303.

58. Ogawa O, Eccles MR, Szeto J, *et al.* Relaxation of insulin-like growth factor II gene imprinting implicated in Wilms tumour. *Nature* 1993; **362**:749–751.

59. Caspary T, Cleary MA, Perlman EJ, *et al.* Oppositely imprinted genes *p57*(Kip2) and *igf2* interact in a mouse model for Beckwith–Wiedemann syndrome. *Genes Dev* 1999; **13**:3115–3124.

60. Weksberg R, Nishikawa J, Caluseriu O, *et al.* Tumor development in the Beckwith–Wiedemann syndrome is associated with a variety of constitutional molecular 11p15 alterations including imprinting defects of *KCNQ1OT1*. *J Hum Mol Genet* 2001; **10**:2989–3000.

61. Bliek J, Maas SM, Ruijter JM, *et al.* Increased tumour risk for BWS patients correlates with aberrant H19 and not KCNQ1OT1 methylation: occurrence of KCNQ1OT1 hypomethylation in familial cases of BWS. *Hum Mol Genet* 2001; **10**:467–476.

62. DeBaun MR, Niemitz EL, McNeil DE, *et al.* Epigenetic alterations of H19 and LIT1 distinguish patients with Beckwith–Wiedemann syndrome with cancer and birth defects. *Am J Hum Genet* 2002; **70**:604–611.

63. Hoyme HE, Seaver LH, Jones KL, *et al.* Isolated hemihyperplasia (hemihypertrophy): report of a prospective multicenter study of the incidence of neoplasia and review. *Am J Med Genet* 1998; **79**:274–278.

64. Wiedemann HR. Tumours and hemihypertrophy associated with Wiedemann–Beckwith syndrome. *Eur J Paediatr* 1983; **141**:129.

65. Veugelers M, DeCat B, Delande M, *et al.* Mutational analysis of the *GPC3/GPC4* glypican gene cluster on Xq26 in patients with Simpson–Golabi–Behmel syndrome: identification of loss-of-function mutations in the *GPC3* gene. *Hum Mol Genet* 2000; **9**:1321–1328.

66. White GR, Kelsey AM, Varley JM, *et al.* Mutations in Wilms tumour. *Br J Cancer* 2002; **86**:1920–1922.

67. Hamel B, Mannens M, Bokkerink J. Perlman syndrome: a report of a case and results of molecular studies. *Am J Hum Genet* 1990; **45**:A48.

68. Neri G, Martini-Neri ME, Katz BE, Opitz JM. The Perlman syndrome: familial renal dysplasia with Wilms tumor, fetal gigantism and multiple congenital anomalies. *Am J Med Genet* 1984; **19**:195–207.

69. Greenberg F, Copeland K, Gresik MV. Expanding the spectrum of the Perlman syndrome. *Am J Med Genet* 1988; **29**:773–776.

70. Perlman M, Levin M, Wittels B. Syndrome of fetal gigantism, renal hamartomas, and nephroblastomatosis with Wilms tumor. *Cancer* 1975; **35**:1212–1217.

71. Grundy RG, Pritchard J, Baraitser M, *et al.* Perlman and Wiedemann–Beckwith syndromes: two distinct conditions associated with Wilms tumour. *Eur J Pediatr* 1992; **151**:895–898.

72. Henneveld HT, Van Lingen RA, Hamel BC, *et al.* Perlman syndrome: four additional cases and review. *Am J Med Genet* 1999; **86**:439–446.

73. Stay EJ, Vawter G. The relationship between nephroblastoma and neurofibromatosis (Von Recklinghausen disease). *Cancer* 1977; **39**:2550–2555.

74. Blatt J, Jaffe R, Deutsch M, Adkins JC. Neurofibromatosis and childhood tumors. *Cancer* 1986; **57**:1225–1229.

75. Perilongo G, Felix CA, Meadows AT, *et al.* Sequential development of Wilms tumor, T-cell acute lymphoblastic leukemia, medulloblastoma and myeloid leukemia in a child with type 1 neurofibromatosis: a clinical and cytogenetic case report. *Leukemia* 1993; **7**:912–915.

76. Hartley AL, Birch JM, Tricker K, *et al.* Wilms tumor in the Li–Fraumeni cancer family syndrome. *Cancer Genet Cytogenet* 1993; **67**:133–135.

77. Varley JM, McGown G, Throncroft M, *et al.* A novel *TP53* splicing mutation in a Li–Fraumeni syndrome family: a patient with Wilms tumour is not a mutation carrier. *Br J Cancer* 1998; **78**:1081–1083.

78. Clericuzio CL. Clinical phenotypes and Wilms tumor. *Med Pediatr Oncol* 1993; **21**:182–187.

79. Pastore G, Carli M, Lemerle J, *et al.* Epidemiological features of Wilms tumor: results of studies by the International Society of Paediatric Oncology (SIOP). *Med Pediatr Oncol* 1988; **16**:7–11.

80. Breslow NE, Olson J, Moksness J, *et al.* Familial Wilms tumour: a descriptive study. *Med Pediatr Oncol* 1996; **27**:398–403.

81. Matsunaga E. Genetics of Wilms tumor. *Hum Genet* 1981; **57**:231–246.

82. Olson JM, Breslow NE, Barce J. Cancer in twins of Wilms tumor patients. *Am J Med Genet* 1993; **47**:91–94.

83. Huff V, Compton DA, Chao LY, *et al.* Lack of linkage of familial tumour to chromosomal band 11p13. *Nature* 1988; **336**:377–378.

84. Schwartz CE, Haber DA, Stanton VP, *et al.* Familial predisposition to Wilms tumor does not segregate with the *WT1* gene. *Genomics* 1991; **10**:927–930.

85. Huff V, Reeve AE, Leppert M, *et al.* Nonlinkage of 16q markers to familial predisposition to Wilms tumor. *Cancer Res* 1992; **52**:6117–6120.

86. Pelletier J, Bruening W, Li FP, *et al.* *WT1* mutations contribute to abnormal genital system development and hereditary Wilms tumour. *Nature* 1991; **353**:431–434.

87. Kaplinsky C, Ghahremani M, Frishberg Y, *et al.* Familial Wilms associated with a *WT1* zinc finger mutation. *Genomics* 1996; **38**:451–453.

88. Pritchard-Jones K, Rahman N, Gerrard M, *et al.* Familial Wilms tumour resulting from *WT1* mutation: intronic polymorphism causing artefactual constitutional homozygosity [letter]. *J Med Genet* 2000; **37**:377–379.

89. Rahman N, Arbour L, Tonin P, *et al.* Evidence for a familial Wilms tumour gene (*FWT1*) on chromosome 17q12–q21. *Nature Genet* 1996; **13**:461–463.

90. Rahman N, Abidi F, Ford D, *et al.* Confirmation of *FWT1* as a Wilms tumour susceptibility gene and phenotypic characteristics of Wilms tumour attributable to *FWT1*. *Hum Genet* 1998; **103**:547–556.

91. Rapley EA, Barfoot R, Bonaiti-Pellie C, *et al.* Evidence for susceptibility genes to familial Wilms tumour in addition to *WT1*, *FWT1* and *FWT2*. *Br J Cancer* 2000; **83**:177–183.

92. Rahman N, Arbour L, Tonin P, *et al.* The familial Wilms tumour susceptibility gene, *FWT1*, may not be a tumour suppressor gene. *Oncogene* 1997; **14**:3099–3102.

93. McDonald JM, Douglass EC, Fisher R, *et al.* Linkage of familial Wilms tumor predisposition to chromosome 19 and a

two-locus model for the etiology of familial tumors. *Cancer Res* 1998; **58**:1387–1390.

94. DeBaun MR, Siegel MJ, Choyke PL. Nephromegaly in infancy and early childhood: a risk factor for Wilms tumor in Beckwith–Wiedemann syndrome. *J Pediatr* 1998; **132**:401–404.

95. Beckwith JB. Children at increased risk for Wilms tumor: monitoring issues [editorial; comment]. *J Pediatr* 1998; **132**:377–379.

96. Coppes MJ, Arnold M, Beckwith JB, *et al.* Factors affecting the risk of contralateral Wilms tumor development: a report from the National Wilms Tumor Study Group. *Cancer* 1999; **85**: 1616–1625.

97. Diller L, Ghahremani M, Morgan J, *et al.* Constitutional *WT1* mutations in Wilms tumor patients. *J Clin Oncol* 1998; **16**:3634–3640.

98. Green DM, Breslow NE, Beckwith JB, *et al.* Screening of children with hemihypertrophy, aniridia, and Beckwith–Wiedemann syndrome in patients with Wilms tumor: a report from the National Wilms Tumor Study. *Med Pediatr Oncol* 1993; **21**:188–192.

99. Choyke PL, Siegel MJ, Craft AW, *et al.* Screening for Wilms tumor in children with Beckwith–Wiedemann syndrome or idiopathic hemihypertrophy. *Med Pediatr Oncol* 1999; **32**:196–200.

100. Porteus MH, Narkool P, Neuberg D, *et al.* Characteristics and outcome of children with Beckwith–Wiedemann syndrome and Wilms tumor: a report from the National Wilms Tumor Study Group. *J Clin Oncol* 2000; **18**:2026–2031.

101. Breslow NE, Takashima IR, Ritchey ML, *et al.* Renal failure in the Denys–Drash and Wilms tumor – aniridia syndromes. *Cancer Res* 2000; **60**:4030–4032.

102. Austin MB, Fechner RE, Roggli VL. Pleural malignant mesothelioma following Wilms tumor. *Am J Clin Pathol* 1986; **86**:227–230.

103. Park S, Schalling M, Bernard A, *et al.* The Wilms tumour gene *WT1* is expressed in murine mesoderm-derived tissues and mutated in a human mesothelioma. *Nature Genet* 1993; **4**:415–420.

104. Pritchard-Jones K, Renshaw J, King-Underwood L. The Wilms tumour (*WT1*) gene is mutated in a secondary leukaemia in a WAGR patient. *Hum Mol Genet* 1994; **3**:1633–1637.

105. Weeks DA, Beckwith JB, Mieran GW, Luckey DW. Rhabdoid tumor of kidney. A report of 111 cases from the National Wilms tumor Study Pathology Center. *Am J Surg Pathol* 1989; **13**:439–458.

106. Versteege I, Sevenet N, Lange J, *et al.* Truncating mutations of *hSNF5/INI1* in aggressive paediatric cancer. *Nature* 1998; **394**:203–206.

107. Savla J, Chen TT, Schneider NR, *et al.* Mutations of the *SNF5/INI1* gene in renal rhabdoid tumors with second primary brain tumors. *J Natl Cancer Inst* 2000; **92**:648–650.

108. Biegel JA, Zhou JY, Rorke LB, *et al.* Germ-line and acquired mutations of *INI1* in atypical teratoid and rhabdoid tumors. *Cancer Res* 1999; **59**:74–79.

109. Taylor MD, Gokgoz N, Andrulis IL, *et al.* Familial posterior fossa brain tumors of infancy secondary to germline mutation of the *SNF5* gene. *Am J Hum Genet* 2000; **66**:1403–1406.

110. Knezevich SR, Garnett MJ, Pysher TJ, *et al.* *ETV6-NTRK3* gene fusions and trisomy 11 establish a histogenetic link between mesoblastic nephroma and congenital fibrosarcoma. *Cancer Res* 1998; **58**:5046–5048.

111. Argani P, Perlman EJ, Breslow NE, *et al.* Clear cell sarcoma of the kidney: a review of 351 cases from the National Wilms Tumor Study Group Pathology Center. *Am J Surg Pathol* 2000; **24**:4–18.

112. Hartman DS, Davis CJ Jr, Madewell JE, *et al.* Primary malignant renal tumors in the second decade of life: Wilms tumor versus renal cell carcinoma. *J Urol* 1982; **127**:888–891.

113. Carcao MD, Taylor GP, Greenberg ML, *et al.* Renal-cell carcinoma in children: a different disorder from its adult counterpart? *Med Pediatr Oncol* 1998; **31**:153–158.

114. Schmidt L, Duh FM, Chen F, *et al.* Germline and somatic mutations in the tyrosine kinase domain of the *MET* proto-oncogene in papillary renal carcinomas. *Nature Genet* 1997; **16**:68–73.

115. Clark J, Lu YJ, Sidhar SK, *et al.* Fusion of splicing factor genes *PSF* and *NonO* (*p54nrb*) to the *TFE3* gene in papillary renal cell carcinoma. *Oncogene* 1997; **15**:2233–2239.

116. Tazi K, Chretien Y, Droz D, *et al.* Renal cell carcinoma in a 14-year-old girl with Von Hippel Lindau disease. *Ann Urol* 1999; **33**:414–417.

10

Genetic susceptibility to renal cell carcinoma

EAMONN R. MAHER AND BERTON ZBAR

INTRODUCTION

Renal cell carcinoma (RCC) is the most common adult kidney tumour and accounts for 2 per cent of all cancers diagnosed. Large epidemiological studies have identified cigarette smoking as the strongest known risk factor in non-occupation-associated RCC, but additional factors include hypertension and obesity, and there is an increased risk in patients with end-stage renal failure.[1] Occupational exposure to hydrocarbons (trichloroethylene) is associated with an increased risk of RCC.

The histopathological classification of RCC has provoked considerable debate. In 1986, a new classification of RCC was proposed with five principal subtypes.[2] The most common form of RCC is clear cell, which accounts for up to 80 per cent of cases. Non-clear-cell types include chromophilic (papillary), chromophobe, oncocytoma and ductus Bellini. The importance of this classification has been the extent to which different histopathological subtypes have correlated with familial causes of RCC and somatic genetic events. Although only 2 per cent of RCC cases are familial (see Table 10.1), the elucidation of

Table 10.1 *Inherited disorders associated with renal cell carcinoma*

Disorder	Histopathology	Gene	Location
Von Hippel–Lindau disease	Clear	*VHL*	3p25
Chromosome 3 translocations	Clear	–	3p14–3q21
Familial clear-cell RCC	Clear	?	?
Hereditary papillary RCC	Type 1 papillary	*MET*	7q31
Familial papillary thyroid cancer and papillar renal neoplasia	Papillary	?	1q21
Birt–Hogg–Dube syndrome	Oncocytoma (but variable)	*BHD*	17p11.2
Tuberous sclerosis	Variable	*TSC1, TSC2*	9q34, 16p13
Hyperparathyroidism–jaw tumour syndrome	Hamartoma, papillary	*HRPT2*	1q21–q31
Hereditary non-polyposis cancer syndrome	Transitional	*MSH2, MLH1, MSH6, PMS1, PMS2, MSH3*	2p27, 3p21, 2p16, 2q31, 7q22, 5q11

Hereditary non-polyposis colorectal cancer (HNPCC) is described in Chapters 24 and 25. In addition, medullary carcinoma of the kidney associated with sickle cell trait is a recently recognized distinct entity that is a rare cause of renal tumours in young African Americans.[65]
RCC, renal cell carcinoma.

inherited causes of RCC has provided important insights into the mechanisms of renal tumorigenesis.

VON HIPPEL–LINDAU DISEASE

Von Hippel–Lindau (VHL) disease is the most common disorder causing genetic susceptibility to clear-cell renal cell carcinoma. This dominantly inherited multisystem familial cancer syndrome has an incidence of ~1 per 30 000.[3] The eponym was coined by Melmon and Rosen[4] in recognition of the seminal contributions of the German ophthalmologist Eugene von Hippel, who described retinal angiomas almost 100 years ago (although familial retinal angioma had been described some 20 years previously by Treacher Collins), and the Swedish pathologist Arvid Lindau, who, in 1926, described the major features of VHL disease and recognized the significance of the association of retinal and cerebellar haemangioblastomas.

Clinical features and diagnosis of VHL disease

The major manifestations of VHL disease in an unselected UK-based series are shown in Table 10.2.[5] Clinical presentation may be in childhood or old age, and variable expression and age-dependent penetrance are striking features. Penetrance is tumour specific with, on average, retinal and cerebellar haemangioblastomas (HABs) presenting earlier than RCC. In an unselected series, penetrance is almost complete by the age of 60 years; however, the advent of molecular diagnosis has demonstrated that specific VHL mutations may be associated with markedly different phenotypes.[6] Thus, while data from unselected series may provide overall estimates of tumour risks, they do not allow for variations in expression and penetrance from allelic heterogeneity. Three subgroups of VHL disease are distinguished: type 1 is characterized by RCC, retinal and central nervous system (CNS) HABs. VHL type 2A is characterized by phaeochromocytomas, retinal and CNS HABs, but a low risk of RCC. Type 2B is characterized by phaeochromocytomas, RCC and CNS haemangioblastomas. Prototypic 2A and 2B mutations are Tyr^{98}His and Arg^{167}Gln, respectively (see Table 10.2). For mutations that occur frequently or in large families, mutation-specific penetrances may be calculated.

In VHL type 1 families, retinal or cerebellar HABs are usually the presenting features. However, in familial cases, routine surveillance of at-risk relatives ensures that most tumour diagnoses are made presymptomatically. Details of specimen surveillance protocols are provided in Table 10.3. The precise follow-up investigations should be individualized to take into account interfamilial genotype-phenotype differences. In addition, intrafamilial

Table 10.2 *Major manifestations of von Hippel–Lindau disease in an unselected series (mainly type 1), and for two prototypic type 2A and 2B mutations*

Lesion	Unselected UK series		
	(Type 1 and Type 2B)[5]	Type 2A (Tyr^{98}His)[11]	Type 2B (Arg^{167}Trp)[11]
Retinal angioma (haemangioblastoma)	59%	47%	71%
Cerebellar haemangioblastoma	59%	9%	33%
Spinal cord haemangioblastoma	13%		
Renal cell carcinoma	28%	0%	31%
Phaeochromocytoma	7%	55%	71%

phenotypic variability can result from stochastic events, genetic modifier effects and mosaicism.[7]

Conventionally, a clinical diagnosis of VHL disease is made in the presence of: (1) a typical VHL tumour, if there is a positive family history; or (2) if there is no family history, the presence of two tumours (e.g. two HABs, or a HAB and a visceral tumour). These criteria are reliable in most circumstances but recognition of isolated cases is delayed because of the need for two tumours to occur. In addition, we have observed patients with multiple HABs only, no family history and no detectable VHL gene mutation. Such cases may have tissue mosaicism. In isolated cases, the involvement of two organs may provide better criteria for the diagnosis of VHL disease (e.g. retinal angioma + CNS HAB, or retinal angioma + renal carcinoma, or CNS HAB + renal carcinoma, or retinal angioma (HAB) + phaeochromocytoma).

The identification of the VHL tumour suppressor gene provided opportunities for the early diagnosis of VHL in patients who do not satisfy the clinical diagnostic criteria.[8] Current VHL mutation analysis using a complete range of techniques can provide a detection rate approaching 100 per cent in non-mosaic patients with classical VHL disease.[9] The uptake of predictive DNA testing by at-risk relatives is high as surveillance can be discontinued in those who are not found to be gene carriers. Predictive testing is usually offered from age 5 years. In addition to establishing carrier status, VHL mutation characterization may also provide clues as to the likely phenotype. Thus, most patients with deletions and truncating mutations will have a type 1 phenotype. Missense mutations associated with phaeochromocytoma usually also predispose to HAB and RCC (type 2B phenotype), but specific mutations (e.g. Tyr^{98}His and Tyr^{112}His) may produce type 2A.[10,11] In families presenting with isolated familial phaeochromocytoma, type 2B or 2A mutations may be identified, but other rare mutations (e.g. Leu188Val) seem likely to only predispose to phaeochromocytoma

Table 10.3 *Example surveillance programmes for von Hippel–Lindau disease (VHL) in asymptomatic affected patients and at-risk relatives*

Protocol 1 – Birmingham, UK (adapted from Maher *et al.,* 1990[5]); and Protocol 2 – National Cancer Institute, USA (see www.vhl.org/meetings/meet98/98efglen.htm). At-risk relatives who are demonstrated not to have inherited the *VHL* mutation identified in the family can be released from surveillance.

Protocol 1

Affected patient

1 Annual physical examination and urine testing
2 Annual direct and indirect ophthalmoscopy
3 MRI brain scan every 3 years to age 50 and every 5 years thereafter
4 Annual renal ultrasound or MRI scan (CT scan may be required if multiple renal or pancreatic cysts are present)
5 Annual 24-hour urine collection for catecholamines from age 11

At-risk relative

1 Annual physical examination and urine testing
2 Annual direct and indirect ophthalmoscopy from age 5 to 60 (fluoroscein angioscopy or angiography may be used from age 10 to increase sensitivity)
3 MRI brain scan every 3 years to from age 15 to 40 years and then every 5 years until age 60 years
4 Annual renal ultrasound scan or MRI scan from age 15 to 65 years
5 Annual 24-hour urine collection for catecholamines from age 11

Protocol 2

From conception	Inform obstetrician of family history of VHL
From birth	Inform paediatrician of family history of VHL
	Eye examinations
Ages 2–10	Annual:

- Eye/retinal examination by ophthalmologist informed about VHL
- Physical examination by physician informed about VHL (physical examinations include scrotal examination in males)
- Test for elevated catecholamines in 24-hour urine collection

Ages 11–19	Annual:

- Eye/retinal examination by ophthalmologist informed about VHL
- Physical examination by physician informed about VHL (physical examinations include scrotal examination in males)
- Test for elevated catecholamines in 24-hour urine collection
- Ultrasound of abdomen (focus on kidneys, pancreas and adrenals)

Every 2 years:

- MRI with gadolinium of brain and spine (annually at onset of puberty or before and after pregnancy, not during)

Age 20 and beyond	Annual:

- CT scan with and without contrast of abdomen (kidneys/pancreas/adrenals)
- Eye/retinal examination by ophthalmologist informed about VHL
- Physical examination by physician informed about VHL
- Test for elevated catecholamines in 24-hour urine collection

Every 2 years:

- MRI with gadolinium of brain and spine (annually before and after, but not during pregnancy, and onset of menopause)

CT, computed tomography; MRI, magnetic resonance imaging.

Notes

1. Slight modifications of screening schedules may sometimes be made by personal physicians familiar with individual patients and with their VHL family history.
2. After age 60, if no children with VHL and still not diagnosed, imaging tests may be every 2 years for CT and every 3 years for MRI.
3. All head MRIs should be examined by radiologists for any suggestion of ELST (endolymphatic sac tumour). If suspicious, or at first sign or symptom of hearing loss, tinnitus or vertigo, MRI or CT of internal auditory canal and audiologic tests are indicated.

(type 2C).[12] False-negative mutation analysis may result from mosaicism.

Molecular investigations for VHL disease should be considered in patients with isolated retinal or CNS HABs and familial, multicentric or young-onset phaeochromocytoma and RCC <40 years. Thus, ~50 per cent of patients with apparently isolated familial phaeochromocytoma or bilateral phaeochromocytoma have germline *VHL* gene mutations, as do ~4 per cent of patients with isolated HAB diagnosed at <50 years with no family history or other evidence of VHL disease.[13,14] Estimates of the risk of VHL disease in patients with isolated retinal angioma have also been provided.[15]

Management and surveillance

VHL disease is a multisystem disorder and so the effective management of families requires a coordinated multidisciplinary approach. In particular, it is important that responsibility for coordination of family ascertainment, screening and DNA testing is assumed. All at-risk relatives are contacted and offered surveillance as outlined in Table 10.3. Lifelong surveillance is offered to affected individuals and unaffected individuals who carry the *VHL* mutation. In the absence of DNA testing, at-risk individuals without clinical or subclinical evidence of VHL should be followed up until at least age 60 years.[5]

KIDNEY

The major renal manifestations of VHL disease are renal cystic disease and multiple, bilateral clear cell RCC. Although mean age at diagnosis of symptomatic RCC is ~40 years, the widespread adoption of surveillance programmes including annual renal imaging (see Table 10.3) has resulted in many renal lesions being detected at an early stage. Thus, the surgical management of RCC in VHL disease has shifted from the treatment of large symptomatic RCC, to the challenges of how best to manage small asymptomatic tumours. Computed tomography (CT) is the most sensitive method for detecting renal tumours (particularly in the presence of renal cysts), but magnetic resonance imaging (MRI) or ultrasound scans are preferred for regular follow-up to avoid a large cumulative radiation load. Most small renal tumours enlarge slowly (mean < 2 cm/year), and after establishing the growth rate, an individual lesion can usually be scanned every 6 months.[16] The risk of distant metastasis from a solid lesion < 3 cm in size is remote and a non-interventional approach is followed until the tumour reaches a diameter of 3 cm.[17] At that stage, the tumour is treated by a limited partial nephrectomy and other smaller encapsulated lesions are removed. Follow-up of VHL patients managed by such a nephron-sparing approach suggests that, although the risk of local recurrence (from new primary tumours) is high, the risk of distant metastasis is low.[18] In contrast, 25 per cent of VHL patients with a RCC > 3 cm (treated by nephron-sparing surgery or nephrectomy) developed metastatic disease.[17] The objective of this nephron-sparing approach is to maintain adequate renal function for as long as possible. However, multicentric and bilateral tumours are frequent in VHL disease and bilateral nephrectomy may be required eventually. Renal transplantation is an option for a VHL patient in end-stage renal failure and experience so far suggests that immunosuppression does not affect adversely the underlying course of VHL disease.[19] Sporadic RCCs (phenocopies) occasionally occur in members of VHL families; the presence of a single renal tumour in a member of a VHL family, in the absence of other manifestations of VHL, is not sufficient to establish an unequivocal diagnosis of VHL.

The identification of renal cysts in VHL patients is a frequent and expected finding. As these do not usually compromise renal function, no treatment is necessary. It is known, however, that the epithelium lining the cysts in VHL kidneys is frequently atypical and may contain carcinoma *in situ*. If renal imaging suggests only simple cysts are present, then annual follow-up is sufficient. However, if complex cysts are detected, these should be reviewed more frequently as they can develop into solid lesions.[16]

EYE

In type 1 and type 2B families, retinal angiomas (HABs) are the commonest presenting feature of VHL disease, are frequently multiple and occur in ~68 per cent of type 1 and 2B cases.[20] Early detection of retinal angiomas allows small lesions to be treated by laser or cryotherapy, reducing the risk of complications and visual loss.

CENTRAL NERVOUS SYSTEM

Within the CNS, the cerebellum is the most frequent site of HAB followed by the spinal cord and brain stem (Table 10.2). Approximately 30 per cent of all patients with cerebellar HAB have VHL disease and the mean age at diagnosis of those with VHL disease is considerably younger than in sporadic cases.[21] Although the results of surgery for single laterally placed cerebellar lesions are usually excellent, the surgical management of spinal, brain stem or multiple HABs may be difficult and has significant morbidity. In some cases, radiosurgery may be an option and the development of effective anti-angiogenesis agents [e.g. vascular endothelial growth factor (VEGF) antagonists] might offer a medical approach to treatment in the future.

ADRENAL AND EXTRADRENAL PHAEOCHROMOCYTOMA

The overall frequency of phaeochromocytoma in VHL disease is ~10 per cent, but wide interfamilial variations reflect allelic heterogeneity (see earlier) and presentation with apparently isolated familial or bilateral phaeochromocytoma is well recognized.[13] Measurement of plasma normetanephrine levels is reported to be the most sensitive test for detecting phaeochromocytoma in VHL disease,[22] although many centres perform routine screening by urine analysis.

PANCREAS

Pancreatic cysts are frequent, but are usually asymptomatic and treatment is not required. In contrast, solid pancreatic tumours (usually non-secretory islet cell neoplasms), occur in only 5–10 per cent of cases but have been associated with a high risk of malignancy.[23] Early surgical intervention has been recommended, such that tumours >3 cm should be resected.[24]

OTHER SITES

Epididymal cysts are very common in males with VHL disease and may, if bilateral, impair fertility. However, their presence in an at-risk individual does not provide unequivocal evidence of carrier status. Endolymphatic sac tumours (ELST) may cause hearing loss, tinnitus and vertigo, and all medical staff dealing with VHL families should be aware of this complication, which can be detected by MRI scanning in up to 11 per cent of cases.[25]

Function of the VHL tumour suppressor gene product

The *VHL* tumour suppressor gene maps to chromosome 3p25 and encodes two proteins. The full-length 212 amino acid VHL protein ($pVHL_{29}$) migrates with an apparent molecular weight of ~29 kDa, but a second product ($pVHL_{19}$) is generated from an internal translation initiation site and lacks the first 53 amino acids.[26] No germline or somatic mutations have been reported in the first 53 codons and VHL_{19} has been shown to possess tumour suppressor activity. The complex genotype-phenotype associations observed in VHL disease suggest that the *VHL* gene product will have multiple and tissue-specific functions.[27] pVHL has been reported to bind directly or indirectly a number of proteins, including elongins B and C, Cul2, Rbx1 and fibronectin, and to regulate cell-cycle progression and expression of target genes, such as vascular endothelial growth factor and carbonic anhydrases (see Kaelin and Maher[27] and references within). Critical insights into a candidate function for pVHL have emanated from the suggestion that there were similarities between the VCBC(R) (VHL–elongin C–elongin B–Cul2–Rbx1) complex and the SCF (Skp-1–Cdc53/Cul1–F box protein) class of E3 ubiquitin ligases.[28] Thus, Maxwell *et al.* (1999) demonstrated that pVHL is critical for targeting the hypoxia-inducible transcription factors HIF-1 and HIF-2 (EPAS) for proteosomal destruction under normoxic conditions.[29] HIF-1 and HIF-2 transcription factors play a key role in the cellular response to hypoxia (oxygen sensing) and the regulation of genes involved in energy metabolism, angiogenesis and apoptosis including VEGF. Inactivation of the *VHL* tumour suppressor gene (as observed in tumours from VHL patients and most sporadic clear-cell RCCs; CCRCCs) results in elevated intracellular levels of HIF-1 and HIF-2, which correlate with the high levels of VEGF expression and hypervascularity observed in these tumours.[30,31] Recently, the VCBC(R) complex has been shown to promote HIF-1 ubiquitylation[32] and pVHL is predicted to act as an adaptor protein that recruits specific protein targets for ubiquitination and proteosomal degradation. The identification of further protein targets or additional non-SCF-like functions for pVHL may provide insights into genotype-phenotype correlations. The three-dimensional structure of VHL bound to elongins B and C has been solved; the locations of mutations have been mapped on the three-dimensional structure of the protein and the impact of mutations on elongin binding, binding of other substrates and VHL protein structure reported. However, the functional effects and phenotypic consequences of missense mutations are dependent on both the nature and position of the substitution so that alternative amino-acid substitutions at a single codon can cause different phenotypes.

CHROMOSOME 3 TRANSLOCATIONS AND CLEAR–CELL RENAL CELL CARCINOMA

The initial report of an association between CCRCC and a chromosome 3 translocation (t(3;8)(p14;q24)) in a large Italian American kindred suggested a RCC susceptibility gene at 3p14.[33] Translocation carriers developed CCRCC, frequently multiple and bilateral, with a penetrance of 67 per cent. Subsequently, an increased risk of thyroid cancer was also reported in the family. The chromosome 3 breakpoint in this family maps to the 3p14 fragile site and disrupts the *FHIT* candidate tumour suppressor gene.[34] However, the involvement of *FHIT* in CCRCC has been questioned and the importance of *FHIT* disruption to CCRCC susceptibility in this translocation family is unclear.

Further reports of chromosome 3 translocations associated with RCC susceptibility have described a variety of chromosome 3 breakpoints, e.g. t(3;6)(p13;q25),[35] t(2;3)(q35;q210[36] and t(3;12)(q35;q21).[37] Thus, there is no consistent involvement of 3p14 and *FHIT*, although chromosome 3 translocations associated with CCRCC are contained within the pericentromeric regions of 3p and 3q.[38] Analysis of tumours from patients with the RCC-associated translocations t(3;8), t(3;6) and t(2;3) has demonstrated loss of the derivative chromosome (an unexpected finding, if the translocation breakpoint disrupted a RCC tumour suppressor gene). Furthermore, the retained chromosome 3 has been found to harbour a somatic *VHL* gene mutation in tumours from individuals with the t(3;8) and t(2;3) (so the tumours had biallelic *VHL* gene inactivation).[36,39] Thus, a model for RCC tumorigenesis in translocation families is: (1) inheritance of a pericentromeric chromosome 3 translocation; (2) loss of the derivative chromosome 3 containing a *VHL* gene by random non-disjunction; and (3) somatic mutation of the *VHL* allele on the normal chromosome 3.

All patients with possible RCC susceptibility should be examined for chromosome 3 translocations. In addition, translocation carriers in kindreds with chromosome 3 translocations and RCC should be offered regular renal surveillance as for VHL disease (see earlier). There are relatively few data available for the risk of RCC in patients ascertained after the finding of a chromosome 3 translocation. However, in one study, there was a substantial increased risk of RCC in translocation carriers.[38] Thus, regular renal ultrasound surveillance may be indicated in chromosome 3 translocation carriers, particularly those with pericentromeric translocations.

FAMILIAL NON–VHL CCRCC

Familial RCC is uncommon and, prior to 1991, there had been 23 reports of 105 patients with familial RCC.[40] Although VHL disease, tuberous sclerosis and RCC associated with chromosome 3 translocations were well recognized then, familial non-clear cell RCC was not well defined until 1994.[41] The definition of subtypes of familial RCC based on histopathology and the availability of molecular genetic testing for germline *VHL* and *MET* gene mutations has led to the recognition of families with dominantly inherited susceptibility to CCRCC who do not have VHL disease or a chromosome 3 translocation.[42,43] The molecular basis of familial non-VHL CCRCC (FCRC) has not been defined except that it is not linked to *VHL*, *MET* or chromosome 3p.[42,43] In the original description of two large kindreds with FCRC, the age at onset was later than in VHL disease (8 out of 9 cases aged >50 years) and usually unilateral. However, a further report identified additional families with FCRC in which there was early onset of RCC (50 per cent diagnosed <50 years of age) and it was suggested that screening by renal imaging should be offered to at-risk relatives from age 20 years.[43] To date, there is no evidence of a significantly increased risk for non-renal cancers in FCRC kindreds.

HEREDITARY PAPILLARY RCC TYPE 1

Hereditary papillary RCC type 1 (HPRC1) is a rare dominantly inherited disorder (minimum prevalence 1 per 10 million) characterized by the development of multiple, bilateral type 1 papillary RCC. HPRC1 is caused by germline mutations in the *MET* proto-oncogene.[41,44,45]

Papillary RCC is the commonest form of non-CCRCC. Recently, it was suggested that papillary RCC can be subdivided into two groups: type 1 tumours, which are usually multiple and low grade; and type 2, which are single of higher grade and have a poorer prognosis.[46] Patients with germline *MET* gene mutations and HPRC1 have type 1 tumours so the histopathological analysis can be used to guide the priority for molecular genetic investigation.[47]

All germline *MET* mutations associated with HPRC1 appear to be activating missense mutations within the tyrosine kinase domain.[44,45] Three HPRC1 *MET* gene mutations (H1112R, V1238I, V1110I) have been reported as probable founder mutations. A striking feature of HPRC1 families is non-penetrance and there is a high frequency of subclinical disease in gene carriers who undergo renal imaging. The penetrance of the H1112R has been estimated as only 30 per cent at age 50 years, despite abdominal CT scanning.[48] Individuals with, or at risk for, HPRC1 should be offered annual renal imaging from age 30 years.

The *MET* proto-oncogene, primarily expressed in epithelial cells, encodes a cell-surface receptor for hepatocyte growth factor (HGF). Under normal circumstances, signalling by the MET receptor tyrosine kinase requires the present of the ligand, HGF. Normal signalling through the MET receptor tyrosine kinase is involved in cell growth, cell movement and cell differentiation. The impact of the *MET* mutations identified in HPRC patients has been studied by introducing these mutations into the mouse *met* gene and testing the impact of these mutations on the growth of indicator cells. The *met* mutations cause malignant transformation of mouse indicator cells.[49] Cells transformed by these mutations show constitutive signalling, constitutive phosphorylation and constitutive activation of downstream signalling pathways. The impact of the different *MET* mutations varies and there is evidence that for some *MET* mutations, different signalling pathways are activated. The three-dimensional structure of the MET tyrosine kinase has been modelled and the location of mutations mapped.

FAMILIAL PAPILLARY THYROID CANCER AND PAPILLARY RENAL NEOPLASIA

Malchoff *et al.* have described a single kindred with familial papillary thyroid cancer susceptibility mapping to chromosome 1q21.[50] Two family members developed papillary renal tumours, suggesting a common link between these tumour types.

FAMILIAL RENAL ONCOCYTOMA AND BIRT–HOGG–DUBE SYNDROME

Familial renal oncocytoma (FRO) is a recently described disorder characterized by two or more family members with renal oncocytomas.[51] Zbar and colleagues noticed that some FRO kindreds contained affected individuals with rare hamartomatous tumours of the hair follicle known as fibrofolliculoma.[52] Fibrofolliculomas are a characteristic feature of the dominantly inherited skin disorder Birt–Hogg–Dube (BHD) syndrome.[53] Typically, fibrofolliculomas in BHD develop after the age of 20 years and affected individuals may have between a few or hundreds of tumours on the face, neck or upper chest. BHD has been associated with spontaneous pneumothorax, lipomas and colorectal polyps and cancer. The risk for development of renal tumours in BHD appears to be increased.[54] Renal tumors in BHD may be single or multiple; the histologic appearance of renal tumors in BHD is variable and they are histologically distinct from those in HRRC1. In view of the elevated risk of RCC in some BHD kindreds, it is suggested that affected individuals should be offered annual renal ultrasound scans from age 25 years.

TUBEROUS SCLEROSIS

This dominantly inherited multiple hamartoma syndrome has been associated with an increased risk of RCC.[55–57] Tuberous sclerosis is caused by germline mutations in the *TSC1* and *TSC2* tumour suppressor genes. In rats, germline mutations in *Tsc2* cause the Eker rat model of familial RCC (Kobayashi *et al.*, 1995) and heterozygous *Tsc1* and *Tsc2* knockout mice develop a renal cystadenoma/carcinoma phenotype.[58,59] However, in humans, angiomyolipomas are by far the most common renal lesion. Although RCC is infrequent in tuberose sclerosis, several reports have described multifocal and bilateral disease in young patients.[55–57] Although the histological appearances of angiomyolipoma are very variable and some lesions could be mistaken for atypical RCC, the consensus opinion is that there is a real association between tuberous sclerosis and RCC (of variable histopathology).[60,61]

HYPERPARATHYROIDISM–JAW TUMOUR SYNDROME

A familial hyperparathyroidism syndrome associated with jaw cysts (HPT-JT) was mapped to chromosome 1q21–q31 by Szabo *et al.*[62] Subsequently, Teh *et al.*

confirmed linkage and reported an association with renal cysts and hamartomas.[63] Furthermore, renal hamartomas demonstrated 1q21–31 allele loss affecting the wild-type allele inherited from the normal parent consistent with HRPT2 functioning as a tumour suppressor gene. Recently, Haven *et al.* described a further family linked to the HPT-JT region in which a variety of tumours, including renal cortical adenoma and papillary RCC, were associated with parathyroid tumours and renal cysts.[64]

KEY POINTS: EVALUATION OF THE FAMILY WITH RENAL CANCER

Proper evaluation of a family with several members affected with renal cancer requires answers to a series of questions as shown below.

- Are the renal tumours single, or multiple – unilateral or bilateral?
- What are the histological appearances of the renal tumours in the different family members? Is the histologic appearance of the renal tumours in the various family members similar or different? In patients with multiple renal tumours, does each tumour nodule have a similar or different histologic appearance? Are there precursor lesions present in the normal parenchyma? The finding of multiple, bilateral, histologically similar renal tumours, combined with the finding of precursor lesions in normal renal parenchyma strongly suggests an inherited renal cancer syndrome.
- Evidence of additional features suggestive of a specific disorder should be sought by clinical enquiry and examination: is there a history of spontaneous pneumothorax, or facial skin bumps? Is there a history compatible with retinal angiomas or CNS hemangioblastomas? Is there a history of papillary thyroid carcinoma? Is there a history of cigarette smoking? Answers to these questions will help pinpoint which inherited renal tumour syndrome accounts for the findings in a referred family.

Mutation analysis of the RCC susceptibility genes, *VHL* and *MET*, facilitates the management of families with several members affected with renal cancer. When performed by a reliable DNA diagnostic laboratory and when proper attention is paid to the possibility of mosaicism, a negative test for a germline *VHL* mutation casts considerable doubt on a clinical diagnosis of VHL disease. Similarly, in the absence of a positive test for *MET* proto-oncogene mutations, doubt is cast on the diagnosis of hereditary papillary renal carcinoma type 1. The schema for clinical screening are shown in Table 10.3.

REFERENCES

1. Chow W-H, Gridley G, Fraumeni JF, Jarvholm B. Obesity, hypertension and the risk of kidney cancer in man. *N Engl J Med* 2000; **343:**1305–1311.

2. Thoenes W, Storkel S, Rumpelt HJ. Histopathology and classification of renal cell tumors (adenomas, oncocytomas and carcinomas). The basic cytological and histopathological elements and their use for diagnostics. *Path Res Pract* 1986; **181:**125–143.

3. Maher ER, Iselius L, Yates JRW, *et al.* Von Hippel–Lindau disease: a genetic study. *J Med Genet* 1991; **28:**443–447.

4. Melmon KL, Rosen SW. Lindau's disease. *Am J Med* 1964; **36:**595–617.

5. Maher ER, Yates JRW, Harries R, *et al.* Clinical features and natural history of von Hippel–Lindau disease. *Q J Med* 1990; **77:**1151–1163.

6. Zbar B, Kishida T, Chen F, *et al.* Germline mutations in the von Hippel–Lindau disease (*VHL*) gene in families from North America, Europe, and Japan. *Hum Mutat* 1996; **8:**348–357.

7. Webster AR, Richards FM, MacRonald FE, *et al.* An analysis of phenotypic variation in the familial cancer syndrome von Hippel–Lindau disease: evidence for modifier effects. *Am J Hum Genet* 1998; **63:**1025–1035.

8. Latif F, Tory K, Gnarra J, *et al.* Identification of the Vonhippel–Lindau disease tumor-suppressor gene. *Science* 1993, **260:**1317–1320.

9. Stolle C, Glenn G, Zbar B, *et al.* Improved detection of germline mutations in the von Hippel–Lindau disease tumor suppressor gene. *Hum Mutat* 1998; **12:**417–423.

10. Brauch H, Kishida T, Glavac D, *et al.* Von Hippel–Lindau (VHL) disease with pheochromocytoma in the Black-Forest Region of Germany – evidence for a founder effect. *Hum Genet* 1995; **95:**551–556.

11. Chen F, Slife L, Kishida T, *et al.* Genotype–phenotype correlation in von Hippel–Lindau disease: identification of a mutation associated with VHL type 2A. *J Med Genet* 1996; **33:**716–717.

12. Neumann HPH, Eng C, Mulligan L, *et al.* Consequences of direct genetic testing for germline mutations in the clinical management of families with multiple endocrine neoplasia type 2. *JAMA* 1995; **274:**1149–1151.

13. Woodward ER, Eng C, McMahon R, *et al.* Genetic predisposition to phaeochromocytoma: analysis of candidate genes *GDNF*, *RET* and *VHL*. *Hum Mol Genet* 1997; **6:**1051–1056.

14. Hes FJ, McKee S, Taphoorn MJB, *et al.* Cryptic Von Hippel–Lindau disease: germline mutations in haemangioblastoma-only patients. *J Med Genet* 2000; **37:**939–943.

15. Webster AR, Maher ER, Bird AC, Moore AT. Risk of multisystem disease in isolated ocular angioma. *J Med Genet* 2000; **37:**62–63.

16. Choyke PL, Glenn GM, Walther MCM, *et al.* The natural-history of renal lesions in von Hippel–Lindau Disease – a serial CT study in 28 patients. *Am J Roentgenol* 1992; **159:**1229–1234.

17. Walther MM, Choyke PL, Glenn G, *et al.* Renal cancer in families with hereditary renal cancer: prospective analysis of a tumor size threshold for renal parenchymal sparing surgery. *J Urol* 1999; **161:**1475–1479.

18. Steinbach F, Novick AC, Zincke H, *et al.* Treatment of renal-cell carcinoma in von Hippel–Lindau disease – a multicenter study. *J Urol* 1995; **153:**1812–1816.

19. Goldfarb DA, Neumann HP, Penn I, Novick AC. Results of renal transplantation in patients with renal cell carcinoma and von Hippel–Lindau disease. *Transplantation* 1997; **64:**1726–1729.

20. Webster AR, Maher ER, Moore AT. Clinical characteristics of ocular angiomatosis in von Hippel–Lindau disease and correlation with germline mutation. *Arch Ophthalmol* 1999; **117:**371–378.

21. Maher ER, Yates JRW, Ferguson-Smith MA. Statistical-analysis of the 2 stage mutation model in von Hippel–Lindau disease, and in sporadic cerebellar hemangioblastoma and renal-cell carcinoma. *J Med Genet* 1990; **27:**311–314.

22. Eisenhofer G, Lenders JW, Linehan WM, *et al.* Plasma normetanephrine and metanephrine for detecting pheochromocytoma in von Hippel–Lindau disease and multiple endocrine neoplasia type 2. *N Engl J Med.* 1999; **340:**1872–1979.

23. Binkovitz LA, Johnson CD, Stephens DH. Islet cell tumors in von Hippel–Lindau Disease – increased prevalence and relationship to the multiple endocrine neoplasias. *Am J Roentgenol* 1990; **155:**501–505.

24. Libutti SK, Choyke PL, Bartlett DL, *et al.* Pancreatic neuroendocrine tumors associated with von Hippel–Lindau disease: diagnostic and management recommendations. *Surgery* 1998; **124:**1153–1159.

25. Manski TJ, Heffner DK, Glenn GM, *et al.* Endolymphatic sac tumors – a source of morbid hearing loss in von Hippel–Lindau disease. *JAMA* 1997; **277:**1461–1466.

26. Schoenfeld A, Davidowitz EJ, Burk RD. A second major native von Hippel–Lindau gene product, initiated from an internal translation start site, functions as a tumor suppressor. *Proc Natl Acad Sci USA* 1998; **95:**8817–8822.

27. Kaelin WG, Maher ER. The *VHL* tumour suppressor gene paradigm. *Trends Genet* 1998; **14:**423–425.

28. Lonergan KM, Iliopoulos O, Ohh M, *et al.* Regulation of hypoxia inducible mRNAs by the von Hippel Lindau tumor suppressor protein requires binding to complexes containing elongins B/C and Cul2. *Mol Cell Biol* 1998; **18:**732–741.

29. Maxwell P, Wiesener M, Chang G-W, *et al.* The von Hippel–Lindau gene product is necessary for oxygen-dependent proteolysis of hypoxia-inducible factor α subunits. *Nature* 1999; **399:**271–275.

30. Siemeister G, Weindel K, Mohrs K, *et al.* Reversion of deregulated expression of vascular endothelial growth factor in human renal carcinoma cells by von Hippel–Lindau tumor suppressor protein. *Cancer Res* 1996; **56:**2299–2301.

31. Leung SK, Ohh M. Playing tag with HIF: the VHL story. *J Biomed Biotechnol* 2002; **2:**131–135.

32. Cockman ME, Masson N, Mole DR, *et al.* Hypoxia inducible factor-alpha binding and ubiquitylation by the von Hippel–Lindau tumor suppressor protein. *J Biol Chem* 2000; **275:**25733–25741.

33. Cohen AJ, Li FP, Berg S, *et al.* Hereditary renal cell carcinoma associated with a chromosomal translocation. *N Engl J Med* 1979; **301:**592–595.

34. Gemmill RM, West JD, Boldog F, *et al.* The hereditary renal cell carcinoma 3;8 translocation fuses *FHIT* to a patched-related gene, TRC8. *Proc Natl Acad Sci USA* 1998; **95:**9572–9577.

35. Kovacs G, Brusa P, De Riese W. Tissue-specific expression of a constitutional 3;6 translocation: development of multiple

bilateral renal-cell carcinomas. *Int J Cancer* 1989; **43:** 422–427.

36. Bodmer D, Eleveld MJ, Ligtenberg MJL, *et al.* An alternative route for multistep tumorigenesis in a novel case of hereditary renal cell cancer and a t(2;3)(q35;q21) chromosome translocation. *Am J Hum Genet* 1998; **62:**1475–1483.

37. Kovacs G, Hoene E. Loss of der(3) in renal carcinoma cells of a patient with constitutional t(3;12). *Hum Genet* 1988; **78:**148–150.

38. van Kessel AG, Wijnhoven H, Bodmer D, *et al.* Renal cell cancer: chromosome 3 translocations as risk factors. *J Natl Cancer Inst* 1999; **91:**1159–1160.

39. Schmidt L, Li F, Brown RS, *et al.* Mechanism of tumorigenesis of renal carcinomas associated with the constitutional chromosome 3;8 translocation. *Cancer J Sci Am* 1995; **1:**191–196.

40. Maher ER, Yates JRW. Familial renal cell carcinoma – clinical and molecular genetic aspects. *Br J Cancer* 1991; **63:**176–179.

41. Zbar B, Glenn G, Lubensky I, *et al.* Hereditary papillary renal carcinoma: clinical studies in 10 families. *J Urol* 1995; **153:**907–912.

42. Teh BT, Giraud S, Sari NF, *et al.* Familial non-VHL non-papillary clear-cell renal cancer. *Lancet* 1997; **349:**848–849.

43. Woodward ER, Clifford SC, Astuti D, *et al.* Familial clear cell renal cell carcinoma (FCRC): clinical features and mutation analysis of the *VHL, MET,* and *CUL2* candidate genes. *J Med Genet* 2000; **37:**348–353.

44. Schmidt L, Duh FM, Chen F, *et al.* Germline and somatic mutations in the tyrosine kinase domain of the MET proto-oncogene in papillary renal carcinomas. *Nature Genet* 1997; **16:**68–73.

45. Schmidt L, Junker K, Weirich G, *et al.* Two North American families with hereditary papillary renal carcinoma and identical novel mutations in the *MET* proto-oncogene. *Cancer Res* 1998; **58:**1719–1722.

46. Delahunt B, Eble JN. Papillary renal cell carcinoma: a clinicopathologic and immunohistochemical study of 105 tumors. *Mod Pathol* 1997; **10:**537–544.

47. Lubensky IA, Schmidt L, Zhuang ZP, *et al.* Hereditary and sporadic papillary renal carcinomas with c-*MET* mutations share a distinct morphologic phenotype. *Am J Pathol* 1999; **155:**517–526.

48. Choyke PL, Walther MM, Glenn GM, *et al.* Imaging features of hereditary papillary renal cancers. *J Comput Assist Tomogr* 1997; **21:**737–741.

49. Jeffers M, Schmidt L, Nakaigawa N, *et al.* Activating mutations for the Met tyrosine kinase receptor in human cancer. *Proc Natl Acad Sci USA* 1997; **94:**11445–11450.

50. Malchoff CD, Sarfarazi M, Tendler B, *et al.* Papillary thyroid carcinoma associated with papillary renal neoplasia: genetic linkage analysis of a distinct heritable tumor syndrome. *J Clin Endocrinol Metab* 2000; **85:**1758–1764.

51. Weirich G, Glenn G, Junker K, *et al.* Familial renal oncocytoma: clinicopathologic study of 5 families. *J Urol* 1998; **160:**335–340.

52. Toro J, Duray P, Glenn G, *et al.* Birt–Hogg–Dube syndrome: a novel marker of renal neoplasia. *Arch Dermatol* 1999; **135:**1195–1202.

53. Birt AR, Hogg GR, Dube WJ. Hereditary multiple fibrofolliculomas and trichodiscomas and acrochordons. *Arch Dermatol* 1977; **113:**1674–1677.

54. Zbar B, Alvord WG, Glenn G, *et al.* Risk of renal and colonic neoplasms and spontaneous pneumothorax in the Birt-Hogg-Dube syndrome. *Cancer Epidemiol Biomarkers Prev* 2002 Apr; **11**(4):393–400.

55. Bjornsson J, Short MP, Kwiatkowski DJ, Henske EP. Tuberous sclerosis-associated renal cell carcinoma: clinical, pathologic and genetic features. *Am J Pathol* 1996; **149:**1201–1208.

56. Sampson JR, Patel A, Mee AD. Multifocal renal cell carcinoma in sibs from a chromosome 9 linked (TSC1) tuberous sclerosis family. *J Med Genet* 1995; **32:**848–850.

57. Al-Saleem T, Wessner LL, Scheitauer BW, *et al.* Malignant tumours of the kidney, brain and soft malignant tissues in children and young adults with the tuberous sclerosis complex. *Cancer* 1998; **83:**2208–2216.

58. Kobayashi T, Hirayama Y, Kobayashi E, *et al.* A germline insertion in the tuberous sclerosis (*Tsc2*) gene gives rise to the Eker rat model of dominantly inherited cancer. *Nature Genet* 1995; **9:**70–74.

59. Onda H, Lueck A, Marks PW, *et al.* Tsc2(+\−) mice develop tumors in multiple sites that express gelsolin and are influenced by genetic background. *J Clin Invest* 1999; **104:**687–695.

60. Pea M, Bonetti F, Martignoni G, *et al.* Apparent renal cell carcinomas in tuberous sclerosis are heterogeneous – the identification of malignant epithelioid angiomyolipoma. *Am J Surg Path* 1998; **22:**180–187.

61. Robertson FM, Cendron M, Klauber GT, Harris BH. Renal cell carcinoma in association with tuberous sclerosis in children. *J Pediatr Surg* 1996; **31:**729–730.

62. Szabo J, Heath B, Hill VM, *et al.* Hereditary hyperparathyroidism-jaw tumor syndrome: the endocrine tumor gene *HRPT2* maps to chromosome 1q21-q31. *Am J Hum Genet* 1995; **56:**944–950.

63. Teh BT, Farnebo F, Kristoffersson U, *et al.* Autosomal dominant primary hyperparathyroidism and jaw tumor syndrome associated with renal hamartomas and cystic kidney disease: linkage to 1q21-q32 and loss of the wild type allele in renal hamartomas. *J Clin Endocrinol Metab* 1996; **81:**4204–4211.

64. Haven CJ, Wong FK, van Dam EW, *et al.* A genotypic and histopathological study of a large Dutch kindred with hyperparathyroidism–jaw tumor syndrome. *J Clin Endocrinol Metab* 2000; **85:**1449–1454.

65. Davis CJ Jr, Mostofi FK, Sesterhenn IA. Renal medullary carcinoma. The seventh sickle cell nephropathy. *Am J Surg Pathol* 1995; **19:**1–11.

11

The Li–Fraumeni syndrome and the role of *TP53* mutations in predisposition to cancer

JILLIAN M. BIRCH

INTRODUCTION AND DEFINITIONS

In 1969, as part of a survey of nearly 650 children with rhabdomyosarcoma in the USA, Li and Fraumeni identified three pairs of siblings affected with the disease when less than one was expected by chance. One pair of affected cousins was also identified.

Information obtained by interview demonstrated a high incidence of breast cancer, sarcomas and other unusual cancers in close relatives of index cases. It is notable that three of the mothers of index children developed breast cancer under 30 years of age.[1] In a more detailed report, a second pair of cousins with childhood soft tissue sarcoma were identified, and the finding of adrenocortical carcinoma and brain tumours in first-degree relatives of children with soft tissue sarcoma suggested that these cancers may also be components of the syndrome.[2]

One family showing a similar pattern of cancers had been published previously,[3] and descriptions of other families, consistent with Li and Fraumeni's findings, were reported subsequently.[4–6] At this time, however, it was uncertain whether these observations were due to inherited predisposition to a range of neoplasms, exposure to a common environmental agent, or whether the reported families simply represented rare chance aggregations of cancers. A series of subsequent systematic studies of families and patient populations provided several pieces of evidence, which strongly supported the notion of inherited susceptibility.

Firstly, Li and Fraumeni carried out a follow-up study of the four families and found that, over a 12-year period, 10 of 31 surviving members had between them developed 16 additional cancers, compared with less than one expected. These cancers showed the same pattern as had been observed originally and included five breast cancers, four soft tissue sarcomas and two brain tumours. The excess was particularly marked for breast cancers, with five observed and only 0.08 expected. Four soft tissue sarcomas occurred within previous radiotherapy fields but, when these were excluded, there was still a highly significant excess of cancers (12 observed, 0.5 expected). The observation that 12 of the cancers occurred as second or subsequent primaries, and were predominantly sarcomas and carcinoma of the breast, added further weight to the idea of genetic susceptibility in these individuals.[7]

Definitive evidence came from two groups who studied cancer incidence in the families of a population-based series of children with soft-tissue sarcoma, and a hospital-based series of survivors of childhood soft tissue sarcoma, respectively.[8–11] The first report was based on an analysis of cancer incidence in mothers of children included in the Manchester Children's Tumour Registry (UK) with a diagnosis of soft tissue sarcoma. There was an increased incidence of cancer among these mothers, particularly premenopausal breast cancer, where the observed to expected ratio was 3.0.[8,9] This group went on to study the cancer experience among all first-degree relatives and showed a statistically significant excess of cancers (relative risk 1.6), which was accounted for by cancers in mothers and siblings, with no excess in the fathers. The excess was mainly due to carcinoma of the breast and paediatric tumours. The risk was highest for cancers diagnosed at younger ages. Multivariate analysis of clinical characteristics in the index patient identified young age at diagnosis, histological subtype of embryonal rhabdomyosarcoma and male sex as independent indicators of increased cancer risk in first-degree relatives.[10]

Among first-degree relatives of a hospital-based series of survivors of childhood soft tissue sarcoma, a similar excess of cancers was also found, with 34 observed compared with 20.7 expected, the excess again being predominantly due to breast cancers and cancers of bone and soft tissue, at young ages. In this series, the relatives of children with multiple primary cancers, soft tissue sarcoma diagnosed at younger ages and histologic type of embryonal rhabdomyosarcoma were at highest risk.[11]

Segregation analysis demonstrated that the cancer distribution in the families was compatible with a rare autosomal dominant gene (gene frequency 0.00002), with a penetrance of almost 50 per cent by age 30 years and 90 per cent by age 60. In children who are gene carriers, the estimated relative risk of developing cancer was 100 times the background rate. Although age-specific penetrance was slightly higher in females, maternal and paternal lineages contributed equally to the evidence favouring a dominant gene.[12,13]

In order to study the characteristic components of the syndrome, Li *et al.* assembled 24 kindreds conforming to standard criteria, as follows: bone or soft tissue sarcoma, diagnosed under the age of 45 years, in an individual designated the proband, one first-degree relative with cancer under 45 years of age, and one first- or second-degree relative in the same lineage, with cancer under 45 or sarcoma diagnosed at any age.[14] These criteria have been widely accepted as a clinical definition of the syndrome and families conforming to these criteria are hereafter referred to as having classic Li–Fraumeni syndrome (LFS). An example of a family with classic LFS is shown in Figure 11.1.

Among the 151 individuals in the cancer lineage of each family who developed cancer, 119 (79 per cent) were affected under the age of 45 years, compared with 10 per cent of all cancers occurring below this age in the general population. Li *et al.* compared the distribution of cancer

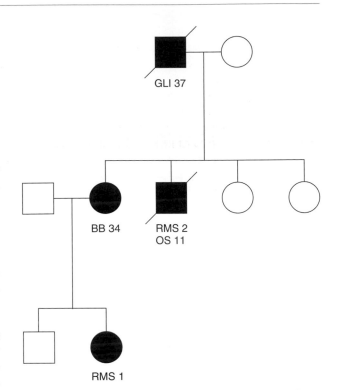

Figure 11.1 *Family conforming to the syndrome criteria of Li et al.[14] – 'Classic Li–Fraumeni syndrome'. BB, bilateral breast carcinoma; GLI, glioma; RMS, rhabdomyosarcoma. Numbers indicate age at diagnosis.*

types below age 45 years with the distribution in this age range in the US population. They found that, in addition to sarcoma and breast cancer, three other cancer types were more frequent in the families. These included brain tumours, leukaemia and adrenocortical carcinoma. Fifteen patients had multiple primary cancers and the types of cancer, which emerged as the principal components of the syndrome on the basis of first primary cancers, also predominated as second and subsequent primaries.[14] The distribution of cancers among the population-based and hospital-based series of families of children with soft tissue sarcoma were consistent with these findings. but also suggested that melanoma, germ cell tumours and Wilms tumour may represent additional syndrome components.[10,11,13,15–17]

IDENTIFICATION OF MUTATIONS IN THE *TP53* GENE AS A CAUSE OF LFS

The above systematic studies provided compelling evidence that, in certain families, there was an inherited predisposition to a diverse but specific range of cancers, but identification of the gene(s) responsible for LFS was problematical. No characteristic constitutional chromosomal aberrations were found and classic genetic linkage analysis was difficult because of the high mortality associated with the component tumours. Furthermore, because some of the component cancers are frequent in the general population (e.g. breast cancer), the problem of phenocopies also arose. For these reasons, Malkin et al. adopted an alternative approach, in choosing to analyse candidate genes.[18] They reasoned that the LFS gene was most likely to be a tumour suppressor gene. Deletions and/or mutations in the *TP53* gene had been found in tumour tissue from sporadic osteosarcomas, soft tissue sarcomas, brain tumours, leukaemias and carcinoma of the breast. In addition, mice with a constitutional *p53* mutation had been shown to develop bone and soft tissue sarcomas, adrenal and lymphoid tumours and other tumours at an increased level.[19] The *TP53* gene, therefore, appeared to be a plausible candidate for LFS. Constitutional samples from members of five families with LFS were analysed and germline mutations in the *TP53* gene were found in all cancer-affected individuals tested.

The *TP53* gene contains five domains within the coding region, which are evolutionarily highly conserved. In sporadic tumours, *TP53* mutations tend to cluster in four of the highly conserved domains in exon 5, encompassing two of these domains, exon 7 and exon 8. Certain codons have emerged as mutational hot spots. The six most commonly affected codons are 175, 245, 249, 248, 273 and 282.[20] The germline mutations in LFS families reported by Malkin et al.[18] affected codons 245, 248 (two families) 252 (later corrected to deletion at codon 184)[21] and 258. Shortly after this report, a sixth LFS family with a germline mutation in codon 245 was published.[22] These germline mutations had apparently all occurred in a stretch of 14 codons within the fourth conserved domain, which resides in exon 7 of the gene. Following these two reports, there was much speculation about the possible significance of this positional clustering and it was suggested that there may be restriction on the types of *TP53* mutations, which could occur in the germline with the possibility that other mutations could be lethal.[23]

Following on from the above work, many groups throughout the world have analysed LFS families, families with cancer clusters suggestive of LFS (LF like or LFL families) and series of patients with LFS-associated cancers, including osteosarcomas, rhabdomyosarcomas, other soft tissue sarcomas, brain tumours, leukaemias and adrenocortical carcinomas. Because of the frequency of premenopausal breast cancer in LFS families, series of breast cancer patients and site-specific familial breast cancer were also studied. In addition, a number of groups have analysed patients with multiple primary tumours. To date, there are 226 published germline *TP53* mutations of confirmed or probable biological significance.[18,21,22,24–121] Reports of sequence variants of uncertain significance[122–125] are not considered in the analyses presented below.

GERMLINE *TP53* MUTATIONS IN FAMILIAL CANCER CLUSTERS

It soon became clear that germline *TP53* mutations are not restricted to families conforming to the criteria for classic LFS. Conversely, germline mutations in *TP53* cannot be detected in all classic LFS families. In total, there are 83 published examples of LFS families with germline *TP53* mutations.[121] However, the majority of these comprise single family reports. Only three groups have published series of LFS families, which provide details of mutation negative as well as mutation positive families. Birch et al.[28] and Frebourg et al.[47] reported germline *TP53* mutations in 6 of 12 and 7 of 15 LFS families, respectively, giving a germline mutation rate of 50 per cent. More recently, Chompret et al.[35] reported mutations in 8 out of 16 LFS families. However, the mutation detection methods used in these studies were likely to miss some mutations. Thus, although Frebourg et al.[47] analysed exons 2–11 by direct sequencing, the intron–exon boundaries were not analysed and some parts of exons were not included. The study by Chompret et al.[35] employed the FASAY,[126] which consistently fails to detect splicing mutations.[107] The estimate of a germline mutation rate of 50 per cent will, therefore, be an underestimate. To overcome these problems Varley et al.[112] extended the series of Birch et al.[28] and used comprehensive, automated methods to sequence exons 1–11 including all splice junctions, the promotor and the 3′-untranslated region. The series was updated by Birch et al.[127] and, in total, 15 of 20 (75 per cent) LFS families were found to carry germline *TP53* mutations.

Numerous reports exist of germline *TP53* mutations in families with clusters of cancers that are suggestive of LFS but do not strictly conform to the criteria.[14] Such families may be designated Li–Fraumeni like (LFL). In order to study the frequency of *TP53* mutations among LFL families systematically, Birch et al.[28] defined LFL syndrome as follows: a proband with any childhood cancer or sarcoma, brain tumour or adrenocortical carcinoma diagnosed under 45 years of age, with one first- or second-degree relative with typical LFS cancer (sarcoma, breast cancer, brain tumour, leukaemia or adrenocortical carcinoma diagnosed at any age, plus one first- or second-degree relative in the same lineage with any cancer diagnosed under 60 years). These criteria are broader than the LFS criteria and allow for non-sarcoma probands, unaffected mutation carriers and a somewhat wider age range. However, site-specific breast cancer families are not included, and the criteria still require a cluster of mainly unusual cancers diagnosed at ages younger than the population average. Birch et al. analysed a series of LFL families conforming to these criteria.[28] The series was extended by Varley et al.[112] and updated by Birch et al.[127] In total, germline *TP53* mutations were detected in 5 of

14 (36 per cent) LFL families. In the literature, there are a further 28 reports of families with germline *TP53* mutations conforming to these criteria, which, therefore, appear to select families at high risk of carrying such mutations.

GERMLINE *TP53* MUTATIONS IN SERIES OF CANCER PATIENTS

Several groups have analysed the frequency of germline *TP53* mutations among patients with bone or soft tissue sarcoma.[25,38,59,73,83,105] The selection criteria varied between studies with respect to age restrictions, family history and presence of multiple primary tumours. Overall, about 3 per cent of early-onset osteosarcoma carry germline *TP53* mutations but with a higher rate (up to 30 per cent) in those cases with a relevant family history or multiple tumours. In childhood rhabdomyosarcoma, approximately 10 per cent appear to be associated with mutations overall but with a higher rate (more than 20 per cent) in those diagnosed at very young age.[38]

A number of groups have studied the frequency of germline *TP53* mutations among patients with brain tumours.[34,36,63,65,104,115,120] Selection criteria varied with respect to type of brain tumour, presence of multi-focal tumours, history of other primary neoplasms and family histories of brain tumours and/or other cancers. Some reports were based on unselected cases. Across all unselected series, 5 per cent of cases were associated with germline *TP53* mutations. In the majority of these patients, the associated brain tumour was high-grade astrocytoma/glioblastoma multiforme. Among the selected patients with significant family histories or multiple tumours, 15 per cent carried germline *TP53* mutations.

Adrenocortical carcinoma (ACC) in children is exceedingly rare but is frequently seen in LFS. Four groups have studied unselected series of childhood ACC to determine the frequency of mutations in apparently sporadic cases. Wagner *et al.* found mutations in three of six cases (50 per cent).[116] However, the mutation detection methods used are likely to have missed a proportion of mutations. Varley *et al.*, using more comprehensive methods, found germline *TP53* mutations in 11 of 14 (85 per cent) cases.[109] In the latter series, cases associated with LFS or LFL were excluded.

Ribeiro *et al.* analysed 36 cases of ACC in Brazilian children.[110] Brazil has an incidence of ACC, which is 10–15 times higher than most other countries worldwide.[110] Remarkably, the same germline *TP53* mutation involving a single base change at codon 337 (Arg to His) in the tetramerization domain was found in 35 of the children. Full family histories were available on 25 families and, in 24 of these, there was no evidence of increased cancer predisposition. In the remaining family, an LFL cancer pattern was seen in second- and higher-degree relatives. However, multiple cases of ACC were observed in four families. These observations were confirmed in an independent series of 55 ACC patients, also from Brazil, including 37 adults and 18 children. The same codon 337 mutation was identified in 19 of the cases, 14 children and 5 adults.[111] It is possible that there may be an environmental determinant present in Brazil, which is responsible for the induction of this mutation, leading to a high incidence of ACC. These 54 cases with mutation at codon 337, in the absence of frank familial predisposition, are not included in the analyses of mutation spectrum below.

Breast cancer is a very common feature in LFS and LFL families. Three groups have now collectively analysed more than 800 unselected breast cancer patients.[30,85,128] Among these cases, germline *TP53* mutations were detected in only 2 (0.25 per cent). Such mutations are clearly rare among apparently sporadic breast cancers. There have been four reports from groups who have analysed series of breast cancers in patients selected because of family history of breast cancer or early-onset (under 40 years of age) disease.[30,99,128,129]

A total of 383 such cases have been analysed and among these four patients with mutations were detected (1 per cent). It is also clear, therefore, that germline *TP53* mutations account for only a small number even among selected cases.

Only one series of childhood leukaemia patients has been analysed.[43] In this study, among the 25 patients, one was found to carry a germline *TP53* mutation. Further studies would be required to assess the proportion of childhood leukaemia cases, which may be due to such mutations. There has been a single study of the frequency of germline *TP53* mutations among ovarian cancer patients,[62] where 2 of 20 patients (10 per cent) were found to carry such mutations. This is a surprisingly high frequency given the low frequency of ovarian malignancies in LFS families. Further studies are required to substantiate this finding.

There have been several single case reports of germline *TP53* mutations in patients with multiple primary cancers, but only one large and one small series of patients with multiple primaries have been analysed.[71,98] Malkin *et al.* originally reported such mutations in 4 of 59 children and young adults with second primary cancers.[71] However, this was later corrected to 3 of 59.[70] Shiseki *et al.* examined five patients, each with three primary cancers, and found a germline *TP53* mutation in one case.[98] It is noteworthy that in the four cases among these two series with mutations, in general, both the first and subsequent primaries were consistent with tumours observed in LFS.

Many of the studies referred to above looked at relatively small series of patients. In addition, some mutation detection methods employed would have missed a proportion of mutations, because only limited regions of the gene were sequenced and/or rapid screening techniques were used. Therefore, the mutation frequencies found must be regarded as uncertain or underestimates of the true mutation frequencies.

DISTRIBUTION OF GERMLINE *TP53* MUTATIONS AND FREQUENCY OF MUTATION TYPES

Analyses of the location and frequency of germline *TP53* mutations are given on the International Agency for Research on Cancer (IARC) *p53* website and database.[121] This database has now been redesigned to take into account family phenotype and data entry has been completed for published mutations up to mid-2002. The analyses presented below are, therefore, based on data abstracted from the 208 published germline *TP53* mutations cited above. Figure 11.2 represents the location and frequency distribution of 189 mutations within the coding region of *TP53* where the affected codons are specified. Where deletion and/or insertion mutations affect more than one codon, the location of the first affected codon is plotted. The figure also shows the exon delineation and the positions of the five conserved domains.[130]

Mutations are found from exon 4 through to exon 10, but are concentrated in exons 5–8, which include almost 90 per cent of all published mutations. To some extent this distribution has been influenced by a large number of studies in which exons 5–9 or 5–8 only have been analysed. However, even in studies employing comprehensive analysis methods that include coding and noncoding regions of the gene, the majority of the detected mutations occurred in exons 5–8. Varley *et al.*[112] employing such methods, described 19 mutations of which 14 (74 per cent) occurred in exons 5–8.

A number of mutational 'hot-spot' codons have emerged and these are individually labelled in Figure 11.2. Five of these, codons 175, 245, 248, 273 and 282, are also mutational 'hot spots' for somatic mutations.[131] Mutations at these five codons account for 34 per cent of all coding mutations in the germline. Other frequently mutated codons are 125,133,152, 213 and 235, each of which includes at least five examples. With the exception of codon 213, these positions do not emerge as 'hot spots' for somatic mutations.

Figure 11.3 shows the distribution of mutation types among the published germline *TP53* mutations. Transitions account for 65 per cent and, of these, 44 per cent were at CpG sites. Transversions account for 22 per cent, and deletions and/or insertions comprise 13 per cent. CpG dinucleotides are common sites of cytosine methylation and transitions can occur as a result of replication errors

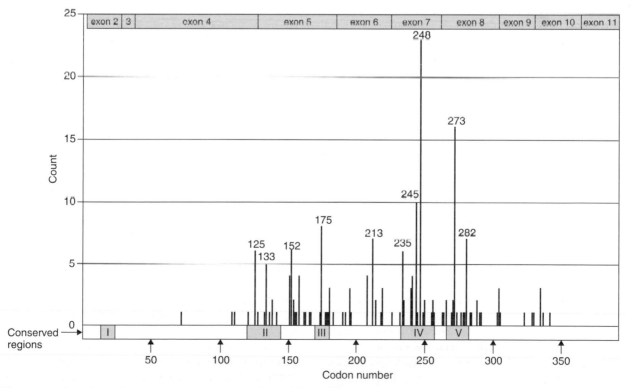

Figure 11.2 *Location and frequency of germline mutations within the* TP53 *coding region.*

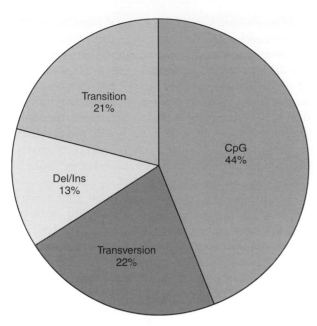

Figure 11.3 *Frequency by type of germline* TP53 *mutation. Del/Ins, deletions and/or insertions.*

following deamination of 5-methylcytosine producing thymine. Such mutations are regarded as endogenous events.[20] Transversions may occur as result of replication errors but could also arise owing to exposure to exogenous carcinogens. It has been noted previously[132] that a statistically significant higher proportion of transversions has been found in patients with no family history of cancer, raising the possibility that some germline mutations, which have arisen recently, may be due to DNA damage following exposure to exogenous carcinogens. The proportion of deletion/insertion mutations, 13 per cent, is exactly the same as that among somatic *TP53* mutations[20] but, whereas deletions or insertions in sporadic tumours occur more frequently in exons 2–4 and 9–11, in the germline, 74 per cent are found in exons 5–8. The possible significance of these differences is unclear at present.

Splicing mutations have been reported relatively infrequently and represent 8 per cent of published germline *TP53* mutations. This will certainly be an underestimate, since most investigators have not analysed splice junctions. The true frequency of splicing mutations is likely to be much higher.[107] It is interesting to note that six of the 17 published splicing mutations affect the same residue, codon 125, at the splice donor site in exon 4.

The frequency of *de novo* germline *TP53* mutations among unselected series of patients cannot be ascertained reliably from the current literature, since often only the index patient and one other person who may not be informative have been tested. Transmission/segregation of the mutant genotype, therefore, cannot be established. Only one study has looked at this issue systematically.[35] In this study, four *de novo* mutations were detected among

a total of 17 germline *TP53* mutations occurring in 268 index cases with malignancies diagnosed during childhood. This represents a surprisingly high *de novo* mutation rate.

FUNCTIONAL SIGNIFICANCE OF GERMLINE *TP53* MUTATIONS

The *TP53* gene possesses a range of properties, including transcriptional activation and repression through sequence-specific DNA binding to specific target sequences. The amino terminus of the protein includes sequences that show transactivation properties when interacting with target sequences through specific DNA interactions.[130,132–136] The first conserved domain (codons 13–23) resides within the transactivation domain (codons 1–50). Conserved domains 2–5 all reside within the central core DNA binding region encompassing codons 102–292. The crystal structure of the DNA binding domain has been determined and consists of a β-sandwich, which acts as a scaffold for two large loops and a loop–sheet–helix motif forming the DNA binding surface of the TP53 protein.[133] It is striking that the elements of the structure involved in DNA binding coincide with conserved regions 3–5.

An important observation followed the elucidation of the crystal structure is that the majority of human germline and somatic *TP53* mutations fall within the three loop motifs. In general, mutations occur most frequently in the regions of the core domain that are closest to the DNA binding region. Residues that are infrequently mutated in general are far from the DNA binding region. The two most frequently mutated residues in both the germline and in tumours, Arg-248 and Arg-273, directly contact DNA, whereas Arg-175, Gly-245 and Arg-282 play a critical role in stabilizing the structure of the DNA binding surface. Thus, two classes of mutation may be defined as; contact mutations, whereby failure to bind DNA may be attributed to loss of critical DNA contacts, and structural mutations, whereby loss of DNA binding may be attributed to structural defects in the mutant product.[133] However, missense mutations at almost every codon in the DNA binding domain have been found in human tumours and amino acid substitution at most, if not all, of the 191 residues in the core domain appears to disrupt or modify respective interactions of the TP53 protein with target DNA.[131]

The TP53 protein functions as a tetramer and codons 323–356 comprise the tetramerization domain.[130] Mutations in the tetramerization domain are relatively infrequent in tumours and in the germline except in cases of ACC from Brazil,[110,111] but such mutations could be predicted to prevent efficient functioning of *TP53*. The codon

337 (Arg to His) mutation frequently found in cases of ACC from Brazil appears to be highly sensitive to pH in the physiological range and is less stable than the wild type.[137]

Wild-type *TP53* functions in checkpoint control following DNA damage, resulting in either a delay in progression through the cell cycle, thus allowing DNA repair to occur, or leading to apoptosis, and *TP53* has been termed the guardian of the genome.[134] A number of approaches have demonstrated that the biochemical and biological properties of naturally occurring mutant TP53 proteins vary under experimental conditions.[135–140] These properties include effects upon *in vitro* cell lines and the tumorigenicity of cell lines expressing p53, when injected into nude mice.[135–139] The four residues within the DNA binding domain representing mutational 'hot spots', codons 175, 245, 248 and 273, have all been shown to exhibit gain of function and/or dominant negative properties in at least some assays,[138] giving rise to the prediction that tumours with mutant missense TP53 proteins may be more aggressive or have a poorer prognosis than tumours with no functional TP53 protein.

The accepted model for a tumour suppressor gene involves mutation of one allele and loss of the remaining wild-type allele (loss of heterozygosity; LOH). It has been demonstrated, however, that only 44 per cent of tumours from members of families carrying germline *TP53* mutations show loss of the wild-type allele.[141] Furthermore, the lowest proportion of LOH occurred in tumours arising in patients with mutations at 'hot spot' codons with a high proportion of tumours showing LOH in patients with protein inactivating mutations. These data would tend to support an oncogenic gain of function in the protein products associated with at least some missense mutations in the core DNA binding domain.

THE *TP53* PHENOTYPE

Germline *TP53* mutations have been detected in about 70 per cent of classic LFS families, but it has not been possible to identify *TP53* mutations in a proportion of such families.[112] Conversely, germline *TP53* mutations have been demonstrated in families displaying clusters of cancers which fall outside of the strict LFS criteria. The question of which cancers constitute the *TP53* phenotype, therefore, arises.

Three systematic analyses have sought to address this question. Studies by Kleihues *et al.*[142] and Nichols *et al.*[143] relied mainly on reviews of the frequency of specific cancers among published families with germline *TP53* mutations. There are a number of problems associated with literature-based analyses. Such an approach does not allow for methods of ascertainment of families, the varying quality of family data, and whether or not the

detected mutations have been shown to segregate with cancers in the families. Factors such as these can influence both the observed and the expected cancers. Additionally, such families have been ascertained over a very wide time span and originate from many different countries. Variations in cancer incidence over time and between populations may influence the pattern of cancers. Furthermore, these two studies included proband cancers in the analysis, which will inevitably result in a distortion of the frequencies of occurrence of certain tumours. The study by Birch *et al.* was based on a large series of families analysed at a single centre and which were fully documented with special histopathological review in the majority of cancers.[144]

All three studies concluded that, numerically, the main cancers to occur in carriers of germline *TP53* mutations are breast cancers, bone and soft tissue sarcomas, and brain tumours, and that adrenocortical carcinoma also occurs to excess. There was agreement that leukaemia does not appear to be a major component of the *TP53* syndrome. Results on other possible components of the syndrome, however, differed between studies. Thus, Nichols *et al.*[143] concluded that carcinomas of lung and gastrointestinal tract, lymphomas and other neoplasms occurred at much earlier ages than expected in the general population, and were, therefore, likely to be associated with the syndrome. This conclusion was based on ages at cancer diagnosis among all families and patients with germline *TP53* mutations published in the literature, compared with the respective median ages at diagnosis for specific cancers in the US population.

Birch *et al.* estimated the expected frequencies of specific cancers among a cohort of individuals from 28 families fulfilling the diagnostic criteria for LFS and segregating germline *TP53* mutations.[144] The estimated cancer frequencies were based on the age, sex, calendar period, site and morphology-specific national cancer incidence rates applied to the cohort. The distribution of cancers in the cohort was highly significantly different from that expected. There were highly significant excesses of carcinoma of the female breast, tumours of brain and spinal cord, soft tissue sarcoma, osteosarcoma and chondrosarcoma, Wilms' tumour, adrenocortical carcinoma and malignant phyllodes tumour. There was a moderate excess of carcinoma of pancreas. Neuroblastoma and leukaemia appeared to be weakly associated. No other cancers occurred to excess, but it is interesting to note that there were deficits of carcinomas of lung and colon. Birch *et al.* concluded that germline *TP53* mutations predispose to a specific spectrum of mainly rare cancers, and that carcinoma of the female breast and carcinoma of pancreas are the only two common cancers that constitute major components of the *TP53* syndrome.

While it is possible that the very early onset cancers of lung, colon and other sites observed in a small number of individuals may have arisen in part due to the presence of germline *TP53* mutation, it is likely that other genetic and/or environmental factors contribute. It should also be recognized that many of the families tested were selected because of a high incidence of early onset cancers and some of these cancers may represent phenocopies. If the risk of other common cancers is elevated at all, then this is only at very early ages and with a low incidence.

ESTIMATION OF CANCER RISKS IN *TP53* MUTATION CARRIERS

Documentation and mutation testing in individual families ascertained because of high incidence of young age of onset cancers provides little information on actual cancer risks. The study by Birch *et al.*[144] goes some way towards addressing these issues in that estimates of the frequencies of various cancers in mutation carriers relative to the expected frequencies in the general population are given. However, only one group has attempted to provide estimates of absolute cancer risks by age and sex. A method employing a maximum likelihood approach that takes account of, and corrects for, various sources of bias was developed.[145] Chompret *et al.*[35] applied the method to 13 families segregating a *TP53* mutation ascertained through a systematic study of the families of more than 2500 children with cancer treated at a single institute. Penetrance was estimated to ages 16, 45 and 85 years and found to be 19 per cent, 41 per cent and 73 per cent, respectively, in males and 12 per cent, 84 per cent and 100 per cent in females. The difference in penetrance between males and females is almost entirely due to breast cancer, which represents 80 per cent of all cancers in the 16–45 year age class. The method would be suitable for estimating risks of specific cancers but a much larger cohort would be required. However, there is some evidence for anticipation in age at onset of cancer in families with *TP53* mutations[146] and some *TP53* mutants may confer a much lower cancer risk than those typically found in LFS families.[109,111] These considerations should be taken into account when estimating cancer risks in individual families.

CORRELATIONS BETWEEN GENOTYPE AND PHENOTYPE

The occurrence of certain families with multiple cases of a particular cancer, for example, breast cancer and brain tumours, suggests the possibility that certain mutations may confer a particularly high risk for specific tumours. This possibility was addressed by Kleihues *et al.*[142] in their analysis of published families and they concluded that there was no evidence for such specific associations.

The observations that gain of function/dominant-negative mutations may have a higher oncogenic potential than loss of function mutations suggests that there may be some phenotypic variation with respect to penetrance depending on the class of mutation segregating in a family. Birch *et al.*[127] applied a formal epidemiological approach to compare cancer incidence and pattern of cancers in families segregating point mutations in the DNA binding domain of *TP53*, with cancer pattern and incidence in families segregating other types of mutation in this gene. The former group of mutations would include the known gain of function/dominant-negative mutations and the latter would largely comprise loss of function mutations. The results of these analyses demonstrated a more highly penetrant cancer phenotype in families with missense mutations in the core DNA binding domain, characterized by a higher cancer incidence in general and earlier ages at diagnosis, particularly of breast cancer and brain tumours.

These observations were supported by a study, which demonstrated that the average age at diagnosis among 40 patients with sporadic glioblastomas was significantly younger in patients with tumours in which dominant-negative mutations had been detected, compared with recessive mutations or no mutations.[147] This suggests that dominant-negative *TP53* mutants accelerate the development and/or growth of such brain tumours. It has also been suggested that certain missense point mutations in the DNA binding domain, which are outside of the conserved regions and affect residues not known to contact DNA or be critical in maintaining protein structure, may be associated with a low-penetrance cancer phenotype.[109] Whether there are variations in penetrance with different classes of mutation, dependent on their effect on protein structure and function, will need to be confirmed in substantially larger series of families and patients.

GENETIC BASIS OF CANCER PREDISPOSITION IN LFS FAMILIES WITH NO DETECTABLE *TP53* MUTATION

In a substantial minority of LFS families, no germline *TP53* mutations have been detected. In these families, the striking clustering of rare and early age of onset cancers is unlikely to be due to chance. In spite of the rigorous mutation detection methods employed by some groups, the possibility of undetected germline *TP53* mutations remains. However, in two families, the involvement of *TP53* has been excluded by linkage analysis.[148,149] Linkage studies to identify loci of possible causative genes in *TP53* negative families remain problematic because families tend to be small owing to the early onset of cancers and the often rapidly fatal outcome. Also genetic heterogeneity among *TP53*-negative families is likely. Therefore, the candidate gene approach is probably most appropriate in attempting to establish the genetic basis of cancer predisposition in these families. One study has excluded *CDKN2* and *PTEN* as the causative genes in a series of 16 LFS and LFL families.[150] Germline mutations in the *hCHEK2* gene have been reported in one classic LFS family and four other families with features of LFS;[151,152] however, other *TP53* negative families were also negative for *hCHEK2* mutations. The significance of *hCHEK2* mutations in *TP53*-negative LFS and LF-like families was called into doubt by the observation of such mutations associated with low-penetrance susceptibility to breast cancer rather than LFS *per se*.[152,153] Further observations on the phenotype associated with specific *hCHEK2* mutations are required. A possible candidate gene in some LFL families is *hMSH2*, as suggested by a report of *hMSH2* deficiency in a family that included two siblings with non-Hodgkin's lymphoma at 15 months of age and glioblastoma at 3 years, respectively.[154]

PREDICTIVE GENETIC TESTING AND CLINICAL MANAGEMENT OF LI–FRAUMENI FAMILIES AND *TP53* MUTATION CARRIERS

Predictive testing in asymptomatic members of families with germline *TP53* mutations presents a number of ethical, technical and clinical difficulties. Present data suggest that the prevalence of germline *TP53* mutations among cancer patients in general is very low, even among patients with LFS-associated cancers. The incidence of such mutations appears to be of the order of 5–10 per cent for bone and soft tissue, sarcomas and high-grade gliomas, but is much lower for breast cancers. Exceptionally, adrenocortical tumours appear to be associated with such mutations in a very high proportion of patients. With this possible exception, it would be inappropriate to screen the generality of patients with these cancers for the presence of mutations.

In common with current practice for other cancer-associated genes, predictive presymptomatic testing should be offered only to individuals judged to be at risk in families where a germline mutation has already been identified. Candidate families in whom it would be appropriate to search for a germline *TP53* mutation with a view to subsequent predictive testing include those fulfilling the criteria for LFS[14] and LFL,[28] families including pairs of individuals with typical LFS-associated cancers in close relatives (incomplete LFS)[35] and patients with multiple primary tumours consistent with LFS (premenopausal breast cancer, bone and soft tissue sarcoma, brain tumours and adrenocortical carcinoma).

In order to maximize the chances of detecting a mutation, comprehensive molecular methods should be applied.[112,155] If a mutation is detected, then certain criteria should be fulfilled before proceeding with predictive tests as follows: (1) it should be demonstrated that the mutation segregates with the cancers in the branch of the family that includes the 'at-risk' individual requesting the predictive test; and (2) the biological significance of the detected mutation should be demonstrated in terms of effect on protein function. The functional significance of many of the common *TP53* mutations has been demonstrated and mutations that truncate the protein may be accepted as affecting key properties of the TP53 protein. However, predictive testing on the basis of missense mutations affecting residues outside the conserved regions of the DNA binding domain or splice site mutations should not be undertaken unless functional studies have demonstrated their probable significance in terms of disruption of the normal protein.[107]

Counselling families on cancer risks is difficult because the morphology, site, age and sex-specific incidence of cancer in mutation carriers are uncertain. Furthermore, as discussed above, it is possible that there may be mutation-specific variations in cancer risks. Currently, the best available risk estimates provide figures for cancers in general but no risk estimates are available for specific cancers.[35] The main spectrum of cancers and their frequencies in specific age groups relative to the expected population frequencies have been defined,[144] and this provides some basis for counselling individual carriers about possible site-specific risks. Furthermore, the estimate of penetrance from Le Bihan *et al.*[145] is useful. However, the occurrence of cancers other than those for which a clear association has been demonstrated cannot be ruled out. Childhood cancers are a common feature in LFS and LFL families, and a further difficulty, therefore, arises as to whether it would be ethical to test healthy children. This could only be justified if it could be demonstrated that screening for early detection of cancers in such children conferred a survival benefit or reduction in morbidity. At present, there is only weak evidence to suggest that this is the case. However, each request should be treated on its own merits and testing may be appropriate in rare cases.[132]

In adult carriers, it is difficult to envisage a programme of screening that would be effective in early detection of associated cancers. Even mammography, aimed at early detection of breast cancer, the most common cancer in *TP53* mutation carriers, is of doubtful benefit and other screening modalities (e.g. magnetic resonance imaging) might be considered. However, while there is no proven way for early detection of tumours in *TP53* mutation carriers, it is essential that such individuals have access to informed clinicians so that early symptoms may be investigated in a thorough and timely fashion. These issues are discussed in more detail elsewhere.[132]

CONCLUSIONS

The study of Li–Fraumeni syndrome and the discovery of germline *TP53* mutations provides a good example of how clinical observations and painstaking epidemiological research, together with biochemical and molecular biological research, initially in a purely experimental system, have come together to yield results of profound scientific interest that are also of great importance in a clinical setting. There are still many unresolved problems. These include the most appropriate therapy protocols for treating cancers in patients with germline *TP53* mutations, provision of reliable morphology, site, sex and age-specific cancer risks in carriers, clarification of genotype–phenotype variations in risk and the biological basis for the tissue specificity of cancers arising in mutation carriers. The coming years should provide some answers to these problems.

KEY POINTS

- The definition of *Classical* Li-Fraumeni Syndrome (LFS) is based upon an epidemiological association.
- To date, germline mutations in the *TP53* gene account for at least 75 per cent of LFS families.
- Li-Fraumeni-like families have some of the features of LFS, but not all and they have a lower proportion of germline *TP53* mutation (36 per cent).
- There appears to be a genotype/phenotype correlation, but further work is needed to refine this.
- The resistance to apoptosis that is seen in cells with a germline *TP53* mutation means that screening modalities that use irradiation should be avoided.

REFERENCES

1. Li FP, Fraumeni JF Jr. Soft-tissue sarcomas, breast cancer, and other neoplasms. A familial syndrome? *Ann Intern Med* 1969; **71**:747–752.
2. Li FP, Fraumeni JF Jr. Rhabdomyosarcoma in children: epidemiologic study and identification of a familial cancer syndrome. *J Natl Cancer Inst* 1969; **43**:1365–1373.
3. Bottomley RH, Trainer AL, Condit PT. Chromosome studies in a 'cancer family'. *Cancer* 1971; **28**:519–528.
4. Lynch HT, Krush AJ, Harlan WL, *et al.* Association of soft tissue sarcoma, leukemia and brain tumors in families affected with breast cancer. *Am Surg* 1973; **39**:199–206.
5. Blattner WA, McGuire DB, Mulvihill JJ, *et al.* Genealogy of cancer in a family. *JAMA* 1979; **241**, 259–261.
6. Pearson ADJ, Craft AW, Ratcliffe JM, *et al.* Two families with the Li-Fraumeni cancer family syndrome. *J Med Genet* 1982; **19**:362–365.
7. Li FP, Fraumeni JF Jr. Prospective study of a family cancer syndrome. *JAMA* 1982; **247**:2692–2694.
8. Birch JM, Hartley AL, Marsden HB, *et al.* Excess risk of breast cancer in the mothers of children with soft tissue sarcomas. *Br J Cancer* 1984; **49**, 325–331.
9. Birch JM, Hartley AL, Blair V, *et al.* Cancer in the families of children with soft tissue sarcoma. *Cancer* 1990; **66**:2239–2248.
10. Birch JM, Hartley AL, Blair V, *et al.* Identification of factors associated with high breast cancer risk in the mothers of children with soft tissue sarcoma. *J Clin Oncol* 1990; **8**:583–590.
11. Strong, LC, Stine M, Norsted TL. Cancer in survivors of childhood soft tissue sarcoma and their relatives. *J Natl Cancer Inst* 1987; **79**:1213–1220.
12. Williams WR, Strong LC. Genetic epidemiology of soft tissue sarcomas in children. In: Muller H, Weber W (eds) *Familial cancer. First International Research Conference on Familial Cancer, Basel, 1985.* Basel: Karger, 1995:151–153.
13. Lustbader ED, Williams WR, Bondy ML. *et al.* Segregation analysis of cancer in families of childhood soft-tissue-sarcoma patients. *Am J Hum Genet* 1992; **51**:344–356.
14. Li FP, Fraumeni JF Jr, Mulvihill JJ, *et al.* A cancer family syndrome in twenty-four kindreds. *Cancer Res* 1988; **48**:5358–5362.
15. Hartley AL, Birch JM, Marsden HB, *et al.* Malignant melanoma in families of children with osteosarcoma, chondrosarcoma and adrenal cortical carcinoma. *J Med Genet* 1987; **24**, 664–668.
16. Hartley AL, Birch JM, Kelsey AM, *et al.* Are germ cell tumours part of the Li-Fraumeni Cancer Family Syndrome? *Cancer Genet Cytogenet* 1989; **42**:221–226.
17. Hartley AL, Birch JM, Tricker K, *et al.* Wilms tumour in the Li Fraumeni cancer family syndrome. *Cancer Genet Cytogenet* 1993; **67**:133–135.
18. Malkin D, Li FP, Strong LC, *et al.* Germline p53 mutations in a familial syndrome of breast cancer, sarcomas and other neoplasms. *Science* 1990; **250**:1233–1238.
19. Lavigueur A, Maltby V, Mock D, *et al.* High incidence of lung, bone and lymphoid tumors in transgenic mice over-expressing mutant alleles of the *p53* oncogene. *Mol Cell Biol* 1989; **9**:3982–3991.
20. Hainaut P, Hollstein M. *p53* and human cancer: the first ten thousand mutations. *Adv Cancer Res* 2000; **77**:81–137.
21. Malkin D, Friend SH. Correction: a Li–Fraumeni syndrome *p53* mutation. *Science* 1993; **259**:878.
22. Srivastava S, Zou Z, Pirollo K, *et al.* Germ-line transmission of a mutated *p53* gene in a cancer-prone family with Li-Fraumeni syndrome. *Nature* 1990; **348**:747–749.
23. Vogelstein B. A deadly inheritance. *Nature* 1990; **348**:681–682.
24. Auer H, Warncke K, Nowak D, *et al.* Variations of p53 in cultured fibroblasts of patients with lung cancer who have a presumed genetic predisposition. *Am J Clin Oncol* 1999; **22**:278–282.
25. Ayan I, Luca JW, Jaffe N, *et al.* De novo germline mutations of the *p53* gene in young children with sarcomas. *Oncology Rep* 1997; **4**:679–683.
26. Bang Y-J, Kang S-H, Kim T-Y, *et al.* The first documentation of Li-Fraumeni syndrome in Korea. *J Korean Med Sci* 1995; **10**:205–210.
27. Bardeesy N, Falkoff D, Petruzzi M-J, *et al.* Anaplastic Wilms tumour, a subtype displaying poor prognosis, harbours *p53* gene mutations. *Nature Genet* 1994; **7**:91–97.

28. Birch JM, Hartley AL, Tricker KJ, et al. Prevalence and diversity of constitutional mutations in the p53 gene among 21 Li–Fraumeni families. Cancer Res 1994; 54:1298–1304.

29. Blau O, Avigad S, Stark B, et al. Exon 5 mutations in the p53 gene in relapsed childhood acute lymphoblastic leukemia. Leuk Res 1997; 21:721–729.

30. Børresen A-L, Andersen TI, Garber J. Screening for germ line TP53 mutations in breast cancer patients. Cancer Res 1992; 52:3234–3236.

31. Bot FJ, Sleddens HFBM, Dinjens WNM. Molecular assessment of clonality leads to the identification of a new germ line TP53 mutation associated with malignant cystosarcoma phyllodes and soft tissue sarcoma. Diagnos Mol Path 1998; 7:295–301.

32. Brugiéres L, Gardes M, Moutou C, et al. Screening for germ line p53 mutations in children with malignant tumors and a family history of cancer. Cancer Res 1993; 53:452–455.

33. Camplejohn RS, Sodha N, Gilchrist R, et al. The value of rapid functional assays of germline p53 status in LFS and LFL families. Br J Cancer 2000; 82:1145–1148.

34. Chen P, Iavarone A, Fick J, et al. Constitutional p53 mutations associated with brain tumors in young adults. Cancer Genet Cytogenet 1995; 82:106–115.

35. Chompret, A, Brugiéres L, Ronsin M, et al. p53 germline mutations in childhood cancers and cancer risk for carrier individuals. Br J Cancer 2000; 82:1932–1937.

36. Chung R, Whaley J, Kley N, et al. TP53 gene mutations and 17p deletions in human astrocytomas. Genes Chromosomes Cancer 1991; 3:323–331.

37. Cornelis RS, van Vliet M, van de Vijver MJ, et al. Three germline mutations in the TP53 gene. Hum Mutat 1997; 9:157–163.

38. Diller L, Sexsmith E, Gottlieb A, et al. Germline p53 mutations are frequently detected in young children with rhabdomyosarcoma. J Clin Invest 1995; 95:1606–1611.

39. Dockhorn-Dworniczak B, Wolff J, Poremba C, et al. A new germline TP53 gene mutation in a family with Li–Fraumeni syndrome. Eur J Cancer 1996; 32A:1359–1365.

40. Eeles RA, Warren W, Knee G, et al. Constitutional mutation in exon 8 of the p53 gene in a patient with multiple primary tumours: molecular and immunohistochemical findings. Oncogene 1993; 8:269–1276.

41. Felix CA, Hosler MR, Provisor D, et al. The p53 gene in pediatric therapy-related leukemia and myelodysplasia. Blood 1996; 87:4376–4381.

42. Felix CA, Megonigal MD, Chervinsky DS, et al. Association of germline p53 mutation with MLL segmental jumping translocation in treatment related leukemia. Blood 1998; 91:4451–4456.

43. Felix CA, Nau MM, Takahashi T, et al. Hereditary and acquired p53 gene mutations in childhood acute lymphoblastic leukemia. J Clin Invest 1992; 89:640–647.

44. Felix CA, Slavc I, Dunn M, et al. p53 gene mutations in pediatric brain tumors. Med Pediat Oncol 1995; 25:431–436.

45. Felix CA, Strauss EA, D'Amico D, et al. A novel germline p53 splicing mutation in a pediatric patient with a second malignant neoplasm. Oncogene 1993; 8:1203–1210.

46. Flaman JM, Frebourg T, Moreau V, et al. A simple p53 functional assay for screening cell lines, blood and tumors. Proc Natl Acad Sci 1995; 92:3963–3967.

47. Frebourg T, Barbier N, Yan Y-X, et al. Germ-line p53 mutations in 15 families with Li–Fraumeni syndrome. Am J Hum Genet 1995; 56:608–615.

48. Gallo O, Sardi I, Pepe G, et al. Multiple primary tumors of the upper aerodigestive tract: is there a role for constitutional mutations in the p53 gene? Int J Cancer 1999; 82:180–186.

49. Garcia AG, Barros F, Bouzas ML, et al. Li–Fraumeni syndrome and osteosarcoma of the maxilla. J Oral Maxillofac Surg 1998; 56:1106–1109.

50. Giunta C, Youil R, Venter D, et al. Rapid diagnosis of germline p53 mutation using the enzyme mismatch cleavage method. Diagnos Mol Path 1996; 5:265–270.

51. Goi K, Takagi M, Iwata S, et al. DNA damage-associated dysregulation of the cell cycle and apoptosis control in cells with germ-line p53 mutation. Cancer Res 1997; 57:1895–1902.

52. Grayson GH, Moore S, Schneider BG, et al. Novel germline mutation of the p53 tumor suppressor gene in a child with incidentally discovered adrenal cortical carcinoma. Am J Pediatr Hematol Oncol 1994; 16:341–347.

53. Güran S, Tunca Y, İmirzalioğlu N. Hereditary TP53 codon 292 and somatic P16 INK4A codon 94 mutations in a Li–Fraumeni syndrome family. Cancer Genet Cytogenet 1999; 113:145–151.

54. Gutierrez M.I, Bhatia KG, Barreiro C, et al. A de novo p53 germline mutation affecting codon 151 in a six year old child with multiple tumors. Hum Mol Genet 1994; 3:2247–2248.

55. Hamelin R, Barichard F, Henry I, et al. Single base pair germ-line deletion in the p53 gene in a cancer predisposed family. Hum Genet 1994; 94:88–90.

56. Horio Y, Suzuki H, Ueda R, et al. Predominantly tumor-limited expression of a mutant allele in a Japanese family carrying a germline p53 mutation. Oncogene 1994; 9:1231–1235.

57. Hung J, Mims B, Lozano G, et al. TP53 mutation and haplotype analysis of two large african american families. Hum Mutat 1999; 14:216–221.

58. Huusko P, Castén, K, Launonen V, et al. Germ-line TP53 mutations in Finnish cancer families exhibiting features of the Li–Fraumeni syndrome and negative for BRCA1 and BRCA2. Cancer Genet Cytogenet 1999; 112:9–14.

59. Iavarone A, Matthay KK, Steinkirchner TM, et al. Germ-line and somatic p53 gene mutations in multifocal osteogenic sarcoma. Proc Natl Acad 1992; 89:4207–4209.

60. Jolly KW, Malkin D, Douglass EC, et al. Splice-site mutation of the p53 gene in a family with hereditary breast ovarian cancer. Oncogene 1994; 9:97–102.

61. Kovar H, Auinger A, Jug G, et al. p53 mosaicism with an exon 8 germline mutation in the founder of a cancer-prone pedigree. Oncogene 1992; 7:2169–2173.

62. Kupryjńczyk J, Thor AD, Beauchamp R, et al. p53 gene mutations and protein accumulation in human ovarian cancer. Proc Natl Acad Sci USA 1993; 90:4961–4965.

63. Kyritsis AP, Bondy ML, Xiao M, et al. Germline p53 gene mutations in subsets of glioma patients. J Natl Cancer Inst 1994; 86:344–349.

64. Law JC, Strong LC, Chidambaram A, et al. A germ line mutation in exon 5 of the p53 gene in an extended cancer family. Cancer Res 1991; 51:6385–6387.

65. Li Y-J, Sanson M, Hoang-Xuan K, *et al*. Incidence of germ-line *p53* mutations in patients with gliomas. *Int J Cancer Pred Oncol* 1995; **64**:383–387.

66. Lomax ME, Barnes DM, Gilchrist R, *et al*. Two functional assays employed to detect an unusual mutation in the oligomerisation domain of *p53* in a Li-Fraumeni like family. *Oncogene* 1997; **14**:1869–1874.

67. Lübbe J, von Ammon K, Watanabe K, *et al*. Familial brain tumour sydrome associated with a *p53* germline deletion of codon 236. *Brain Path* 1995; **5**:15–23.

68. Luca JW, Strong LC, Hansen MF. A germline missense mutation R337C in exon 10 of the human *p53* gene. *Hum Mutat* 1998; (Suppl. 1):S58–S61.

69. MacGeoch C, Turner G, Bobrow LG, *et al*. Heterogeneity in Li-Fraumeni families: *p53* mutation analysis and immunohistochemical staining. *J Med Genet* 1995; **32**:186–190.

70. Malkin D, Friend SH, Li FP, *et al*. Germ-line mutations of the *p53* tumor-suppressor gene in children and young adults with second malignant neoplasms. *N Engl J Med* 1997; **336**:734.

71. Malkin D, Jolly KW, Barbier N, *et al*. Germline mutations of the *p53* tumor-suppressor gene in children and young adults with second malignant neoplasms. *N Engl J Med* 1992; **326**:1309–1315.

72. Mazoyer S, Lalle P, Moyret-Lalle, *et al*. Two germ-line mutations affecting the same nucleotide at codon 257 of *p53* gene, a rare site for mutations. *Oncogene* 1994; **9**:1237–1239.

73. McIntyre JF, Smith-Sorensen B, Friend SH, *et al*. Germline mutations of the *p53* tumor suppressor gene in children with osteosarcoma. *J Clin Oncol* 1994; **12**:925–930.

74. Metzger AK, Sheffield VC, Duyk G, *et al*. Identification of a germ-line mutation in the *p53* gene in a patient with an intracranial ependymoma. *Proc Natl Acad Sci USA* 1991; **88**:7825–7829.

75. Moutou C, Le Bihan C, Chompret A, *et al*. Genetic transmission of susceptibility to cancer in families of children with soft tissue sarcomas. *Cancer* 1996; **78**:1483–1491.

76. Murakawa Y, Yokoyama A, Kato S, *et al*. Astrocytoma and B-cell lymphoma development in a man with a *p53* germline mutation. *Jpn J Clin Oncol* 1998; **28**:631–637.

77. Nadav Y, Partorino U, Nicholson AG. Multiple synchronous lung cancers and atypical adenomatous hyperplasia in Li-Fraumeni syndrome. *Histopathology* 1998; **33**:52–54.

78. Orellana C, Martinez F, Hernandez-Marti M, *et al*. A novel *TP53* germ-line mutation identified in a girl with a primitive neuroectodermal tumor and her father. *Cancer Genet Cytogenet* 1998; **105**:103–108.

79. Panizo C, Patĩno A, Calasanz J, *et al*. Emergence of secondary acute leukemia in a patient treated for osteosarcoma: implications of germline *TP53* mutations. *Med Pediatr Oncol* 1998; **30**:165–169.

80. Pivnick EK, Furman WL, Velagaleti GVN, *et al*. Simultaneous adrenocortical carcinoma and ganglioneuroblastoma in a child with Turner syndrome and germline *p53* mutation. *J Med Genet* 1998; **35**:328–332.

81. Plummer SJ, Santiáñez-Koref M, Kurosaki T, *et al*. A germline 2.35 kb deletion of *p53* genomic DNA creating a specific loss of the oligomerization domain inherited in a Li-Fraumeni syndrome family. *Oncogene* 1994; **9**:3273–3280.

82. Ponten F, Berg C, Ahmadian A, *et al*. Molecular pathology in basal cell cancer with *p53* as a genetic marker. *Oncogene* 1997; **15**:1059–1067.

83. Porter DE, Holden ST, Steel CM, *et al*. A significant proportion of patients with osteosarcoma may belong to Li-Fraumeni cancer families. *J Bone Joint Surg* 1992; **74-B**:883–886.

84. Pratt CB, Meyer WH, Luo X, *et al*. Second malignant neoplasms occurring in survivors of osteosarcoma. *Cancer* 1997; **80**:960–965.

85. Prosser J, Porter D, Coles C, *et al*. Constitutional *p53* mutation in a non-Li-Fraumeni cancer family. *Br J Cancer* 1992; **65**:527–528.

86. Quesnel S, Verselis S, Portwine C, *et al*. *p53* compound heterozygosity in a severely affected child with Li-Fraumeni syndrome. *Oncogene* 1999; **18**:3970–3978.

87. Rapakko K, Allinen M, Syrjakoski K, *et al*. Germline *TP53* alterations in Finnish breast cancer families are rare and occur at conserved mutation-prone sites. *Br J Cancer* 2001; **84**:116–119.

88. Reifenberger J, Janssen G, Weber R, *et al*. Primitive neuroectodermal tumors of the cerebral hemispheres in two siblings with *TP53* germline mutation. *J Neuropathol Exp Neurol* 1998; **57**:179–187.

89. Rines RD, van Orsouw NJ, Sigalas I, *et al*. Comprehensive mutational scanning of the *p53* coding region by two-dimensional gene scanning. *Carcinogenesis* 1998; **19**:979–984.

90. Russo CL, McIntyre J, Goorin AM, *et al*. Secondary breast cancer in patients presenting with osteosarcoma: possible involvement of germline *p53* mutations. *Med Paediatr Oncol* 1994; **23**:354–358.

91. Saeki Y, Tamura K, Yamamoto Y, *et al*. Germline *p53* mutation at codon 133 in a cancer-prone family. *J Mol Med* 1997; **75**:50–56.

92. Sameshima Y, Tsunematsu Y, Watanabe S, *et al*. Detection of novel germ-line *p53* mutations in diverse-cancer-prone families identified by selecting patients with childhood adrenocortical carcinoma. *J Natl Cancer Inst* 1992; **84**:703–707.

93. Scott RJ, Krummenacher F, Mary JL, *et al*. Vererbbare *p53*-Mutation bei einem Patienten mit Mehrfachtumoren: Bedeutung für die genetische Beratung. *Schweiz Med Wochenschr* 1993; **123**:1287–1292.

94. Sedlacek Z, Kodet R, Kriz V, *et al*. Two Li-Fraumeni syndrome families with novel germline *p53* mutations: loss of the wild-type *p53* allele in only 50 per cent of tumours. *Br J Cancer* 1998; **77**:1034–1039.

95. Sedlacek Z, Kriz V, Seemanova E, *et al*. Methodological detection of germinal mutations in the tumour suppressing gene *p53*. *Casopis Lekaru Ceskych* 1996; **135**:762–767.

96. Shay JW, Tomlinson G, Piatyszek MA, Gollahon LS. Spontaneous in vitro immortalization of breast epithelial cells from a patient with Li-Fraumeni syndrome. *Mol Cell Biol* 1995; **15**:425–432.

97. Shibata A, Tsai YC, Press MF, *et al*. Clonal analysis of bilateral breast cancer. *Clin Cancer Res* 1996; **2**:743–748.

98. Shiseki M, Nishikawa R, Yamamoto H, *et al*. Germ-line *p53* mutation is uncommon in patients with triple primary cancers. *Cancer Lett* 1993; **73**:51–57.

99. Sidransky D, Tokino T, Helzlsouer K, *et al*. Inherited *p53* gene mutations in breast cancer. *Cancer Res* 1992; **52**:2984–2986.

100. Speiser P, Gharehbaghi-Schnell E, Eder S, *et al*. A constitutional *de novo* mutation in exon 8 of the *p53* gene in

a patient with multiple primary malignancies. *Br J Cancer* 1996; **74**:269–273.

101. Stolzenberg M-C, Brugéres L, Gardes M, *et al.* Germ-line exclusion of a single *p53* allele by premature termination of translation in a Li–Fraumeni syndrome family. *Oncogene* 1994; **9**:2799–2804.

102. Strauss EA, Hosler MR, Herzog P, *et al.* Complex replication error causes *p53* mutation in a Li–Fraumeni family. *Cancer Res* 1995; **55**:3237–3241.

103. Sugano K, Taniguchi T, Saeki M, *et al.* Germline *p53* mutation in a case of Li–Fraumeni syndrome presenting gastric cancer. *Jpn J Clin Oncol* 1999; **29**:513–516.

104. Tachibana I, Smith JS, Sato K, *et al.* Investigation of germline *PTEN*, *p53*, $p16^{INK4A}/p14^{ARF}$ and *CDK4* alterations in familial glioma. *Am J Med Genet* 2000; **92**:136–141.

105. Toguchida J, Yamaguchi T, Dayton SH, *et al.* Prevalence and spectrum of germline mutations of the *p53* gene among patients with sarcoma. *N Engl J Med* 1992; **326**:1301–1308.

106. Vahteristo P, Tamminen A, Karvinen P, *et al.* p53, *CHK2*, and *CHK1* Genes in Finnish families with Li–Fraumeni syndrome: further evidence of *CHK2* in inherited cancer predisposition. *Cancer Res* 2001; **61**:5718–5722.

107. Varley JM, Attwooll C, White G, *et al.* Characterization of germline *TP53* splicing mutations and their genetic and functional analysis. *Oncogene* 2001; **20**:2647–2654.

108. Varley JM, McGown G, Thorncroft M, *et al.* A previously undescribed mutation within the tetramerisation domain of *TP53* in a family with Li–Fraumeni syndrome. *Oncogene* 1996; **12**:2437–2442.

109. Varley JM, McGown G, Thorncroft M, *et al.* Are there low-penetrance *tp53* alleles? Evidence from childhood adrenocortical tumors. *Am J Hum Genet* 1999; **65**:995–1006.

110. Ribeiro RC, Sandrini F, Figueiredo B, *et al.* An inherited *p53* mutation that contributes in a tissue-specific manner to pediatric adrenal cortical carcinoma. *Proc Natl Acad Sci USA* 2001; **98**:9330–9335.

111. Latronico AC, Pinto EM, Domenice S, *et al.* An inherited mutation outside the highly conserved DNA-binding domain of the p53 tumor suppressor protein in children and adults with sporadic adrenocortical tumors. *J Clin Endocrinol Metab* 2001; **86**:4970–4973.

112. Varley JM, McGown G, Thorncroft M, *et al.* Germ-line mutations of *TP53* in Li–Fraumeni families: an extended study of 39 families. *Cancer Res* 1997; **57**:3245–3252.

113. Varley JM, Thorncroft M, McGown G, *et al.* A novel deletion within exon 6 of *TP53* in a family with Li Fraumeni-like syndrome, and LOH in a benign lesion from a mutation carrier. *Cancer Genet Cytogenet* 1996; **90**:14–16.

114. Verselis S, Rheinwald JG, Fraumeni JF, *et al.* Novel *p53* splice site mutations in three families with Li–Fraumeni syndrome. *Oncogene* 2000; **19**:4230–4235.

115. Vital A, Bringuier P-P, Huang H, *et al.* Astrocytomas and choroid plexus tumors in two families with identical *p53* germline mutations. *J Neuropathol Exp Neurol* 1998; **57**:1061–1069.

116. Wagner J, Portwine C, Rabin K, *et al.* High frequency of germline *p53* mutations in childhood adrenocortical cancer. *J Natl Cancer Inst* 1994; **86**:1707–1710.

117. Warneford SG, Witton LJ, Townsend ML, *et al.* Germ-line splicing mutation of the *p53* gene in a cancer-prone family. *Cell Growth Different* 1992; **3**:839–846.

118. Wilkin F, Gagne N, Paquette J, *et al.* Pediatric adrenocortical tumors: molecular events leading to insulin-like growth factor II gene overexpression. *J Clin Endocrinol Metab* 2000; **85**:2048–2056.

119. Yonemoto T, Tatezaki S-I, Ishii T, *et al.* Two cases of osteosarcoma occurring as second malignancy of childhood cancer. *Anticancer Res* 1999; **19**:5563–5566.

120. Zhou X-P, Sanson M, Hoang-Xuan K, *et al.* Germline mutations of *p53* but not *p16/cdkn2* or *pten/mmac1* tumor suppressor genes predispose to gliomas. *Ann Neurol* 1999; **46**:913–916.

121. Olivier M, Eeles R, Hollstein M, *et al.* The IARC database: new online mutation analysis and recommendations to users. *Hum Mutat* 2002; **19**:607–614.

122. Sun X-F, Johannsson O, Hakansson S, *et al.* A novel *p53* germline alteration identified in a late onset breast cancer kindred. *Oncogene* 1996; **13**:407–411.

123. Avigad S, Barel D, Blau O, *et al.* A novel germ line *p53* mutation in intron 6 in diverse childhood malignancies. *Oncogene* 1997; **14**:1541–1545.

124. Barel D, Avigad S, Mor C, *et al.* A novel germ-line mutation in the noncoding region of the *p53* gene in a Li–Fraumeni family. *Cancer Genet Cytogenet* 1998; **103**:1–6.

125. Lehman TA, Haffty BG, Carbone CJ, *et al.* Elevated frequency and functional activity of a specific germ-line *p53* intron mutation in familial breast cancer. *Cancer Res* 2000; **60**:1062–1069.

126. Ishioka C, Frebourg T, Yan Y, *et al.* Screening patients for heterozygous *p53* mutations using a functional assay in yeast. *Nature Genet* 1993; **5**:124–129.

127. Birch JM, Blair V, Kelsey AM, *et al.* Cancer phenotype correlates with constitutional *TP53* genotype in families with the Li–Fraumeni syndrome. *Oncogene* 1998; **17**:1061–1068.

128. Rapakko K, Allinen M, Syrjakoski K, *et al.* Germline *TP53* alterations in Finnish breast cancer families are rare and occur at conserved mutation prone sites. *Br J Cancer* 2001; **84**:116–119.

129. Zelada-Hedman M, Børresen-Dale A-L, Claro A, *et al.* Screening for *TP53* mutations in patients and tumours from 109 Swedish breast cancer families. *Br J Cancer* 1997; **75**:1201–1204.

130. May P, May E. Twenty years of *p53* research: structural and functional aspects of the p53 protein. *Oncogene* 1999; **18**:7621–7636.

131. Hollstein M, Hergenhahn M, Yang Q, *et al.* New approaches to understanding *p53* gene tumor mutation spectra. *Mutat Res* 1999; **431**:199–209.

132. Varley JM, Evans DGR, Birch JM. Li–Fraumeni syndrome – a molecular and clinical review. *Br J Cancer* 1997; **76**:1–14.

133. Cho Y, Gorina S, Jeffrey PD, *et al.* Crystal structure of a p53 tumor suppressor-DNA complex: understanding tumorigenic mutations. *Science* 1994; **265**:346–355.

134. Lane DP. p53, guardian of the genome. *Nature* 1992; **358**:15–16.

135. Frebourg T, Kassel J, Lam KT, *et al.* Germ-line mutations of the *p53* tumor suppressor gene in patients with high risk for cancer inactivate the p53 protein. *Proc Natl Acad Sci USA* 1992; **89**:6413–6417.

136. Milner J, Medcalf EA. Cotranslation of activated mutant *p53* with wild type drives the wild-type p53 protein into the mutant conformation. *Cell* 1991; **65**:765–774.

137. DiGiammarino EL, Lee AS, Cadwell C, *et al*. A novel mechanism of tumorigenesis involving pH-dependent destabilization of a mutant *p53* tetramer. *Nature Struct Biol* 2002; **9**:12–16.

138. Dittmer D, Pati S, Zambetti G, *et al*. Gain of function mutations in *p53*. *Nature Genet* 1993; **4**:42–46.

139. Chen J-Y, Funk WD, Wright WE, *et al*. Heterogeneity of transcriptional activity of mutant p53 proteins and p53 DNA target sequences. *Oncogene* 1993; **8**:2159–2166.

140. Kawamura M, Yamashita T, Segawa K, *et al*. The 273rd codon mutants of *p53* show growth modulation activities not correlated with *p53*-specific transactivation activity. *Oncogene* 1996; **12**:2361–2367.

141. Varley JM, Thorncroft M, McGown G, *et al*. A detailed loss of heterozygosity on chromosome 17 in tumours from Li–Fraumeni patients carrying a mutation to the *TP53* gene. *Oncogene* 1997; **14**:865–871.

142. Kleihues P, Schäuble B, Hausen, A, *et al*. Tumors associated with *p53* germline mutations: a synopsis of 91 families. *Am J Pathol* 1997; **150**:1–13.

143. Nichols KE, Malkin D, Garber JE, *et al*. Germ-line *p53* mutations predispose to a wide spectrum of early-onset cancers. *Cancer Epidemiol Bio Prev* 2001; **10**:83–87.

144. Birch JM, Alston RD, McNally RJQ, *et al*. Relative frequency and morphology of cancers in carriers of germline *TP53* mutations. *Oncogene* 2001; **20**:4621–4628.

145. Le Bihan C, Moutou C, Brugiéres L, *et al*. ARCAD: a method for estimating age-dependent disease risk associated with mutation carrier status from family data. *Genet Epidemiol* 1995; **12**:13–25.

146. Trkova M, Hladikova M, Kasal P, *et al*. Is there anticipation in the age at onset of cancer in families with Li–Fraumeni syndrome? *J Hum Genet* 2002; **47**:381–386.

147. Marutani M, Tonoki H, Tada M, *et al*. Dominant-negative mutations of the tumor suppressor *p53* relating to early onset of glioblastoma multiforme. *Cancer Res* 1999; **59**:4765–4769.

148. Birch JM, Heighway J, Teare MD, *et al*. Linkage studies in a Li–Fraumeni family with increased expression of p53 protein but no germline mutation in *p53*. *Br J Cancer* 1994; **70**:1176–1181.

149. Evans SC, Mims B, McMasters KM, *et al*. Exclusion of a *p53* germline mutation in a classic Li–Fraumeni syndrome family. *Hum Genet* 1998; **102**:681–686.

150. Burt EC, McGown G, Thorncroft M, *et al*. Exclusion of the genes *CDKN2* and *PTEN* as causative gene defects in Li–Fraumeni syndrome. *Br J Cancer* 1999; **80**:9–10.

151. Bell DW, Varley JM, Szydlo TE, *et al*. Heterozygous germ line *hCHK2* mutations in Li–Fraumeni syndrome. *Science* 1999; **286**:2528–2531.

152. The *CHEK2*-Breast Cancer Consortium. Low penetrance susceptibility to breast cancer due to *CHEK2**1100del C in noncarriers of *BRCA1* or *BRCA2* mutations. *Nature Genet* 2002; **31**:55–59.

153. Sodha N, Houlston RS, Bullock S, *et al*. Increasing evidence that germline mutations in *CHEK2* do not cause Li–Fraumeni syndrome. *Human Mutat* 2002; **20**:460–462.

154. Bougeard G, Charbonnier F, Moerman A, *et al*. Early-onset brain tumor and lymphoma in *MSH2*-deficient children. *Am J Hum Genet* 2003; **72**:213–216.

155. Evans DGR, Birch JM, Thorncroft M, *et al*. Low rate of *TP53* germline mutations in breast/sarcoma families not fulfilling classical criteria for Li–Fraumeni syndrome. *J Med Genet* 2002; **39**:941–944.

Cowden syndrome

CHARIS ENG

INTRODUCTION

Cowden syndrome (CS; MIM* 158350) is an under-recognized, under-diagnosed autosomal dominant disorder characterized by multiple hamartomas affecting tissues derived from all three germ layers and a high risk of breast, thyroid and endometrial tumours. Germline mutations of *PTEN*, localized to 10q23. 3 and encoding a tumour suppressor dual-specificity phosphatase, cause CS.[1,2] Further, *PTEN* is also the susceptibility gene for at least a proportion of cases with Bannayan Riley–Ruvalcaba syndrome (BRR; MIM 153480), characterized by macrocephaly, lipomatosis and speckled penis[3,4] and a Proteus-like syndrome.[5] In addition, somatic mutations and deletions occur in a variety of benign and malignant tumours.

The complete function of *PTEN* is not yet fully understood. However, over the past 3 years, overexpression and null experiments involving *PTEN* have revealed that it plays a significant role in the cell cycle, apoptosis and, possibly, cell adhesion, cell migration and cell–cell interaction.[6–16]

CLINICAL ASPECTS

Incidence

Because CS is under-recognized and under-diagnosed, the true incidence is unknown. As of 1993, there were

approximately 160 reported cases in the world literature.[17] Prior to gene identification, the incidence of CS was estimated to be one in a million,[18] although after gene identification, this figure was revised to one in 200 000,[19] which is still likely to be an underestimate. Because of frequencies such as these, this syndrome is often listed as rare, but exponents of the field suspect that it is much more common than believed. Because of the variable, protean and often subtle external manifestations of CS, many cases remain[20,21] (C. Eng et al., unpublished). Indeed, between two centres in the USA dedicated to the study of Cowden syndrome, over 80 cases have been ascertained (C. Eng and M. Peacocke, unpublished). These cases are not included in those reported prior to 1993. Further, each of the features of CS could occur in the general population as well, thus confounding recognition of this disease. Despite the apparent rarity of CS, the syndrome is worthy of note from both scientific and clinical viewpoints.

Because CS is likely to be underdiagnosed, a true count of the fraction of isolated cases (defined as no obvious family history) and familial cases (defined as two or more related affected individuals) cannot be performed. From the literature and the experience of both major US CS centres, the majority of CS cases are isolated. As a broad estimate, perhaps 10–50 per cent of CS cases are familial.

Diagnostic criteria

Cowden syndrome usually presents by the late 20s. It has variable expression and, probably, an age-related

---

*Mendelian Inheritance in Man Catalogue Number

Table 12.1 *Common manifestations of Cowden syndrome*

Mucocutaneous lesions (90–100%)
  Trichilemmomas
  Acral keratoses
  Verucoid or papillomatous papules

Thyroid abnormalities (50–67%)
  Goitre
  Adenoma
  Cancer (3–10%)

Breast lesions
  Fibroadenomas/fibrocystic disease (76% of affected
    females)
  Adenocarcinoma (25–50% of affected females)

Gastrointestinal lesions (40%)
  Hamartomatous polyps

Macrocephaly (38%)

Genitourinary abnormalities (44% of females)
  Uterine leiomyoma (multiple, early onset)

Table 12.2 *International Cowden Syndrome Consortium operational criteria for the diagnosis of Cowden syndrome (Version 2000)* [a]

Pathognomonic criteria
Mucocutanous lesions:
  Trichilemmomas, facial
  Acral keratoses
  Papillomatous papules
  Mucosal lesions

Major criteria
  Breast carcinoma
  Thyroid carcinoma (non-medullary), especially follicular
    thyroid carcinoma
  Macrocephaly (megalencephaly) (say, ⩾97%ile)
  Lhermitte–Duclos disease (LDD)
  Endometrial carcinoma

Minor criteria
  Other thyroid lesions (e.g, adenoma or multinodular goitre)
  Mental retardation (say, IQ ⩽ 75)
  Gastrointestinal hamartomas
  Fibrocystic disease of the breast
  Lipomas
  Fibromas
  Genitourinary tumors (e.g. renal cell carcinoma, uterine
    fibroids) or malformation

Operational diagnosis in an individual

1 Mucocutanous lesions alone if:
  (a) there are six or more facial papules, of which three or
      more must be trichilemmoma, or
  (b) cutaneous facial papules and oral mucosal
      papillomatosis, or
  (c) oral mucosal papillomatosis and acral keratoses, or
  (d) palmo plantar keratoses, six or more
2 Two major criteria, but one must include macrocephaly or
  LDD
3 One major and three minor criteria
4 Four minor criteria

*Operational diagnosis in a family where one individual is
diagnostic for Cowden*

1 The pathognomonic criterion/criteria
2 Any one major criterion with or without minor criteria
3 Two minor criteria

[a] Operational diagnostic criteria are reviewed and revised on a continuous basis as new clinical and genetic information becomes available. The 1995 version and 2000 version have been accepted by the US-based National Comprehensive Cancer Network High Risk/Genetics Panel.

penetrance, although the exact penetrance is unknown. Most investigators acknowledge that penetrance is >90 per cent after the age of 20.[18] By the third decade, 99 per cent of affected individuals would have developed the mucocutaneous stigmata, although any of the features could be present already (Tables 12.1 and 12.2). Because the clinical literature on CS consists mostly of reports of the most florid and unusual families, or case reports by subspecialists interested in their respective organ systems, the spectrum of component signs is unknown. Despite this, the most commonly reported manifestations are mucocutaneous lesions, thyroid abnormalities, fibrocystic disease and carcinoma of the breast, gastrointestinal hamartomas, multiple, early-onset uterine leiomyoma, macrocephaly (specifically, megencephaly) and mental retardation (Table 12.1).[22–25] Pathognomonic mucocutaneous lesions are trichilemmomas and papillomatous papules (Table 12.2). Because of the lack of uniform diagnostic criteria for CS prior to 1995, a group of individuals, the International Cowden Consortium, interested in studying this syndrome systematically, arrived at a set of consensus operational diagnostic criteria, which has been revised recently in the context of new data and these criteria are reflected by the practice guidelines of the US-based National Comprehensive Cancer Network Genetics/High Risk Panel (Table 12.2).[26]

The two most commonly recognized cancers in CS are carcinoma of the breast and thyroid.[22] By contrast, in the general population, lifetime risks for breast and thyroid cancers are approximately 11 per cent (in women), and 1 per cent, respectively. In women with CS, lifetime risk estimates for the development of breast cancer range from 25 to 50 per cent.[22,23,25,27] The mean age at diagnosis is likely to be 10 years earlier than breast cancer occurring in the general population.[22,25] Although Rachel Cowden died of breast cancer at the age of 31[28,29] and the earliest recorded age of diagnosis of breast cancer is 14,[22] the majority of CS breast cancers are diagnosed after the age of 30–35 years (range 14–65).[25] Until genotype–phenotype analyses were performed with the discovery of the susceptibility gene, it was thought that male breast cancer was

Table 12.3 *Reported malignancies in patients with Cowden syndrome*

Central nervous system
Glioblastoma multiforme

Mucocutaneous
Squamous cell carcinoma
Basal cell carcinoma
Malignant melanoma
Merkel cell carcinoma

Breast
Adenocarcinoma

Endocrine
Non-medullary thyroid carcinoma (classically of follicular histology)

Pulmonary
Non-small-cell carcinoma

Gastrointestinal
Colorectal carcinoma
Hepatocellular carcinoma
Pancreatic carcinoma

Genitourinary
Uterine carcinoma
Ovarian carcinoma
Transitional cell carcinoma of the bladder
Renal cell carcinoma

Other
Liposarcoma

Table 12.4 *Non-cutaneous benign lesions reported in Cowden syndrome*

Nervous system
Lhermitte–Duclos disease
Megencephaly
Glioma
Meningioma
Neuroma
Neurofibroma
Bridged sella turcica
Mental retardation

Breast
Fibrocystic disease
Fibroadenoma
Hamartoma
Gynaecomastia of male breast

Thyroid
Goitre
Adenoma
Thyroiditis
Thyroglossal duct cyst
Hyperthyroidism
Hypothyroidism

Gastrointestinal
Hamartomatous polyposis of entire tract
Diverticuli of colon and sigmoid
Ganglioneuroma
Leiomyoma
Hepatic hamartoma

Genitourinary (female)
Leiomyomas
Ovarian cysts
Vaginal and vulvar cysts
Various developmental anomalies (e.g. duplicated collecting system)

Genitourinary (male)
Hydrocoele
Varicocoele
Hypoplastic testes

Skeletal
Craniomegaly
Adenoid facies
High arched palate
Hypoplastic zygoma
Kyphoscoliosis
Pectus excavatum
Bone cysts
Rudimentary sixth digit

Other
Hypoplastic vulva
Atrial septal defect
Ateriovenous malformations
Eye cataracts
Retinal angioid streaks

not a component of CS. However, male breast cancer does occur in CS but with unknown frequency.[2]

The lifetime risk for thyroid cancer can be as high as 10 per cent in males and females with CS. Because of small numbers, it is unclear if the age of onset is truly earlier than that of the general population. Histologically, the thyroid cancer is predominantly follicular carcinoma, although papillary histology has also been rarely observed[22,23,25] (C. Eng, unpublished observations). Medullary thyroid carcinoma has yet to be observed in patients with CS.

Benign tumours are also common in CS. Apart from those of the skin, benign tumors or disorders of breast and thyroid are the most frequently noted and likely represent true component features of this syndrome (Table 12.1). Fibroadenomas and fibrocystic disease of the breast are common signs in CS, as are follicular adenomas and multinodular goitre of the thyroid. An unusual central nervous system tumour, cerebellar dysplastic gangliocytoma or Lhermitte–Duclos disease, has only recently been associated with CS.[30,31]

Other malignancies and benign tumors have been reported in patients or families with CS (Tables 12.3 and 12.4). Given the availability of new data with the discovery of the gene, exponents of this field believe that endometrial carcinoma is a true component tumour of CS as well (Table 12.2). Whether malignant tumours other than those in the breast, thyroid and endometrium are true components of CS, or whether some are coincidental findings is as yet unknown.

Histology

Like other inherited cancer syndromes, multifocality and bilateral involvement is the rule. Hamartomas are the hallmark of CS. These are classic hamartomas in general, and are benign tumours comprising all the elements of a particular organ but in a disorganized fashion. Of note, the hamartomatous polyps found in this syndrome are different in histomorphology from Peutz–Jeghers polyps, which have a distinct appearance. A preliminary report examining the gastrointestinal manifestations of nine patients from six unrelated CS kindreds found that all patients examined had colonic non-adenomatous hamartomatous polyps.[32] Additionally, a majority had acanthosis of the esophagus.[32]

With regard to the individual cancers, even of the breast and thyroid, as of mid-2000, there has yet to be a systematic study published. One study has attempted to look at benign and malignant breast pathology in CS patients. Although these are preliminary studies without true matched controls, it is, to date, the only study that examines breast pathology in a series of CS cases. Breast histopathology from 59 cases belonging to 19 CS women was systematically analysed.[21] Thirty-five specimens had some form of malignant pathology. Of these, 31 (90 per cent) had ductal adenocarcinoma, one tubular carcinoma and one lobular carcinoma *in situ*. Sixteen of the 31 had both invasive and *in situ* (DCIS) components of ductal carcinoma, while 12 had DCIS only and two only invasive adenocarcinoma. Interestingly, it was noted that 19 of these carcinomas appeared to have arisen in the midst of densely fibrotic hamartomatous tissue.

Benign thyroid pathology is more common in CS than malignant. Multinodular goitre and thyroid adenomas are often noted. Follicular thyroid carcinomas are much more common than papillary, although mixed follicular and papillary histology can be observed.[22,24,27] No systematic studies on thyroid pathology in CS have been performed.

GENETICS

CS is inherited as an autosomal dominant disorder, with age-related penetrance. Using linkage analysis and 12 unrelated CS families, members of the International Cowden Consortium mapped the CS-susceptibility gene to 10q22–23.[18] Fine structure genetic analysis, somatic genetics on component tumours and candidate gene analysis identified *PTEN*, which is virtually ubiquitously expressed, as the CS susceptibility gene.[1] That *PTEN* is the CS gene has been confirmed by other groups.[33–35]

Genotype–phenotype associations in Cowden syndrome

A series of 37 unrelated CS probands was ascertained by the strict operational diagnostic criteria of the International Cowden Consortium (Version 1995–96)[36] for purposes of genotype-phenotype analyses.[2] Of the 37 CS probands, 30 (81 per cent) were found to carry germline *PTEN* mutations.[2] Among the 30 mutation positive probands were two males with breast cancer. Approximately two-thirds of all mutations were found in exons 5, 7 or 8. Although exon 5, which encodes the phosphatase core motif, represents 20 per cent of the coding sequence, it harbours 40 per cent of all *PTEN* mutations in CS. Association analyses revealed that CS families with germline *PTEN* mutations are more likely to develop malignant breast disease when compared to *PTEN* mutation-negative families.[2] Further, non-truncating mutations and those within the phosphatase core motif and 5′ of it appeared to be associated with involvement of five or more organs, a surrogate phenotype for severity of disease.[2] Another group examined families for germline *PTEN* mutations and found mutations in only 13 probands.[19] They could not find any clear genotype–phenotype associations, most likely due to their small sample size.

When germline *PTEN* mutations were found in the Bannayan–Riley–Ruvalcaba syndrome, which is an autosomal dominant disorder characterized by macrocephaly, hamartomas, telangiectasias, lipomatosis and speckled penis,[37–40] it suggested that CS and BRR are allelic.[3] A series of 43 unrelated BRR probands were ascertained to examine their mutation spectrum in the context of the CS spectrum and to examine genotype–phenotype association in BRR.[4] In contrast to CS, 60 per cent of BRR were found to have germline *PTEN* mutations. Further, two of these mutations included one with a cytogenetically detectable deletion of 10q23, encompassing *PTEN*, and another with a translocation involving 10q23. The mutational spectra of BRR and CS seemed to overlap, thus lending formal proof that CS and BRR, at least a subset, are allelic.[4] There was no difference in mutation frequencies between isolated BRR and familial BRR. Of interest, >90 per cent of CS–BRR overlap families were found to have germline *PTEN* mutations. The presence of *PTEN* mutation in BRR was found to be associated with the development of any cancer as well as tumours of the breast and lipomas. Therefore, the presence of *PTEN* mutations in BRR may have implications for cancer surveillance in this syndrome previously not believed to be associated with malignancy.

Cryptic Cowden syndrome

Because CS is difficult to diagnose, *PTEN* mutation frequencies in 'CS' have ranged from a low of 10 per cent[33] to a high of 81 per cent.[2] The highest mutation frequencies are obtained when CS is strictly defined by the operational diagnostic criteria of the International Cowden Consortium (Table 12.2).[1,2] A study was performed, which purposefully ascertained CS-like probands in which the subjects must not meet the Consortium criteria, but must minimally have breast cancer and thyroid disease in a single individual or in two first-degree relatives.[41] Sixty-four probands were enrolled, and one germline mutation was found in a family with follicular thyroid cancer, bilateral breast cancer and endometrial cancer. This study concluded that the Consortium criteria were robust, even at the molecular level, and that endometrial carcinoma might be an important component cancer of CS. Another recent study, a nested cohort comprising 103 eligible women with multiple primary cancers within the 32 826-member Nurses' Health Study were examined for the occult presence of germline *PTEN* mutations.[42] Among 103 cases, five (5 per cent) were found to have germline missense mutations, all of which have been shown to cause some loss of function. Of these five cases, two cases themselves had endometrial cancer. This study, therefore, suggests that occult germline mutations of *PTEN* and by extrapolation, CS, occur with a higher frequency than previously believed. Further, these data confirm the previous observations[41] that endometrial carcinoma is an important component cancer of CS and, indeed, its presence in a case or family that is reminiscent of CS but does not quite meet Consortium criteria might actually help increase the prior probablity of finding *PTEN* mutation.

When 62 unrelated women with breast cancer diagnosed under the age of 40 were examined for the occult presence of germline *PTEN* mutations, two (3.2 per cent) were found to have missense mutations.[43] Despite all these studies, site-specific breast cancer families without CS features not linked to *BRCA1* or *BRCA2* were found not to be linked to 10q23[44] and were not found to have germline *PTEN* mutations.[45]

Genetic differential diagnosis

With the variable expression of Cowden syndrome, this disorder can be considered a great imitator of many syndromes. BRR could be considered in the differential diagnosis, although with the identification of *PTEN* mutations in this syndrome, most believe that CS and at least a subset of BRR should be considered a single genetic entity, with the proposed name of PTEN Hamartoma Tumour Syndrome, or PHTS.[4] The PHTS entity is particularly germane because there are currently over 14 families with an overlap of both CS and BRR features[4] (C. Eng, unpublished observations). Natural differential diagnoses to consider include the other hamartoma syndromes, especially juvenile polyposis (JPS; MIM 174900) and Peutz–Jeghers syndrome (PJS; MIM 174900). JPS is an autosomal dominant disorder characterized by hamartomatous polyps in the gastrointestinal tract and a high risk of colorectal cancer, and in a sense, may be viewed as a clinical diagnosis of exclusion. A single report claimed that germline *PTEN* mutations can occur in JPS.[46] However, closer inspection of these probands revealed that one likely has CS and the other was too young to exclude CS clinically, given that the penetrance under the age of 20 for classic CS is <10 per cent. Indeed, when Kurose *et al.* ascertained a series of patients with the diagnosis of juvenile polyposis, he found one with germline *PTEN* mutation and, unlike the previous series, these investigators were able to recall that patient for re-examination, and discovered clinical stigmata of CS.[47] Thus, finding a germline *PTEN* mutation in a presumed JPS case alters the diagnosis to CS.[48] Subsequently, a major *JPS* locus was identified on 18q and germline mutations in *SMAD4* have been found in a subset of JPS.[49–51] PJS, which carries a high risk of intestinal carcinomas and breast cancers, should be clinically quite distinct. The pigmentation of the peroral region in this autosomal dominant hamartoma syndrome is pathognomonic.[52,53] The hamartomatous polyp in PJS has a diagnostic appearance as well, and is referred to as the Peutz–Jeghers polyp. They are unlike the hamartomatous polyps seen in CS and JPS. Clinically, while Peutz–Jeghers polyps are often symptomatic (interssuception, rectal bleeding), CS polyps are rarely so. Germline mutations in *LKB1/STK11*, on 19p, have been found in isolated and familial PJS cases,[54–56] although some believe that there is a minor susceptibility gene on 19q as well.[57]

Proteus syndrome (MIM 176920) could be considered in the differential diagnosis of CS because of the common theme of overgrowth (e.g. hemihypertrophy, macrocephaly, connective tissue naevi and lipomatosis).[58] Like CS, Proteus syndrome can have a broad spectrum of phenotypic expression, and so its diagnosis is also made by consensus operational criteria as well.[59] Mandatory diagnostic criteria include mosaic distribution of lesions, progressive course and sporadic occurrence.[59] Connective tissue naevi are pathognomonic for this syndrome. In a small pilot study to determine if Proteus syndrome is part of PHTS, an apparently isolated case of a Proteus-like syndrome comprising hemihypertrophy, macrocephaly, lipomas, connective tissue naevi and multiple arteriovenous malformations was found to have a germline *PTEN* mutation R335X.[5] Interestingly, a naevus, a lipomatous region and arteriovenous malformation tissue were found to harbour a 'second-hit' non-germline *PTEN* mutation R130X, possibly representing a germline mosaic. Both these mutations have been previously described in classic CS and BRR.

Thus, this Proteus-like case may be classified as PHTS at the molecular level, with all its implications for development of malignancies characteristic of CS/BRR. What proportion of clinical Proteus syndrome or Proteus-like cases will be reclassified as PHTS at the molecular level is being investigated.

Other minor differential diagnoses to consider include neurofibromatosis type 1 (NF1), basal cell naevus (Gorlin) syndrome and Darier–White disease. In NF1, the only two consistent features are café au lait macules and fibromatous tumors of the skin. The plexiform neuroma is highly suggestive of NF1. The susceptibility gene for this syndrome has been isolated.[60,61] Because of the large size of the gene, direct mutation analysis is still not practical. In informative families, linkage analysis is feasible for predictive testing purposes and is 98 per cent accurate.[62] Basal cell naevus syndrome is an autosomal dominant condition characterized by basal cell naevi, basal cell carcinoma and diverse developmental abnormalities. In addition, affected individuals can develop other tumors and cancers, such as fibromas, hamartomatous gastric polyps and medulloblastomas. However, the dermatologic findings and developmental features in CS and basal cell naevus syndrome are markedly different. For instance, the palmar pits together with the characteristic facies of the latter are never seen in CS. The susceptibility gene for basal cell naevus syndrome is also distinct from CS/BRR, and is the human homologue of the *Drosophila patched* gene, *PTC* on 9q22–31.[63] Linkage analysis and mutation analysis are (technically) possible. However, since it is not known what proportion of patients with this syndrome will actually turn out to have mutations in *PTC*, predictive testing based on mutation analysis alone should be deferred until more data become available. Finally, Darier–White disease is an autosomal dominant disorder characterized by keratotic, often oozing, papules in the 'seborrhoeic areas' of the skin and sometimes can be confused with CS. Nonetheless, the dermatologic findings of these two syndromes, especially at the microscopic level, are distinct. The susceptibility locus for Darier–White disease has been mapped to 12q23–24.1 and so this syndrome is genetically distinct from PHTS.[64,65]

CLINICAL CANCER GENETIC MANAGEMENT

The key to proper genetic counselling in CS is recognition of the syndrome. Families with CS should be counselled as for any autosomal dominant trait with high penetrance. What is unclear, however, is the variability of expression between and within families. We suspect that there are CS families who have nothing but trichilemmomas and, therefore, never come to medical attention.

The three most serious, and established, component tumours in CS are breast cancer for affected females and males, non-medullary thyroid cancer and endometrial cancer. Patients with CS or those who are at risk for CS should undergo surveillance for these three cancers. Beginning in their teens, these individuals should undergo annual physical examinations paying particular attention to the thyroid examination. Beginning in their mid-20s, women with CS or those at risk for it should be encouraged to perform monthly breast self-examinations and to have careful breast examinations during their annual physicals. The value of annual imaging studies is unclear because there are no objective data available. Nonetheless, we usually recommend annual mammography and/or breast ultrasounds performed by skilled individuals in women at risk beginning at age 30 or 5 years earlier than the earliest breast cancer case in the family, whichever is younger. Some women with CS develop severe, sometimes disfiguring, fibroadenomas of the breasts well before age 30. This situation should be treated individually. For example, if the fibroadenomas cause pain or if they make breast cancer surveillance impossible, then some have advocated prophylactic mastectomies.[29] Careful annual physical examination of the thyroid and neck region beginning at age 18 or 5 years younger than the earliest diagnosis of thyroid cancer in the family (whichever is earlier) should be sufficient, although a single baseline thyroid ultrasound in the early 20s might be considered as well. Surveillance for endometrial carcinoma is recommended perhaps beginning at the age of 35–40 (no data for age at onset) or 5 years younger than the earliest onset case in the family. For premenopausal women, annual blind repel (suction) biopsies of the endometrium should be performed. In the postmenopausal years, uterine ultrasound should suffice.

Whether other tumours are true components of CS is unknown. It is believed, however, that skin cancers, for instance, might be true features of CS as well. For now, therefore, surveillance for other organs should follow the American Cancer Society guidelines, although proponents of CS will advise routine skin surveillance as well.

A preliminary study has demonstrated that the presence of germline *PTEN* mutation in BRR is associated with cancer development.[4] Until additional data become available, it might be conservative to manage all BRR families, especially with germline *PTEN* mutations, like CS cases with respect to cancer formation and surveillance. Given the enormous amount of genetic data that has accumulated regarding *PTEN* mutations and PHTS, it would seem that routine clinical laboratory testing for *PTEN* mutations, both as a molecular diagnostic tool and as a predictive tool, might become commonplace. In the USA, at least one academic centre offers clinical *PTEN* testing with the molecular diagnostics laboratory working very closely with the Clinical Cancer Genetics Program.

The key to successful management of CS and/or BRR, and all PHTS patients and their families, is a multidisciplinary team. There should always be a primary care provider, usually a general internist, who orchestrates the care of such patients, some of whom will need the care of surgeons, gynaecologists, dermatologists, oncologists and geneticists at some point.

PTEN EXPRESSION AND FUNCTION

Somatic *PTEN* mutations and *PTEN* expression in sporadic neoplasia

Somatic *PTEN* mutations occur at a broad range of frequencies depending on tumour type. The sporadic CS-component tumours, those of the breast, thyroid and endometrium, will be presented here as an illustration of somatic mutation and PTEN silencing in sporadic neoplasia. Initial cell line work for a broad range of tumour types revealed a high frequency of intragenic *PTEN* mutations and homozygous deletions.[66,67] However, when non-cultured tumours were examined, the frequency of intragenic mutation and two clear somatic genetic 'hits' occurred in the minority. In non-cultured primary breast carcinomas, the high mutation and deletion frequency observed in breast cancer cell lines has not been borne out.[68–71] In one study of 54 unselected primary breast carcinomas, only one true somatic mutation was noted.[68] Even when selected for 10q23 hemizygous deletion, only 1 of 14 samples had a somatic intragenic mutation.[71] However, the 10q region has not previously shown prominent loss of heterozygosity in breast cancers. Yet, deletions in the region of *PTEN* occur in 30–40 per cent of primary breast carcinomas.[69–71] In one study, hemizygous deletion of *PTEN* and the 10q23 region occurred with any frequency only in invasive carcinomas of the breast but not in *in situ* cancers, and appeared to be associated with loss of oestrogen receptor.[71] In order to gather evidence of mechanisms of *PTEN* inactivation other than genetic, 33 well-characterized primary invasive breast adenocarcinomas without intragenic *PTEN* mutations[70] were examined for *PTEN* deletion and PTEN expression by immunohistochemistry.[72] Of these cancers, 11 had hemizygous deletion of *PTEN*. Five of these 11 with hemizygous deletion had complete PTEN silencing, while the remainder had markedly decreased PTEN expression. These observations argue that the second 'hit' in breast cancers is epigenetic.

To date, three early series have demonstrated somatic *PTEN* mutation in 34–50 per cent of apparently sporadic endometrial carcinoma.[73–75] From these three early series, it was noted that the frequency of intragenic mutation was much higher (86 per cent) in those of endometrioid histology with microsatellite instability.[73] Recently, however, 83 per cent of endometrioid endometrial carcinomas were shown to have somatic intragenic mutations and the frequency was equivalently high irrespective of microsatellite stability status.[76] Interestingly, only 33 per cent had deletions or mutations involving both *PTEN* alleles, yet 61 per cent expressed no protein.[76] In matched precancers, 55 per cent had intragenic mutation, while 75 per cent had no expression. Hence, *PTEN* mutation is an early event initiating endometrial precancers and epigenetic PTEN silencing can precede genetic alteration in the earliest precancers.

Deletions, represented by loss of heterozygosity of anonymous polymorphic markers residing on chromosome 10, have been prominent among both benign and malignant epithelial thyroid tumors.[77] Three studies, based mainly on thyroid tumours of European origin, have demonstrated that hemizygous deletion of *PTEN* occurs with a higher frequency in follicular adenomas (20–25 per cent) compared to follicular carcinomas (5–10 per cent).[78–80] The only intragenic point mutation was a somatic frameshift mutation in a single papillary thyroid carcinoma.[79] This observation suggests that the pathogenesis of adenomas and carcinomas may proceed along two different pathways, and that the adenoma–carcinoma sequence is not the rule in epithelial thyroid neoplasia.[80] The data were initially surprising in that epithelial thyroid malignancy does occur in 3–10 per cent of CS patients,[22,27] and one would expect that a larger proportion of sporadic thyroid carcinomas are associated with somatic *PTEN* alteration. It was rationalized that benign thyroid disease occurs in 50–67 per cent of CS individuals, far outnumbering the frequency of thyroid carcinomas. However, a recent expression and genetic analysis of 139 benign and malignant non-medullary thyroid tumours yielded some interesting data that may begin to address this apparent paradox.[81] In this series, follicular adenomas, follicular carcinomas and papillary thyroid carcinomas all had a 20–30 per cent frequency of hemizygous deletion, while almost 60 per cent of undifferentiated carcinomas had hemizygous *PTEN* deletion. Of note, hemizygous deletion and decreased PTEN expression were associated. Decreasing PTEN expression was observed with declining degree of differentiation. Decreasing nuclear PTEN expression seemed to precede that in the cytoplasm. The thyroid data suggest that, in addition to structural deletion, inappropriate subcellular compartmentalization might also contribute to PTEN inactivation. These observations are corroborated by the observations in endocrine pancreatic tumours where 10q loss is not associated with immunostaining intensity.[82] Instead, 10q loss was associated with malignant status. More interestingly, PTEN expression was predominantly cytoplasmic in the endocrine pancreatic tumours, whereas expression was predominantly nuclear in normal islet cells.[82]

When the first studies of PTEN in sporadic neoplasia were performed, it was believed that somatic *PTEN* mutations, and by inference, inactivation, occurred predominantly in advanced cancers, as illustrated by glioblastoma multiforme[83–86] and prostate cancer.[87] However, with further study at the genetic and recently, expressional level, it has become clear that somatic *PTEN* mutation can occur as an early event as well, as illustrated by endometrial carcinoma and precancers.[76] It would also appear that, depending on the tissue, there seems to be a predominant mechanism of PTEN inactivation. For example, in the endometrial neoplasia system, either two genetic 'hits', or one genetic 'hit' and one epigenetic silencing 'hit' can occur, although the latter predominates. In malignant melanoma, both inactivating 'hits' for PTEN are epigenetic.[88] In contrast, PTEN might also be inactivated by differential subcellular compartmentalization as illustrated by thyroid neoplasia and endocrine pancreatic tumours. This mechanism is somewhat puzzling, as PTEN has no obvious nuclear localization signal. The precise mechanisms of epigenetic inactivation have to be explored in further detail.

PTEN function

The rudimentary function of PTEN, affecting the cell cycle and apoptosis, was predicted from the manifestations of CS even before the gene was identified.[18] At that time, it was also predicted from the phenotype of CS that PTEN would play a fundamental role in shaping all three germ-cell layers during human development, an idea which has been borne out by expression studies during human development and in non-human pten null models.[9,15,89,90]

Despite intensive study since 1997 and much knowledge gained, little is known about every detail of PTEN's function, all its downstream targets and its upstream molecules. From nucleotide sequence alone, it was suggested that PTEN would be a phosphatase, most likely a dual-specificity phosphatase, that is, one that removes phosphates from both tyrosine and serine/threonine.[66,91,92] Initially thought to be a protein phosphatase,[6] it has been shown that PTEN is the major 3-phosphatase for phosphoinositide-3,4,5,-triphosphate[7,8,10] and signals down the AKT/ PKB apoptotic pathway.[7,10,11,13,93] Accordingly, when PTEN was transiently ectopically expressed in *PTEN*-null breast cancer lines, only apoptosis occurred.[11] When PTEN was expressed in endogenously wild-type breast lines, no differences were observed.[11] In contrast, when PTEN was transiently expressed in glioma lines, only G1 cell-cycle arrest was observed.[12,13,94] However, when wild-type PTEN was stably expressed in endogenous wild-type PTEN breast cancer lines, a time-dependent G1 arrest followed by apoptosis was observed.[14] Most likely, apoptosis occurs through PTEN's lipid phosphatase activity via AKT because downstream of AKT lies BAD, Bcl, 14-3-3 sigma

and FKRLH, which presumably could act as the transcription factor for the death factor FAS.[95] The mediators of G1 arrest are unknown. Whether it is RB-dependent or independent remains controversial.

Because of PTEN's sequence homology to tensin and auxilin, it was postulated that PTEN would play some role in cell adhesion. It was also shown that PTEN dephosphorylated focal adhesion kinase (FAK) and inhibits cell migration and spreading.[16] This result must be considered preliminary, however, because no other studies have been able to confirm these observations.

Non–human PTEN null models

PTEN is conserved from human and mouse down to *C. elegans* and yeast. There are three murine *pten* knockout models, targeted in three different ways.[9,15,90] The homozygous null status leads to embryonic death in all three models. All three *pten* ± mouse models, despite similar background (129SV), resulted in three different phenotypes. Initially, none of the models were similar to human CS or BRR. The closest resemblance was the model generated by Podsypanina *et al.* in which the *pten* ± mice developed hyperplastic polyps in the colon, endometrial hyperplasia and follicular thyroid cancer.[15] With subsequent ageing, the mouse generated by Suzuki *et al.*, which was initially characterized predominantly by thymic lymphomas,[90] began to develop breast and endometrial carcinomas, but also phaeochromocytomas.[96] Interestingly, neuroendocrine neoplasia has not been a prominent feature of human CS or BRR, despite strong expression of PTEN in the developing human neural crest and its derivatives.[89]

The PTEN homologue in *C. elegans* is daf-18, which is one of the proteins that controls dauer (larval) formation.[97–99] daf-18 is a key element in the insulin-like signalling pathway that controls entry into dispause, which is related to longevity. Interestingly, the equivalents of the PI3-K/Akt pathways downstream of daf-18 are also conserved. The yeast homologue TEP-1 was isolated while looking for genes regulated by transforming growth factor β.[92]

SUMMARY AND CONCLUSIONS

Cowden syndrome (CS) is named after Rachel Cowden, who died of bilateral breast cancer at the age of 33.[28,29] In the last 37 years since the discovery of this syndrome, so much has been uncovered, particularly in the last 4 years. Prior to 1996, nothing about the genetic basis of the inherited hamartoma tumour syndromes was known. In 1996, CS was linked to 10q22–23,[18] followed rapidly the next year by the identification of the susceptibility gene,

$PTEN$,[1] and the delineation of other allelic conditions, Bannayan–Riley–Ruvalcaba syndrome and a Proteus-like syndrome.[2–5] Given these and the genotype-phenotype data, it was proposed that those syndromes characterized by germline $PTEN$ mutation be collectively referred to as PHTS.[4] The PHTS categorization is important because of individual and familial risk of developing the cancers associated with CS, with implications for DNA-based predictive testing, medical management, surveillance and even prophylactic surgeries.

At the fundamental level, the protean intracellular molecular pathways affected by PTEN and its function are only just beginning to be elucidated. PTEN will likely affect multiple pathways several times over, and full understanding is necessary before targeting of molecules in these pathways is safe and effective.

ACKNOWLEDGEMENTS

I would like to acknowledge the members of my laboratory: Patricia Dahia, Heather Dziema, Oliver Gimm, Jennifer Kum, Keisuke Kurose, Debbie Marsh, Margaret Ginn-Pease, Aurel Perren, Wendy M. Smith, Liang-Ping Weng, Zimu Zheng and Xiao-Ping Zhou, who, over the course of the last four and a half years, have contributed to some of the work described in this chapter. No comprehensive human genetic studies would have been possible without the assistance of the many cancer genetic counsellors, especially Heather Hampel and Kathy Schneider, and collaborators and clinicians, especially George Mutter and Monica Peacocke.

Work in my laboratory is funded by the National Institutes of Health, Bethesda, MD, USA, the American Cancer Society, the US Army Breast Cancer Research Program, the Susan G. Komen Breast Cancer Research Foundation and the Mary Kay Ash Charitable Foundation.

KEY POINTS

- Cowden syndrome is named after a patient, Rachel Cowden.
- It has diagnostic criteria (Table 12.1).
- It consists of multiple hamartomas.
- There is an increased cancer risk in the breast, thyroid and endometrium. The colon cancer risk is debated.
- A large proportion of cases is due to germline mutations in the $PTEN$ gene on 10q.
- A spectrum of conditions are due to germline mutations in $PTEN$ (Cowden syndrome, Proteus, Bannayan–Riley–Ruvalcaba or BRR).

REFERENCES

1. Liaw D, Marsh DJ, Li J, et al. Germline mutations of the PTEN gene in Cowden disease, an inherited breast and thyroid cancer syndrome. Nature Genet 1997; 16:64–67.
2. Marsh DJ, Coulon V, Lunetta KL, et al. Mutation spectrum and genotype–phenotype analyses in Cowden disease and Bannayan–Zonana syndrome, two hamartoma syndromes with germline PTEN mutation. Hum Mol Genet 1998; 7:507–715.
3. Marsh DJ, Dahia PLM, Zheng Z, et al. Germline mutations in PTEN are present in Bannayan–Zonana syndrome. Nature Genet 1997; 16:333–334.
4. Marsh DJ, Kum JB, Lunetta KL, et al. PTEN mutation spectrum and genotype–phenotype correlations in Bannayan–Riley–Ruvalcaba syndrome suggest a single entity with Cowden syndrome. Hum Mol Genet 1999; 8:1461–1472.
5. Zhou XP, Marsh DJ, Hampel H, et al. Germline and germline mosaic mutations associated with a Proteus-like syndrome of hemihypertrophy, lower limb asymmetry, arterio-venous malformations and lipomatosis. Hum Mol Genet 2000; 9:765–768.
6. Myers MP, Stolarov J, Eng C, et al. PTEN, the tumor suppressor from human chromosome 10q23, is a dual specificity phosphatase. Proc Natl Acad Sci USA 1997; 94:9052–9057.
7. Myers MP, Pass I, Batty IH, et al. The lipid phosphatase activity of PTEN is critical for its tumor suppressor function. Proc Natl Acad Sci USA 1998; 95:13513–13518.
8. Maehama T, Dixon JE. The tumor suppressor, PTEN/MMAC1, dephosphorylates the lipid second messenger phosphoinositol 3,4,5-triphosphate. J Biol Chem 1998; 273:13375–13378.
9. Di Cristofano A, Pesce B, Cordon-Cardo C, Pandolfi PP. Pten is essential for embryonic development and tumour suppression. Nature Genet 1998; 19:348–355.
10. Stambolic V, Suzuki A, de la Pompa JL, et al. Negative regulation of PKB/Akt-dependent cell survival by the tumor suppressor PTEN. Cell 1998; 95:1–20.
11. Li J, Simpson L, Takahashi M, et al. The PTEN/MMAC1 tumor suppressor induces cell death that is rescued by the AKT/protein kinase B oncogene. Cancer Res 1998; 58:5667–5672.
12. Li DM, Sun H. PTEN/MMAC1/TEP1 suppresses the tumorigenecity and induces G1 cell cycle arrest in human glioblastoma cells. Proc Natl Acad Sci USA 1998; 95:15406–15411.
13. Furnari FB, SuHuang H-J, Cavanee WK. The phosphoinositol phosphatase activity of PTEN mediates a serum-sensitive G1 growth arrest in glioma cells. Cancer Res 1998; 58:5002–5008.
14. Weng L-P, Smith WM, Dahia PLM, et al. PTEN suppresses breast cancer cell growth by phosphatase function-dependent G1 arrest followed by apoptosis. Cancer Res 1999; 59:5808–5814.
15. Podsypanina K, Ellenson LH, Nemes A, et al. Mutation of Pten/Mmac1 in mice causes neoplasia in multiple organ systems. Proc Natl Acad Sci USA 1999; 96:1563–1568.
16. Tamura M, Gu J, Matsumoto K, et al. Inhibition of cell migration, spreading and focal adhesions by tumor supressor PTEN. Science 1998; 280:1614–1617.
17. Lyons CJ, Wilson CR, Horton JC. Association between meningioma and Cowden's disease. Neurology 1993, 43:1436–1437.

18. Nelen MR, Padberg GW, Peeters EAJ, et al. Localization of the gene for Cowden disease to 10q22–23. Nature Genet 1996; 13:114–116.

19. Nelen MR, Kremer H, Konings IBM, et al. Novel PTEN mutations in patients with Cowden disease: absence of clear genotype- phenotype correlations. Eur J Hum Genet 1999; 7:267–273.

20. Haibach H, Burns TW, Carlson HE, et al. Multiple hamartoma syndrome (Cowden's disease) associated with renal cell carcinoma and primary neuroendocrine carcinoma of the skin (Merkel cell carcinoma). Am J Clin Pathol 1992; 97:705–712.

21. Schrager CA, Schneider D, Gruener AC, et al. Clinical and pathological features of breast disease in Cowden's syndrome: an under-recognised syndrome with an increased risk of breast cancer. Hum Pathol 1997; 29:47–53.

22. Starink TM, van der Veen JPW, Arwert F, et al. The cowden syndrome: a clinical and genetic study in 21 patients. Clin Genet 1986; 29:222–233.

23. Hanssen AMN, Fryns JP. Cowden syndrome. J Med Genet 1995; 32:117–119.

24. Mallory SB. Cowden syndrome (multiple hamartoma syndrome). Dermatol Clin 1995; 13:27–31.

25. Longy M, Lacombe D. Cowden disease. Report of a family and review. Ann Genet 1996; 39:35–42.

26. NCCN. NCCN Practice guidelines: genetics/familial high risk cancer. Oncology 1999; 13(11A):161–186.

27. Eng C. Cowden syndrome. J Genet Counsel 1997; 6:181–191.

28. Lloyd KM, Denis M. Cowden's disease: a possible new symptom complex with multiple system involvement. Ann Intern Med 1963; 58:136–142.

29. Brownstein MH, Wolf M, Bilowski JB. Cowden's disease. Cancer 1978; 41:2393–2398.

30. Padberg GW, Schot JDL, Vielvoye GJ, et al. Lhermitte–Duclos disease and Cowden syndrome: a single phakomatosis. Ann Neurol 1991; 29:517–523.

31. Eng C, Murday V, Seal S, et al. Cowden syndrome and Lhermitte–Duclos disease in a family: a single genetic syndrome with pleiotropy? J Med Genet 1994; 31:458–461.

32. Weber HC, Marsh D, Lubensky I, et al. Germline PTEN/MMAC1/TEP1 mutations and association with gastrointestinal manifestations in Cowden disease. Gastroenterology 1998; 114S:G2902.

33. Tsou HC, Teng D, Ping XL, et al. Role of MMAC1 mutations in early onset breast cancer: causative in association with Cowden's syndrome and excluded in BRCA1-negative cases. Am J Hum Genet 1997; 61:1036–1043.

34. Nelen MR, van Staveren CG, Peeters EAJ, et al. Germline mutations in the PTEN/MMAC1 gene in patients with Cowden disease. Hum Mol Genet 1997; 6:1383–1387.

35. Lynch ED, Ostermeyer EA, Lee MK, et al. Inherited mutations in PTEN that are associated with breast cancer, Cowden syndrome and juvenile polyposis. Am J Hum Genet 1997; 61:1254–1260.

36. Eng C, Parsons R. Cowden syndrome. In: Vogelstein B, Kinzler KW (eds) The genetic basis of human cancer. New York: McGraw-Hill, 1998: 519–526.

37. Higginbottom MC, Schultz P. The Bannayan syndrome: an autosomal dominant disorder consisting of macrocephaly, lipomas and hemangiomas, and risk for intracranial tumours. Pediatrics 1982; 69:632–634.

38. Halal F, Silver K. Slowly progressive macrocephaly with hamartomas: a new syndrome? Am J Med Genet 1989; 33:182–185.

39. Bannayan GA. Lipomatosis, angiomatosis, and macrencephalia: a previously undescribed congenital syndrome. Arch Pathol 1971; 92:1–5.

40. Zonana J, Rimoin DL, Davis DC. Macrocephaly with multiple lipomas and hemangiomas. J Pediatr 1976; 89:600–603.

41. Marsh DJ, Caron S, Dahia PLM, et al. Germline PTEN mutations in Cowden syndrome-like families. J Med Genet 1998; 35:881–885.

42. DeVivo I, Gertig DM, Nagase S, et al. Novel germline mutations in the PTEN tumour suppressor gene found in women with multiple cancers. J Med Genet 2000; 37:336–341.

43. FitzGerald MG, Marsh DJ, Wahrer D, et al. Germline mutations in PTEN are an infrequent cause of genetic predisposition to breast cancer. Oncogene 1998; 17:727–731.

44. Shugart YY, Cour C, Renard H, et al. Linkage analysis of 56 multiplex families excludes the Cowden disease gene PTEN as a major contributor to familial breast cancer. J Med Genet 1999; 36:720–721.

45. Chen J, Lindblom P, Lindblom A. A study of the PTEN/MMAC1 gene in 136 breast cancer families. Hum Genet 1998; 102:124–125.

46. Olschwang S, Serova-Sinilnikova OM, Lenoir GM, Thomas G. PTEN germline mutations in juvenile polyposis coli. Nature Genet 1998; 18:12–14.

47. Kurose K, Araki T, Matsunaka T, et al. Variant manifestation of Cowden disease in Japan: hamatomatous polyposis of the digestive tract with mutation of the PTEN gene. Am J Hum Genet 1999; 64:308–310.

48. Eng C, Ji H. Molecular classification of the inherited hamartoma polyposis syndromes: clearing the muddied waters. Am J Hum Genet 1998; 62:1020–1022.

49. Howe JR, Ringold JC, Summers RW, et al. A gene for familial juvenile polyposis maps to chromosome 18q21. 1. Am J Hum Genet 1998; 62:1129–1136.

50. Howe JR, Roth S, Ringold JC, et al. Mutations in the SMAD4/DPC4 gene in juvenile polyposis. Science 1998; 280:1086–1088.

51. Houlston R, Bevan S, Williams A, et al. Mutations in DPC4 (SMAD4) cause juvenile polyposis syndrome, but only account for a minority of cases. Hum Mol Genet 1998; 7:1907–1912.

52. Eng C, Blackstone MO. Peutz–Jeghers syndrome. Med Rounds 1988; 1:165–171.

53. Rustgi AK. Medical progress – hereditary gastrointestinal polyposis and nonpolyposis syndromes. N Engl J Med 1994; 331:1694–1702.

54. Hemminki A, Tomlinson I, Markie D, et al. Localisation of a susceptibility locus for Peutz–Jeghers syndrome to 19p using comparative genomic hybridization and targeted linkage analysis. Nature Genet 1997; 15:87–90.

55. Hemminki A, Markie D, Tomlinson I, et al. A serine/threonine kinase gene defective in Peutz–Jeghers syndrome. Nature 1998; 391:184–187.

56. Jenne DE, Reimann H, Nezu J-i, et al. Peutz–Jeghers syndrome is caused by mutations in a novel serine threonine kinase. Nature Genet 1998; 18:38–44.

57. Mehenni H, Blouin JL, Radhakrishna U, *et al*. Peutz–Jeghers syndrome: confirmation of linkage to chromosome 19p13. 3 and identification of a potential second locus on 19q13. 4. *Am J Hum Genet* 1997; **61**:1327–1334.

58. Gorlin RJ. Proteus syndrome. *J Dysmorphol* 1984; **2**:8–9.

59. Biesecker LG, Happle R, Mulliken JB, *et al*. Proteus syndrome: diagnostic criteria, differential diagnosis and patient evaluation. *Am J Med Genet* 1999; **84**:389–395.

60. Viskochil D, Buchberg AM, Xu G, *et al*. Deletions and translocation interrupt a cloned gene at the neurofibromatosis type 1 locus. *Cell* 1990; **62**:187–192.

61. Wallace MR, Marchuk DA, Anderson LB, *et al*. Type 1 neurofibromatosis gene: identification of a large transcript disrupted in three NF1 patients. *Science* 1990; **249**:181–186.

62. Ward K, O'Connell P, Carey J, *et al*. Diagnosis of neurofibromatosis 1 by using tightly linked, flanking DNA markers. *Am J Hum Genet* 1990; **46**:943–949.

63. Johnson RL, Rothman AL, Xie J, *et al*. Human homolog of patched, a candidate gene for the basal cell nevus syndrome. *Science* 1996; **272**:1668–1671.

64. Bashir R, Munro CS, Mason S, *et al*. Localisation of a gene for Darier's disease. *Hum Mol Genet* 1993; **2**:1937–1939.

65. Craddock N, Dawson E, Burge S, *et al*. The gene for Darier's disease maps to chromosome 12q23–24. 1. *Hum Mol Genet* 1993; **2**:1941–1943.

66. Li J, Yen C, Liaw D, *et al*. PTEN, a putative protein tyrosine phosphatase gene mutated in human brain, breast and prostate cancer. *Science* 1997; **275**:1943–1947.

67. Teng DH-F, Hu R, Lin H, *et al*. MMAC1/PTEN mutations in primary tumor specimens and tumor cell lines. *Cancer Res* 1997; **57**:5221–5225.

68. Rhei E, Kang L, Bogomoliniy F, *et al*. Mutation analysis of the putative tumor suppressor gene PTEN/MMAC1 in primary breast carcinomas. *Cancer Res* 1997; **57**:3657–3659.

69. Singh B, Ittman MM, Krolewski JJ. Sporadic breast cancers exhibit loss of heterozygosity on chromosome segment 10q23 close to the Cowden disease locus. *Genes Chrom Cancer* 1998; **21**:166–171.

70. Feilotter HE, Coulon V, McVeigh JL, *et al*. Analysis of the 10q23 chromosomal region and the PTEN gene in human sporadic breast carcinoma. *Br J Cancer* 1999; **79**:718–723.

71. Bose S, Wang SI, Terry MB, *et al*. Allelic loss of chromosome 10q23 is associated with tumor progression in breast carcinomas. *Oncogene* 1998; **17**:123–127.

72. Perren A, Weng LP, Boag AH, *et al*. Immunohistochemical evidence of loss of PTEN expression in primary ductal adenocarcinomas of the breast. *Am J Pathol* 1999; **155**:1253–1260.

73. Tashiro H, Blazes MS, Wu R, *et al*. Mutations in PTEN are frequent in endometrial carcinoma but rare in other common gynecological malignancies. *Cancer Res* 1997; **57**:3935–3940.

74. Kong D, Suzuki A, Zou T-T, *et al*. PTEN1 is frequently mutated in primary endometrial carcinomas. *Nature Genet* 1997; **17**:143–144.

75. Risinger JI, Hayes AK, Berchuck A, Barrett JC. PTEN/MMAC1 mutations in endometrial cancers. *Cancer Res* 1997; **57**: 4736–4738.

76. Mutter GL, Lin M-C, Fitzgerald JT, *et al*. Altered PTEN expression as a diagnostic marker for the earliest endometrial precancers. *J Natl Cancer Inst* 2000; **92**:924–931.

77. Zedenius J, Wallin G, Svensson A, *et al*. Allelotyping of follicular thyroid tumors. 1995; **96**:27–32.

78. Marsh DJ, Zheng Z, Zedenius J, *et al*. Differential loss of heterozygosity in the region of the Cowden locus within 10q22–23 in follicular thyroid adenomas and carcinomas. *Cancer Res* 1997; **57**:500–503.

79. Dahia PLM, Marsh DJ, Zheng Z, *et al*. Somatic deletions and mutations in the Cowden disease gene, PTEN, in sporadic thyroid tumors. *Cancer Res* 1997; **57**:4710–4713.

80. Yeh JJ, Marsh DJ, Zedenius J, *et al*. Fine structure deletion analysis of 10q22–24 demonstrates novel regions of loss and suggests that sporadic follicular thyroid adenomas and follicular thyroid carcinomas develop along distinct parallel neoplastic pathways. *Gene Chrom Cancer* 1999; **26**:322–328.

81. Gimm O, Perren A, Weng LP, *et al*. Differential nuclear and cytoplasmic expression of PTEN in normal thyroid tissue, and benign and malignant epithelial thyroid tumors. *Am J Pathol* 2000; **156**:1693–1700.

82. Perren A, Komminoth P, Saremaslani P, *et al*. Mutation and expression analyses reveal differential subcellular compartmentalization of PTEN in endocrine pancreatic tumors compared to normal islet cells. *Am J Pathol* 2000; **157**: 1097–1103.

83. Dürr E-M, Rollbrocker B, Hayashi Y, *et al*. PTEN mutations in gliomas and glioneuronal tumours. *Oncogene* 1998; **16**:2259–2264.

84. Wang SI, Puc J, Li J, *et al*. Somatic mutations of PTEN in glioblastoma multiforme. *Cancer Res* 1997; **57**:4183–4186.

85. Rasheed BKA, Stenzel TT, McLendon RE, *et al*. PTEN gene mutations are seen in high-grade but not in low-grade gliomas. *Cancer Res* 1997; **37**:4187–4190.

86. Maier D, Zhang ZW, Taylor E, *et al*. Somatic deletion mapping on chromosome 10 and sequence analysis of PTEN/MMAC1 point to the 10q25–26 region as the primary target in low-grade and high-grade gliomas. *Oncogene* 1998; **16**:3331–3335.

87. Wang SI, Parsons R, Ittman M. Homozygous deletion of the PTEN tumor suppressor gene in a subset of prostate adenocarcinomas. *Clin Cancer Res* 1998; **4**:811–815.

88. Zhou XP, Gimm O, Hampel H, *et al*. Epigenetic PTEN silencing in malignant melanomas without PTEN mutation. *Am J Pathol* 2000; **157**:1123–1128.

89. Gimm O, Attè-Bitach T, Lees JA, *et al*. Expression of PTEN in human embryonic development. *Hum Mol Genet* 2000; **9**:1633–1639.

90. Suzuki A, de la Pompa JL, Stambolic V, *et al*. High cancer susceptibility and embryonic lethality associated with mutation of the PTEN tumor suppressor gene in mice. *Curr Biol* 1998; **8**:1169–1178.

91. Steck PA, Pershouse MA, Jasser SA, *et al*. Identification of a candidate tumour suppressor gene, MMAC1, at chromosome 10q23. 3 that is mutated in multiple advanced cancers. *Nature Genet* 1997; **15**:356–362.

92. Li D-M, Sun H. TEP1, encoded by a candidate tumor suppressor locus, is a novel protein tyrosine phosphatase regulated by transforming growth factor B. *Cancer Res* 1997; **57**:2124–2129.

93. Dahia PLM, Aguiar RCT, Alberta J, *et al*. PTEN is inversely correlated with the cell survival factor PKB/Akt and is

inactivated by diverse mechanisms in haematologic malignancies. *Hum Mol Genet* 1999; **8:**185–193.

94. Furnari FB, Lin H, Huang H-JS, Cavanee WK. Growth suppression of glioma cells by *PTEN* requires a functional catalytic domain. *Proc Natl Acad Sci USA* 1997; **94:**12479–12484.

95. Di Cristofano A, Kotsi P, Peng YF, *et al.* Impaired Fas response and autoimmunity in *Pten +/−* mice. *Science* 1999; **285:** 2122–2125.

96. Stambolic V, Tsao MS, MacPherson D, *et al.* High incidence of breast and endometrial neoplasia resembling human Cowden syndrome in *pten +/−* mice. *Cancer Res* 2000; **60:**3605–3611.

97. Ogg S, Ruvkun G. The C. elegans *PTEN* homolog, DAF-18, acts in the insulin receptor-like metabolic signaling pathway. *Mol Cell* 1998; **2:**887–893.

98. Gil EB, Malone Link E, Liu LX, *et al.* Regulation of the insulin-like developmental pathway of Caenorhabditis elegans by a homolog of the *PTEN* tumor suppressor gene. *Proc Natl Acad Sci USA* 1999; **96:**2925–2930.

99. Rouault JP, Kuwabara PE, Sinilnikova OM, *et al.* Regulation of dauer larva development in Caenorhabditis elegans by daf-18, a homologue of the tumour suppressor *PTEN*. *Curr Biol* 1999; **9:**329–332.

PART 3

Chromosome fragility syndromes and the Gorlin syndrome

13

Clinical, cellular and mutational variations in ataxia telangiectasia

A. MALCOLM R. TAYLOR, G. STEWART, T. STANKOVIC, S. MAN AND P.J. BYRD

INTRODUCTION

Ataxia telangiectasia (A-T) is a progressive neurological disorder with a birth incidence of approximately 1 in 300 000.[1,2] The major neurological features include progressive cerebellar ataxia presenting in infancy, oculomotor dyspraxia and dysarthria. Immunodeficiency is an important feature of this disorder, although it is not usually severe. A majority of patients, if not all, have a deficiency of cell-mediated immunity, whereas deficiencies in humoral immunity are more variable. The resulting predisposition to infection is very variable between patients with some not noticeably affected and others showing frequent episodes of severe infection. In addition, patients show thymic hypoplasia, hypogonadism, a high level of serum alpha-fetoprotein (AFP), growth retardation and an abnormality of blood vessels (telangiectasia). The *ATM* gene also confers an increased radiosensitivity, which can be observed both in patients and in cultured cells from patients.

Phenotypic variations have been observed in a number of patients with A-T. The variations are mainly in the degree of neurological deterioration, levels of immunodeficiency, levels of cellular radiosensitivity and in the presence or absence of tumours.[3–5] Both the age of onset of cerebellar features and its rate of progress has been reported to be variable. Families have been reported with either unusual genetic features,[1] or both unusual genetic and clinical features.[6–10] The occurrence of a particular type of lymphoid tumour in more than one sibling in a significant number of families and concordance of tumour type in these cases[3,8] suggests strongly that cancer predisposition may be greater for some A-T patients than for others. There is, therefore, a need for elucidating the underlying molecular mechanism of phenotypic heterogeneity in the disorder. We discuss the heterogeneity which is seen to result either from the presence of different *ATM* mutations or from mutations in a further gene, *MRE11*.

Although phenotypically normal, *ATM* mutation carriers in A-T families may also be at a higher risk of developing breast cancer.[1,11] This observation may have wide implications as the frequency of the A-T carriers varies between 0.5 and 1 per cent depending on the population (reviewed by Easton[12]).

THE ATM PROTEIN

The *ATM* gene spans 150 kb of genomic DNA and encodes a ubiquitously expressed transcript of approximately 13 kb consisting of 66 exons. The main promoter of *ATM* is bidirectional[13] and the single open reading frame of the *ATM* gene gives a 350 kDa protein of 3056 amino acids. This protein shows similarity at its carboxyl-terminal end to the catalytic domain of phosphatidylinositol-3 (PI-3) kinases.[14,15] The PI-3 kinase motif is common to a group of proteins including *Drosophila melanogaster* mei41, *Saccharomyces cerevisiae* TOR1 and TOR2 and their human homologues FRAP and rRAFT, *Schizosaccharomyces pombe* rad3, MEC I and a DNA-dependent protein kinase catalytic subunit,[14,15] which is involved in cell-cycle regulation, response to DNA damage, interlocus recombination and control of telomere length.

ATM is principally a nuclear protein. Its expression level and localization is not affected by the stage of the cell cycle nor whether there has been prior exposure of the cell to ionizing radiation.[16] Some ATM protein may also be located in the cytoplasm.[17] Although the complete inventory of ATM functions is still to be established, it is known that it has a role in activating the G1/S, S and G2/M cell-cycle checkpoints following exposure to DNA damage.[18] ATM-deficient cells also have a defect in stress response pathways, so that, for example, c-Jun N-terminal kinase (JNK) activation following exposure of cell to ionizing radiation is defective.[19] The triggering of cell death (apoptosis) is a normal physiological response to eliminate cells with levels of genetic damage too high to be repaired. Cells defective in ATM appear to be more resistant to ionizing radiation-induced apoptosis, although this appears to be a cell-type-specific response.[20,21]

ATM is a serine/threonine protein kinase that is activated by exposure of cells to ionizing radiation.[22,23] A major role of ATM is to regulate the p53 protein. Following exposure of normal cells to ionizing radiation, p53 is stabilized and accumulates leading to activation of p21, inhibition of cyclin-dependent kinases and cell-cycle arrest. ATM can directly bind and phosphorylate p53 at ser-15.[22,23] This probably enhances the ability of p53 to transactivate downstream responsive genes like p21. Accumulation of p53 probably results from the ATM dependent phosphorylation of p53 by CHEK1 and CHEK2 at ser-20.[24] This prevents binding of MDM2 to p53 allowing accumulation of p53 instead of it being targeted for degradation. In the absence of ATM, there is no stabilization of p53 and, therefore, no cell-cycle arrest. In addition to p53, several other substrates for ATM have been identified including B-adaptin, c-Abl, Nbsl and BRCA1. An amino-acid consensus phosphorylation sequence has been compiled and various other putative substrates identified.[25]

ATM is reported to be part of a large complex of proteins.[26] This has been given the name BRCA1-associated genome surveillance complex (BASC). As the name implies, this is a group of proteins that associate with the BRCA1 (breast cancer 1) protein. In addition to ATM, the MRE11/RAD50/NBS1 complex and BRCA1, at least five other proteins are reported to be in this large complex. What does all this do? An important class of genes serves to maintain the integrity of the genetic material of our cells and prevent the occurrence of mutations. *ATM* is one of the genes that is part of the BASC super complex, which, in turn, appears to act in recognizing damage to the genetic material and also in repairing it.

Of particular importance is the function of the ATM protein in the central nervous system and especially the cerebellum, which is most affected in A-T. During the development of the normal fetus, some cells are selected to die, and this is important for normal tissue modelling and also for the development of the immune system. There is no indication that this is abnormal in A-T. Programmed cell death, however, may also be triggered by damage, generated intrinsically or extrinsically, to the genome. In experiments on a-t mice, lacking any functional atm protein, programmed cell death did not occur when the mouse brain cells were exposed to ionizing radiation. This abnormality was seen in different parts of the brain including the cerebellum. In normal mice, radiation-induced programmed cell death occurred normally. It has been proposed that this function of ATM in programmed cell death is necessary in normal cells to remove spontaneously occurring damage that has accumulated in the genetic material of developing neurons. The damaged neurones that are not removed in the developing fetus, later could affect the function of that part of the brain. Failure to remove particular damaged neurones might contribute to the neurodegeneration in A-T.[27]

ATM MUTATIONS IN A-T PATIENTS

Types and location of mutations

Approximately 120 A-T families are known in the UK. With a few exceptions, patients are compound heterozygotes. Approximately 70 per cent of mutations are predicted to lead to the premature termination of the protein, 14 per cent of mutations are frame deletions and 15 per cent are missense mutations predicted to cause exchange of one amino acid by another. Mutations are scattered across the whole coding sequence of the *ATM* gene, although there appears to be some clustering of the mutations within the 3' end of the gene. Approximately one-third of all mutations occur between exons 54 and

60 (about 15 per cent of the coding region) corresponding to the PI-3 kinase domain and the region 5′ adjacent to this.[8]

Founder mutations

Eleven mutations identified in more than one UK family have been confirmed as founder mutations by the presence of a common haplotype within the families.[8] Approximately one-quarter of families carry one of these founder mutations. Patients with either founder mutation FM7 or FM9 show a milder clinical phenotype. One of these (FM7) is a splicing mutation (5762ins137)[7] and the other (FM9) is a missense mutation (7271T > G) (see later). In addition, three mutations, 2125del126nt, 7630del159 and 9139C > T, are believed to be recurrent mutations in the UK A-T population as no evidence of a founder effect was observed in patients with these mutations. Founder mutations are also reported in other populations.

ATM protein expression

Expression of ATM protein was investigated in lymphoblastoid cell lines (LCLs) from 74 A-T patients in the British Isles.[8] Patients with the founder mutations, 5762ins137 and 7636del9, showed some expression of normal and mutant ATM, respectively.[16] In addition, patients from a further 12 families showed some expression and patients from another five families showed a very low level of expression of mutant ATM. All mutant ATM proteins detected were either full or nearly full length. ATM proteins predicted to be prematurely terminated were not identified in any patient, indicating that such proteins are unstable, and 40 A-T patients showed no detectable ATM protein at all.

FEATURES OF CLASSICAL A-T

Sedgwick and Boder[4] described classical A-T in the following way:

> The cardinal features of A-T are progressive cerebellar ataxia beginning in infancy, progressive oculocutaneous telangiectasia first noted in the exposed bulbar conjunctivae, simulating conjunctivitis; susceptibility to neoplasia and sinopulmonary infection, including bronchiectasis; progressive apraxia of eye movements, simulating ophthalmoplegia; characteristic facies and posture.

To this can be added the observation that all classical A-T patients show an increased level of chromosome translocations involving chromosomes 7 and 14 in peripheral blood T cells; they also all show an increased radiosensitivity, which can also be measured in lymphocyte chromosomes. The opinion of Sedgwick and Boder[4] was that the diagnostic *sine qua non* was an early-onset progressive cerebellar ataxia with later onset oculocutaneous telangiectasia. They also suggested that the disease may exist without the telangiectasia but not without the cerebellar ataxia. This is interesting in the light of the recently described A-T-like disorder (ATLD) (see later).

Classical A-T will result from the total absence of any functional ATM protein and, at the gene level, this is the consequence of homozygosity or compound heterozygosity for *ATM* null alleles so that no functional ATM protein is produced. Interestingly *ATM*, therefore, is not an essential gene, and there must be redundancy with at least one and possibly more than one other protein. This begs the question of the identity of these other proteins and the consequences at the clinical level of mutations in these genes. It is possible, therefore, that there are other genes that, when mutated, will give an A-T-like phenotype (see later).

A–T WITH MILDER CLINICAL AND CELLULAR PHENOTYPE

The following examples of particular *ATM* mutations show how these can result in a modified A-T phenotype.

A–T and mutation at *ATM* 5762ins137

Patients heterozygous for this mutation have a later mean age of onset of A-T compared with classical patients (approximately 4 years of age compared with 1.5 years). Comparing A-T patients >16 years of age, the 5762ins137 individuals are less severely affected in all their neurological features than age-matched classical A-T patients.[7] The implication is that these patients have a slower rate of progress. None have had serious problems with infection and none have developed lymphoid tumours. At the cellular level, all these patients were initially classified as having a variant A-T phenotype on the basis of reduced radiosensitivity following exposure of cells to gamma-rays.[28] Indeed, at the chromosomal level, the amount of induced damage could be almost normal.

The A-T patients in 14 families have a 137 bp insertion in their cDNA caused by a point mutation in a sequence resembling a splice-donor site. The predicted consequence of this mutation is to produce a truncated protein but, in practice, no protein at all is produced, indicating the instability of such truncations. It is, therefore, paradoxical that such a major disruption of the ATM protein should be associated with a milder clinical and cellular phenotype.

An explanation is that the mutation affects the efficiency of correct exon splicing, resulting in the production of both normal and aberrant transcripts from the mutant allele.[7] The ratio of normal to mutant product may vary between patients and this may account for the variable clinical picture between patients carrying this mutation. Indeed, the level of the 137 bp polymerase chain reaction product containing the insertion was lowest in two patients with the latest onset of cerebellar ataxia. At the protein level, it can be shown that cells from these patients express a low level of, presumably, normal ATM protein and this has been shown to retain some normal function.[29] In summary, it appears that there is sufficient expression of normal ATM protein to moderate the phenotype.

A–T and mutation at 7271T > G

Three UK families (referred to as 46, 109 and 136) have been reported to carry in common a 7271T > G transversion and a common haplotype. The 7271T > G mutation is predicted to produce a change in codon 2424, with replacement of valine by glycine. The presence of this mutation is associated with a mild clinical phenotype and lower radiosensitivity, compared with classical A-T. Family 109, where the mutation is present in the homozygous state, contains the oldest patients in the British Isles with proven A-T and, with one patient in his seventh decade, possibly the oldest patient reported with A-T. This family also shows one further remarkable feature, which is that one of the affected daughters has a son, indicating the widespread effects of this milder mutation.[8]

Three members of a sibship of four, in family 109, have longstanding ataxia. The affected individuals have minimal telangiectasia and no obvious increased tendency to infections. Aged 48 years, the proband had had truncal ataxia and progressive dysarthia from her early 20s. A computed tomography scan at the age of 33 years showed cerebellar degeneration but she was able to work in a factory to the age of 34 years. She has minimal telangiectasia, dysarthric but comprehensible speech, and is of normal intelligence. Despite severe truncal ataxia, she can still just walk with aids. Peripheral ataxia is evident but less severe. Oculomotor apraxia is marked. An affected sister (50 years) has had a similar neurological course to the proband. She had normal periods and has borne one child after many years of trying to conceive. The brother, eldest of the sibship, had abnormal head movements from 3 years. Ataxia was first recognized when he was 9. His neurological course has been similar to his sisters but with an earlier onset, and has been slightly more severe (see Stankovic et al.[8] for further details).

The two affected brothers from family 46 are compound heterozygotes for the ATM gene.[8] In addition to the 7271T > G transversion, the second ATM mutation in this family is 3910del7nt, which is predicted to lead to the premature truncation of the ATM protein. The older brother (28 years) had a longstanding ataxia. He had complex nystagmus with very broken saccades but no frank oculomotor apraxia. He also had peripheral neuropathy. However, he was still able to walk short distances with support. He had frequent ear and chest infections. His younger, 16-year-old, brother could still walk unaided. Like his brother, he also had frequent infections. Both patients had typical oculocutaneous telangiectasia.

Based on the level of damage in lymphocytes from these two families, it appears that lymphocytes from two siblings in family 46 are less radiosensitive than those from the siblings in family 109. Western blot analysis using ATM-specific antibodies revealed the presence of full-length ATM in the parents from both families as well as from the five affected individuals. Remarkably, the level of mutated ATM protein in the affected siblings of family 109 is similar to the level of ATM in both the carrier mother and normal individuals, while the levels in both A-T siblings heterozygous for mutation 7271T > G (46, II-I and 46, II-2) is reduced compared with normal. This suggests that the 350 kDa protein identified in the five affected individuals in families 46 and 109 is the protein that genetic analysis predicted to be full length but with a single amino-acid change. The fact that the abundance of mutated ATM in homozygotes is similar to wild-type ATM shows that the stability of the protein is also not affected.

In a third family, 136 with the 7271T > G mutation the age of onset of A-T features was 18 years. The second mutation in this family has not been identified yet but may also be a missense mutation.

A–T caused by mutation in the MRE11 gene

Occasionally, mutations in the ATM gene cannot be detected in patients who have ataxia telangiectasia. This can be for technical reasons or because there is, in fact, no ATM mutation. We encountered two families in which the affected individuals presented with many clinical features of A-T, especially progressive cerebellar degeneration. Although none of the affected individuals from either family exhibited ocular telangiectasia, their clinical presentations were otherwise consistent with the diagnosis of A-T. Previously, we reported the increased cellular and chromosomal radiosensitivity of two cousins in one of these families.[30] Approximately 8 per cent of peripheral lymphocytes carried translocations including t(7;14)(p15;q32) and t(7;14)(q35;q11) seen in A-T patients. Chromosomal radiosensitivity in lymphocytes was increased to the level seen in classical A-T patients.[30] Haplotype data, however, indicated the presence of different haplotypes in the cousins in the region of the *ATM* gene consistent with the A-T in this family not being due to an *ATM* mutation.[30,31] In family 1, two brothers had clinical features of ataxia telangiectasia.[32] They also showed an increased level of chromosome translocations (1 per cent of cells with t(7;14)(q35;q11) and an increased chromosomal radiosensitivity intermediate between classical A-T and normal (indicated as patients 53, II-I and II-2 in).[33] Their parents were unrelated. We searched for *ATM* mutations in the affected individuals in both families but found none.[7] Consistent with the failure to detect mutations in *ATM*, normal ATM protein levels were present in all four patients from both families supporting the notion that perhaps mutation in another gene was responsible for this disorder. We have called this condition ATLD for ataxia telangiectasia-like disorder.

We were able to show that these individuals had mutations in the *MRE11* gene. Interestingly, MRE11 is a DNA double-strand break repair protein and part of the MRE11/RAD50/NBS1 protein complex acting in the same DNA damage-response pathway as ATM. In one family, we showed that two brothers were compound heterozygotes for mutations in the *MRE11* gene. DNA sequence analysis of ATLD3 and 4 *MRE11* cDNA revealed one missense mutation, 350 A > G, resulting in an N 117 S amino acid change, which was of paternal origin. The maternally derived mutation was 1714 C > T, 572 R > STOP.[31] In the second (consanguineous) family, two affected cousins (ATLD1 and 2) were homozygous for a 1897C > T change in *MRE11*, creating a truncated protein (R633X). Three of the four parents were shown to be heterozygous for the same mutation (the father of ATLD1 was deceased).

In ATLD1 and 2 there was total loss of full-length MRE11 protein expression, with truncated MRE11 being observed in these patients. In addition, there was a marked decrease in the levels of RAD50 and NBS1 in these cells. In the parents, MRE11 levels were reduced compared with normal cells. In the patients, ATLD3 and 4, reduced levels of MRE11, RAD50, and NBS1 were observed, but none of these proteins was present in a truncated form. Cells from the mother, but not the father of the boys, also showed reduced MRE11 levels. It appears that alteration in one member of a multiprotein complex can destabilize some or all of its protein components.

Attempts to create *mre11* and *rad50* knockout mice resulted in lethality,[35,36] which indicates that, unlike *ATM*, both of these genes are essential. It is, therefore, unlikely that individuals with two null alleles of *MRE11* or *RAD50* will be found in the human population. The mutations described in the present families result in mutant MRE11 protein with some residual function as shown by the fact that the truncated protein produced by ATLD1 and 2 and the full-length mutated protein expressed by ATLD3 and 4 is capable of complexing with both RAD50 and NBS1.

CLINICAL FEATURES OF A-T PATIENTS COMPARED WITH ATLD

A-T and ATLD patients cannot easily be distinguished at the clinical level. For example, patient ATLD1 was unsteady from the age of 3–4 years and her walking was ataxic. She was short for her age, had vertical nystagmus, slow saccadic eye movements, slight choreiform movements of the arms, intention tremors, absent ankle reflexes and flexor plantars. Dysarthria developing in the teenage years was present, but there was no cutaneous or ocular telangiectasia. Serum immunoglobulins and AFP levels were normal. There was no intellectual impairment. Her seven siblings and mother were normal (father is deceased). Her male cousin, ATLD2, presented at age 3–4 years with an ataxic gait and constant drooling. At age 20, he had progressive unsteadiness in walking, dysarthria, vertical nystagmus and loss of pursuit movements, choreiform movements of the hands and moderate peripheral ataxia. Again, there was no intellectual impairment. No cutaneous or ocular telangiectasia was present, and serum immunoglobulins and AFP levels were normal. The remaining sibling and parents were normal (see Hernandez *et al.*[30] for further details).

In the second such family, two of three sons (ATLD3 and ATLD4), born to non-consanguineous parents, developed choreic movements at about the age of 12 months. Both had additional mild dystonia at 4 years, which progressively became more marked. By the age of 13, they both had many of the features of A-T, including oculomotor apraxia with slow saccades and head thrusts, cerebellar dysarthria, gait and limb ataxia, mild lower limb spasticity and distal wasting. There was no evidence of telangiectasia in either brother. The older brother appeared to have more severe features (for further details see Klein *et al.*[32]). Their disorder was described as 'ataxia without telangiectasia masquerading as benign hereditary chorea' (see Klein *et al.*[32] for further details). None of these ATLD patients showed any evidence of immune deficiency or any cancer.

CLINICAL FEATURES OF A-T PATIENTS COMPARED WITH NIJMEGEN BREAKAGE SYNDROME PATIENTS

For some time, A-T was the only disorder in which increased radiosensitivity was a recognized part of the disorder. Subsequently, patients were described with the Nijmegen breakage syndrome (NBS),[37] who also show increased radiosensitivity.[38] These two disorders show similar features at the cellular level, based mainly on their increased sensitivity to ionizing radiation. This observation led to the suggestion that the genes causing the two disorders were likely to be involved in the same damage response pathway. Clinical overlap, however, between A-T and NBS is only partial. In most cases, it is not difficult to distinguish between classical A-T and NBS clinically. The similarities between A-T and NBS1 include an immuno-deficiency and an increased risk of lymphoid malignancies, although in NBS patients there is a predilection for B-cell tumours.[37] Patients with NBS show a microcephaly and frequently a borderline mental retardation, but do not develop cerebellar degeneration or telangiectasia. They also show chromosome translocations in peripheral lympho-cytes with breaks at the sites of the T-cell receptor genes.

A clear biochemical link between double-strand break (DSB) repair and mammalian cellular responses to DNA damage was revealed by the observation that the gene (*NBS1*) for NBS functions in a complex with the highly conserved DSB repair proteins MRE11 and RAD50.[39–41] The subsequent finding that *MRE11* mutations are associated with the clinical features of ataxia telangiectasia further links A-T to the NBS. More recent work has shown that *ATM* is linked more directly to this repair complex because the ATM protein phosphorylates NBS1 follow-ing exposure of cells to damage (see Lim *et al.*).[42]

Interestingly, a variant form of A-T called AT$_{FRESNO}$, combines a typical A-T phenotype with microcephaly and mental retardation,[9] two of the features associated with NBS. Cells from these patients had no ATM protein and were shown to be homozygous for an *ATM* mutation predicted to result in loss of protein expression.[10] The A-T component of this disorder, therefore, is caused by the homozygous *ATM* mutation, but the NBS-like fea-tures have some other unknown cause, either genetic or environmental.[10]

CELLULAR FEATURES OF ATLD PATIENTS COMPARED WITH A-T AND NBS

NBS, A-T and ATLD cells can be distinguished from each other by the levels of MRE11, RAD50, NBS1 and ATM pro-tein expression as well as by mutation analysis. Increased sensitivity to ionizing radi-ation as measured either chro-mosomally or by colony-forming assays is a feature of A-T, ATLD and NBS. Failure to suppress DNA synthesis upon treatment with ionizing radiation (radioresistant DNA synthesis; RDS) is a hallmark of cells from all three dis-orders. The suppression of DNA inhibition in fibroblasts from ATLD patients 2, 3 and 4 is somewhat less pro-nounced than in A-T cell strains. However, none of the ATLD cells suppressed DNA synthesis to the same level as the wild-type control. In this regard, ATLD 2, 3 and 4 resemble the RDS phenotype seen in NBS fibroblasts.[31] Two aspects of the A-T phenotype distinct from S-phase checkpoint defects are the failure of A-T cells to effect the

c-Abl-mediated induction of stress-activated protein kinases (SAPKs – c-Jun N-terminal kinases),[19] and the fail-ure of these cells to stabilize p53 in response to gamma-irradiation. We have examined ATLD cells for their ability to activate JNK following ionizing radiation (IR) treat-ment. Whereas JNK activity in normal cells was stimulated approximately sixfold by IR, this activity was essentially unaffected by IR treatment of A-T, ATLD and NBS cells.[31] In contrast, both the timing and the magnitude of the p53 response in ATLD2, 3 and 4 fell within the range defined by two control lymphoblastoid cell lines (LCLs). An NBS cell line was also tested and found to have a similarly normal p53 response. Hence, although the cellular phenotypes of ATLD and classical A-T are very similar, they can be distin-guished from one another on the basis of the p53 response as well as by the severity of the RDS phenotype.[31] The sta-bility of inter-actions of MRE11 with RAD50 and NBS1, as measured by co-immunoprecipitation procedures, in cells from ATLD patients, is compromised but not abolished by the ATLD mutations. As observed previously in NBS cells,[39] the subcellular distribution of the MRE11/RAD50/NBS1 protein complex, as measured by irradiation-induced focus formation (IRIF), is aberrant in ATLD cells, irrespective of prior gamma-irradiation. Whereas MRE11 and NBS1 immunoreactivity is exclusively nuclear in wild-type cells, MRE11 and NBS1 staining is much more diffuse in the ATLD cells. Thus, the IRIF response of ATLD cells express-ing both *MRE11* alleles is essentially lost.[31]

LABORATORY AIDS FOR THE DIAGNOSIS OF A-T

The increased radiosensitivity of cells and the increased level of translocation chromosomes remains the quickest way of initially confirming the diagnosis of A-T, NBS or ATLD. Differentiating between these disorders is fairly straightforward at the level of protein expression in LCLs derived from the patients, although, rarely, the presence of two missense mutations for *ATM* or *MRE11* may result in normal levels of protein expression. The final resort is to sequence for the mutations themselves, although there is no guarantee of detecting these in cDNA (e.g. if there is no transcript from one of the alleles) in which case genomic sequencing is required. A screen for MRE11 pro-tein levels or an *MRE11* mutation screen of *ATM* muta-tion-negative cases may reveal mutations in *MRE11*. Such individuals could also be screened for possible mutations in the *RAD50* locus, where hitherto no mutations have so far been described.

Bearing in mind the fact that different *bona fide* A-T patients can show one or more cellular variations from classical A-T including (1) no increased radiosensitivity, (2) almost normal levels of ATM protein, (3) no mutation in *ATM* (but in *MRE11* instead), and this can be accompanied clinically by, for example, (1) a much slower rate of cerebellar degeneration, (2) increased longevity, (3) fertility and (4) possible absence of predisposition to lymphoid tumours, the question must be asked what other clinical presentation might be expected. A note of caution is required concerning expectations of the phenotypes of patients with mutations in DNA damage response genes. It is curious that patients with an *MRE11* mutation have a clinical picture similar to A-T, rather than NBS (since the MRE11 protein is part of the RAD50/NBS1 complex). The clinical picture of a patient with an *RAD50* mutation may not be A-T like. Nor is it clear what the clinical picture might be of a patient with, say, two *ATM* missense mutations or two *MRE11* missense mutations. Are there patients with mutations in *RAD50* or *DNA-PK* or other genes involved in the DNA damage response? How do we confirm the presence of a defect in the absence of any other distinguishing cellular feature? DNA sequencing of a range of genes in such patients may be the only way to detect the gene defect.

MALIGNANT DISEASE IN A-T PATIENTS

Lymphoid tumours

An increased risk of developing malignant disease is an important feature of A-T. Indeed, approximately 10–15 per cent of all A-T patients develop a malignancy in childhood with the majority of these tumours being lymphoid in origin, including both B- and T-cell lymphoid tumours as well as Hodgkin's disease. Our limited number of observations suggest that A-T patients with T-cell tumours can be grouped into either an older or a younger category. Older patients with a mean age of about 33 years develop T cell prolymphocytic leukaemia (T-PLL). Two of the patients we studied with T-PLL showed proliferation of a t(X;14)(q28;q11) containing lymphocyte clone to 100 per cent of T cells, while a third patient showed a large inv(14)(q11q32) clone and a fourth patient showed a complex rearrangement of chromosome 14. In all cases the tumour arose from the clone following the appearance of additional chromosome translocations. There are several other examples in the literature showing the association between T-PLL and translocation clone proliferation in A-T patients in early adulthood.[5] In some patients with leukaemia of mature post-thymic lymphocytes, progress of the disease may be as rapid as in T cell acute lymphocytic leukaemia (T-ALL). Therefore, a pre-existing large clone in the peripheral blood lymphocytes of A-T patients is associated with a high risk of development of T-PLL.

Younger patients in our group tended to develop T-cell acute leukaemia or T-cell lymphoma. There are far fewer

observations on the chromosomal changes associated with these tumour types in A-T patients but inv(14) and t(4;14) translocations are seen. The *ATM* gene defect appears to allow either a higher level of formation of illegitimate chromosome translocations, involving recombination of T-cell receptor (TCR genes), in T lymphocytes compared with non A-T individuals or a lower rate of removal of these translocations. The wide range of translocations associated with T-ALL in non A-T patients presumably also occurs in A-T patients because of a likely defect in recombination in A-T cells. The presence of this variety of initial chromosome translocations explains the potential for the development of the several forms of T-cell tumour in a population of A-T patients. In some patients, a translocation that affects a gene at the top of the regulatory cascade will be associated with the development of T-ALL; in other patients, the translocation may activate a gene that allows a steady proliferation of lymphocytes in which further mutational events accumulate to give the eventual transformation to, say, T-PLL.

ATM mutations in A-T patients with leukaemia and lymphoma

In order to establish the relationship between the type and localization of *ATM* mutations and the risk of developing leukaemia or lymphoma, we have analysed *ATM* mutations in A-T patients who developed these tumours or exhibited pre-leukaemic features, such as T-cell clonal proliferation, and compared them with the mutations in A-T patients without tumours.

Mutations were scattered across the *ATM* gene, suggesting that a single position within the *ATM* coding sequence was unlikely to be associated with occurrence of leukaemia or lymphoma in A-T patients. Although one might expect that, within families, the development of different forms of T-cell tumour might occur at random, there are reports of concordance within families for the development of either T-PLL or T-ALL. While the number of families is small, this may be an indication of the effect of allele specificity and, therefore, heterogeneity. It might also indicate the importance of the presence of modifying genes in these families.

Breast cancer

Two families, 46 and 109, sharing the founder mutation 7271T > G, described in the previous section, both had a history of familial breast cancer.[8] In family 109, the carrier mother was 82 when she developed breast cancer, which may have been sporadic, but the two A-T daughters had breast cancers diagnosed at the ages of 44 and 50, and in both daughters it was bilateral. The remaining daughter is a carrier and as yet unaffected by breast cancer. Interestingly, two out of three of the sisters of the paternal carrier of the 7271T > G mutation in family 46 have also had breast cancer at ages 50 and 55, respectively. We have confirmed that one sister with breast cancer is a carrier but the second sister is deceased. The youngest sister without breast cancer is 50 years old.

One further A-T patient, 47-3 from a different family, with only one mutation identified, (7630del159) an in-frame deletion, also developed breast cancer. Cells from this patient also showed a high level of mutant ATM protein expression. In addition, a carrier of an *ATM* missense mutation, 5228C > T also developed a breast cancer at the age of 29 years, although this *ATM* allele expressed mutant ATM protein at a very low level in cells from her A-T son.

Other tumours

Other tumours seen in A-T patients at a higher frequency include various epithelial cell tumours and brain tumours.[3]

CANCER RISKS IN NBS AND ATLD PATIENTS

The importance of NBS1 and ATM in the maintenance of genomic stability is well established. Disruption of the MRE11/RAD50/NBS1 complex through mutations in the *NBS1* gene in patients with NBS also results in a high frequency of lymphoma in these individuals.[37] In 40 per cent of patients, cancer (mainly lymphoid) was confirmed before the age of 21 years. Although the role of inherited and acquired *MRE11* mutations in the development of tumours is currently unknown, disruption of the MRE11/ RAD50/NBS1 complex through mutations in the *MRE11* gene may also be associated with an increased risk of lymphoid tumour development. Clearly, disruption of the DNA damage response pathway in which these proteins function leads to decreased genome stability and strongly potentiates the malignant process.

CANCER RISKS OF *ATM* MUTATION CARRIERS

Although *ATM* mutations in A-T patients predispose to lymphoid tumours, the effect of the mutations may be numerically more important in the heterozygous state. Approximately 0.5–1 per cent of the population carry an *ATM* mutation and carriers have been reported to have an increased risk of breast cancer. In a prospective study, Swift *et al.*[11] estimated that women in A-T families, heterozygous for the *ATM* gene, were 5.5 (95 per cent confidence interval 1.5–16.9) times more likely to develop breast cancer than non-carriers of an *ATM* mutation. Other studies have reported an excess of breast cancer in

individuals in A-T families heterozygous for *ATM* mutations, but the numbers have been small. A meta-analysis of these studies to 1994[12] estimated a relative risk of breast cancer to A-T heterozygotes to be 3.9-fold. More recent studies have tended to confirm this small increased risk for carriers in A-T families.[43–45] There is also the possibility that the risk may be higher for certain mutations, including missense mutations expressing abnormal ATM protein. Therefore, involvement of *ATM* gene mutations in breast cancer may be very significant in particular families.

What is the contribution of *ATM* mutations to breast cancer overall? FitzGerald *et al.*[46] showed that germline *ATM* mutations were found to be present in only 2 out of 401 women with early onset of breast cancer compared with 2 out of 202 controls. They concluded that heterozygous mutations do not confer genetic predisposition to early-onset beast cancer. This study, however, would still be consistent with a moderate risk of breast cancer because the confidence interval in this study is large.[47] In addition, the authors used a method that will only detect truncated ATM protein. These results contrast with those in A-T families. Broeks *et al.*,[48] screening a selected group of Dutch patients with breast cancer, reported that *ATM* heterozygotes in this population had an approximately ninefold increased risk of developing breast cancer. The contribution of *ATM* mutations to breast cancer incidence remains the subject of further investigation.

ATM mutations have a role in the development of some sporadic tumours. *ATM* mutations have been described in sporadic T-cell prolymphocytic leukaemia,[49–51] B-cell chronic lymphocytic leukaemia[51–54] and mantle cell lymphoma.[55]

DISCUSSION

The majority of patients have classical A-T resulting from homozygosity or compound heterozygosity for *ATM* null alleles. Approximately, 70 per cent of all *ATM* mutations are predicted to lead to truncation of the ATM protein. Loss of all ATM function would be expected to result in homogeneity in clinical features in such patients, irrespective of the individual mutations present. Loss of all ATM function is not a lethal event in man or in the knockout mouse model. However, some crosses with the *Atm* knockout mouse result in lethality, indicating that other genes can carry out some functions of ATM. If this is the case, then some subtle heterogeneity may be expected within the group of classical A-T patients as a result of the modifying effect of other genes. A possible example of this is the observation of concordance for the tumour type in some families. For example, both affected siblings from family 10, compound heterozygous for the truncating mutations 2639del200 and 8206de1AA, developed acute T-cell leukaemia at a similar age. In addition, both affected siblings from the family 39, compound heterozygous for the mutations 136del4 and 7636de19, developed T-cell lymphoma at a similar age.[8] Since the allelic complexity among A-T patients is very large in comparison to that of NBS and ATLD, it is also a reasonable hypothesis that some differences in the clinical and cellular phenotypes observed are allele-specific.

An important conclusion is that there is clearly variation in the clinical and cellular features shown by a group of *bona fide* A-T patients with *ATM* mutations. This is seen particularly in terms of the severity of the cerebellar features, the level of immunodeficiency, longevity, and also the age of onset and type of leukaemia or lymphoma these patients develop. This can result from expression of a small amount of normal ATM protein or a larger amount of mutant protein. Up to 29 per cent of *ATM* mutations in some populations[8] may be in-frame deletions and point mutations predicted to allow expression of some protein and, in some cases, this can lead to some milder features of A-T. Some mutations were recurrent as they occur in different haplotypes. In addition, the same mutations have also been reported in the literature in quite different populations.

Although it is possible that all expressed mutant proteins are null functionally and, in terms of risk of tumour occurrence, there is no difference between patients expressing these proteins and patients with no protein at all, evidence from families with the 7271T > C mutation suggests that this is not correct and some residual normal catalytic function can remain in mutated ATM protein to confer the less severe clinical phenotype. This mutation is localized several hundred basepairs upstream to the catalytic PI3-kinase domain and, although important functions of ATM may reside in this kinase domain,[56] the 7271T > G mutation seems to cause a sufficient alteration to the ATM protein to produce a mild A-T phenotype. This would imply that the resulting amino acid exchange is within a region that is crucial for some functions of the ATM protein.

Even when families have in common the presence of the same mutation and expression of the same mutant protein, as in the case of the 7271T > G missense mutation, there may be variation of the clinical and cellular phenotype. Affected individuals from two UK families with 7271T > G mutation showed a milder A-T phenotype than is seen in classical A-T patients, but individuals in family 109 homozygous for the 7271T > G *ATM* mutation showed the milder phenotype of the two, including fertility.

In addition, mutation in a second gene, *MRE11*, can give the features of ataxia telangiectasia apart from the presence of telangiectasia. This ataxia telangiectasia-like disorder is difficult to distinguish clinically from A-T and will account for only a small proportion of A-T patients. The fact that mutation of *MRE11*, a second member of the MRE11/RAD50/NBS1 protein complex, leads to both the clinical and cellular phenotypes of A-T, provides compelling evidence that this complex acts in the same pathway as the *ATM* gene. The data demonstrate that ATM and members of the MRE11/RAD50/NBS1 protein complex are not functionally redundant.

The link between defects in the cellular DNA damage response and the progressive neurodegeneration in A-T is presently unclear. The progressive neuronal degeneration in A-T and ATLD patients, as well as the severe neuro-developmental abnormalities in NBS patients have not been specifically associated with genomic instability. It is not known what component of the cellular response to damage (defective DNA repair, or other responses, such as defective induction of p53 leading to cell-cycle arrest or apoptosis) are important in causing the neuronal degeneration. Interestingly, mice deficient in DNA ligase IV and its cofactor, Xrcc4, exhibit defects in neuronal development.[57,58] In contrast to the gene mutations in A-T, ATLD and NBS, *DNA ligase IV* and *Xrcc4* gene mutations result only in gross DNA repair deficiency, apparently without perturbing cell-cycle checkpoint functions, which are observed in A-T cells. This suggests that some deficient DNA repair functions might be important in contributing to the neuronal degeneration seen in A-T and ATLD. Finally, it is not clear whether the neurological features of A-T are solely a consequence of a neuronal degeneration. They may also be, in part, the consequence of an ATM-dependent developmental abnormality. Some evidence for this may be the presence of ectopic Purkinje cells in the cerebellum.[4]

Much has been learned in recent years about the clinical, cellular and genetic heterogeneity of ataxia telangiectasia. The role of ATM function and its interactions with other protein complexes, particularly with respect to DNA damage responses, has also received much attention. Some features of A-T, most importantly, the basis of the neurodegeneration, are still poorly understood and, at present, little can be offered by way of helping patients. Understanding the basis of the neurodegeneration and being able to offer some treatment to control its progressive nature is a goal for the immediate future.

ELECTRONIC DATABASE INFORMATION

- Ataxia-Telangiectasia Society UK: http://www.atsociety.org.uk/
- The A-T Appeal: http://www.atsociety.org.uk/
- A-T Childrens project (USA): http://www.atcp.org/
- Ataxia telangiectasia mutation database: http://www.vmresearch.org/atm.htm
- Online Mendelian Inheritance in Man (OMIM): http://www3.ncbi.nlm.nih.gov/omim/

KEY POINTS

- Classical Ataxia Telangiectasia (A-T) is an autosomal recessive disorder characterized by cerebellar ataxia, oculocutaneous telangiectasia, susceptibility to sinopulmonary infections and neoplasia. They are radiation sensitive.
- Heterozygous mutation carriers are now thought to have an increased cancer risk, especially breast cancer in women. There is no definite evidence that they are radiation sensitive.
- A-T is due to mutations in the *ATM* gene on 11q, a few families are due to mutations in another DNA repair gene, *MRE11*.

REFERENCES

1. Swift M, Morell D, Cromartie E, *et al.* The incidence and gene frequency of ataxia telangiectasia in the United States. *Am J Hum Genet* 1986; **39:**573–583.
2. Woods CG, Bundey SE, Taylor AMR. Unusual features in the inheritance of ataxia telangiectasia. *Hum Genet* 1990; **84:**555–562.
3. Spector BD, Filipovich AM, Perry GS, Kersey KS. Epidemiology of cancer in ataxia-telangiectasia In: Bridges BA, Harnden DG (eds) *Ataxia-telangiectasia – a cellular and molecular link between cancer, neuropathology and immune deficiency.* Chichester: John Wiley, 1982:103–138.
4. Sedgwick RP, Boder E. Ataxia telangiectasia. In: de Jong JMBV (ed.) *Handbook of clinical neurology. hereditary neuropathies and spinocerebellar atrophies,* Vol 16. Amsterdam: Elsevier Science Publishers BV, 1991:347–423.
5. Taylor AMR, Metcalfe JA, Thick J, Mak Y-F. Leukaemia and lymphoma in ataxia telangiectasia. *Blood* 1996; **87:**423–438.
6. Ying KL, DeCoteau WE. Cytogenetic anomalies in a patient with ataxia, immune deficiency and high alpha-fetoprotein in the absence of telangiectasia. *Cancer Genet Cytogenet* 1981; **4:**311–317.
7. McConville CM, Stankovic T, Byrd PJ, *et al.* Mutations associated with variant phenotypes in ataxia telangiectasia. *Am J Hum Genet* 1996; **59:**320–330.
8. Stankovic T, Kidd AMJ, Sutcliffe A, *et al. ATM* mutations and phenotypes in ataxia telangiectasia families in the British Isles: Expression of mutant *ATM* and the risk of leukaemia, lymphoma and breast cancer. *Am J Hum Genet* 1998; **62:**334–345.
9. Curry CJ, O'Lague P, Tsai J, *et al.* ATFresno: a phenotype linking ataxia-telangiectasia with the Nijmegen breakage syndrome. *Am J Hum Genet* 1989; **45:**270–275.
10. Gilad S, Chessa L, Khosravi R, *et al.* Genotype–phenotype relationships in ataxia-telangiectasia and variants. *Am J Hum Genet* 1998; **62:**551–561.
11. Swift M, Morell D, Massey RB, Chase CL. Incidence of cancer in 161 families affected by ataxia-telangiectasia. *N Engl J Med* 1991; **325:**1831–1836.
12. Easton DF. Cancer risk in A-T heterozygotes. *Int J Radiat Biol* 1994; **66:**S177–S182.
13. Byrd PJ, Cooper P, Stankovic T, *et al.* A gene transcribed from the bidirectional ATM promoter coding for a serine rich protein: amino acid sequence, structure and expression. *Hum Mol Genet* 1996; **5:**1785–1791.
14. Savitsky K, Bar-Shira A, Gilad S, *et al.* A single ataxia telangiectasia gene with a product similar to PI-3 kinase. *Science* 1995; **268:**1749–1753.
15. Savitsky K, Sfez S, Tagle DA, *et al.* The complete sequence of the coding region of the *ATM* gene reveals similarity to cell cycle regulators in different species. *Hum Mol Genet* 1995; **4:**2025–2032.
16. Lakin ND, Weber P, Stankovic T, *et al.* Analysis of the ATM protein in wild type and ataxia telangiectasia cells. *Oncogene* 1996; **13:**2707–2716.
17. Watters D, Khanna KK, Beamish H, *et al.* Cellular localisation of the ataxia-telangiectasia (ATM) gene product and discrimination between mutated and normal forms. *Oncogene* 1997; **14:**1911–1921.
18. Shiloh Y. Ataxia-telangiectasia and the Nijmegen breakage syndrome: related disorders but genes apart. *Ann Rev Genet* 1997; **31:**635–662.
19. Shafman TD, Saleem A, Kyriakis J, *et al.* Defective induction of stress-activated protein kinase activity in ataxia telangiectasia cells exposed to ionizing radiation. *Cancer Res* 1995; **55:**3242–3245.
20. Barlow C, Brown KD, Deng C-X, *et al.* Atm selectively regulates distinct p53-dependent cell cycle checkpoint and apoptotic pathways. *Nature Genet* 1997; **17:**453–456.
21. Chong MJ, Murray MR, Gosink EC, *et al.* Atm and Bax cooperate in ionizing radiation-induced apoptosis in the central nervous system. *Proc Natl Acad Sci USA* 2000; **97:**889–894.
22. Banin S, Moyal L, Shieh S-Y, *et al.* Enhanced phosphorylation of p53 by ATM in response to DNA damage. *Science* 1998; **281:**1674–1677.
23. Canman CE, Lim D-S, Cimprich KA, *et al.* Activation of the ATM kinase by ionizing radiation and phosphorylation of p53. *Science* 1998; **281:**1677–1679.
24. Chehab NH, Malikzay A, Appel M, Halazonetis TD. *Chk2/Cds1* functions as a DNA damage checkpoint in G(1) by stabilizing p53. *Genes Dev* 2000; **14:**278–288.
25. Kim S-T, Lim D-S, Canman CE, Kastan MB. Substrate specificities and identification of putative substrates of ATM kinase family members. *J Biol Chem* 1999; **274:** 37538–37543.
26. Wang Y, Cortez D, Yazdi P, *et al.* BASC, a super complex of BRCA1-associated proteins involved in the recognition and repair of aberrant DNA structures. *Genes Dev* 2000; **14:**927–939.
27. Herzog KH, Chong MJ, Kapsetaki M, *et al.* Requirement for Atm in ionizing radiation-induced cell death in the developing central nervous system. *Science* 1998; **280:**1089–1091.
28. Taylor AMR, McConville CM, Rotman G, *et al.* A haplotype common to intermediate radiosensitivity variants of ataxia telangiectasia in the UK. *Int J Radiat Biol* 1994; **66:**S35–S41.
29. Stewart GS, Last JI, Stankovic T, *et al.* Residual ataxia telangiectasia mutated protein function in cells from ataxia telangiectasia patients, with 5762ins137 and 7271T->G mutations, showing a less severe phenotype. *J Biol Chem.* 2001; **276:**30133–30144.

30. Hernandez D, McConville CM, Stacey M, *et al.* A family showing no evidence of linkage between the ataxia telangiectasia gene and chromosome 11q22–23. *J Med Genet* 1993; **30:**135–140.

31. Stewart GS, Maser RS, Stankovic T, *et al.* The DNA double-strand break repair gene *MRE11* is mutated in individuals with an ataxia-telangiectasia-like disorder. *Cell* 1999; **99:**577–587.

32. Klein C, Wenning GK, Quinn NP, Marsden CD. Ataxia without telangiectasia masquerading as benign hereditary chorea. *Mov Disord* 1996; **11:**217–220.

33. Taylor AMR, Hernandez D, McConville CM, *et al.* Malignant disease and variations in radiosensitivity in ataxia telangiectasia patients In: Eeles RA, Ponder BAJ, Easton DF, Horwich D (eds) *Genetic predisposition to cancer.* London: Chapman and Hall, 1996:138–151.

34. Pitts SA, Kullar HS, Stankovic T, *et al.* hMRE11: genomic structure and a null mutation identified in a transcript protected from nonsense-mediated mRNA decay. *Hum Mol Genet.* 2001; **10:**1155–1162.

35. Xiao Y, Weaver DT. Conditional gene targeted deletion by Cre recombinase demonstrates the requirement for the double-strand break repair MRE11 protein in murine embryonic stem cells. *Nucl Acids Res* 1997; **25:**2985–2991.

36. Luo G, Yao MS, Bender CF, *et al.* Disruption of mRAD50 causes embryonic stem cell lethality, abnormal embryonic development, and sensitivity to ionising radiation. *Proc Natl Acad Sci USA* 1999; **96:**7376–7381.

37. Hiel JA, Weemaes CM, van Engelen BG, *et al.* The International Nijmegen Breakage Syndrome Study Group. Nijmegen Breakage Syndrome. *Arch Dis Child* 2000; **82:**400–406.

38. Taalmann RDFM, Jaspers NGJ, Scheres JMJC, *et al.* Hypersensitivity, in vitro, to ionizing radiation in a new chromosomal instability syndrome, the Nijmegen Breakage Syndrome. *Mutation Res* 1983; **112:**23–32.

39. Carney JP, Maser RS, Olivares H, *et al.* The MRE11/RAD50 protein complex and Nijmegen Breakage Syndrome; linkage of double-strand-break repair to the cellular DNA damage response. *Cell* 1998; **93:**477–486.

40. Varon R, Vissinga C, Platzer M, *et al.* Nibrin, a novel DNA double-strand break repair protein, is mutated in Nijmegen breakage syndrome. *Cell* 1998; **93:**467–476.

41. Matsuura S, Tauchi H, Nakamura A, *et al.* Positional cloning of the gene for Nijmegen breakage syndrome. *Nature Genet* 1998; **19:**179–181.

42. Lim DS, Kim ST, Xu B, *et al.* ATM phosphorylates p95/nbs1 in an S-phase checkpoint pathway. *Nature* 2000; **404:**613–617.

43. Athma P, Rappaport R, Swift M. Molecular genotyping shows that ataxia telangiectasia heterozygotes are predisposed to breast cancer. *Cancer Genet Cytogenet* 1996; **42:**130–134.

44. Janin N, Andrieu N, Ossian K, *et al.* Breast cancer risk in ataxia telangiectasia (AT) heterozygotes: haplotype study in French AT families. *Br J Cancer* 1999; **80:**1042–1045.

45. Inskip HM, Kinlen LJ, Taylor AM, *et al.* Risk of breast cancer and other cancers in heterozygotes for ataxia-telangiectasia. *Br J Cancer* 1999; **79:**1304–1307.

46. FitzGerald MG, Bean JM, Hegde SR, *et al.* Heterozygous ATM mutations do not contribute to early onset of breast cancer. *Nature Genet* 1997; **15:**307–310.

47. Bishop DT, Hopper J. AT-tributable risks? *Nature Genet* 1997; **15:**276.

48. Broeks A, Urbanus JH, Floore AN, *et al.* ATM-heterozygous germline mutations contribute to breast cancer-susceptibility. *Am J Hum Genet* 2000; **66:**494–500.

49. Vorechovsky I, Luo L, Dyer MJ, *et al.* Clustering of missense mutations in the ataxia-telangiectasia gene in a sporadic T-cell leukaemia. *Nature Genet* 1997; **17:**96–99.

50. Stilgenbauer S, Schaffner C, Litterst A, *et al.* Biallelic mutations in the ATM gene in T-prolymphocytic leukemia. *Nat Med* 1997; **3:**1155–1159.

51. Stoppa-Lyonnet D, Soulier J, Lauge A, *et al.* Inactivation of the ATM gene in T-cell prolymphocytic leukemias. *Blood* 1998; **91:**3920–3926.

52. Stankovic T, Weber P, Stewart G, *et al.* Inactivation of ataxia telangiectasia mutated gene in B-cell chronic lymphocytic leukaemia. *Lancet* 1999; **353:**26–29.

53. Bullrich F, Rasio D, Kitada S, *et al.* ATM mutations in B-cell chronic lymphocytic leukemia. *Cancer Res* 1999; **59:**24–27.

54. Schaffner C, Stilgenbauer S, Rappold GA, Dohner H, Lichter P. Somatic ATM mutations indicate a pathogenic role of ATM in B-cell chronic lymphocytic leukemia. *Blood* 1999; **94:**748–753.

55. Schaffner C, Idler I, Stilgenbauer S, *et al.* Mantle cell lymphoma is characterized by inactivation of the ATM gene. *Proc Natl Acad Sci USA* 2000; **97:**2773–2778.

56. Morgan SE, Lovly C, Pandita TK, *et al.* Fragments of ATM which have dominant-negative or complementing activity. *Mol Cell Biol* 1997; **17:**2020–2029.

57. Barnes DE, Stamp G, Rosewell I, *et al.* Targeted disruption of the gene encoding DNA ligase IV leads to lethality in embryonic mice. *Curr Biol* 1998; **8:**1395–1398.

58. Gao Y, Sun Y, Frank KM, *et al.* A critical role for DNA end-joining proteins in both lymphogenesis and neurogenesis. *Cell* 1998; **95:**891–902.

14

Fanconi anaemia

PIA A.J. HUBER AND CHRISTOPHER G. MATHEW

THE FANCONI ANAEMIA SYNDROME

Fanconi anaemia (FA) is an autosomal recessive inherited disorder characterized by progressive aplastic anaemia, multiple congenital abnormalities and predisposition to malignancies, including leukaemia and solid tumours.[1–5] The developmental abnormalities include radial aplasia, hyperpigmentation of the skin, growth retardation, micropthalmia and malformation of the kidneys (Table 14.1).[6,7] The disorder generally presents as aplastic anaemia between the ages of 5 and 10 years, but the diagnosis may be made much earlier if characteristic developmental abnormalities are present, or if there is a family history. However, the diagnosis may also be made much later, some cases having presented as young adults with acute myeloid leukaemia (AML).[8] The variability in the clinical phenotype of FA is independent of geographical and racial background, and is evident even among siblings with consanguineous parents.[3,9] This suggests that embryonic development can be affected at different stages, without precise targeting of a particular organ system.[10–12] FA is a rare disease with an incidence of 1 in 200 000–400 000 live births,[10,13] and the heterozygote frequency is estimated to be 1 in 200. However, it is more common in some populations, with carrier frequencies of about 1 in 90 reported in South African Afrikaners and Ashkenazi Jews.[14,15] The disorder is genetically heterogeneous, with eight complementation groups (A, B, C, D1, D2, E, F and G) having been described (see later section on genetic heterogeneity).

Diagnosis

During a period of almost 40 years from the first case report in 1927,[16] FA was diagnosed by the concurrence of aplastic anaemia with physical abnormalities (see details in Table 14.1). In 1964, increased chromosomal breakage was observed in lymphoblasts and fibroblasts derived from FA patients,[17,18] and later it was discovered that cells

Table 14.1 *Physical abnormalities in Fanconi anaemia*[6,7]

Physical abnormalities	Occurrence (%)
Skin abnormalities (pigmentation, café au lait spots)	73
Short stature	60
Upper limb defects (radial ray, i.e. thumb abnormalities)	48
Urogenital defects (hypogonadism)	12 (male 40%, female 3%)
Head abnormalities (including eyes, microcephaly)	56
Renal abnormalities	23
Lower limb abnormalities	17
Deafness	10
Gastrointestinal abnormalities	8
Cardiopulmonary defects	8
Neurological (hyper-reflexivity, mental retardation, central nervous system)	15
Short stature and/or skin only	8
None	6

from FA patients were hypersensitive to DNA interstrand cross-linking agents (ICLs).[19–22] This discovery provided the basis for sensitive and specific laboratory tests for FA, using DNA ICLs, such as diepoxybutane (DEB) and mitomycin C (MMC), to induce chromosome breakage.[23,24] In view of the highly variable clinical presentation of FA, this test, in conjunction with the assessment of haematological and physical abnormalities and family history, is important in confirming the diagnosis of FA. Assessment of the chromosome breakage test result may be complicated by the presence of two cell populations, one sensitive and one resistant to the cross-linker. At least some of these cases arise as a result of somatic mosaicism (see later section on genotype/phenotype correlations). The cloning of seven genes mutated in FA has recently led to the development of two additional diagnostic procedures. One of these takes advantage of the observation that the FANCD2 protein is monoubiquitinated in normal but not in FA cells. Primary lymphocytes are analysed for FANCD2 monoubiquination by immunoblotting. The absence of the monoubiquitinated FANCD2 isoform has been found to correlate with the diagnosis of FA by DEB testing.[25] Subtyping of the complementation groups can now be achieved by transfection of retroviral vectors containing the cDNA of the various FA genes into primary T cells from FA patients, which are then tested for correction of ICL hypersensitivity.[26]

Clinical management

The primary manifestation of the disease, aplastic anaemia, is treated with androgens (oxymetholone with prednisone) to stimulate blood cell production. Androgen therapy can reverse the pancytopenia for a period of several years.[27] At present, the anaemia can only be cured by stem cell transplantation from cord blood or bone marrow, with unrelated transplants having a lower success rate.[28] General transplant preconditioning protocols with clastogenic agents, such as cyclophosphamide, are highly toxic in FA patients. This has led to the development of special preconditioning regimens, with greatly improved survival rates.[20,29–33] Because of a lack of suitable donors, haematological complications result in the death of 81 per cent of FA patients before the age of 40. Other causes of death include infections and solid tumours. In the longer term, gene therapy may become possible, since haematopoietic stem cells are accessible for gene transduction, and corrected cells would be expected to have a growth advantage over uncorrected cells. One pilot clinical trial of three FA patients has been reported,[34] in which bone marrow enriched for stem cells was transfected with the FA complementation group C gene inserted into a retrovirus. Only transient improvement in bone marrow cellularity was observed in the three patients. Promising longer term results were achieved in knockout mice using lentiviral vectors.[35,36]

CANCER IN FANCONI ANAEMIA

Homozygotes

It has long been known that FA patients are at high risk of developing leukaemia. In a study of 700 cases, leukaemia (mainly AML) or myelodysplastic syndrome (MDS) was observed in about 10 per cent of subjects, with a mean age at diagnosis of 14.8 years and a mean age at death in these patients of 15.5 years.[37] Variable chromosomal abnormalities were detected in these cases, most commonly monosomy 7, and translocations or duplications of chromosome 1q. Another study indicated a 52 per cent combined risk of developing AML or MDS by the age of 40 years.[38] In a recent literature survey of 1301 FA cases, hepatocellular carcinoma was reported in 2.8 per cent of affected individuals,[4] which may reflect the combination of a premalignant condition and long-term androgen therapy. The same study found solid tumours, most frequently of the head and neck, oesophagus, vulva and uterine cervix, in 5.3 per cent of affected individuals (Table 14.2). A study of malignancy after stem cell transplantation estimated that FA patients had a 42 per cent risk of developing any malignancy by 20 years after transplant.[39] In summary, FA is associated with a high risk of haematological malignancy in older children and young adults, and a high risk of an unusual spectrum of solid tumours in long-term survivors of the haematological complications.

Heterozygotes

The possibility that FA heterozygotes might be at increased risk of cancer was first suggested by Swift et al.,[40] but this was not confirmed in a later study by the same author.[41]

Table 14.2 *Malignancies in Fanconi anaemia*[4]

Type of malignancy	Incidence (%)[a]	Cumulative incidence (%)[b]
Leukaemia	8.9	37 (by age 29)
MDS	6.8	50 (by age 45)
Head and neck	2.9	
Oesophagus	0.7	
Vulva/anus	0.8	
Cervix	0.2	
Brain	0.5	
Liver (possibly iatrogenic)	2.8	46 (by age 50)
All solid tumours	5.2	76 (by age 45)

MDS = myelodysplastic syndrome.
[a] Incidence in 1301 cases of Fanconi anaemia reported in the literature 1927–2001.[4]
[b] Cumulative probability of developing the cancer in the absence of competing risks.[4]

The number of families included in these studies was relatively small and would thus be unlikely to have sufficient power to detect a modest effect. The issue could be resolved by larger studies and a study design that involved molecular testing for carrier status in relatives with a diagnosis of cancer. This is feasible now that the genes for the major FA complementation groups have been identified (see later section on gene cloning). The recent finding that FANCD1 is identical to BRCA2 raises the possibility that heterozygotes from the FA-D1 complementation group may have an increased risk of breast cancer, but this group accounts for less than 1 per cent of all FA families (Table 14.3).

GENETICS OF FANCONI ANAEMIA

Genetic heterogeneity

Fusion of cell lines from different FA patients, followed by analysis of heterokaryons for MMC sensitivity, suggested the existence of multiple complementation groups in FA gene defects. The number of complementation groups rose to 8,[42–44] which were designated FA-A to FA-H. Although FA-H has been reclassified as FA-A,[45] there are still at least eight complementation groups owing to an additional reclassification of FA-D, which was found to consist of two complementation groups, FA-D1 and FA-D2.[46] The proportion of FA patients belonging to a particular complementation group is variable (see Table 14.3), with FA-A accounting for about two-thirds of cases worldwide.[47] The proportion of FA patients belonging to a particular complementation group also varies in different populations: almost all Ashkenazi Jewish patients, for instance, belong to FA-C (see later). Unlike the situation in ataxia telangiectasia, where most complementation groups have been shown to result from mutations in the same gene (Chapter 13), at least seven of the FA groups are associated with mutations in different genes (see following section).

Gene cloning

The genes for FA groups A–G are now denoted FANCA–FANCG, superseding the older nomenclature (e.g. FAA, FAC, etc.). FANCC was the first gene to be isolated.[48] An Epstein–Barr virus-based cDNA expression library, which was derived from lymphoblasts treated with DNA cross-linkers, was used for transfection of a FA-C cell line. Transfected cDNAs were recovered from MMC- and DEB-resistant cells, and the identity of the gene confirmed by detection of mutations in several FA-C patients. This elegant approach was subsequently applied successfully to the cloning of the FANCA, FANCG, FANCF and FANCE genes.[47,49–51] The more traditional approach of linkage mapping and positional cloning also proved useful in the initial mapping of the FANCA and FANCE genes,[52,53] and the cloning of the FANCA gene.[54] The FANCD2 gene was cloned by a combination of functional complementation and positional cloning,[46,55,56] and FANCD1 has been found to be identical with BRCA2 by mutation screening of BRCA2 as a candidate gene.[57] Of the existing complementation groups, therefore, only the location and identity of FANCB is unknown. The chromosomal locations and genomic structures of the known FA genes are summarized in Table 14.3. None of these genes is homologous to any of the others, and, with the exception of FANCD2, show limited evolutionary conservation in vertebrates (Table 14.3).

Gene inactivation studies in mice

Inactivation of the Fancc gene in mice is characterized by chromosomal instability and reduced fertility, but no haematological or congenital abnormalities have been observed.[58,59] Fanca knockout mice showed hypogonadism and impaired fertility, and embryonic fibroblasts exhibited spontaneous chromosomal instability and were hyper-responsive to the clastogenic effect of the cross-linker MMC.[60] Reduced fertility and hypersensitivity to MMC were also characteristics of Fancg/Xrcc9 null mice, but no haematopoietic failure was found.[61,62] Overall, Fancg(−/−) mice closely resembled those reported for Fancc and Fanca as well as Fancc/Fanca double null mice,[63] supporting a tight interdependence of the corresponding gene products in a common pathway.

FA gene mutations

The mutation spectra of the FA genes have proved to be highly heterogeneous. In the FANCC gene, most mutations are frameshifts or stop codons, which lead to premature truncation of translation.[48,64–67] However, two missense mutations (L554P and L496R) have been shown to abrogate the function of the FANCC protein.[68,69] The most important mutation, in molecular diagnostic terms, is IVS4 + 4A > T,[64] which accounts for almost all cases of FA in Ashkenazi Jews, and has a carrier frequency of about 1 in 90 in that population.[14,70] The mutation spectrum in FANCA is extremely varied,[71–73] and includes a high proportion of large intragenic deletions, which remove from 1 to 43 exons from the gene.[72,74] Most FANCA mutations are predicted to be null mutations, resulting in total absence of the FANCA protein, but some missense mutations, such as H1110P, are clearly pathogenic.[75] FANCG mutations are also mostly null mutations and include several splice site mutations.[76] The few mutations described for FANCE and FANCF are also predicted to result in total absence of their protein products.[50,51]

Table 14.3 *Gene/protein properties*

	FANCA	FANCB	FANCC	FANCD1/BRCA2	FANCD2	FANCE	FANCF	FANCG/XRCC9
Prevalence (of complementation group)[71]	70%	>1%	14%	>1%	>1%	2%	2.5%	10%
Chromosomal location	16q24.3	n.k.	9q22.3	13q12–q13	3p25.3	6p21.3	11p15	9p13
Exons (gene size)	43 (80 kb)	n.k.	14 (>150 kb)	27	44	10 (15 kb genomic)	1	14 (72 kb)
Amino acids	1455	n.k.	558	3418	1471	536	374	622
Molecular weight (kDa)	162.8	n.k.	63.3	384.3	~166.5	58.7	42.3	68.5
Predicted pI	6.6	n.k.	6.1	6.3	5.8	5.2	9.2	5.4
Leucine content (average: 7.4 mol%)	Leu 14.6%	n.k.	Leu 14.9%	Leu 16.8%	Leu 13.7 %	Leu 19.2%	Leu 16.8%	Leu 19.5%
Putative motifs/special features	NLS Leucine zipper Region similar to haemperoxidase[84]	n.k.	8 conserved cysteines Exon 8 similar to MEC1 (=yeast checkpoint gene)[83]	NLS Coiled-coil region BRC motif[144]	NLS	NLS Interferon α,β,δ family region	Region with ROM similarity[50]	Leucine zipper Region similar to MCM family
Evolutionary conservation[a] (farthest removed from human with significant conservation)	Fish (*Tetraodon nigroviridis*)[145] *D. melanogaster*	n.k.	Fish (*Takifugu rubripes*)[145]	*A. thaliana* Pufferfish Mosquito Trypanosome	*A. thaliana* *C. elegans* *D. melanogaster*	Fish[145] (*Tetraodon nigroviridis*) *D. melanogaster* *C. elegans*	Fish[145] (*Tetraodon nigroviridis*) *C. elegans*	Fish (*Danio rerio*)[145]

[a] Evolutionary information also from http://www.ncbi.nlm.nih.gov/UniGene/

FANCD2 mutations include a nucleotide insertion predicting a severely truncated protein and a splice site mutation.[46] A splice site mutation and nucleotide insertions were also identified within *FANCD1* (*BRCA2*).[57]

Genotype–phenotype correlations

One possible explanation for the variable clinical phenotype in FA is that different complementation groups or specific mutations are associated with different clinical outcomes. Initial studies of FA-C patients found that individuals with the IVS4 + 4A > T mutation in *FANCC* had a more severe phenotype than those with the 322delG mutation.[77,78] Our European collaborative group, EUFAR, studied 245 FA patients from all seven complementation groups, and found more severe cytopaenia and a higher incidence of AML or MDS in FA-G, and a lower prevalence of somatic abnormalities in FA-C.[7] Also, FA-A patients who were homozygous for null mutations had an earlier onset of anaemia and a higher incidence of leukaemia than those with mutations producing an altered protein. The extent of the aberrations in the FA pathway was found to be related to the nature of the mutation in a study where *FANCA*-deficient fibroblasts were transfected with 21 different *FANCA* mutants.[79] Some mutants showed an apparently normal reconstitution of the FA pathway, while others showed various defects in functions so far identified. These mutation-dependent defects may account for the phenotypic variation seen in FA patients. A possible contribution of modifier genes or environmental factors to the clinical phenotype has been proposed by Futaki *et al.*,[80] who found that Japanese FA patients with the IVS4 + 4A > T mutation in *FANCC* had a much less severe phenotype than Ashkenazi Jewish patients with the same mutation.

Somatic mosaicism

Recently, a molecular explanation has been found for the observation that a substantial minority of FA patients have two cell populations, one that is hypersensitive and one with a normal response to DNA cross-linking agents. In several patients who were compound heterozygotes for mutations in *FANCC*, intragenic recombination or gene conversion has occurred, which has restored wild-type sequence to one allele.[73] Remarkably, several patients who were homozygous for mutations in *FANCA* or *FANCC* had acquired a compensatory secondary mutation in *cis*, which restored the function of the mutant allele.[68] For example, the frameshift mutation 1615delG in *FANCA* was compensated for by two additional single base deletions, 1637delA and 1641delT. Although the predicted proteins were slightly different from wild type, they were still capable of correcting the MMC hypersensitivity in a functional assay. Lymphoblastoid cell lines derived from such patients are generally MMC resistant, since reverted cells are preferentially immortalized.[81]

FANCONI ANAEMIA PROTEINS

Properties

Some properties of the FA proteins are summarized in Table 14.3. The proteins range in size from 42 kDa (FANCF) to 384 kDa (FANCD1 = BRCA2). An unusual feature of their primary structure is a very high content of leucine residues, of between 13.7 and 19.5 per cent, compared to an average of 7.4 per cent in all proteins.[82] There are no striking homologies between the FA proteins and any other known protein, but some regions with similarities have been found. A region (exon 8) in FANCC with high conservation through four species is similar to the yeast checkpoint gene MEC1.[83] FANCA contains a peroxidase domain.[84] There are small regions of similarity between FANCE and the interferon α, β, δ family, between FANCF and the RNA binding protein ROM,[50] and between FANCG and the initiator of DNA replication, MCM. Further analysis for functional motifs using Block, PSORTII and InterPro Search detected nuclear localization signals (NLS) in FANCA, FANCG, FANCE, FANCD1 and FANCD2, and leucine zippers in FANCA and FANCG. Mutagenesis of the putative NLS in FANCA suggests that it does contribute to the nuclear localization of this protein.[85,86] Further biological studies are required to clarify these predictions and similarities.

Protein interactions and cellular localization

Initial studies located a major proportion of FANCC in the cytoplasm,[87–90] which would be consistent with a role in the catabolism of genotoxic agents. A cytoplasmic location was supported by the finding that transfer of FANCC to the nuclear compartment, by fusion of the protein to a nuclear localization signal, abolished its ability to correct MMC sensitivity when overexpressed in FA-C cells.[89] However, other studies found that FANCA and FANCC co-localized, and were present in both cytoplasm and nucleus.[91–95] The localization of FANCA was found to be predominantly nuclear.[86,96] More recently, studies have revealed that a nuclear multiprotein complex is formed by the proteins FANCA, -C, -E, -F and -G.[97–99] This complex was found to be essential for the activation of FANCD2 into a monoubiquitinated isoform, which co-localizes with BRCA1 in nuclear foci.[100] Direct interaction was also detected between FANCA and BRCA1, but the functional consequence of this interaction have to be determined.[101] BRCA1 is a component of the mRNA-synthesizing machine known as the RNA polymerase II

(PolII) holoenzyme complex,[102] and of the chromatin remodelling complex SWI/SNF.[103] BRCA1 also interacts with BRCA2,[104] now shown to be identical with FANCD1, and this in turn interacts with RAD51, amongst many other proteins.[105] Cells from complementation group D1 and other FA groups have reduced DNA damage-induced nuclear RAD51 focus formation,[106,107] and cells from several FA groups were unable to form foci of the RAD50/NBS1/MRE11 complex in response to ICLs.[108] Also, FANCD2 co-localizes with NBS1 and MRE11 after DNA damage.[109] These studies link at least part of the FA pathway very clearly to a DNA repair mechanism (see also later section on DNA repair). However, a multitude of other protein interactions have been described that link the FA proteins to several seemingly distinct pathways, including transcriptional regulation, control of the cell cycle, oxidative metabolism and cell signalling. Table 14.4 summarizes the interactions described and their putative functional implications.

FA gene expression patterns

FANCA and *FANCC* gene expression patterns have been studied in mice. Both genes were found to be ubiquitously expressed but at different levels in different tissues. High expression of *FANCA* was noted in testis, ovary and lymphoid tissues, such as the thymus, spleen, mesenteric lymphoid tissue and lymph nodes.[110] Developmental studies showed some overlap between the expression profiles of *FANCA* and *FANCC*, but this was not complete. Both proteins were detected in the developing kidney, brain, liver and whisker follicles. However, only FANCC was expressed in developing lung and gut, suggesting that expression of FANCA and FANCC is not necessarily coupled in development.[111,112] The intracellular concentration of FANCC has recently been found to be controlled by post-translational processes, such as protein stabilization and degradation mechanisms.[113]

THE FUNCTIONAL PATHWAY IN FANCONI ANAEMIA

The cellular phenotype in FA is one of genomic instability. This is consistent with most of the varied clinical manifestations of FA. Chromosomal breaks in rapidly dividing cells could lead to progressive depletion of the haematopoietic stem cell population and to gene rearrangements, which initiate oncogenic transformation in blood and other tissues. It is also possible that chromosome breakage in genes critical for development could occur during embryogenesis, thus leading to congenital abnormalities. It has become apparent that part of the endpoint of genomic instability in FA is caused by a defect in the DNA repair process.

However, FA proteins may also be further involved in metabolizing potentially genotoxic agents. At least four possible functional pathways have been implicated in the molecular mechanism of FA protein function: (1) cell cycle control, (2) regulation of cytokines and apoptosis, (3) oxygen metabolism, and (4) DNA repair (see also Table 14.4).

Cell–cycle control

Cell-cycle disturbance is found in FA cells exposed to DNA cross-linking agents as a prolongation of the G2 phase. Some FA cells enter a second growth phase without prior completion of the delayed S and G2/M segments of the cell cycle. Renewed replication ensues in these cells without prior passage through mitosis and cytokinesis, leading to endoreduplication.[114,115] Since it was found that G2/M accumulation was similar in normal and FA-C cells when the cross-linker dosage was adjusted to produce a similar cytotoxic effect, it was argued that FA cells show normal checkpoint function.[116] Indeed, a delay in G2 is precisely what would be expected from cells with substantial chromosomal damage.

Cytokine regulation and defects in apoptosis

Several studies have shown abnormal cytokine regulation in FA cells. These include the presence of high levels of tumour necrosis factor α (TNFα) in FA lymphoblasts,[117,118] and a markedly diminished colony-forming capacity in bone marrow progenitor cells from *Fancc* −/− mice after exposure to interferon γ (INFγ).[59] Inhibitory cytokines, such as IFNγ, TNFα and macrophage inflammatory protein-1α (MIP1α) were found to induce deregulated progenitor growth and apoptosis in haematopoietic cells from *Fancc* −/− mice.[119] Disturbance in normal apoptotic function was deduced from the inability of FA-C cells to activate caspase-3 after ionizing radiation.[120] Apoptosis deregulation in FA was also implicated because FA cells were found to be resistant to apoptosis,[121,122] and FANCC overexpression induced apoptosis.[123] Pang *et al.*, however, found that FANCC is involved in the activation of STAT1 via growth factors, and proposed that FA-C cells are excessively apoptotic as a consequence of the resulting imbalance between survival and apoptotic stimuli.[124] They further observed that FANCC binds Hsp70, and prevents apoptosis in haematopoietic cells exposed to IFNγ and TNFα.[125]

Oxygen metabolism

It has been known for many years that chromosome breakage in FA cells increases with increasing oxygen

Table 14.4 *Proteins found to interact with Fanconi anaemia proteins*

Functional class	Specific function	Protein name	Interacts with	Description	References
Transcription involvement	Transcription regulators	FAZF	FANCC	Fanconi anaemia zinc finger protein	Hoatlin et al. (1999)[146]
	Stress induced (heat shock)	Hsp70	FANCC	Heat shock protein 70	Pang et al. (2001)[125]
		GRP94	FANCC	Glucose regulated family of proteins, homology to HSP90	Hoshino et al. (1998)[147]
	Chromatin modifiers	BRG1	FANCA	Brm-related gene 1; subunit of SWI/SNF;	Otsuki et al. (2001)[148]
Cell cycle	Kinase	Cdc2	FANCC	Cyclin-dependent kinase (p34)	Kupfer et al. (1997)[91]
		ATM	FANCD2	Ataxia telangiectasia mutated (kinase)	Taniguchi et al. (2002)[149]
DNA repair		BRCA1	FANCD2/FANCD1 (=BRCA2)	Breast cancer-associated protein 1	Garcia-Higuera et al. (2001)[100] Folias et al. (2002)[101]
		XPF	FANCA/FANCC	Xeroderma pigmentosum factor F	McMahon et al. (2001)[150]
	Structural proteins	Alpha spectrin	FANCA/FANCC	Participant of cytoskeleton and membrane skeleton	McMahon et al. (1999)[151]
Oxidative metabolism		RED	FANCC	NADPH cytochrome 450 reductase, catalyses conjugation of glutathiones to xenobiotics	Kruyt et al. (1998)[152]
		GSTP1	FANCC	Pi glutathione S-transferase; catalyses detoxification of xenobiotics and by-products of oxidative stress; suppresses apoptosis	
		CYP2E1	FANCG	Cytochrome P450 2E1, role in redox mechanism	Cumming et al. (2001)[153] Futaki et al. (2002)[154]
Signalling	Interferon/cytokine-induced or related genes	Stat 1	FANCC	Signal transducer and activator of transcription-1	Pang et al. (1998)[155]
		IκB kinase	FANCA	Activates NFκB	Otsuki et al. (1998)[156], Otsuki et al. (2002)[157]
	Secondary modification	Akt kinase	FANCA	Negative regulator of FANCA phosphorylation	Otsuki et al. (2002)[158]
Transporter function	Cytoplasmic	SNX5	FANCA	Sorting nexin 5; trafficking, sorting activity	Waisfisz (1999),[159] Otsuki et al. (1999)[160]

tension, and it was proposed that the primary defect was a failure to tolerate oxidative stress.[126,127] It was also shown that G2 arrest in FA cells is reduced at lower oxygen levels.[112] These features could result from a failure to metabolize reactive oxygen species (ROS) or from failure to repair the DNA damage that they induce. It was also found that antioxidants such as superoxide dismutase (SOD) and thioredoxin have a protective effect on FA lymphocytes in culture,[128,129] and that the mean value of SOD activity in FA patients was significantly lower than in healthy donors.[130] In addition, $Sod1^{-/-}/Fancc^{-/-}$ mice showed a haematological phenotype that was strongly reminiscent of FA patients.[131] However, none of the known free-radical scavenging pathways were grossly defective in FA cells,[132,133] and FA cells are not hypersensitive to superoxide radical-generating agents, such as paraquat.[134] Recently, it was shown that culture of FA cells in 5 per cent oxygen normalizes their MMC sensitivity, whereas they are hypersensitive to MMC at a 20 per cent oxygen concentration.[135] Since MMC is oxidized to an inactive form at high oxygen concentrations, the authors argue that the MMC hypersensitivity is more likely to be due to the production of ROS. A role in oxidative metabolism for FA genes is an attractive proposition, because it would provide an explanation for the spontaneous chromosomal damage that occurs in FA cells. Several redox regulatory proteins have been shown to interact with FANCC (see Table 14.4). However, it is difficult to explain the marked and specific sensitivity of FA cells to DNA cross-linking agents purely on the basis of oxidative damage.

DNA repair

FA cells were shown to be defective in endonuclease activities, and a damage recognition protein that binds to DNA containing interstrand cross links was absent or defective in FA-A cells.[136,137] This protein was identified as α spectrin II, and it was proposed that it forms a complex with FANCA and FANCC that associates with regions of DNA damage. FA-A cells were further found to be defective in the execution of particular incisions at sites of interstrand cross-links.[138] Several studies have shown that nuclear extracts from FA cells are deficient in their capacity to repair plasmid substrates *in vitro*, which suggests a defect in non-homologous end-joining.[139–141] The discovery that FANCD1 is, in fact, BRCA2 links the FA pathway strongly to the process of double-strand break repair, since BRCA2 has a now well-established role in homologous recombination repair.[142] A role for FA proteins in DNA repair is also strongly suggested by their interaction or co-localization with other known repair proteins in DNA damage-induced nuclear foci

(see earlier section on protein interactions and cellular localization).

CONCLUSION

The identification of FANCD1 as BRCA2, and the reported interactions of FANCA with BRCA1, and FANCD2 with BRCA1 and the RAD50/NBS1/MRE11 complex, provide strong support for a role for the FA complex in aspects of DNA repair. However, whether the FA proteins are involved in DNA damage recognition, signalling to the repair machinery or the repair itself is far from clear. The BRCA2 connection implies a direct role in homologous recombination repair, and it will be important to establish whether there are direct interactions between this protein and other parts of the FA complex. The evidence for a DNA repair function does not preclude involvement in other cellular functions as well, such as oxidative metabolism. The profusion of proteins that have been found to interact with one or other of the FA proteins (Table 14.4) has led to more confusion than clarity in our understanding of function in FA, and it will be important to resolve which of these interactions have biological relevance. Finally, the genes for several more FA complementation groups remain to be cloned[143] and these may shed further light on the functional pathways involved.

ACKNOWLEDGEMENTS

Work in the authors' laboratory was supported by the Leukaemia Research Fund and Fanconi Anaemia Breakthrough (UK).

KEY POINTS

- Fanconi anaemia (FA) is an autosomal recessive disorder with developmental abnormalities and an associated risk of leukaemia in homozygous mutation carriers. There is no convincing evidence of an increased cancer risk in heterozygous gene carriers, but the amount of data is small.
- There are several complementation groups. One of these is due to homozygous mutations in the *BRCA2* gene. Others have been found to be due to mutations in the *FANC* genes which are involved in DNA repair.
- FA is a chromosome breakage syndrome; individuals are sensitive to chemotherapy and radiation.

REFERENCES

1. Fanconi G. Familial constitutional panmyelocytopathy, Fanconi's anemia (F.A.). I. Clinical aspects. *Semin Hematol* 1967; **4**:233–240.

2. Alter BP. Leukemia and preleukemia in Fanconi's anemia. *Cancer Genet Cytogenet* 1992; **58**:206–208.

3. Auerbach AD, Buchwald M, Joenje H. Fanconi anemia. In: Kinzler V (ed.) *The genetic basis of human cancer.* New York: McGraw-Hill Inc., 1998:317–331.

4. Alter BP. Cancer in Fanconi anemia, 1927–2001. *Cancer* 2003; **97**:425–440.

5. Tischkowitz MD, Hodgson SV. Fanconi anaemia. *J Med Genet* 2003; **40**:1–10.

6. Alter BP. Fanconi's anaemia and its variability. *Br J Haematol* 1993; **85**:9–14.

7. Faivre L, Guardiola P, Lewis C, *et al.* Association of complementation group and mutation type with clinical outcome in Fanconi anemia. *Blood* 2000; **96**:4064–4070.

8. Dokal I, Chase A, Morgan NV, *et al.* Positive diepoxybutane test in only one of two brothers found to be compound heterozygotes for Fanconi's anaemia complementation group C mutations. *Br J Haematol* 1996; **93**:813–818.

9. Poole SR, Smith AC, Hays T, *et al.* Monozygotic twin girls with congenital malformations resembling Fanconi anemia. *Am J Med Genet* 1992; **42**:780–784.

10. Alter BP. Fanconi's anemia. Current concepts. *Am J Pediatr Hematol Oncol* 1992; **14**:170–176.

11. Chaganti RS, Houldsworth J. Fanconi anemia: a pleotropic mutation with multiple cellular and developmental abnormalities. *Ann Genet* 1991; **34**:206–211.

12. Ebell W, Friedrich W, Kohne E. Therapeutic aspects of Fanconi's anaemia. In: Schroeder-Kurth TM, Auerbach AD, Obe G (eds) *Fanconi anaemia: clinical, cytogenetic and experimental aspects.* Berlin: Springer-Verlag, 1989:47–59.

13. Swift M. Fanconi's anaemia in the genetics of neoplasia. *Nature* 1971; **230**:370–373.

14. Verlander PC, Kaporis A, Liu Q, *et al.* Carrier frequency of the IVS4 + 4 A → T mutation of the Fanconi anemia gene *FAC* in the Ashkenazi Jewish population. *Blood* 1995; **86**:4034–4038.

15. Rosendorff J, Bernstein R, Macdougall L, Jenkins T. Fanconi anemia: another disease of unusually high prevalence in the Afrikaans population of South Africa. *Am J Med Genet* 1987; **27**:793–797.

16. Fanconi G. Familiaere infantile perniziosaartige Anaemie (pernizioeses Blutbild und Konstitution). *Jahrbuch Kinderheil* 1927; **117**:257–280.

17. Schroeder TM, Anschutz F, Knopp A. Spontaneous chromosome aberrations in familial panmyelopathy. *Humangenetik* 1964; **1**:194–196.

18. Schmid W, Scharer K, Baumann T, Fanconi G. Chromosomal fragility in familial panmyelopathy (Fanconi type). *Schweiz Med Wochenschr* 1965; **95**:1461–1464.

19. Sasaki MS, Tonomura A. A high susceptibility of Fanconi's anemia to chromosome breakage by DNA cross-linking agents. *Cancer Res* 1973; **33**:1829–1836.

20. Berger R, Bernheim A, Gluckman E, Gisselbrecht C. In vitro effect of cyclophosphamide metabolites on chromosomes of Fanconi anaemia patients. *Br J Haematol* 1980; **45**:565–568.

21. Auerbach AD, Wolman SR. Susceptibility of Fanconi's anaemia fibroblasts to chromosome damage by carcinogens. *Nature* 1976; **261**:494–496.

22. Auerbach AD, Wolman SR. Carcinogen-induced chromosome breakage in Fanconi's anaemia heterozygous cells. *Nature* 1978; **271**:69–71.

23. Schroeder-Kurth TM, Zhu TH, Hong Y, Westphal I. Variation in cellular sensitivities among Fanconi anemia patients, non-Fanconi anemia patients, their parents and siblings, and control probands. In: Schroeder-Kurth TM, Auerbach AD, Obe G (eds) *Fanconi anaemia: clinical, cytogenetic and experimental aspects.* Heidelberg: Springer-Verlag, 1989:105.

24. Auerbach AD. Fanconi anemia diagnosis and the diepoxybutane (DEB) test. *Exp Hematol* 1993; **21**:731–733.

25. Shimamura A, De Oca RM, Svenson JL, *et al.* A novel diagnostic screen for defects in the Fanconi anemia pathway. *Blood* 2002; **100**:4649–4654.

26. Hanenberg H, Batish SD, Pollok KE, *et al.* Phenotypic correction of primary Fanconi anemia T cells with retroviral vectors as a diagnostic tool. *Exp Hematol* 2002; **30**:410–420.

27. dos Santos CC, Gavish H, Buchwald M. Fanconi anemia revisited: old ideas and new advances. *Stem Cells* 1994; **12**:142–153.

28. Guardiola P, Pasquini R, Dokal I, *et al.* Outcome of 69 allogeneic stem cell transplantations for Fanconi anemia using HLA-matched unrelated donors: a study on behalf of the European Group for Blood and Marrow Transplantation. *Blood* 2000; **95**:422–429.

29. Gluckman E, Broxmeyer HA, Auerbach AD, *et al.* Hematopoietic reconstitution in a patient with Fanconi's anemia by means of umbilical-cord blood from an HLA-identical sibling. *N Engl J Med* 1989; **321**:1174–1178.

30. Auerbach AD, Adler B, O'Reilly RJ, *et al.* Effect of procarbazine and cyclophosphamide on chromosome breakage in Fanconi anemia cells: relevance to bone marrow transplantation. *Cancer Genet Cytogenet* 1983; **9**:25–36.

31. Gluckman E. Radiosensitivity in Fanconi anemia: application to the conditioning for bone marrow transplantation. *Radiother Oncol* 1990; **18**(Suppl. 1):88–93.

32. de Medeiros CR, Silva LM, Pasquini R. Unrelated cord blood transplantation in a Fanconi anemia patient using fludarabine-based conditioning. *Bone Marrow Transplant* 2001; **28**:110–112.

33. McCloy M, Almeida A, Daly P, *et al.* Fludarabine-based stem cell transplantation protocol for Fanconi's anaemia in myelodysplastic transformation. *Br J Haematol* 2001; **112**:427–429.

34. Liu JM, Kim S, Read EJ, *et al.* Engraftment of hematopoietic progenitor cells transduced with the Fanconi anemia group C gene (*FANCC*). *Hum Gene Ther* 1999; **10**:2337–2346.

35. Galimi F, Noll M, Kanazawa Y, *et al.* Gene therapy of Fanconi anemia: preclinical efficacy using lentiviral vectors. *Blood* 2002; **100**:2732–2736.

36. Noll M, Bateman RL, D'Andrea AD, Grompe M. Preclinical protocol for in vivo selection of hematopoietic stem cells corrected by gene therapy in Fanconi anemia group C. *Mol Ther* 2001; **3**:14–23.

37. Auerbach AD, Allen RG. Leukemia and preleukemia in Fanconi anemia patients. A review of the literature and report of the International Fanconi Anemia Registry. *Cancer Genet Cytogenet* 1991; **51**:1–12.

38. Butturini A, Gale RP, Verlander PC, *et al.* Hematologic abnormalities in Fanconi anemia: an International Fanconi Anemia Registry study. *Blood* 1994; **84**:1650–1655.

39. Deeg HJ, Socie G, Schoch G, *et al.* Malignancies after marrow transplantation for aplastic anemia and Fanconi anemia: a joint Seattle and Paris analysis of results in 700 patients. *Blood* 1996; **87**:386–392.

40. Swift M, Zimmerman D, McDonough ER. Squamous cell carcinomas in Fanconi's anemia. *JAMA* 1971; **216**:325–326.

41. Swift M, Caldwell RJ, Chase C. Reassessment of cancer predisposition of Fanconi anemia heterozygotes. *J Natl Cancer Inst* 1980; **65**:863–867.

42. Duckworth-Rysiecki G, Cornish K, Clarke CA, Buchwald M. Identification of two complementation groups in Fanconi anemia. *Somat Cell Mol Genet* 1985; **11**:35–41.

43. Strathdee CA, Duncan AM, Buchwald M. Evidence for at least four Fanconi anaemia genes including FACC on chromosome 9. *Nature Genet* 1992; **1**:196–198.

44. Joenje H, Oostra AB, Wijker M, *et al.* Evidence for at least eight Fanconi anemia genes. *Am J Hum Genet* 1997; **61**:940–944.

45. Joenje H, Levitus M, Waisfisz Q, *et al.* Complementation analysis in Fanconi anemia: assignment of the reference FA-H patient to group A. *Am J Hum Genet* 2000; **67**:759–762.

46. Timmers C, Taniguchi T, Hejna J, *et al.* Positional cloning of a novel Fanconi anemia gene, *FANCD2*. *Mol Cell* 2001; **7**:241–248.

47. Lo Ten Foe JR, Rooimans MA, Bosnoyan-Collins L, *et al.* Expression cloning of a cDNA for the major Fanconi anaemia gene, *FAA*. *Nature Genet* 1996; **14**:320–323.

48. Strathdee CA, Gavish H, Shannon WR, Buchwald M. Cloning of cDNAs for Fanconi's anaemia by functional complementation. *Nature* 1992; **356**:763–767 (correction: *Nature* **358**:434).

49. de Winter JP, Waisfisz Q, Rooimans MA, *et al.* The Fanconi anaemia group G gene *FANCG* is identical with XRCC9. *Nature Genet* 1998; **20**:281–283.

50. de Winter JP, Rooimans MA, van Der Weel L, *et al.* The Fanconi anaemia gene *FANCF* encodes a novel protein with homology to ROM. *Nature Genet* 2000; **24**:15–16.

51. de Winter JP, Leveille F, van Berkel CG, *et al.* Isolation of a cDNA representing the Fanconi anemia complementation group E gene. *Am J Hum Genet* 2000; **67**:1306–1308.

52. Pronk JC, Gibson RA, Savoia A, *et al.* Localisation of the Fanconi anaemia complementation group A gene to chromosome 16q24.3. *Nature Genet* 1995; **11**:338–340.

53. Waisfisz Q, Saar K, Morgan NV, *et al.* The Fanconi anemia group F gene, *FANCE*, maps to chromosome 6p. *Am J Hum Genet* 1999; **64**:1400–1405.

54. The Fanconi anaemia/breast cancer consortium. Positional cloning of the Fanconi anaemia group A gene. *Nature Genet* 1996; **14**:324–328.

55. Whitney M, Thayer M, Reifsteck C, *et al.* Microcell mediated chromosome transfer maps the Fanconi anaemia group D gene to chromosome 3p. *Nature Genet* 1995; **11**:341–343.

56. Hejna JA, Timmers CD, Reifsteck C, *et al.* Localization of the Fanconi anemia complementation group D gene to a 200-kb region on chromosome 3p25.3. *Am J Hum Genet* 2000; **66**:1540–1551.

57. Howlett NG, Taniguchi T, Olson S, *et al.* Biallelic inactivation of BRCA2 in Fanconi anemia. *Science* 2002; **297**:606–609.

58. Chen M, Tomkins DJ, Auerbach W, *et al.* Inactivation of Fac in mice produces inducible chromosomal instability and reduced fertility reminiscent of Fanconi anaemia. *Nature Genet* 1996; **12**:448–451.

59. Whitney MA, Royle G, Low MJ, *et al.* Germ cell defects and hematopoietic hypersensitivity to gamma-interferon in mice with a targeted disruption of the Fanconi anemia C gene. *Blood* 1996; **88**:49–58.

60. Cheng NC, van De Vrugt HJ, van Der Valk MA, *et al.* Mice with a targeted disruption of the fanconi anemia homolog fanca. *Hum Mol Genet* 2000; **9**:1805–1811.

61. Koomen M, Cheng NC, van De Vrugt HJ, *et al.* Reduced fertility and hypersensitivity to mitomycin C characterize *Fancg/Xrcc9* null mice. *Hum Mol Genet* 2002; **11**:273–281.

62. Yang Y, Kuang Y, De Oca RM, *et al.* Targeted disruption of the murine Fanconi anemia gene, Fancg/Xrcc9. *Blood* 2001; **98**:3435–3440.

63. Noll M, Battaile KP, Bateman R, *et al.* Fanconi anemia group A and C double-mutant mice. Functional evidence for a multi-protein Fanconi anemia complex. *Exp Hematol* 2002; **30**:679–688.

64. Whitney MA, Saito H, Jakobs PM, *et al.* A common mutation in the *FACC* gene causes Fanconi anaemia in Ashkenazi Jews. *Nature Genet* 1993; **4**:202–205.

65. Gibson RA, Hajianpour A, Murer-Orlando M, *et al.* A nonsense mutation and exon skipping in the Fanconi anaemia group C gene. *Hum Mol Genet* 1993; **2**:797–799.

66. Verlander PC, Lin JD, Udono MU, *et al.* Mutation analysis of the Fanconi anemia gene *FACC*. *Am J Hum Genet* 1994; **54**:595–601.

67. Gibson RA, Morgan NV, Goldstein LH, *et al.* Novel mutations and polymorphisms in the Fanconi anemia group C gene. *Hum Mutat* 1996; **8**:140–148.

68. Waisfisz Q, Morgan NV, Savino M, *et al.* Spontaneous functional correction of homozygous Fanconi anaemia alleles reveals novel mechanistic basis for reverse mosaicism. *Nature Genet* 1999; **22**:379–383.

69. Gavish H, dos Santos CC, Buchwald M. A Leu554-to-Pro substitution completely abolishes the functional complementing activity of the Fanconi anemia (FACC) protein. *Hum Mol Genet* 1993; **2**:123–126.

70. Whitney MA, Jakobs P, Kaback M, *et al.* The Ashkenazi Jewish Fanconi anemia mutation: incidence among patients and carrier frequency in the at-risk population. *Hum Mutat* 1994; **3**:339–341.

71. Levran O, Erlich T, Magdalena N, *et al.* Sequence variation in the Fanconi anemia gene *FAA*. *Proc Natl Acad Sci USA* 1997; **94**:13051–13056.

72. Wijker M, Morgan NV, Herterich S, *et al.* Heterogeneous spectrum of mutations in the Fanconi anaemia group A gene. *Eur J Hum Genet* 1999; **7**:52–59.

73. Tachibana A, Kato T, Ejima Y, *et al.* The *FANCA* gene in Japanese Fanconi anemia: reports of eight novel mutations and analysis of sequence variability. *Hum Mutat* 1999; **13**:237–244.

74. Morgan NV, Tipping AJ, Joenje H, Mathew CG. High frequency of large intragenic deletions in the Fanconi anemia Group A gene. *Am J Hum Genet* 1999; **65**:1330–1341.

75. Kupfer G, Nat D, Garcia-Higuera I, *et al.* A patient-derived mutant form of the Fanconi anemia protein, FANCA, is

defective in nuclear accumulation. *Exp Hematol* 1999; **27**:587–593.

76. Yamada T, Tachibana A, Shimizu T, *et al*. Novel mutations of the *FANCG* gene causing alternative splicing in Japanese Fanconi anemia. *J Hum Genet* 2000; **45**:159–166.

77. Yamashita T, Wu N, Kupfer G, *et al*. Clinical variability of Fanconi anemia (type C) results from expression of an amino terminal truncated Fanconi anemia complementation group C polypeptide with partial activity. *Blood* 1996; **87**:4424–4432.

78. Gillio AP, Verlander PC, Batish SD, *et al*. Phenotypic consequences of mutations in the Fanconi anemia *FAC* gene: an International Fanconi Anemia Registry study. *Blood* 1997; **90**:105–110.

79. Adachi D, Oda T, Yagasaki H, *et al*. Heterogeneous activation of the Fanconi anemia pathway by patient-derived *FANCA* mutants. *Hum Mol Genet* 2002; **11**:3125–3134.

80. Futaki M, Yamashita T, Yagasaki H, *et al*. The IVS4 + 4 A to T mutation of the Fanconi anemia gene *FANCC* is not associated with a severe phenotype in Japanese patients. *Blood* 2000; **95**:1493–1498.

81. Lo Ten Foe JR, Kwee ML, Rooimans MA, *et al*. Somatic mosaicism in Fanconi anemia: molecular basis and clinical significance. *Eur J Hum Genet* 1997; **5**:137–148.

82. Klapper MH. The independent distribution of amino acid near neighbor pairs into polypeptides. *Biochem Biophys Res Commun* 1977; **78**:1018–1024.

83. Ching Ying Wong J, Alon N, Buchwald M. Cloning of the bovine and rat Fanconi anemia group C cDNA. *Mamm Genome* 1997; **8**:522–525.

84. Mian IS, Moser MJ. The Fanconi anemia complementation group A protein contains a peroxidase domain. *Mol Genet Metab* 1998; **63**:230–234.

85. Garcia-Higuera I, Kuang Y, Näf D, *et al*. Fanconi anemia proteins FANCA, FANCC, and FANCG/XRCC9 interact in a functional nuclear complex. *Mol Cell Biol* 1999; **19**:4866–4873.

86. Lightfoot J, Alon N, Bosnoyan-Collins L, Buchwald M. Characterization of regions functional in the nuclear localization of the Fanconi anemia group A protein. *Hum Mol Genet* 1999; **8**:1007–1015.

87. Youssoufian H. Localization of Fanconi anemia C protein to the cytoplasm of mammalian cells. *Proc Natl Acad Sci USA* 1994; **91**:7975–7979.

88. Youssoufian H, Auerbach AD, Verlander PC, *et al*. Identification of cytosolic proteins that bind to the Fanconi anemia complementation group C polypeptide in vitro. Evidence for a multimeric complex. *J Biol Chem* 1995; **270**:9876–9882.

89. Youssoufian H. Cytoplasmic localization of FAC is essential for the correction of a prerepair defect in Fanconi anemia group C cells. *J Clin Invest* 1996; **97**:2003–2016.

90. Yamashita T, Barber DL, Zhu Y, *et al*. The Fanconi anemia polypeptide FACC is localized to the cytoplasm. *Proc Natl Acad Sci USA* 1994; **91**:6712–6716.

91. Kupfer GM, Näf D, Suliman A, *et al*. The Fanconi anaemia proteins, FAA and FAC interact to form a nuclear complex. *Nature Genet* 1997; **17**:487–490.

92. Kupfer GM, Yamashita T, Näf D, *et al*. The Fanconi anemia polypeptide, FAC, binds to the cyclin-dependent kinase, cdc2. *Blood* 1997; **90**:1047–1054.

93. Näf D, Kupfer GM, Suliman A, *et al*. Functional activity of the Fanconi anemia protein FAA requires FAC binding and nuclear localization. *Mol Cell Biol* 1998; **18**:5952–5960.

94. Hoatlin ME, Christianson TA, Keeble WW, *et al*. The Fanconi anemia group C gene product is located in both the nucleus and cytoplasm of human cells. *Blood* 1998; **91**:1418–1425.

95. Savoia A, Garcia-Higuera I, D'Andrea AD. Nuclear localization of the Fanconi anemia protein FANCC is required for functional activity. *Blood* 1999; **93**:4025–4026.

96. Walsh CE, Yountz MR, Simpson DA. Intracellular localization of the Fanconi anemia complementation group A protein. *Biochem Biophys Res Commun* 1999; **259**:594–599.

97. de Winter JP, van Der Weel L, de Groot J, *et al*. The Fanconi anemia protein FANCF forms a nuclear complex with FANCA, FANCC and FANCG. *Hum Mol Genet* 2000; **9**:2665–2674.

98. Medhurst AL, Huber PA, Waisfisz Q, *et al*. Direct interactions of the five known Fanconi anaemia proteins suggest a common functional pathway. *Hum Mol Genet* 2001; **10**:423–429.

99. Pace P, Johnson M, Tan WM, *et al*. FANCE: the link between Fanconi anaemia complex assembly and activity. *EMBO J* 2002; **21**:3414–3423.

100. Garcia-Higuera I, Taniguchi T, Ganesan S, *et al*. Interaction of the Fanconi anemia proteins and BRCA1 in a common pathway. *Mol Cell* 2001; **7**:249–262.

101. Folias A, Matkovic M, Bruun D, *et al*. BRCA1 interacts directly with the Fanconi anemia protein FANCA. *Hum Mol Genet* 2002; **11**:2591–2597.

102. Neish AS, Anderson SF, Schlegel BP, *et al*. Factors associated with the mammalian RNA polymerase II holoenzyme. *Nucl Acids Res* 1998; **26**:847–853.

103. Bochar DA, Wang L, Beniya H, *et al*. BRCA1 is associated with a human SWI/SNF-related complex: linking chromatin remodeling to breast cancer. *Cell* 2000; **102**:257–265.

104. Chen J, Silver DP, Walpita D, *et al*. Stable interaction between the products of the *BRCA1* and *BRCA2* tumor suppressor genes in mitotic and meiotic cells. *Mol Cell* 1998; **2**:317–328.

105. Scully R, Chen J, Plug A, *et al*. Association of BRCA1 with RAD51 in mitotic and meiotic cells. *Cell* 1997; **88**:265–275.

106. Godthelp BC, Arwert F, Joenje H, Zdzienicka MZ. Impaired DNA damage-induced nuclear RAD51 foci formation uniquely characterizes Fanconi anemia group D1. *Oncogene* 2002; **21**:5002–5005.

107. Digweed M, Rothe S, Demuth I, *et al*. Attenuation of the formation of DNA-repair foci containing RAD51 in Fanconi anaemia. *Carcinogenesis* 2002; **23**:1121–1126.

108. Pichierri P, Averbeck D, Rosselli F. DNA cross-link-dependent RAD50/MRE11/NBS1 subnuclear assembly requires the Fanconi anemia C protein. *Hum Mol Genet* 2002; **11**:2531–2546.

109. Nakanishi K, Taniguchi T, Ranganathan V, *et al*. Interaction of FANCD2 and NBS1 in the DNA damage response. *Nature Cell Biol* 2002; **4**:913–920.

110. van de Vrugt HJ, Cheng NC, de Vries Y, *et al*. Cloning and characterization of murine Fanconi anemia group A gene: Fanca protein is expressed in lymphoid tissues, testis, and ovary. *Mamm Genome* 2000; **11**:326–331.

111. Abu-Issa R, Eichele G, Youssoufian H. Expression of the Fanconi anemia group A gene (Fanca) during mouse embryogenesis. *Blood* 1999; **94**:818–824.

112. Krasnoshtein F, Buchwald M. Developmental expression of the Fac gene correlates with congenital defects in Fanconi anemia patients. *Hum Mol Genet* 1996; **5**:85–93.

113. Heinrich MC, Silvey KV, Stone S, *et al.* Posttranscriptional cell cycle-dependent regulation of human FANCC expression. *Blood* 2000; **95**:3970–3977.

114. Kubbies M, Schindler D, Hoehn H, *et al.* Endogenous blockage and delay of the chromosome cycle despite normal recruitment and growth phase explain poor proliferation and frequent edomitosis in Fanconi anemia cells. *Am J Hum Genet* 1985; **37**:1022–1030.

115. Johnstone P, Reifsteck C, Kohler S, *et al.* Fanconi anemia group A and D cell lines respond normally to inhibitors of cell cycle regulation. *Somat Cell Mol Genet* 1997; **23**:371–377.

116. Heinrich MC, Hoatlin ME, Zigler AJ, *et al.* DNA cross-linker-induced G2/M arrest in group C Fanconi anemia lymphoblasts reflects normal checkpoint function. *Blood* 1998; **91**:275–287.

117. Schultz JC, Shahidi NT. Tumor necrosis factor-alpha overproduction in Fanconi's anemia. *Am J Hematol* 1993; **42**:196–201.

118. Rosselli F, Sanceau J, Gluckman E, *et al.* Abnormal lymphokine production: a novel feature of the genetic disease Fanconi anemia. II. In vitro and in vivo spontaneous overproduction of tumor necrosis factor alpha. *Blood* 1994; **83**:1216–1225.

119. Haneline LS, Broxmeyer HE, Cooper S, *et al.* Multiple inhibitory cytokines induce deregulated progenitor growth and apoptosis in hematopoietic cells from *Fac−/−* mice. *Blood* 1998; **91**:4092–4098.

120. Guillouf C, Vit JP, Rosselli F. Loss of the Fanconi anemia group C protein activity results in an inability to activate caspase-3 after ionizing radiation. *Biochimie* 2000; **82**:51–58.

121. Monti D, Macchioni S, Guido M, *et al.* Resistance to apoptosis in Fanconi's anaemia. An ex vivo study in peripheral blood mononuclear cells. *FEBS Lett* 1997, **409**:365–369

122. Ridet A, Guillouf C, Duchaud E, *et al.* Deregulated apoptosis is a hallmark of the Fanconi anemia syndrome. *Cancer Res* 1997; **57**:1722–1730.

123. Marathi UK, Howell SR, Ashmun RA, Brent TP. The Fanconi anemia complementation group C protein corrects DNA interstrand cross-link-specific apoptosis in HSC536N cells. *Blood* 1996; **88**:2298–2305.

124. Pang Q, Fagerlie S, Christianson TA, *et al.* The Fanconi anemia protein FANCC binds to and facilitates the activation of STAT1 by gamma interferon and hematopoietic growth factors. *Mol Cell Biol* 2000; **20**:4724–4735.

125. Pang Q, Keeble W, Christianson TA, *et al.* FANCC interacts with Hsp70 to protect hematopoietic cells from IFN-gamma/TNF-alpha-mediated cytotoxicity. *EMBO J* 2001; **20**:4478–4489.

126. Joenje H, Arwert F, Eriksson AW, *et al.* Oxygen-dependence of chromosomal aberrations in Fanconi's anaemia. *Nature* 1981; **290**:142–143.

127. Joenje H, Oostra AB. Effect of oxygen tension on chromosomal aberrations in Fanconi anaemia. *Hum Genet* 1983; **65**:99–101.

128. Nordenson I. Effect of superoxide dismutase and catalase on spontaneously occurring chromosome breaks in patients with Fanconi's anemia. *Hereditas* 1977; **86**:147–150.

129. Ruppitsch W, Meisslitzer C, Hirsch-Kauffmann M, Schweiger M. Overexpression of thioredoxin in Fanconi anemia fibroblasts prevents the cytotoxic and DNA damaging effect of mitomycin C and diepoxybutane. *FEBS Lett* 1998; **422**:99–102.

130. Malorni W, Straface E, Pagano G, *et al.* Cytoskeleton alterations of erythrocytes from patients with Fanconi's anemia. *FEBS Lett* 2000; **468**:125–128.

131. Hadjur S, Ung K, Wadsworth L, *et al.* Defective hematopoiesis and hepatic steatosis in mice with combined deficiencies of the genes encoding Fancc and Cu/Zn superoxide dismutase. *Blood* 2001; **98**:1003–1011.

132. Joenje H, Gille JJP. Oxygen metabolism and chromosomal breakage in Fanconi anaemia. In: Schroeder-Kurth TM, Obe G, Auerbach AD (eds) *Fanconi anaemia: clinical, cytogenetic and experimental aspects*. Berlin: Springer-Verlag, 1989:174–182.

133. Hoehn H, Kubbies M, Schindler D, *et al.* BrdU-Hoechst flow cytometry links the cell kinetic defect of Fanconi anaemia to oxygen hypersensitivity. In: Schroeder-Kurth TM, Obe G, Auerbach AD (eds) *Fanconi anaemia, clinical, cytogenetic and experimental aspects*. Berlin: Springer-Verlag, 1989:162–173.

134. Poot M, Gross O, Epe B, *et al.* Cell cycle defect in connection with oxygen and iron sensitivity in Fanconi anemia lymphoblastoid cells. *Exp Cell Res* 1996; **222**:262–286.

135. Clarke AA, Philpott NJ, Gordon-Smith EC, Rutherford TR. The sensitivity of Fanconi anaemia group C cells to apoptosis induced by mitomycin C is due to oxygen radical generation, not DNA crosslinking. *Br J Haematol* 1997; **96**:240–247.

136. Hang B, Yeung AT, Lambert MW. A damage-recognition protein which binds to DNA containing interstrand cross-links is absent or defective in Fanconi anemia, complementation group A, cells. *Nucl Acids Res* 1993; **21**:4187–4192.

137. Lambert MW, Tsongalis GJ, Lambert WC, Parrish DD. Correction of the DNA repair defect in Fanconi anemia complementation groups A and D cells. *Biochem Biophys Res Commun* 1997; **230**:587–591.

138. Kumaresan KR, Lambert MW. Fanconi anemia, complementation group A, cells are defective in ability to produce incisions at sites of psoralen interstrand cross-links. *Carcinogenesis* 2000; **21**:741–751.

139. Escarceller M, Rousset S, Moustacchi E, Papadopoulo D. The fidelity of double strand breaks processing is impaired in complementation groups B and D of Fanconi anemia, a genetic instability syndrome. *Somat Cell Mol Genet* 1997; **23**:401–411.

140. Escarceller M, Buchwald M, Singleton BK, *et al.* Fanconi anemia C gene product plays a role in the fidelity of blunt DNA end-joining. *J Mol Biol* 1998; **279**:375–385.

141. Lundberg R, Mavinakere M, Campbell C. Deficient DNA end joining activity in extracts from Fanconi anemia fibroblasts. *J Biol Chem* 2001; **276**:9543–9549.

142. West SC. Cross-links between Fanconi anaemia and BRCA2. *DNA Repair* 2003; **2**:231–234.

143. Levitus M, Rooimans MA, Steltenpool J, *et al.* Heterogeneity in Fanconi anemia: evidence for two new genetic subtypes. *Blood* 2003; **103**:2498–2503.

144. Jasin M. Homologous repair of DNA damage and tumorigenesis: the BRCA connection. *Oncogene* 2002; **21**:8981–8993.

145. Joenje H, Patel KJ. The emerging genetic and molecular basis of Fanconi anaemia. *Nature Rev Genet* 2001; **2**:446–457.

146. Hoatlin ME, Zhi Y, Ball H, *et al.* A novel BTB/POZ transcriptional repressor protein interacts with the Fanconi anemia group C protein and PLZF. *Blood* 1999; **94**:3737–3747.

147. Hoshino T, Wang JX, Devetten MP, *et al.* Molecular chaperone GRP94 binds to the Fanconi anemia group C protein and regulates its intracellular expression. *Blood* 1998; **91**:4379–4386.

148. Otsuki T, Furukawa Y, Ikeda K, *et al.* Fanconi anemia protein, FANCA, associates with BRG1, a component of the human SWI/SNF complex. *Hum Mol Genet* 2001; **10**:2651–2660.

149. Taniguchi T, Garcia-Higuera I, Xu B, *et al.* Convergence of the fanconi anemia and ataxia telangiectasia signaling pathways. *Cell* 2002; **109**:459–472.

150. McMahon LW, Sangerman J, Goodman SR, *et al.* Human alpha spectrin II and the FANCA, FANCC, and FANCG proteins bind to DNA containing psoralen interstrand cross-links. *Biochemistry* 2001; **40**:7025–7034.

151. McMahon LW, Walsh CE, Lambert MW. Human alpha Spectrin II and the Fanconi anemia proteins FANCA and FANCC interact to form a nuclear complex. *J Biol Chem* 1999; **274**:32904–32908.

152. Kruyt FAE, Hoshino T, Liu JM, *et al.* Abnormal microsomal detoxification implicated in Fanconi anemia group C by interaction of the FAC protein with NADPH cytochrome P450 reductase. *Blood* 1998; **92**:3050–3056.

153. Cumming RC, Lightfoot J, Beard K, *et al.* Fanconi anemia group C protein prevents apoptosis in hematopoietic cells through redox regulation of GSTP1. *Nature Med* 2001; **7**:814–820.

154. Futaki M, Igarashi T, Watanabe S, *et al.* The FANCG Fanconi anemia protein interacts with CYP2E1: possible role in protection against oxidative DNA damage. *Carcinogenesis* 2002; **23**:67–72.

155. Pang Q, Fagerlie S, Christianson TA, *et al.* The Fanconi anemia (FA) protein FAC is required for recruitment of stat 1 to the IFNγ receptor complex. *Am J Hum Genet* 1998; **63**(Suppl. 4):476a.

156. Otsuki T, Mercurio F, Liu JM. The Fanconi anemia group A gene product is a component of the IκB kinase signalsome complex involved in NF-κ-B activation. *Am J Hum Genet* 1998; **63**(Suppl. 4):692a.

157. Otsuki T, Young DB, Sasaki DT, *et al.* Fanconi anemia protein complex is a novel target of the IKK signalsome. *J Cell Biochem* 2002; **86**:613–623.

158. Otsuki T, Nagashima T, Komatsu N, *et al.* Phosphorylation of Fanconi anemia protein, FANCA, is regulated by Akt kinase. *Biochem Biophys Res Commun* 2002; **291**:628–634.

159. Waisfisz Q. Towards a molecular understanding of the Fanconi anemia defect. PhD thesis, Academisch Proefschrift, Vrije Universiteit, 1999.

160. Otsuki T, Kajigaya S, Ozawa K, Liu JM. SNX5, a new member of the sorting nexin family, binds to the Fanconi anemia complementation group A protein. *Biochem Biophys Res Commun* 1999; **265**:630–635.

15

The Gorlin (nevoid basal cell carcinoma) syndrome

PETER A. FARNDON

THE GORLIN SYNDROME

Introduction

Gorlin syndrome (MIM number 109400, gene symbol *NBCCS*) is a fully penetrant autosomal dominant disorder with over one hundred recognized features. The most frequent and clinically important components are nevoid basal cell carcinomas and odontogenic keratocysts, each affecting about 90 per cent of patients. The non-progressive skeletal anomalies present in a high proportion of cases are helpful diagnostically, as is the presence of ectopic calcification, particularly of the falx, which is present in 90 per cent of cases over the age of 20, and bone cysts. About 70 per cent of individuals have a recognizable appearance, which includes macrocephaly, frontal bossing, hypertelorism and facial milia. Congenital malformations (in 5 per cent of patients) occur at an increased frequency. Ovarian fibromas, medulloblastoma with a peak incidence at 2 years of age and cardiac fibromas are also important components of the syndrome.

The syndrome, therefore, offers a paradigm for understanding the cellular relationships between developmental malformations and cancer.

Following localization of the syndrome to chromosome 9q22.3–31,[1-3] evidence of allele loss from the unaffected parent in basal cell carcinomas (BCCs)[4] confirmed

that the gene acts as a tumour suppressor gene. Loss of heterozygosity was also demonstrated in syndromic jaw cysts,[5] which present from late childhood.

The syndrome was subsequently shown to be caused by mutations in the patched gene *PTCH*.[6,7] There is no evidence for genetic heterogeneity. The congenital malformations are predicted to be caused by a different mechanism – haploinsufficiency, resulting in gene dosage alterations in the sensitive hedgehog-patched-Gli pathway during development.[8]

History

The first reported cases appear to be those of Jarisch and White in 1894, but mummies from early Egyptian times have been found with skeletal signs of the syndrome. Gorlin and Goltz's description of two patients and literature review in 1960[9] drew the condition to wide attention. However, Howell and Caro had introduced the term 'basal cell nevus syndrome' in 1959,[10] proposing that the tumours were a unique type of BCC, which was capable of aggressive behaviour in adults, and were associated with developmental anomalies. They noted that the harmless clinical appearance of the nevi, especially in childhood, contrasted strikingly with the microscopic appearance and the destructive behaviour of tumours in adulthood. They cautioned against the use of ionizing radiation in treatment because of concern over new BCCs erupting in the irradiated area. Gorlin presented extensive reviews of the syndrome in 1987[11] and 1995.[12]

The information in this chapter is taken from a review of the literature and the author's own observations in a series of over 150 patients.

Nomenclature

The syndrome has been given many names, reflecting the multiplicity of presenting signs and symptoms, and include basal cell naevus syndrome, nevoid basal cell carcinoma syndrome (NBCCS), epitheliomatose multiple generalizee, fifth phakomatosis, hereditary cutaneomandibular polyoncosis, multiple basalioma syndrome and Gorlin syndrome.

The term basal cell naevus syndrome is inappropriate because histologically the naevi are BCCs, although not all behave aggressively. Throughout Europe, the condition is known as Gorlin syndrome, reflecting Professor Robert Gorlin's contributions to the understanding of the condition. He has suggested that it be known as the nevoid basal cell carcinoma syndrome, although this too may not be the most appropriate name because 10 per cent of adults do not develop BCCs. In addition, patients seem to prefer an eponymous title rather than one that contains the word 'carcinoma'.

Prevalence

The prevalence in a population-based study in North West England in 1991 was 1 in 55 600,[13] the latest prevalence figure from that continuing study is 1 in 40 000. A study in Australia gave a minimum prevalence of 1 in 164 000.[14]

FREQUENCY OF THE SYNDROME AMONGST PATIENTS WITH ONE OR MORE BCCs

In a group of 49 children under the age of 19 with a histologically proven BCC, 13 (26 per cent) had features of the Gorlin syndrome.[15] Two other children were developing a second BCC but they had no signs of the syndrome on X-ray or examination.

In 1904 cases with one or more BCCs, Summerly[16] found that 198 (10.4 per cent) were under 45 years. Two unequivocal cases of the syndrome were found in 125 of these patients available for study – 1.9 per cent of patients under 45. However, this may be an underestimate, because an additional 21 patients in this group had facial milia, two had cervical ribs and two had jaw cysts. A Russian study found five cases amongst 122 patients with multiple and/or early-onset BCCs.[17] In a series of 105 patients with an eyelid BCC, four had Gorlin syndrome, all of whom had a family history.[18]

FREQUENCY OF THE SYNDROME AMONGST PATIENTS WITH ODONTOGENIC KERATOCYSTS

In a series of 122 patients,[19] 113 had single cysts, and 9 (7 per cent) had multiple cysts. Gorlin syndrome was diagnosed in three out of nine patients who had more than one odontogenic keratocyst. The minimum estimate is, therefore, 2.5 per cent of patients with one or more cysts.

It has been suggested that an isolated odontogenic keratocyst may represent the 'least complete' form of the syndrome. No family member at risk of the syndrome in the North West of England longitudinal study is known to have an odontogenic keratocyst in the absence of other signs or symptoms. In addition, there appears to be no evidence that there is a familial tendency to develop odontogenic keratocysts in the absence of other features of the syndrome. Loss of heterozygosity for markers around the patched gene has been demonstrated in cysts from patients who do not have the syndrome,[20] suggesting that an isolated keratocyst is also likely to be due to homozygous inactivation of the patched gene.

Inheritance, penetrance and variability in expression

The syndrome is inherited as an autosomal dominant, with a one in two chance that a child of an affected parent will inherit the mutated gene. There is wide variability in expression both between and within families. The variability manifests itself not only in the presence or absence of a particular feature, but also in its severity.

New mutation rate

A new mutation rate of 40 per cent has been suggested from a review of the literature;[21] in an Australian series 37 out of 64 (58 per cent) were apparently isolated cases.[14]

In the author's personal series, several patients were referred as isolated cases, but physical and X-ray examinations revealed that one of the parents also had the syndrome. Parents of apparently isolated cases should, therefore, be examined and investigated carefully, being mindful of the variation in expression. The condition appeared to be the result of a new mutation in 17 per cent of the fully investigated families in the author's series.

A paternal age effect was reported in a study of 12 sporadic cases[22] – the mean paternal age was 36.9 (control population 29.9) and maternal age 31.7 (control 26.5).

FEATURES OF THE SYNDROME

The major features shown in Table 15.1 are adapted from 53 patients reported by Professor Gorlin in his review,

Table 15.1 *Features of Gorlin syndrome*[a]

Multiple basal cell carcinomas	90%
Odontogenic keratocysts of jaws	90%
Calcified falx cerebri	>85%
Characteristic face	70%
Palmar and/or plantar pits	65%
Rib anomalies (splayed, fused, partially missing, bifid, etc.)	60%
Spina bifida occulta of cervical or thoracic vertebrae	60%
Calcified diaphragma sellae (bridged sella, fused clinoids)	60–80%
Hyperpneumatization of paranasal sinuses	60%
Epidermoid cysts of skin	>50%
Enlarged occipitofrontal circumference	>50%
Mild ocular hypertelorism	>50%
Calcification of tentorium cerebelli	40%
Lumbarization of sacrum	40%
Kyphoscoliosis or other vertebral anomalies	30–40%
Pseudocystic lytic lesion of bones (hamartomas)	35%
Facial milia	30%
Calcified ovarian fibromas	24%
Calcification of petroclinoid ligament	20%
Short fourth metacarpals	20%
Pectus excavatum or carinatum	15–49%
Strabismus (exotropia)	14%
Cataract, glaucoma, coloboma of iris, retina, optic nerve, medullated retinal nerve fibres	7%
Grand mal seizures	6%
Sprengel deformity of scapula	5–25%
Cleft lip and/or palate	5.7%
Medulloblastoma	5%
Cardiac fibroma	2.5%
Meningioma	1%

Less than 5% – but not random
Lymphomesenteric cysts
Inguinal hernia
Fetal rhabdomyoma
Marfanoid build
Agenesis of corpus callosum
Cyst of septum pellucidum
Postaxial polydactyly – hands or feet
Subcutaneous calcifications of skin
Minor kidney malformations
Hypogonadism in males
Undescended testes
Mental retardation 0/80 had moderate or severe retardation

[a] Features are arranged in order of approximate frequency, and figures given where available. Features where a more precise figure is unavailable are listed together at the end of the appropriate part of the table. In addition, many other features have been reported, but it is difficult to know whether these are truly related to the syndrome, or have occurred in an affected patient by chance.

information from the literature and the author's own observations of over 150 patients, many of whom have been followed for more than 10 years. Some features are described in more detail below. Several large studies all give similar results.[13,14,23,24]

Skin

MILIA, EPIDERMOID AND MEIBOMIAN CYSTS

Small keratin filled cysts (milia) are found on the face in 30 per cent, most commonly in the infraorbital areas but they can also occur on the forehead. Larger epidermoid cysts (usually 1–2 cm in diameter) occur on the limbs and trunk in over 50 per cent of cases. In a survey of the UK Gorlin Syndrome Group, 15 out of 33 respondents had developed meibomian cysts on the eyelids.

PALMAR/PLANTAR PITS

The distinctive pits found on the palms and soles appear to be pathognomonic.[25] They increase in number with age, are permanent and, when found in a child, are a strong diagnostic indicator. Their number may vary from only a few to greater than a hundred. Basal cell carcinomas have very rarely arisen in the base of the pits.

In the author's series, 65 per cent had palmar pits by the age of 10 rising to 80 per cent by age 15. They were present in 85 per cent cases over the age of 20 years. The pits are small (1–2 mm), often asymmetric, shallow depressions, with the colour of the base being white flesh-coloured or pale pink (Figure 15.1). They are found more commonly on the palms (77 per cent) than on the soles (50 per cent). Pits can also appear independently on the sides of the fingers, when they are tiny, bright red pinpricks. They are easier to see in patients who undertake manual labour and may be better visualized if the patient's hands are soaked in warm water for about 10 minutes.

The pits appear to be caused by premature desquamation of horny cells along the intercellular spaces but they are not due to degeneration of the horny cells themselves. Light microscopy reveals a lack of keratinization of pit tissue and a proliferation of basaloid cells in irregular rete ridges.[26]

CAFÉ AU LAIT PATCHES

A few café au lait patches are commonly present, usually on the trunk, which may lead to consideration of a diagnosis of neurofibromatosis, especially in those patients with a large head circumference. Axillary freckling, however, is not found.

NAEVI AND BASAL CELL CARCINOMAS

As 'naevi' and the BCCs found in the syndrome are histologically identical, they can both be classified as naevoid basal cell carcinomas (NBCCs). Clinically, however, the 'naevi' often develop first and behave differently from the BCCs, which can appear to arise from naevi. For the clinical description that follows, however, it can be helpful to consider 'naevi' and 'naevoid basal cell carcinomas' as though they were separate entities.

The naevi are flesh coloured, reddish brown or pearly, resembling moles, skin tags, ordinary naevus cell naevi or haemangiomas. The naevi tend to occur multiply in crops, their numbers increasing with time, although they can appear as individual lesions. Some grow rapidly for a few days to a few weeks, but then most remain static. A patient may develop no naevi, a few, or many hundreds. Ordinary naevus cell naevi, found in about 4 per cent of the general population, are present from birth.

'Naevi' may arise in any area of the skin, affecting the face, neck and upper trunk in preference to the abdomen, lower trunk and extremities. The areas around the eyes, the nose, the malar regions and the upper lip are the most frequently affected sites on the face, leading to a widespread view in the literature that sun exposure is an important factor.

Although naevi are found in 53 per cent of cases under the age of 20 years, only 14 per cent present clinically with a rapidly growing BCC, and it is even more unusual to develop aggressive BCCs before puberty. Seventy four per cent of patients over the age of 20 years have developed a BCC, rising to 90 per cent of white Caucasians by the age of 40. Note that 10 per cent of patients do not develop BCCs: lifestyle, environmental or other genetic factors affording this protection are not known. However, skin pigmentation is known to be protective. Thirty per cent of Italian patients developed BCCs,[24] a figure similar to the 28 per cent (4 out of 11) already established in African Americans.[27] Skin pigmentation does not protect from the adverse events of ionizing radiation.[28]

Only a few naevi may subsequently become aggressive, when they may be locally invasive and behave like ordinary BCCs. Evidence of aggressive transformation of an individual lesion includes, as expected, an increase in size,

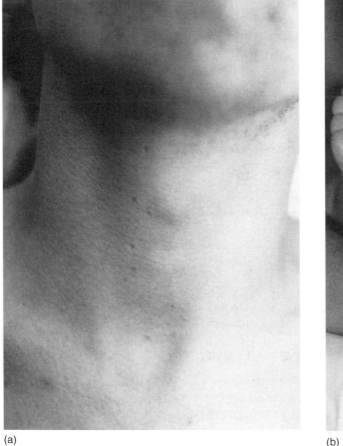

(a)

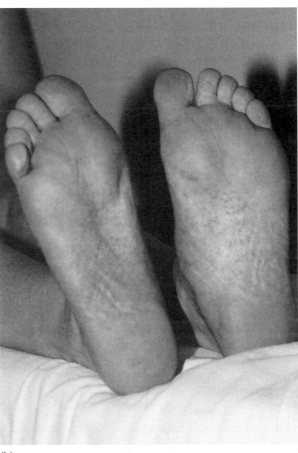

(b)

Figure 15.1 *Palmar/plantar pits [a]. The typical 'white' pits associated with the syndrome, most commonly found on the palms. As palmar pits can be difficult to photograph, shown here are typical pits on the neck of a 21-year-old man, although it is very unusual to develop the pits elsewhere other than the palms and soles. (b). A large number of small pink pits of pinprick size on the soles. These are found more often on the soles than the larger 'white' pits as shown in (a). The pink pits are also often found on the sides of fingers.*

ulceration, bleeding or crusting. It is rare for metastasis to occur. About one-third of patients have two or more types of BCCs, including superficial, multicentric, solid, cystic, adenoid and lattice-like.[29] NBCCs are more commonly associated with melanin pigmentation and foci of calcification than ordinary BCCs.

The clinical behaviour of the skin lesions may suggest that inactivation of the remaining *PTCH* gene in a cell causes a 'naevus' with additional subsequent cellular events causing aggressive behaviour.

Jaw cysts

Cysts of the jaws are a major feature of the syndrome. They are termed odontogenic keratocysts because a great deal of evidence suggests that their origin is the primordial odontogenic epithelium and their linings keratinize.

Some odontogenic keratocysts appear on X-rays to be dentigerous cysts, that is, a cyst that encloses the crown of an unerupted tooth and is attached at its neck. However, the majority of these are not true dentigerous cysts when examined histologically: a layer of fibrous tissue separates the crown from the adjacent cyst cavity. A cyst may impede the eruption of a related tooth or envelop an unerupted tooth to produce a dentigerous appearance.

The cysts may develop during the first decade of life, usually after about the seventh year, with a peak incidence in the second or third decade. This peak is about 10 years earlier than that associated with isolated odontogenic keratocysts. In one series,[13] 82 per cent of patients had developed a cyst by the age of 20 and only 10 per cent of patients over the age of 40 had not developed a cyst.

SITE

The mandible is involved far more frequently (75 per cent) than the maxilla. About one-half of odontogenic keratocysts occur at the angle of the mandible. The cysts also occur mainly in the canine to premolar area, in the mandibular retromolar–ramus area and in the region of the maxillary second molar. They may form in the midline of the mandible and maxilla, and may cross the midline. Asymptomatic, relatively small, single unilocular lesions may be detected by screening but large bilateral multilocular cysts involving both jaws are more often found when investigation follows clinical symptoms.

CLINICAL PRESENTATION

Most cysts are diagnosed on X-ray examination in the absence of symptoms (Figure 15.2). Occasionally, they become infected and cause pain or discharge, or cause swelling by expansion of the jaws. Patients are usually remarkably free of symptoms until the cysts have reached a large size, especially when the ascending ramus is involved, because the cyst extends into the medullary cavity. The enlarging cyst may cause displacement or loosening of teeth. It is rare for a cyst to cause a pathological fracture but they can cause swelling by extending into the soft tissues after perforating the cortex.

RECURRENCES

The odontogenic keratocyst has a tendency to recur after surgical treatment, with reported rates as high as 62 per cent. New cysts may form from satellite cysts associated with the original or from the dental lamina. True recurrences may be the result of incomplete surgical eradication.

PATHOLOGY

The histological features are characteristic.[30] The cysts are lined by a parakeratotic stratified squamous epithelium, which is usually about 5–8 cell layers thick and without rete ridges. Rarely, the form of keratinization is orthokeratotic. The basal layer is well defined with regularly orientated palisaded cells. Satellite cysts, epithelial rests and proliferating dental lamina are sometimes seen in the cyst capsules.

Immunocytochemical staining for Ki67 expression can differentiate between keratocysts associated with the

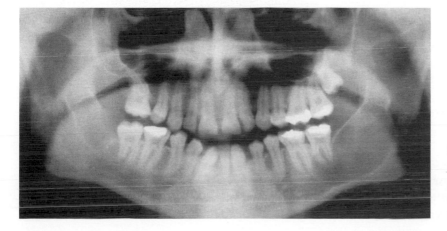

Figure 15.2 *Orthopantogram of the jaws of a 16-year-old male showing a large cyst beginning in the posterior body of the left mandible, extending into the ramus.*

syndrome and non-syndromic simple and recurrent keratocysts.[31]

Musculoskeletal system

Musculoskeletal features may be readily apparent on clinical examination. X-ray investigation may be helpful when the syndrome is suspected but physical signs are equivocal.[32]

HEIGHT

Patients tend to be very tall. Their heights are usually over the 97 centile, often in marked contrast to unaffected siblings. Some patients exhibit a marfanoid build.

SHAPE AND SIZE OF CRANIUM

One of the most striking features is the increased head size, which is present from birth. All children and adults in the author's series had a head circumference on or above the 97th centile, and above the corresponding centile line for height. The head gives the appearance of being long in the anterior–posterior (AP) plane, with a prominent and low occiput. The calvarium is usually large, with frontal and biparietal bossing. The occiput is low and the interorbital distance increased (usually in proportion to the head circumference). Platybasia is frequent.

SPINE AND CHEST

As rib and spine anomalies are present at birth, they are helpful diagnostic signs but 14 per cent of cases do not have anomalies of cervicothoracic spine and/or ribs. Bifid, anteriorly splayed, fused, partially missing or hypoplastic ribs are found in 60 per cent (Figure 15.3) and may give an unusual shape to the chest, including a characteristic downward sloping of the shoulders. The rib anomalies, together with kyphoscoliosis may cause pectus excavatum or carinatum in about 30–40 per cent of patients.

Abnormalities of the cervical or thoracic vertebrae are helpful diagnostic signs, being found in about 60 per cent. C6, C7, T2 and T1 are most frequently involved. Spina bifida occulta of the cervical vertebrae or malformations at the occipitovertebral junction are common. In addition to lack of fusion of the cervical or upper thoracic vertebrae, fusion or lack of segmentation has been documented in about 40 per cent. A defective medial portion of the scapula is occasionally found. Bifid ribs, cervical ribs and synostosis of ribs occur in 6.25, 1.7 and 2.6 per 1000, respectively, of the normal population.[33]

BONE CYSTS

Bone cysts are found in about 35 per cent of patients. There may be just one or two small pseudocystic lytic lesions, most often affecting the phalanges, metapodial,

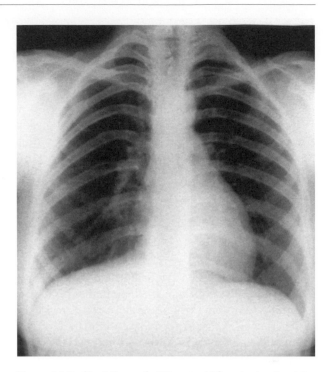

Figure 15.3 *Chest X-ray of a 25-year-old female showing spina bifida occulta of T1 and T2, bifid right fourth and fifth ribs, and variation in thickness of the anterior ends of the ribs, particularly the right second rib.*

and carpal and tarsal bones, but they can be multiple. Occasionally, they are large and involve an entire long bone or the pelvis, generating diagnostic uncertainty and resulting in multiple investigations. Lesions in the calvarium may raise concern that a medulloblastoma has extended into bone. Histology reveals that the lesions are hamartomas composed of fibrous connective tissue, blood vessels and nerves.[34,35]

OTHER BONE ANOMALIES

Thumb anomalies (short terminal phalanges and/or small stiff thumbs) occur in about 10 per cent. Preaxial or postaxial polydactyly of hands or feet is found in about 5 per cent. Syndactyly of second and third fingers is occasionally found. The fourth metacarpal is short in 15–45 per cent of patients but is not a good diagnostic sign, as it is found in about 10 per cent of the normal population. Hallux valgus can be severe, requiring operation. A defective medial portion of the scapula has been reported occasionally.

Ectopic calcification

Calcification of the falx cerebri occurs in at least 85 per cent patients by the age of 20, rising to 95 per cent soon after this age, and should be regarded as an extremely important diagnostic sign. The calcification can appear

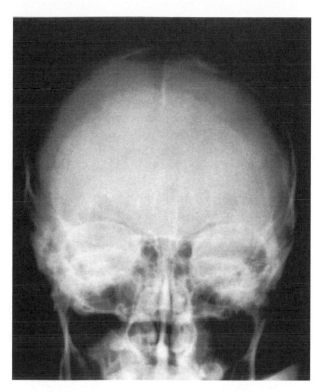

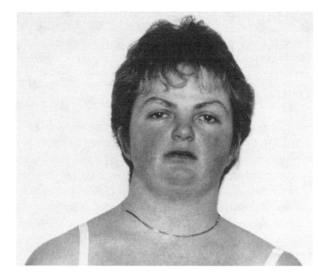

Figure 15.5 *A patient showing many of the facial features associated with the syndrome: arched eyebrows, down-slanting palpebral fissures, prominent jaw, naevi on the neck and chest, sloping shoulders. The frontal bossing is disguised by the cut of the hair.*

Figure 15.4 *Skull X-ray of a 17-year-old male showing calcification of the upper falx, with the typical lamellar appearance.*

very early in life and is often strikingly apparent from late childhood. It has a characteristic lamellar appearance (Figure 15.4), in comparison with the single sheet of calcification found in 7 per cent of the normal older population. Calcification of the falx cerebri in a child should strongly raise Gorlin syndrome as a diagnosis. A normal variant of the skull, a prominent frontal crest, can simulate falx calcification on the AP skull film and should be considered if the calcification appears to be a single line beginning inferiorly. Conversely, the diagnosis should be reconsidered if an adult with non-mosaic Gorlin syndrome does not have calcification of the falx.[36]

Ectopic calcification also occurs in other membranes: the tentorium cerebelli (40 per cent) and petroclinoid ligaments (20 per cent), the dura, pia and choroid plexus. Calcification of the diaphragma sellae causing the appearance of bridging of the sella turcica is found in 80 per cent and is an early sign; this is found in 4 per cent of the normal population in later life.

Calcification may occur subcutaneously in apparently otherwise normal skin of the fingers and scalp.

Craniofacial features

FACIES

About 70 per cent of patients have a characteristic facies (Figure 15.5) but there is intrafamilial variation. Some members of a sibship may have the typical shape to the skull, for instance, while others do not. One of the most striking features is the increased head size (in all adults in our series the head circumference was over 60 cm and above the corresponding centile line for height). The head gives the appearance of being long in the AP plane, with a prominent and low occiput. Frontal, temporal and biparietal bossing give a prominent appearance to the upper part of the face and patients often adopt hairstyles that disguise the bossing. There is often facial asymmetry. Some patients have well developed supraorbital ridges, giving the eyes a sunken appearance. The eyebrows are often heavy, fused and arched. There is a broad nasal root and hypertelorism. The inner canthal, interpupillary and outer canthal distances are all generally above the 97th centile, but appear to be in proportion with the head circumference. The mandible is long and often prominent with the lower lip protruding in front of the upper.

OPHTHALMIC PROBLEMS

In a personally examined series, 26 per cent of cases had ophthalmic problems. Of these 18 patients, ten had a convergent strabismus and three members of a family had rotatory nystagmus. Cataracts were present in four cases and microphthalmia in a single case. A total of 10–15 per cent of patients reported in the literature have ophthalmic abnormalities, including congenital blindness due to corneal opacity, congenital glaucoma, coloboma of the iris, choroid or optic nerve, convergent or divergent strabismus and nystagmus. Medullated nerve fibres and retinal hamartomas have also been noted.

CLEFT LIP AND PALATE

There is a well-established association with cleft lip/palate, which occurs in 5–6 per cent.

Central nervous system

Medulloblastoma (now often called primitive neuroectodermal tumour; PNET) is a well-recognized complication of the syndrome, with an incidence of about 5 per cent. Gorlin syndrome is found in about 3 per cent of children with medulloblastoma and in 10 per cent of those under the age of 2 years.[37,38] The average age of presentation is 2 years, about 5 years before the average age of presentation in children with isolated medulloblastoma. Patients with medulloblastoma associated with Gorlin syndrome are likely to have long-term survival, perhaps associated with the desmoplastic nature of the lesion, but there is a high chance that craniospinal irradiation will result in hundreds of BCCs appearing in the irradiated field.[39–42] There is an additional concern that there may be an increased risk of other second cancers in the radiation field.[43] Meningioma, glioblastoma multiforme and craniopharyngioma have also been described.

In the literature 'mental retardation' has been reported in about 3 per cent. In the population study in the North West of England (apart from treated cases of medulloblastoma), there were no cases of moderate or severe mental retardation in 84 cases.[13] About 6 per cent of patients in that study required prolonged anticonvulsant therapy for grand mal seizures.

Developmental history

Sixty two per cent of children in a personal series had an operative delivery. The average birth weight was 4.1 kg, and head circumference 38 cm, both greatly increased when compared with siblings. Walking was delayed until an average of 18 months; siblings walked at 12–13 months. Several children had investigations for hydrocephalus because of macrocephaly – the head circumference was above the 97th centile but growth continued parallel with the centile lines. Many children initially have a mild motor delay but appear to catch up. All children known to the author have attended mainstream school, a few needing additional help.

Genitourinary system

OVARIAN FIBROMA

In a population study,[13] 25 asymptomatic women with the syndrome underwent abdominal ultrasound and pelvic X-ray examination and 24 per cent had evidence of an ovarian fibroma. Fibromas were found at caesarian section in a woman in whom no abnormality had been detected with imaging.

Ovarian fibromas do not seem to reduce fertility; the main concern is that they may undergo torsion. They may be mistaken for calcified uterine fibroids, especially if they overlap medially. There is no evidence to suggest that they should be removed prophylactically. If operative treatment is required, preservation of ovarian tissue is recommended.[44]

Ovarian fibromas that are bilateral, calcified and multinodular should suggest a search for other features of Gorlin syndrome. Ovarian fibromas, in general, usually form a single mass replacing one ovary, and less than 10 per cent are bilateral or demonstrate calcification. Ovarian fibrosarcoma and other ovarian tumours have been reported, but these are extremely rare.

HYPOGONADOTROPHIC HYPOGONADISM IN MALES

Gorlin estimates that perhaps 5–10 per cent of males show such signs of hypogonadotrophic hypogonadism as anosmia, cryptorchidism, female pubic escutcheon, and scanty facial or body hair.[21] The author has only one case with abnormal endocrinological results in his series.

RENAL MALFORMATIONS

Kidney malformations (horseshoe kidney, unilateral renal agenesis, renal cysts) have been described in isolated case reports but detailed information is not available.

Other findings

MESENTERY

Just as cysts of the skin and jaws are integral parts of the syndrome, so are chylous or lymphatic cysts of the mesentery, although these are rare. They may present, if large, as painless movable masses in the upper abdomen or, rarely, may cause symptoms of obstruction. In most cases, however, they are discovered at laparotomy or on X-ray, if calcified.

CARDIOVASCULAR SYSTEM

In the North West England population study, cardiac fibroma was found to have a frequency of 2.5 per cent.[13] One child died at 3 months of age from multiple cardiac fibromas, while another case has been followed for over 20 years with a single 2 cm cardiac fibroma in the interventricular septum and this has remained unchanged. Long-term prognosis is generally good, but resection may be necessary. The incidence in childhood of an isolated cardiac fibroma is between 0.027 and 0.08 per cent, affecting most frequently the interventricular septum.

NEOPLASIA IN OTHER ORGANS

Tumours in many other organs have been reported in patients with the syndrome. They include renal fibroma, melanoma, leiomyoma, rhabdomyosarcoma, adenoid cystic carcinoma, adrenal cortical adenoma, seminoma, fibroadenoma of the breast, thyroid adenoma, carcinoma of the bladder, Hodgkin's disease and chronic leukaemia. In a personal series, affected people died from Hodgkin's disease, myeloma, renal cell carcinoma, seminoma and lung cancer. There does not appear to be a particular neoplasm occurring at a frequency which would warrant selective screening.

RESPONSE OF PATIENTS TO ULTRAVIOLET AND IONIZING RADIATION

Clinical response to therapeutic radiation

Clinical experience confirms that some patients are extremely sensitive to treatment by radiation, developing new lesions in the irradiated field, while others do not appear to be as clinically radiosensitive. Radiosensitive patients may develop more long-term complications from this treatment than from the original BCCs (Figure 15.6).[45,46] The molecular basis has not been delineated yet and, until the susceptibility of individuals can be identified, avoidance of treatment by radiotherapy is strongly recommended for all patients.

Children who received craniospinal irradiation as part of the treatment for a medulloblastoma[39–42] or Hodgkin's disease[47] have developed thousands of BCCs in the irradiated area. The BCCs often develop within an extremely short latent period of 6 months to 3 years. This is earlier than, and in a distribution different from, other affected family members.[45] NBCCS patients treated for eczema by irradiation to the hands have developed multiple BCCs on the palms.

Increased skin pigmentation may be protective against ultraviolet but not ionizing radiation, as an African-American boy treated with craniospinal irradiation for a medulloblastoma developed numerous BCCs in the irradiated area.[28]

Ultraviolet (UV) radiation

Circumstantial evidence that exposure to sunlight may be deleterious comes from population studies: 14 per cent of cases in a North West England study[13] developed a BCC before the age of 20, compared with 47 per cent in Australia (G. Chenevix-Trench, personal communication). However, the genetic background of the population itself may influence sensitivity to skin cancer.[47] A questionnaire study of 16 NBCCS families in the USA[48] did not find a strong relation between numbers of BCCs in white-skinned people and a history of lifetime sun exposure. In agreement with the literature, only two of their eight black-skinned patients reported a BCC.

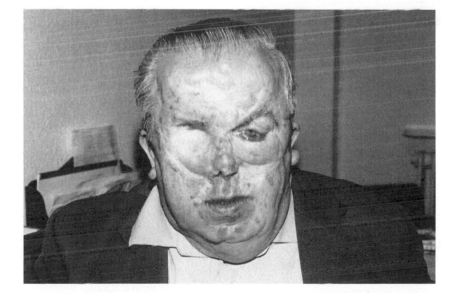

Figure 15.6 *A patient aged 63 showing the effects of multiple facial basal cell carcinomas (BCCs) and treatment. Facial BCCs appeared when he was 28; at the age of 40, multiple BCCs, involving the whole of his right and left lower eyelids, and extending on to the upper eyelids, were treated with excision and radiotherapy. Although new lesions continued to appear in areas not previously irradiated, at the age of 46 he developed multiple recurrences in the area previously treated by radiotherapy. These BCCs behaved extremely aggressively so that, at the age of 47, his right eye had to be enucleated because of carcinomatous invasion of the cornea. The BCCs in the irradiated area were multifocal and cicatricial with diffuse dermal infiltration.*

The distribution of BCCs in white-skinned patients differed from the general population: 35 per cent of BCCs occurred on the trunk, compared with 10.5 per cent in the general population. It was suggested that either frequent sun exposure is not essential for the development of BCCs or patients may be susceptible to low levels of sun exposure.

Variations in DNA repair ability could be a contributing factor based on evidence from patients with xeroderma pigmentosum and otherwise normal patients who had BCCs under the age of 30. *PTCH* mutations occur frequently in sporadic BCCs and in BCCs associated with xeroderma pigmentosum,[49] but less than 50 per cent of patched mutations in sporadic BCCs have the typical UVB signature caused by photodimers.[50] This contrasts with UV-specific *PTCH* mutations in 90 per cent of BCCs from six patients with xeroderma pigmentosum.[51] The inability of xeroderma pigmentosum patients to repair UV-induced *PTCH* mutations appears likely to contribute to the early and frequent BCCs in that syndrome and raises the possibility that the difference in clinical numbers of BCCs in Gorlin syndrome may be due to differences in repair mechanisms.

Ultraviolet-specific nucleotide changes, demonstrated in the *TP53* and *PTCH* genes in BCCs from otherwise clinically normal patients under the age of 30, led Zhang[52] to speculate that such young individuals might have decreased DNA repair ability and that, in such people, UV exposure is, indeed, an important risk factor.

Laboratory findings

In vitro studies of cellular ionizing and ultraviolet radiation hypersensitivity have been undertaken to try to understand the sensitivity to therapeutic irradiation shown by some patients. They continue to give conflicting results. Whether these reflect small sample size and perhaps suboptimal choice of controls, or true disease heterogeneity in cellular responses[53] remains to be determined. Important clinical information (whether or not a patient shows clinical hypersensitivity to the induction of BCCs by irradiation) is not given in most reports.

There may also be differences between different cell types: keratinocytes, for instance, from both Gorlin syndrome and normal donors are more resistant to UVC and X-rays than skin-derived fibroblasts.[54] In one patient with unilateral Gorlin syndrome where fibroblasts from the unaffected side could be used as control cells, there was no difference in X-ray, UV-B or UV-C radiation sensitivity compared with the affected side.[55]

Ionizing radiation

Little found that, overall, the X-ray response of cells from affected individuals showed no systematic difference from that of cells from non-affected relatives, or cell-bank controls for either cytotoxicity or chromosome breakage.[53] One of four affected Gorlin syndrome patients showed a moderate degree of radiation hypersensitivity, whereas the remaining affected and non-affected individuals from the same family responded normally. The response of cells from four other patients who had developed radiation-induced tumours also fell within the normal range. They suggested that isolated cases of *in vitro* radiation hypersensitivity probably do not relate to the underlying genetic disorder.

Gamma-irradiation resulted in deregulation of cell-cycle control and apoptosis in lymphoblastoid cell lines from three patients (two of whom were siblings) with NBCCS.[56] The fraction of apoptotic cells was lower in the NBCCS cells compared with controls, as was the level of p27 expression, but p53, p21 and Rb expression was similar to the controls.

It does appear that the cancer susceptibility is neither caused by nor manifested as chromosome instability,[57] nor that increased cell killing is a major effect of the gene.

ULTRAVIOLET RADIATION

Laboratory experiments with UV radiation have also been inconclusive. Fibroblasts have been found to have no differences in sensitivity[58] following UVC, while others were more sensitive to UVC.[59] The majority of experiments have been conducted with UVC radiation (254 nm), but epidemiological and clinical studies indicate that UVB radiation (280–320 nm) in sunlight is responsible for the induction of most skin cancers in humans.

Gorlin syndrome fibroblasts have been shown to be hypersensitive to killing by UVB but not UVC radiation[60,61] compared with skin fibroblasts from normal individuals. This was not due to a defect in the excision repair of pyrimidine dimers.[62]

Mouse model

There is supporting evidence in an animal model for the adverse effects of radiation. Mice heterozygous for an inactivating *ptc* mutation showed features associated with Gorlin syndrome.[62] They were larger than normal, and a subset developed extra digits, syndactyly, soft tissue tumours and cerebellar medulloblastomas. Homozygous mice died during embryogenesis, and had open and overgrown neural tubes.

With age, the mice heterozygous for an inactivating *ptc* mutation spontaneously developed BCC-like tumours.[63] However, the BCCs were of far greater number and size in mice that had received UV irradiation. A single dose of ionizing radiation markedly enhanced development of BCCs.

DIAGNOSIS AND DIFFERENTIAL DIAGNOSIS

Diagnosis

Confirming or refuting the diagnosis of Gorlin syndrome is vital for appropriate surveillance and treatment, not only for the affected patient but also for other family members, who may be completely asymptomatic at the time of diagnosis. Diagnosis depends on a detailed family history, and physical and X-ray examinations. Direct mutation analysis, or gene tracking when a mutation has not been determined, may also be helpful. Families are increasingly asking for mutation analysis after birth to aid in management, particularly to determine whether protective measures against excessive sunlight should be instituted.

Family history

The different presentations of the syndrome, especially the variability in severity between family members, should be borne in mind while taking the family history. A detailed physical examination and X-ray investigations of the parents of an apparently isolated case should be obligatory before concluding that the patient's condition is the result of a new mutation.

Physical examination

Examination should particularly seek physical signs in the skeletal system and skin, and note any congenital anomalies, such as clefting or polydactyly. Measurements should include height, head circumference, and inner- and outer-canthal and interpupillary distances. The head circumference should be plotted on a chart that takes height into account.[64] Examination should include a search for palmar/plantar pits. Features that may otherwise be disregarded should be specifically noted: frontal bossing, rib cage and spinal anomalies, milia, skin cysts, short stiff thumbs and hallux valgus.

X-ray investigations

X-ray signs may aid diagnosis in family members who have equivocal physical signs.[32,36] X-rays recommended include:

- panoramic views of the jaws (plain films may miss lesions);
- skull – AP;
- skull – lateral;
- chest X-ray;
- thoracic spine – AP and lateral;
- hands (for pseudocysts).

Table 15.2 *Diagnostic criteria for naevoid basal cell carcinoma syndrome. A diagnosis can be made when two major, or one major and two minor, criteria are fulfilled*

Major criteria
1 Multiple (>2[a]) basal cell carcinomas or one under the age of 30 years or >10 basal cell naevi
2 Odontogenic keratocyst (proven on histology) or polyostotic bone cyst
3 Palmar or plantar pits (three or more)
4 Ectopic calcification
   lamellar or early (<20 years) falx calcification
5 First-degree relative affected

Minor criteria
1 Congenital skeletal anomaly
   bifid, fused, splayed or missing rib or fused vertebrae
2 OFC > 97 centile with bossing
3 Cardiac or ovarian fibroma
4 Medulloblastoma (primitive neuroectodermal tumour, PNET)
5 Lymphomesenteric or pleural cysts
6 Congenital malformation
   cleft lip and/or palate, polydactyly, eye anomaly (cataract, coloboma, microphthalmia)

[a]Note that the numbers of basal cell carcinomas (BCCs) given were based on a study carried out in England; the numbers of BCCs for diagnosis will be inappropriate for sunnier climes!
OFC, occipito-frontal circumference

ULTRASOUND EXAMINATION

Ultrasound examinations for ovarian and cardiac fibromas may be helpful.

DIAGNOSTIC CRITERIA

Diagnostic criteria are given in Table 15.2 based on the most frequent and/or specific features of the syndrome. These criteria were based on examination of family cases in England, a land not noted for excessive sunlight. The numbers of BCCs acceptable as a major criterion will vary according to the climate, and will need adaptation for countries such as Australia.

DIAGNOSIS BY MOLECULAR TECHNIQUES

In some children, clinical examination may not be conclusive because of age-dependent features of the syndrome, and mutation analysis for the familial mutation can be justified to institute surveillance and sun-screening precautions. The demand for prenatal diagnosis has been low.

Identifying a pathogenic mutation (nonsense, frameshift, deletion/insertion, splice site) in *PTCH* will of course confirm a clinical diagnosis. Because of technical limitations, a negative mutation screen cannot rule out NBCCS but, in an individual falling short of clinical diagnostic criteria, it will at least be partially reassuring as long as a comprehensive analysis has been performed. Missense mutations are relatively common but, in an isolated patient falling short of diagnostic criteria, they may be difficult to interpret.

Diagnosis by gene tracking using closely linked or intragenic markers may be possible depending on the family structure. Locus heterogeneity has not been reported in studies from central Europe and the UK,[1,2] the USA[3] and Australasia,[65] despite the wide range of features of the syndrome both between and within families.

Mutation detection appears to be less sensitive in the first affected individual in a family owing to somatic mosaicism. Evidence for mosaicism includes the finding of an identical *PTCH* mutation in two or more tumours not present in lymphocyte DNA.

Differential diagnosis

The following conditions may need to be considered when a patient presents with only some of the features of the syndrome.

- Patients with somatic mosaicism for a *PTCH* mutation usually show milder features of the syndrome or only one or two of its signs.
- Localized mosaicism for a *PTCH* somatic mutation is likely to be the cause of multiple basal cell carcinomas, comedones and epidermoid cysts in a unilateral distribution.[66]
- Multiple BCCs, follicular atrophoderma on the dorsum of hands and feet, hypohydrosis and hypotrichosis are features of Bazex syndrome (OMIM 301845). The pitting on the backs of the hands is reminiscent of orange peel and quite unlike the pits of Gorlin syndrome. The inheritance pattern is uncertain: either autosomal or X-linked dominant.[67]
- A dominantly inherited condition similiar to Bazex syndrome was reported in a single family. Rombo syndrome (OMIM 180730) is characterized by vermiculate atrophoderma, milia, hypotrichosis, trichoepitheliomas, BCCs and peripheral vasodilation with cyanosis. The skin is normal until later childhood, BCCs develop later and there is no reduction in sweating.[68]
- A single family with another autosomal or X-linked dominant syndrome of coarse sparse scalp hair, basal cell carcinomas, milia and excessive sweating was reported by Oley *et al.* (OMIM 109390).[69]
- The differential diagnosis of the palmar pitting is porokeratosis of Mantoux,[25] which is a rare form of non-hereditary papular keratosis of the hands and feet, with a few lesions occasionally sprinkled over the ankles. The lesions are changeable and usually disappear with time. The depressions are always found on the summit of the papillary excrescences, resembling

an enlarged sudoriferous pore. Older lesions show a blackish vegetation with a finely lobulated or mulberry-like surface at the bottom of the depression, which is eventually shed, leaving a small depression with a slightly raised margin and a red base. The material resembles a cornified comedone. The characteristic lesion is a translucent papule, which erupts in recurring crops over months or years.

- Two families with multiple infundibulocystic BCCs showed no other signs of NBCCS, but *PTCH* mutation analysis was not performed. The behaviour of the BCCs was less aggressive than those of other types of pathological variants of BCCs – most of the lesions remained small and showed little tendency to ulcerate, very similar to some patients with NBCCS.[70]
- Rasmussen reported a family with trichoepitheliomas, milia and cylindromas presenting in the second and third decades.[71] Inheritance was autosomal dominant. The milia were miniature trichoepitheliomas and appeared only in sun-exposed areas. Cylindromatosis (Turban tumour syndrome) may be the same condition;[72] it shows considerable variation within families in the size and extent of distribution, and age of onset.
- Pseudohypoparathyroidism may be considered because of ectopic calcification and short fourth metacarpals.
- In Cowden syndrome (multiple hamartoma syndrome) mucocutaneous changes develop in the second decade.[73] Multiple facial papules, both smooth and keratotic, are associated with hair follicles and concentrated around the orifices. Small hyperkeratotic and verrucous growths are numerous on the dorsal aspect of the hands and feet, and round translucent palmoplantar keratoses are also common. Similar lesions, including verrucous papules, occur on the oral mucosa. Multiple skin tags are also frequent. Most patients have a broad forehead and a large head circumference. Neoplasms occur in the gastrointestinal system, thyroid and breast.
- Arsenic exposure may cause multiple BCCs.
- Cardiac fibromas are also found in tuberous sclerosis and Beckwith–Wiedemann syndrome.

PREVENTION AND SURVEILLANCE

It is recommended that families are offered regular screening, with perhaps one clinician or a genetic department monitoring and coordinating the programme.[13] Predictive testing by DNA analysis may be justified to identify family members for surveillance. Screening programmes may include the following.

During pregnancy

Ultrasound scans during pregnancy may detect cardiac tumours and developmental malformations, which may require early decisions about neonatal surgery, and extreme macrocephaly, which may necessitate operative delivery.

Neonatal

A detailed neonatal examination may confirm the physical signs of a large head, cleft palate or eye anomaly. X-rays may confirm bifid ribs or vertebral abnormalities. An echocardiogram is best performed early as at least two cases have presented before 3 months of age with fibromas.

Childhood

Six-monthly neurological examination may detect a deficit indicative of a medulloblastoma; computed tomography (CT) scanning in an asymptomatic child is not recommended because of concerns about inducing skin malignancies. At 3 years, the examinations could be reduced to annually until 7 years, after which a medulloblastoma is very unlikely. Although these physical examinations are of low sensitivity and specificity, a parent will have contact with a specialist department should suspicious symptoms develop.

Annual dental screening should commence from about 8 years, usually including a panoramic X-ray of the jaw. Orthopantograms are justified because of complications of untreated jaw cysts, but regular screening by CT scans is strongly to be avoided because of potential skin radiosensitivity resulting in multiple BCCs.

Regular examination of the skin from puberty is recommended, at least yearly, but more usually every 3 months. As a lesion may suddenly become aggressive, however, the patient needs open access to the specialist taking responsibility for treatment of the skin. It is especially important to offer early treatment for lesions of the eyelids, nose, ears and scalp. Patients must be warned to inspect all areas of the body – BCCs have been reported on the vulva and the mucosa of the anal sphincter.

Exposure to sunlight

As sunlight may be one of the environmental agents promoting the appearance of BCCs,[48] sun-screening precautions should be strongly recommended. These should include the wearing of a wide-brimmed hat to offer some protection to the areas around the eyes.

TREATMENT AND SUPPORT

Treatment may seem overwhelming and hopeless to patients with many hundreds of BCCs and multiple jaw cysts. A great deal of support may, therefore, be required, not least to encourage attendance at follow-up clinics and to accept early treatment. This support may need to extend to the whole family, including carers. Support groups specific for the syndrome are active in the UK and USA.

Basal cell carcinomas

LOCAL TREATMENT

Some patients have many naevi that remain symptomless for long periods, which can be kept under frequent review. Others have hundreds of aggressive BCCs. The molecular basis for the difference in behaviour is not known: this could be due to the effects of different genetic backgrounds or exposure to a potentiating environmental factor. Some practitioners urge treatment of all lesions, while others reserve treatment for those with evidence of progression.

The most suitable form of treatment may vary depending on the type, size and site of the NBCC. Surgical excision, cryotherapy, curettage and diathermy, topical 5-fluorouracil, Moh's microsurgery and carbon dioxide laser vaporization have all been used.[74] Radiotherapy should be avoided as discussed earlier. The priorities are to ensure complete eradication of aggressive BCCs and to preserve normal tissue to prevent disfigurement.

A systematic review could not recommend evidence-based guidelines[75] but, regarding recurrence rates, surgical excision was the treatment of first choice. For larger BCCs, especially on the face and those with aggressive behaviour, Moh's microsurgery[76] gives the best results. However, because of the potential for many hundreds of BCCs in Gorlin syndrome, patients wish to have non-surgical treatment modalities to preserve tissue whenever possible, several of which (imiquimod and photodynamic therapy) are under review. A concern of both is that nests of BCCs could remain and cause a recurrence, and long-term results are awaited.

Imiquimod is an immune response modifier, which induces cytokines, including interferons, and stimulates cell-mediated immunity. Its use as a patient administered treatment is promising.[77] A patient with NBCCS, who had three biopsy-proven non-facial BCCs, was treated with 5 per cent imiquimod cream for 18 weeks. Two that were felt to be treated adequately showed no residual tumour on removal. Although the patient tolerated the inflammatory response, he would not wish to have further treatment by imiquimod.[78]

SYSTEMIC RETINOIDS

There are a few reports of oral synthetic retinoids (etretinate, isotretinoin and 13-cis-retinoic acid) preventing the development of new tumours, inhibiting the growth of existing tumours and causing the regression of superficially invasive BCCs.

In a series of reports, Peck et al. followed the progress of 12 adult patients with multiple BCCs, five of whom had

Gorlin syndrome. Oral isotretinoin was given at 1 mg/kg per day increasing to an average maximum dose of 4.6 mg/kg per day for an average of 8 months. Approximately 8 per cent of 270 selected BCCs underwent complete clinical and histological remission. Twenty per cent of tumours showed partial regression and a further 44 per cent minimal regression. Five patients withdrew because of the side effects associated with retinoids. The dose of isoretinoin was reduced to 0.25–1.5 mg/kg per day in the seven remaining patients. Partial regression of tumours was shown in only one patient. New tumours started to develop in a patient with Gorlin syndrome when on a chemopreventative dose of isotretinoin of 0.25 mg/kg per day. He developed 29 new BCCs in the 13 months following discontinuation of treatment.[79]

In two reports,[80,81] etretinate at a dose of 1 mg/kg per day resulted in regression of 76 per cent and 83 per cent of lesions. Less aggressive surgery was required in a female patient, who received treatment with oral etretinate, initially at 1 mg/kg per day.[82]

Isoretinoin in a dose of 0.4 mg/kg per day prevented the formation of the majority of new BCCs and reduced the rate of growth of existing lesions in twin males who had hundreds of lesions.[83]

A child was managed for 10 years with a combination of topical 5-fluorouracil and tretinoin.[84] The hundreds of tumours disappeared after initiation of the combined therapy; most of the remaining tumours did not grow. The patient was examined every 3 months and lesions that demonstrated signs of growth or appeared to be deeply invasive were managed by shave excision and curettage. Development appeared normal and she showed neither clinical nor laboratory evidence of toxicity.

Potential teratogenicity and side effects, such as chelitis, pruritis, peeling of the palms and soles, eczema and diffuse idiopathic skeletal hyperostosis,[85] dictate that retinoids should be used in carefully controlled circumstances. Their long-term role in the management of the condition is still being assessed.

Experience in a chemoprevention study in xeroderma pigmentosum suggests that the retinoid is acting late in the pathogenesis of malignancy, and not in correcting the underlying defect in DNA repair.

TREATMENT BY RADIATION

Radiotherapy should be avoided because of clinical evidence that new lesions can appear in the irradiated field; this is reviewed in the earlier section on the response of patients to radiation.

PHOTODYNAMIC THERAPY

Photodynamic therapy (PDT) involves systemic or topical administration of a photosensitizer followed by exposure of the target area to light to produce activated oxygen species, which promote tumour destruction.[86] In 1984, Tse treated 40 BCCs in three NBCCS adult patients in whom conventional treatments had failed or were no longer possible, with 82.5 per cent complete and 17.5 per cent partial clinical response.[87] There was a 10.8 per cent recurrence rate. A 74-year-old patient with unilateral BCCs responded well to PDT;[88] a 26-year-old man had 13 lesions treated following intravenous SnET2, with no evidence of recurrence after 6 months.[89]

This approach is also being evaluated in Gorlin syndrome by the Roswell Park Cancer Institute in Buffalo, New York, USA (A.R. Roseroff, personal communication, 1997).[90] Although complete clinical BCC response rate was high (93 per cent) in 796 nodular and superficial lesions in 20 adults with 1 mg/kg systemic Photofrin, the results in three children were less satisfactory with a poorer response and scarring. Systemic PDT is, therefore, not recommended for prepubertal children. A major disadvantage of Photofrin is that it can produce a generalized photosensitivity for 4–8 weeks and so new-generation photosensitizers are being developed. Topical treatment with 5-aminolevulinic acid (ALA) has given a 95 per cent initial clinical response rate on treatment of 150 BCCs in two children with Gorlin syndrome who developed multiple lesions in fields irradiated for Hodgkin's disease and medulloblastoma. The healing response was better than with systemic administration of photosensitizer and left no scarring. This approach may prove to be especially useful in such cases where there are thousands of superficial BCCs.

At the Christie Hospital, Manchester, UK, a portable non-laser lamp has been used with topical ALA. Twenty-seven NBCCS patients have been treated with no difference in response rate from non-syndromic BCCs (96 per cent after 24 months) (E. Allan, personal communication, 2002).

Lesions less than 2 mm thick on diagnostic biopsy achieve a superior outcome[91] but a second-generation systemic photosensitizer, meta-tetrahydroxyphenylchlorin (mTHPC), used systemically may prove especially useful for nodular BCCs, as it can achieve tumour necrosis to a depth of 1 cm.[92]

Jaw cysts

As proliferating dental lamina and satellite cysts may occur in the fibrous wall of the primary cyst cavity, marsupialization may be successful only if no satellite cysts are left behind. Small single lesions with regular spherical outlines can usually be completely enucleated provided access is good. Stoelinga has recommended that the overlying mucoperiosteum should be excised for cysts close to the surface because of the possible origin of the cyst from basal cell proliferations.[93] For the large multilocular lesions, excision and immediate bone grafting is the treatment of choice at the first operation.

THE FUNCTION OF THE *PATCHED* GENE AND ITS ROLE IN DEVELOPMENT AND CANCER

The human gene was isolated by positional cloning.[94,95] It has strong homology with the *Drosophila patched* gene, which is involved in establishing segment polarity in embryos and which binds a secreted protein, hedgehog (hh), the interaction being conserved in vertebrates. The hh signalling pathway as demonstrated in *Drosophila* is complex, involving a large number of genes, the human homologues of which have not all been characterized. Indeed, a single gene in *Drosophila* often corresponds to a family of vertebrate homologues. An overview of the pathway (Figure 15.7), chiefly from information from studies in *Drosophila*, but incorporating information from the mouse and human, is given below.

PTCH associates with caveolin 1 (as well as hedgehog and smoothened) in the plasma membrane, which is believed to target PTCH to a specific area of the membrane. Caveolins do not appear to be involved in the mediation of the SHH signal. In the presence of SHH (Figure 15.7b), PTCH–SHH and SMO are rapidly internalized, and SMO segregated from the SHH–PTCH complex. SMO is recycled, during which a phosphorylation event occurs, to appear in the plasma membrane in a compartment free of PTCH. The PTCH– SHH complex is thought to be degraded. Smoothened activates a signal transduction cascade involving cubitus interruptus, ci, in *Drosphila* (vertebrate homologue GLI), which results in

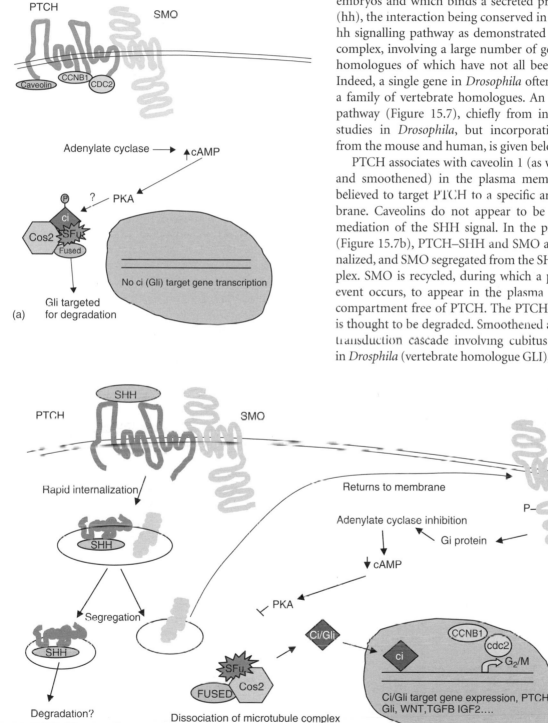

Figure 15.7 *The hedgehog signalling pathway in the absence (a) and presence (b) of SHH. See text for explanation.*

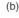

the transcription of a number of genes including decapentaplegic (transforming growth factor β), bone morphogenetic protein (BMP) and wingless (WNT) families, as well as PTCH itself, which takes part in a negative feedback mechanism of autoregulation. In vertebrates, the role of ci is achieved by complex interactions involving three Gli genes. It is not yet clear how SMO achieves its signalling, but it may act to negate PKA (cAMP-dependent protein kinase) activity through the inhibition of adenylate cyclase to reduce cytosolic cAMP levels.

In *Drosophila* cells not exposed to hh, ci forms a tetrameric complex with costal-2, fused and suppressor of fused at the microtubules (Figure 15.7a). Costal 2 and suppressor of fused inhibit the activation of ci and are negative regulators of the pathway. In this form, ci can be cleaved to a fragment retaining the zinc finger domain, which can translocate to the nucleus and repress downstream target genes. In the presence of hedgehog, the complex dissociates and full-length ci is thought to mature into a short-lived transcriptional activator. Within the tetrameric complex, Fused is believed to be activated by hedgehog signalling leading to release of active ci. PKA independently inhibits the activity of the hh pathway and is believed to act directly on ci, probably contributing to its degradation. Activation of the pathway results in PTCH protein being presented at the cell membrane, which sequesters hh and limits its spread beyond the cells in which it is produced (Figures 15.7a and b).

THE HUMAN *PATCHED* GENES, TRANSCRIPTIONAL REGULATION AND THE CELL CYCLE

The human *PTCH* gene consists of 23 exons covering 62 kb of genomic DNA. It encodes an integral membrane protein of 1500 amino acids with 12 transmembrane regions and two extracellular loops, which are required for hedgehog binding (Figure 15.8). Patched (PTCH) is probably the major receptor molecule for all three forms of human hedgehog.

A second *PTCH* gene, *PTCH2*, highly homologous to *PTCH*, was isolated from chromosome 1p32.1–32.2.[96] It is a transmembrane protein of 1203 amino acids, with 22 coding exons. It has low expression in adult tissues and its normal function is not known. A deletion of 2 bp was found in one sporadic medulloblastoma (germline DNA was not available) and a change in a splice donor site not present in germline DNA in one sporadic BCC. No mutations were found in 11 sporadic and 11 familial NBCCS patients in whom *PTCH* screening by SSCP had been negative, 8 families solely with multiple BCCs, 92 medulloblastoma samples and 21 BCCs.

Of the three vertebrate homologues of hh, sonic hedgehog (SHH) is the most widely expressed with major effects on development of the brain, spinal cord, axial skeleton and limbs. PTCH is also associated with smoothened (SMO), a seven-span transmembrane protein with structural similarity to G-protein-coupled receptors. It is an activator of transcription. In the absence of SHH, PTCH inhibits the SMO signalling, thereby resulting in repression of transcription of downstream genes. No direct interaction between PTCH and SMO has been detected, the evidence being that PTCH acts substoichiometrically on SMO.[97] The similarities between PTCH and bacterial transport proteins have led to the speculation that PTCH may transport small molecules that inhibit SMO.

When extracellular SHH binds to PTCH, patched is lost, but there is an increase in smoothened in the cell membrane[98] with an alteration in its phosphorylation status. As the inhibition of SMO is released, the signalling pathway is activated and transcription of downstream target genes ensues.

Human PTCH has three alternatively spliced first exons (1B, 1 and 1A), which are differentially regulated in normal tissues. All three transcripts encode proteins, which interact with smoothened but confer different levels of inhibition.[99] Exon 1B is expressed at low levels in normal tissues but is upregulated in BCCs.

PTCH has also been shown to be involved in cell-cycle regulation. It binds cyclin B1 and CDC2, which, after HH

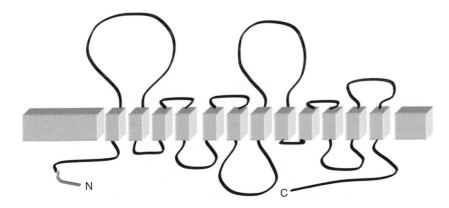

Figure 15.8 *Predicted human PTCH protein structure.*
PATCHED encodes a 12-pass transmembrane glycoprotein with two large extracellular domains and a smaller intracellular domain.

binding, are able to enter the nucleus where they are involved in the G2 → M phase transition.[100]

Mutations in components of the pathway and human diseases

Inherited or sporadic mutations in SHH-pathway genes have been implicated in a number of human birth defects and adult cancers.[8,101] Defects at several steps in the pathway lead to similar clinical phenotypes, presumably through functional effects on target genes downstream. For instance, the syndromes associated with mutations in the GLI genes particularly demonstrate skeletal features also found as components of the Gorlin syndrome. Holoprosencephaly is caused by sporadic and inherited mutations in *SHH*.

As inactivating *PTCH* mutations have been demonstrated in BCCs and medulloblastomas, it would be expected that activating *SMO* mutants might have the same effect. Indeed, these have been demonstrated in BCCs and medulloblastomas.

In the human there are three *GLI* genes, which encode transcription factors. Of the polydactyly syndromes associated with GLI3 gene anomalies, Greig syndrome has amongst its features several of the skeletal system hallmarks of Gorlin syndrome – polydactyly, broad thumbs and toes, hypertelorism and frontal bossing.

Inactivation of PTCH or oncogenic activation of SMO occurs in almost all BCCs, suggesting that dysregulation of SHH signalling is a prerequisite for BCC formation. Additional cellular events are then likely to be required – whether these will prove to be additional mutations or the upregulation of a normal process remains to be elucidated. For instance, additional mutations may be related to the effects of UV and ionizing radiation in some patients (and in a mouse model); enhanced hedgehog signalling would be predicted to increase the replicative capacity of cells and oppose cell cycle arrest.[102]

Phenotypic variability

The SHH-PTCH-GLI pathway appears to be sensitive to the levels of its various proteins. Any mutation or polymorphism in one or more of the genes may affect the amount of functional protein with consequent effects on the activation or repression of downstream genes. This mechanism – with levels of activity ranging from zero in truncating mutations or gene deletions to levels just below normal with other types of mutations – has the potential to produce a wide range of variation in transcription, so generating a spectrum of clinical presentation, as seen between and within families in Gorlin syndrome.

Complete inactivation of one allele results in the features of Gorlin syndrome, as shown in mice heterozygous for an inactivating ptc mutation. They were larger than normal, and a subset developed extra digits, syndactyly, soft tissue tumours and cerebellar medulloblastomas. Homozygous mice died during embryogenesis and had open and overgrown neural tubes.[103]

Human jaw cysts and BCCs are associated with loss of function of the wild-type allele releasing the cell from the remaining control of the SHH–PTCH–GLI pathway exerted by that allele. The majority of PTCH mutations in Gorlin syndrome cause truncation of the protein, adding further support to this hypothesis.

PTCH mutational spectrum in Gorlin syndrome

PTCH is the only gene currently known to be associated with Gorlin syndrome. Screening of the coding region has revealed a wide spectrum of mutations, the majority predicted to result in premature termination of the protein. Mutations are spread through the whole gene with no apparent clustering.

Mutations are detected in about 85 per cent of patients meeting diagnostic criteria. Experience shows that the detection rate is lowest in people who are the first affected individual in their family most probably because of somatic mosaicism as discussed earlier. The mutation may often be more easily detected if an affected child is tested. For patients in whom there is a clinical suspicion of mosaicism, detecting the same *PTCH* mutation in several tumours but not in lymphocyte DNA may confirm this.

The frequency of classes of mutations, obtained from the literature[94,95,104–107] and 120 mutations from the DNA Diagnostic Laboratory at Birmingham Women's Hospital, UK (August 2001) are:

- 65 per cent truncating mutations;
- 16 per cent missense mutations;
- 13 per cent splice site mutations;
- 6 per cent intragenic or large-scale deletions or rearrangements.

Early reports of mutations, which were mostly truncations, did not find a genotype–phenotype correlation.[107] However, a clinical suspicion is accumulating (P Farndon, unpublished data) that missense mutations may be associated with a milder phenotype.

A suggestion that reductions in PTCH activity below normal but at a level above that associated with haploinsufficiency could be sufficient for the development of some tumours and clinical features came from an experiment in mice. Three *PTCH* missense mutations, which had been identified clinically, were shown to have activities reduced by between 1.8- and 3.7-fold when introduced into murine ptc-deficient cells.[108]

However, it is not yet possible to make predictions about clinical severity for developmental and neoplastic features associated with specific mutations, as their effects are also likely to be modified by other genes and environmental factors.

Mutations in *PTCH* in conditions other than Gorlin syndrome

PTCH germline mutations cause a range of severity in Gorlin syndrome but they have not been associated with any other heritable syndromes.

Somatic mutations in *PTCH* have been reported in a range of sporadically occurring tumours, including those observed in Gorlin syndrome: non-syndromic BCC, skin trichoepithelioma, medulloblastoma, ovarian fibroma and keratocysts. UV-specific *PTCH* somatic mutations are a characteristic feature of BCCs from patients with xeroderma pigmentosum.[109]

Missense mutations of *PTCH* have been reported in holoprosencephaly, in five of 100 unrelated probands.[110] The authors hypothesized that the missense mutations would lead to enhanced *PTCH* repressive activity on the hedgehog signalling pathway, unlike the mechanism in NBCCS in which the pathway is activated, usually by haploinsufficiency for *PTCH*.

KEY POINTS

- Gorlin syndrome or nevoid basal cell carcinoma syndrome is an autosomal dominant condition with over 100 features.
- The most common features are nevoid basal cell carcinomas, odontogenic cysts, falx calcification, and pitting of the palms and soles.
- It is associated with ovarian fibromas, medulloblastoma, and cardiac fibromas.
- It is caused by mutations in the patched gene, *PTCH* on 9q22.

REFERENCES

1. Farndon PA, Del Mastro RD, Evans DGR, Kilpatrick MW. Location of gene for Gorlin syndrome. *Lancet* 1992; **339**:581–582.
2. Reis A, Kuster W, Gebel E, *et al.* Localisation of the gene for the naevoid basal cell carcinoma syndrome. *Lancet* 1992; **339**:617.
3. Gailani MR, Bale SJ, Leffell DJ, *et al.* Developmental defects in Gorlin syndrome related to a putative tumor suppressor gene on chromosome 9. *Cell* 1992; **69**:111–117.
4. Bonifas JM, Bare JW, Kerschmann RL, *et al.* Parental origin of chromosome 9q22.3–q31 lost in basal cell carcinomas from basal cell nevus syndrome patients. *Hum Mol Genet* 1994; **3**:447–448.
5. Levanat S, Gorlin RJ, Fallet S, *et al.* A two-hit model for developmental defects in Gorlin syndrome. *Nature Genet* 1996; **12**:85–87.
6. Hahn H, Wicking C, Zaphiropoulos PG, *et al.* Mutations of the human homolog of Drosophila patched in the nevoid basal cell carcinoma syndrome. *Cell* 1996; **85**:841–851.
7. Johnson RL, Rothman AL, Xie J, *et al.* Human homolog of *patched*, a candidate gene for the basal cell nevus syndrome. *Science* 1996; **272**:1668–1671.
8. Villavicencio EH, Walterhouse DO, Iannaccone PM. The sonic hedgehog-patched-Gli pathway in human development and disease. *Am J Hum Genet* 2000; **67**:1047–1054.
9. Gorlin RJ, Goltz RW. Multiple nevoid basal-cell epithelioma, jaw cysts and bifid rib: a syndrome. *N Engl J Med* 1960; **262**:908–912.
10. Howell JB, Caro MR. The basal cell nevus: its relationship to multiple cutaneous cancers and associated anomalies of development. *Arch Dermatol* 1959; **79**:67–80.
11. Gorlin RJ. Nevoid basal-cell carcinoma syndrome. *Medicine* 1987; **66**:96–113.
12. Gorlin RJ. Nevoid basal cell carcinoma syndrome. *Dermatol Clin* 1995; **13**:113–125.
13. Evans DGR, Ladusans EJ, Rimmer S, *et al.* Complications of the naevoid basal cell carcinoma syndrome: results of a population based study. *J Med Genet* 1993; **30**:460–464.
14. Shanley S, Ratcliffe J, Hockey A, *et al.* Nevoid basal cell carcinoma syndrome: review of 118 affected individuals. *Am J Med Genet* 1994; **50**:282–290.
15. Rahbari H, Mehregan AH. Basal cell epithelioma (carcinoma) in children and teenagers. *Cancer* 1982; **49**:350–353.
16. Summerly R. Basal cell carcinoma. An aetiological study of patients aged 45 and under with special reference to Gorlin's syndrome. *Br J Dermatol* 1965; **77**:9–15.
17. Chudina AP, Savluchinskaia LA, Mikhailovskii, Briuzgin VV. Detection of basal-cell nevus syndrome in patients with multiple skin basiliomas. *Voprosy Onkologii* 1989; **35**:1166–1169.
18. Honavar SG, Shields JA, Shields CL, *et al.* Basal cell carcinoma of the eyelid associated with Gorlin–Goltz syndrome. *Ophthalmology* 2001; **108**:1115–1123.
19. Shear M. *Cysts of the oral regions*, 2nd edn. A dental practitioner handbook, no 23. Bristol: Wright, 1983; 11.
20. Lench NJ, High AS, Markham AF, *et al.* Investigation of chromosome 9q22.3–q31 DNA marker loss in odontogenic keratocysts. *Oral Oncol Eur J Cancer* 1996; **32B**:202–206.
21. Gorlin RJ, Cohen MM, Hennekam RCM. *Syndromes of the head and neck*, 4th edn. Oxford: Oxford University Press, 2001; 444–453.
22. Jones KL, Smith DW, Harvey MA, *et al.* Older paternal age and fresh gene mutation: data on additional disorders. *J Pediatr* 1975; **86**:84–88.
23. Kimonis VE, Goldstein AM, Pastakia B, *et al.* Clinical manifestations in 105 persons with nevoid basal cell carcinoma syndrome. *Am J Med Genet* 1997; **69**:299–308.
24. Lo Muzio L, Nocini PF, Savoia A, *et al.* Nevoid basal cell carcinoma syndrome: clinical findings in 37 Italian affected individuals. *Clin Genet* 1999; **55**:34–40.
25. Howell JB, Mehregan AH. Pursuit of the pits in the nevoid basal cell carcinoma syndrome. *Arch Dermat* 1970; **102**:586–597.

26. Howell JD, Freeman RG. Structure and significance of the pits with their tumors in the nevoid basal cell carcinoma syndrome. *J Am Acad Dermatol* 1980; **2**:224–238.

27. Goldstein AM, Pastakia B, DiGiovanna JJ, et al. Clinical findings in two African–American families with nevoid basal cell carcinoma syndrome (NBCC). *Am J Med Genet* 1994; **50**:272–281.

28. Korczak JF, Brahim JS, DiGiovanna JJ, et al. Nevoid basal cell carcinoma syndrome with medulloblastoma in an African–American boy: a rare case illustrating gene–environment interaction. *Am J Med Genet* 1997; **69**:309–314.

29. Gorlin RJ, Vickers RA, Klein E, Williamson JJ. The multiple basal cell nevi syndrome. *Cancer* 1965; **18**:89–104.

30. Ahlfors E, Larsson A, Sjogren S. The odontogenic keratocyst: a benign cystic tumor? *J Oral Maxillofac Surg* 1984; **42**:10–19.

31. Li TJ, Browne RM, Matthews JB. Epithelial cell proliferation in odontogenic keratocysts: a comparative immunocytochemical study of Ki67 in simple, recurrent and basal cell naevus syndrome (BCNS) – associated lesions. *J Oral Pathol Med* 1995; **24**:221–226.

32. Ratcliffe JF, Shanley S, Chenevix-Trench G. The prevalence of cervical and thoracic congenital skeletal abnormalities in basal cell naevus sydnrome; a review of cervical and chest radiographs in 80 patients with BCNS. *Br J Radiol* 1995; **68**:596–599.

33. Etter LE. Osseous abnormalities of the thoracic cage seen in 40,000 consecutive chest photoroentgenograms. *Am J Roentgenol* 1944; **51**:359–363.

34. Blinder G, Barki Y, Pezt M et al. Widespread osteolytic lesions of the long bones in basal cell nevus syndrome. *Skeletal Radiol* 1984; **12**:195–198.

35. Dunnick NR, Head GL, Peck GL et al. Nevoid basal cell carcinoma syndrome: radiographic manifestations including cystlike lesions of the phalanges. *Radiology* 1978; **127**:331–334.

36. Ratcliffe JF, Shanley S, Ferguson J, Chenevix-Trench G. The diagnostic implication of falcine calcification on plain skull radiographs of patients with basal cell naevus syndrome and the incidence of falcine calcification in their relatives and two control groups. *Br J Radiol* 1995; **68**:361–368.

37. Evans DGR, Farndon PA, Burnell LD, et al. The incidence of Gorlin syndrome in 173 consecutive cases of medulloblastoma. *Br J Cancer* 1991; **64**:959–961.

38. Cowan R, Hoban P, Kelsey A, Birch JM, et al. The gene for the naevoid basal cell carcinoma syndrome acts as a tumour-suppressor gene in medulloblastoma. *Br J Cancer* 1997; **76**:141–145.

39. Walter AW, Pivnick EK, Bale AE. Complications of the nevoid basal cell carcinoma syndrome: a case report. *J Pediatr Hematol Oncol* 1997; **19**:258–262.

40. O'Malley S, Weitman D, Olding M, Sekhar L. Multiple neoplasms following crandiospinal irradiation for medulloblastoma in a patient with nevoid basal cell carcinoma syndrome. *J Neurosurg* 1997; **86**:286–288.

41. Atahan IL, Vildiz F, Ozyar E, et al. Basal cell carcinomas developing in a case of medulloblastoma associated with Gorlin's syndrome. *Pediatr Hematol Oncol* 1998; **15**:187–191.

42. Evans DGR, Birch J, Orton C. Brain tumours and the occurrence of severe invasive basal cell carcinomas in first degree relatives with Gorlin syndrome. *Br J Neurosurg* 1991: **5**:643–646.

43. Goldstein AM, Yuen J, Tucker MA. Second cancers after medulloblastoma: population-based results from the United States and Sweden. *Cancer Causes Control* 1997; **8**:865–871.

44. Seracchioli R, Bagnoli A, Colombo FM, et al. Conservative treatment of recurrent ovarian fibromas in a young patient affected by Gorlin syndrome. *Hum Reprod* 2001; **6**:1261–1263.

45. Strong LC. Genetic and environmental interactions. *Cancer* 1977; **40**:1861–1866.

46. Southwick GJ, Schwartz RA. The basal cell nevus syndrome: disasters occurring among a series of 36 patients. *Cancer* 1979; **44**:2294–2305.

47. Zvulunov A, Strother D, Zirbel G. Nevoid basal cell carcinoma syndrome: report of a case with associated Hodgkin's disease. *J Pediatr Hematol Oncol* 1995; **17**:66–70.

48. Goldstein AM, Bale SJ, Peck GL, DiGiovanna JJ. Sun exposure and basal cell carcinomas in the nevoid basal cell carcinoma syndrome. *J Am Acad Derm* 1993; **29**:34–41.

49. Bodak N, Queille S, Avril MF, et al. High levels of *patched* gene mutations in basal-cell carcinomas from patients with xeroderma pigmentosum. *Proc Natl Acad Sci USA* 1999; **96**:5117–5122.

50. Gailani MR, Stahle-Backdahl M, Leffell DJ, et al. The role of the human homologue of Drosophila patched in sporadic basal cell carcinomas. *Nature Genet* 1996; **14**:78–81.

51. D'Errico M, Calcagnile A, Canzona F, et al. UV mutation signature in tumour suppressor genes involved in skin carcinogenesis in xeroderma pigmentosum patients. *Oncogene* 2000; **19**:463–467.

52. Zhang H, Li Ping X, Lee PK, et al. Role of *PTCH* and *p53* genes in early-onset basal cell carcinoma. *Am J Path* 2001; **158**:381–385.

53. Little JB, Nichols WW, Troilo P, et al. Radiation sensitivity of cell strains from families with genetic disorders predisposing to radiation-induced cancer. *Cancer Res* 1989; **49**:4705–4714.

54. Stacey M, Thacker S, Taylor AM. Cultured skin keratinocytes from both normal individuals and basal cell naevus syndrome patients are more resistant to gamma-rays and UV light compared with cultured skin fibroblasts. *Int J Radiat Biol* 1989; **56**:45–58.

55. Sharpe GR, Cox NH. Unilateral naevoid basal cell carcinoma syndrome – an individually controlled study of fibroblast sensitivity to radiation. *Clin Exp Dermatol* 1990; **15**:352–355.

56. Fujii K, Miyashita T, Takanashi J, et al. Gamma-irradiation deregulates cell cycle control and apoptosis in nevoid basal cell carcinoma syndrome-derived cells. *Jpn J Cancer Res* 1999; **90**:1351–1357.

57. Bale AE, Bale SJ, Murli H, et al. Sister chromatid exchange and chromosome fragility in the nevoid basal cell carcinoma syndrome. *Cancer Genet Cytogenet* 1989; **42**:273–279.

58. Lehmann AR, Kirk-Bell S, Arlett CF, et al. Repair of UV light damage in a variety of human fibroblast cell strains. *Cancer Res* 1977; **37**:904–910.

59. Naqawaswa F, Little FF, Burke MJ, et al. Study of basal cell nevus fibroblasts after treatment with DNA damaging agents. *Basic Life Sci* 1984; **29B**:775–785.

60. Ananthaswamy HN, Applegate IA, Goldberg LH, et al. Skin fibroblasts from basal cell nevus patients are hypersensitive to killing by solar UVB radiation. *Photochem Photobiol* 1989; **49**:60S.

61. Applegate LA, Goldberg LH, Ley RD, Ananthaswamy HN. Hypersensitivity of skin fibroblasts from basal cell nevus syndrome patients to killing by ultraviolet B but not by ultraviolet C radiation. *Cancer Res* 1990; **50**:637–641.

62. Goodrich LV, Milenkovic L, Higgins KM, Scott MP. Altered neural cell fates and medulloblastoma in mouse *patched* mutants. *Science* 1997; **277**:1109–1113.

63. Aszterbaum MA, Epstein J, Oro A, *et al.* A mouse model of human basal cell carcinoma: ultraviolet and gamma radiation enhance basal cell carcinoma growth in patched heterozygote knock-out mice. *Nature Med* 1999; **5**:1285–1291.

64. Bushby KMD, Cole T, Matthews JNS, Goodship JA. Centiles for adult head circumference. *Arch Dis Child* 1992; **67**:1286–1287.

65. Chenevix-Trench G, Wicking C, Berkman J, *et al.* Further localization of the gene for nevoid basal cell syndrome in 15 Australasian families: linkage and loss of heterozygosity. *Am J Hum Genet* 1993; **53**:760–767.

66. Bleiberg J, Brodkin RH. Linear unilateral basal cell nevus with comedones. *Arch Dermatol* 1969; **100**:187–90.

67. Viksnins P, Berlin A. Follicular atrophoderma and basal cell carcinomas: the Basex syndrome. *Arch Dermatol* 1977; **113**:948–951.

68. Michaelsson G, Olsson E, Westermark P. The Rombo syndrome. *Acta Dermatovener* 1981; **61**:497–503.

69. Oley CA, Sharpe H, Chenevix-Trench G. Basal cell carcinomas, coarse sparse hair, and milia. *Am J Med Genet* 1992; **43**:799–804.

70. Requena L, del Carmen Farin M, Robledo M, *et al.* Multiple hereditary infundibulocystic basal cell carcinomas. *Arch Dermatol* 1999; **135**:1227–1235.

71. Rasmussen JE. A syndrome of trichoepitheliomas, milia and cylindromas. *Arch Dermatol* 1975; **111**:610–614.

72. Welch JP, Wells RS, Kerr CB. Ancell–Spiegler cylindromas (turban tumours) and Brooke–Fordyce trichoepitheliomas: evidence for a single genetic entity. *J Med Genet* 1968; **5**:29–35.

73. Starink TM, van der Veen JPW, Arwert F, *et al.* The Cowden syndrome: a clinical and genetic study in 21 patients. *Clin Genet* 1986; **29**:222–233.

74. Kopera D, Cerroni L, Fink-Puches R, Kerl H. Different treatment modalities for the management of a patient with nevoid basal cell carcinoma syndrome. *J Am Acad Dermatol* 1996; **34**:937–939.

75. Thissen MRTM, Neumann MHA, Schouten LJ. A systematic review of treatment modalities for primary basal cell carcinomas. *Arch Dermatol* 1999; **135**:1177–1183.

76. Mohs FE, Jones DL, Koranda FC. Microscopically controlled surgery for carcinomas in patients with nevoid basal cell carcinoma syndrome. *Arch Dermatol* 1980; **116**:777–779.

77. Marks R, Gebauer K, Shumack S, *et al.* Imiuimod 5 per cent cream in the treatment of superficial basal cell carcinoma: results of a multicenter 6-week dose-response trial. *J Am Acad Dermatol* 2001; **44**:807–813.

78. Kagy MK, Amonette R. The use of imiquimod 5 per cent cream for the treatment of superficial basal cell carcinomas in a basal cell nevus syndrome patient. *Dermatol Surg* 2000; **26**:577–578.

79. Peck GL, DiGiovanna JJ, Sarnoff DS, *et al.* Treatment and prevention of basal cell carcinoma with oral isotretinoin. *J Am Acad Dermatol* 1988; **19**:176–185.

80. Cristofolini M, Zumiani G, Scappni P, *et al.* Aromatic retinoid in chemoprevention of the progression of nevoid basal cell carcinoma syndrome. *J Dermatol Surg Oncol* 1984; **10**:778–781.

81. Hodak E, Ginzburg A, David M, *et al.* Etretinate treatment of the nevoid basal cell carcinoma syndrome. *Int J Dermatol* 1987; **26**:606–609.

82. Sanchez-Conejo-Mir J, Camacho F. Nevoid basal cell carcinoma syndrome: combined etretinate and surgical treatment. *J Dermatol Surg Oncol* 1989; **15**:868–871.

83. Goldberg LH, Hsu SH, Alcalay J. Effectiveness of isotretinoin in preventing the appearance of basal cell carcinomas in basal cell nevus syndrome. *J Am Acad Dermatol* 1989; **21**:144–145.

84. Strange PR, Lang PG Jr. Long-term management of basal cell nevus syndrome with topical tretinoin and 5-fluorouracil. *J Am Acad Dermatol* 1992; **27**:842–845.

85. Theiler R, Hubscher E, Wagenhauser FJ, *et al.* Diffuse idiopathic skeletal hyperostosis (DISH) and pseudo-coxarthritis following long-term etretinate therapy. *Schweiz Med Wochenschrift* 1993; **123**:649–653.

86. Henderson BW, Dougherty T. How does photodynamic therapy work? *Photochem Photobiol* 1992; **55**:145–157.

87. Tse DT, Kersten RC, Anderson RL. Hematoporphyrin derivative photoradiation therapy in managing nevoid basal cell carcinoma syndrome. A preliminary report. *Arch Ophthalmol* 1984; **102**:990–994.

88. Karrer S, Hohenleutner U. Unilateral localized basaliomatosis: treatment with topical photodynamic therapy after application of 5-amniolevulinic acid. *Dermatology* 1995; **190**:218–222.

89. Rifkin R, Reed B, Hetzel F, *et al.* Photodynamic therapy using SnET2 for basal cell nevus syndrome: a case report. *Clin Ther* 1997; **19**:639–641.

90. Zeitouni NC, Shieh S, Oseroff, AR. Laser and photodynamic therapy in the management of cutaneous malignancies. *Clinics Dermatol* 2001; **19**:328–339.

91. Morton CA, Whitehurst C, McColl JH, *et al.* Photodynamic therapy for basal cell carcinoma – effect of tumour thickness and duration of photosensitizer application on response. *Arch Dermatol* 1998; **134**:248–249.

92. Baas P, Saarnak AE, Oppelaar H, *et al.* Photodynamic therapy with meta-tetrahydroxyphenylchlorin for basal cell carcinoma: a phase I/II study. *Br J Dermatol* 2001; **145**:75–78.

93. Stoelinga PJ, Peters JH, van de Staak WJ, Cohen MM. Some new findings in the basal cell nevus syndrome. *Oral Surg* 1973; **36**:686–692.

94. Hahn H, Wicking C, Zaphiropoulos PG, *et al.* Mutations of the human homolog of *Drosophila patched* in the nevoid basal cell carcinoma syndrome. *Cell* 1996; **85**:841–851.

95. Johnson RL, Rothman AL, Xie J, *et al.* Human homolog of *patched*, a candidate gene for the basal cell nevus syndrome. *Science* 1996; **272**:1668–1671.

96. Smyth I, Narang MA, Evans T, *et al.* Isolation and characterisation of human *Patched 2 (PTCH2)*, a putative tumour suppressor gene in basal cell carcinoma and medulloblastoma on chromosome 1p32. *Hum Molec Genet* 1999; **8**:291–297.

97. Taipale J, Cooper MK, Maiti T, Beachy PA. *Patched* acts catalytically to suppress the activity of smoothened. *Nature* 2002; **418**:892–897.

98. Denef N, Neubuser D, Perez L, *et al.* Hedgehog induces opposite changes in turnover and subcellular localization of patched and smoothened. *Cell* 2000; **102**:521–531.

99. Kogerman P, Krause D, Rahnama F, *et al.* Alternative first exons of PTCH1 are differentially regulated in vivo and may confer different functions of the PTCH1 protein. *Oncogene* 2002; **21**: 6007–6016.

100. Barnes EA, Kong M, Ollendorff V, Donoghue DJ. Ptch interacts with cyclin B1 to regulate cell cycle progression. *EMBO J* 2001; **20**:2214–2223.

101. Bale AE, Yu K-P. The hedgehog pathway and basal cell carcinomas. *Hum Molec Genet* 2001; **10**:757–762.

102. Fan H, Khavari PA. Sonic hedgehog opposes epithelial cell cycle arrest. *J Cell Biol* 1999; **147**:71–76.

103. Goodrich LV, Milenkovic L, Higgins KM, Scott MP. Altered neural cell fates and medulloblastoma in mouse patched mutants. *Science* 1997; **277**:1109–1113.

104. Aszterbaum M, Rothman A, Johnson RL, *et al.* Identification of mutations in the human *PATCHED* gene in sporadic basal cell carcinomas and in patients with the basal cell nevus syndrome. *J Invest Dermatol* 1998; **110**: 885–888.

105. Lench NJ, Telford EAR, High AS, *et al.* Characterisation of human *patched* germ line mutations in naevoid basal cell carcinoma syndrome. *Hum Genet* 1997; **100**:497–502.

106. Wicking C, Gillies S, Smyth I, *et al.* De novo mutations of the *patched* gene in nevoid basal cell carcinoma syndrome help to define the clinical phenotype. *Am J Med Genet* 1997; **73**:304–307.

107. Wicking C, Shanley S, Smyth I, *et al.* Most germ-line mutations in the nevoid basal cell carcinoma syndrome lead to a premature termination of the PATCHED protein, and no genotype–phenotype correlations are evident. *Am J Hum Genet* 1997; **60**:21–26.

108. Bailey EC, Milenkovic L, Scott MP, *et al.* Several *PATCHED1* missense mutations display activity in patched-1 deficient fibroblasts. *J Biol Chem* 2002; **37**:33632–33640.

109. D'Errico M, Calcagnile A, Canzona F, *et al.* UV mutation signature in tumour suppressor genes involved in skin carcinogenesis in xeroderma pigmentosum patients. *Oncogene* 2000; **19**:463–467.

110. Ming JE, Kaupas ME, Roessler E, *et al.* Mutations in *PATCHED-1*, the receptor for SONIC HEDGEHOG, are associated with holoprosencephaly. *Hum Genet* 2002; **110**:297–301.

Xeroderma pigmentosum, Cockayne syndrome and trichothiodystrophy: sun sensitivity, DNA repair defects and skin cancer

COLIN F. ARLETT AND ALAN R. LEHMANN

INTRODUCTION

Xeroderma pigmentosum (XP) is a rare, autosomal recessive disease[1] with a combination of clinical, cellular and molecular features that initially generated an intellectually satisfying and simple association between defects in DNA repair, increased mutability and cancer proneness. As the study of XP patients has proceeded, however, interesting anomalies and unanticipated complexities have been uncovered. In particular, as a consequence of using XP as a model, two other rare but not cancer-prone, autosomal recessive diseases, Cockayne syndrome (CS) and trichothiodystrophy (TTD) have extended the apparent relationship of DNA repair defects to a wide spectrum of associated clinical features.[1] The relationship between the three conditions is complex – there are a few individuals with the features of both XP and CS, and mutations in one of the XP genes can give rise to individuals with XP, TTD, cerebro-oculofacioskeletal syndrome (COFS), XP with CS, or XP with TTD. In order to understand the relationship between DNA damage/repair and cancer revealed in XP, it is necessary to study all three conditions at the clinical, cellular and molecular levels.

CLINICAL OBSERVATIONS

Xeroderma pigmentosum

Comprehensive reviews of the clinical characteristics of XP are available.[1,2] The individuals are sun sensitive, and this is coupled with an abnormal erythemal response.[3] The dermatological features in unprotected individuals include, in sun-exposed areas, pigmented macules, achromic spots and telangiectasia, followed, ultimately, by basal cell carcinoma (BCC), squamous cell carcinoma (SCC) and malignant melanoma. The survey by Kraemer et al. of 830 published cases showed that: (1) individuals with the disease die about 30 years earlier than the US population as a whole; (2) 50 per cent of patients in the 10–14 year age group had skin cancers; and (3) the median age for first skin neoplasms is approximately 50 years lower than in the normal population.[2]

The role of sunlight in the induction of skin cancer in the normal human population is unambiguous: 97 per cent of the BCC plus SCC are found on regions of the body that receive most direct sunlight.[4] Conversely, protection by avoidance of sunlight can materially reduce the extent of cutaneous damage. Thus patients with the cellular characteristics of XP (see later) but with no tumours or reduced skin damage may have been exposed to relatively little sunlight. There are, however, well-documented examples of such individuals who do not attempt to protect themselves from sunlight. The explanation for their relatively mild skin damage is not clear. In addition to increased skin cancer, XP patients have also been reported to have an increased incidence of some internal tumours,[5] but this is much less marked than the dramatically increased incidence of skin cancer.

Neurological defects were described in 20 per cent of the patients reviewed by Kraemer et al.[2] Here, of course, no direct involvement of sunlight can be inferred. Progressive neurological degeneration results from premature neuronal death.

A number of other clinical abnormalities have been associated with XP. Impaired immune status has been reported. This includes a reduced response to recall antigens and dinitrochlorobenzene (DNCB) antigens, a reduction in the ratio of T-helper/suppressor cells and a reduced response to phytohaemagglutinin stimulation of lymphocytes. There is considerable variation amongst patients with regard to these effects. Natural killer (NK) cell number and function have been found to be reduced in some but not all XP patients.[6,7] Indeed, in one interesting case, an individual aged 65 years with self-healing melanomas had reduced NK function on a per-cell basis but greatly increased numbers of NK cells.[8] Turner et al. reported a case where intralesional α-interferon injection was effective in the treatment of melanomas in an XP patient.[9] This is consistent with the concept that such patients have a reduced capacity to mount a γ-interferon stimulation of intercellular adhesion molecule 1 (ICAM-1) expression in comparison with normal individuals.[10]

Cockayne syndrome

This rare disorder shows a pattern of inheritance consistent with a recessive status. In a review of 140 published cases, Nance and Berry suggested that the primary clinical hallmarks included neurodevelopmental delay and dwarfism together with any three of the following: hearing loss, dental caries, pigmentary retinopathy (with or without cataract), characteristic facial appearance and photosensitivity[11] (see also Lehmann et al.[12]). No increased incidence of skin cancer has been recorded.

There have been only limited investigations of their immunological status. In two patients, adaptive cell-mediated immunity and NK cell function were within normal limits.[6] Surprisingly, in the light of the rarity of both CS and XP, there are reports of individuals with features of both syndromes. This provides a strong indication of a causal connection between these disorders.

Trichothiodystrophy

This rare autosomal recessive condition is characterized by sulphur-deficient brittle hair, ichthyosis, physical and mental retardation and abnormal facies.[13] The condition is extremely heterogeneous, and various forms have been given different acronyms, e.g. BIDS, IBIDS, PIBIDS, the latter denoting P(hotosensitivity), I(chthyosis), B(rittle hair), I(mpaired intelligence), D(ecreased fertility) and S(hort stature). The brittle hair is caused by a reduction in the levels of cysteine-rich matrix proteins, leading to a 'tiger-tail' appearance of the hair in polarized light microscopy.[13] Patients can be severely affected leading to their death as early as 36 months, but there are also patients that have reached their 30s.[14] In many, but not all, cases photosensitivity is recorded, but the ichthyosis precludes any attempt to assess monochromator tests. There are no reports of skin cancer in association with TTD. No defects were observed in the immune system of one patient studied.[6]

CELLULAR AND BIOCHEMICAL REPAIR STUDIES

Xeroderma pigmentosum

The first indication of a cellular defect was recorded by Gartler, who reported hypersensitivity to the lethal effects of ultraviolet C (UVC) irradiation.[15] In 1968, Cleaver made the major discovery that XP fibroblasts were defective in excision repair of UV-C damage.[16] This was followed shortly by the recognition of a so-called 'variant' form of XP (comprising about 20 per cent of all XPs), which was indistinguishable at the clinical level but competent in excision repair.[17] Variant fibroblasts were shown subsequently to be defective in daughter strand repair[18] and are minimally hypersensitive to the lethal effects of UV light.

Excision-defective XP fibroblasts are also hypersensitive to the lethal action of many chemical carcinogens, such as benzo(a)pyrene diol-epoxide or 4-nitroquinoline-1-oxide, which produce bulky lesions in DNA.[19] Hypersensitivity to the lethal action of 254 nm UV light is not limited to XP fibroblasts, but has been recorded for lymphoblastoid lines and both unstimulated and stimulated T-lymphocytes.[20]

Nucleotide excision repair (NER) involves several steps, which will be discussed in more detail in the later section on XP genes:

1 the recognition of a lesion;
2 opening out of the DNA around the damaged site;
3 incision of the damaged DNA strand on both sides of the lesion;

4 removal of the oligonucleotide containing the damage;
5 synthesis of new, replacement, DNA using the intact complementary strand as a template; and, finally,
6 ligation.

The synthesis step 5 of NER can be monitored conveniently by incorporation of ^{3}[H]thymidine into non-S-phase or non-dividing cells. This is defined as unscheduled DNA synthesis (UDS). Excision-defective XP cells have reduced UDS compared with normal cells at comparable UV dose levels.

NER can be divided into two different branches. Damage in the transcribed strands of active genes is repaired most rapidly (transcription-coupled repair; TCR), whereas the rest of the genome is repaired relatively slowly (global genome repair; GGR). These different branches of NER are under the control of different genes.

COMPLEMENTATION GROUPS

The ability of cell cultures from different XP patients to complement each other can be determined by fusing pairwise combinations and measuring levels of UDS in response to UV radiation. This has been used extensively as the basis of a genetic complementation test and to date seven excision-defective complementation groups, A–G, have been assigned to this disease.[21] The excision-proficient XP variants appear to fall into a single complementation group.

When complementation studies were first performed, there was much discussion as to whether the various complementation groups represented separate genes or whether intragenic complementation was occurring. Subsequent investigations have identified chromosomal locations for the XP complementing genes (see Table 16.1) and show unequivocally that they represent different genes. The structure and function of these genes is described in the later section on XP genes. There is an uneven distribution of the complementation groups both on the basis of their frequency and worldwide occurrence. Groups A, C, D and variant are the most common in Europe and the USA, while in Japan, groups A and variant are the most common, and groups C and D are rarely observed. The patients in the two known XP families in group B have the features of both XP and CS, and other individuals with XP and CS are known, two in group D and several in group G.[21]

As reviewed in detail elsewhere[21] cell strains from XPs of different complementation groups have different repair characteristics. XP-A cells, in general, have very low levels of UDS and are most sensitive to killing by UV. XP-D and XP-C cells have significant levels of UDS but XP-C cells are more resistant than XP-D cells. Although the overall level of UDS is severely reduced in XP-C cells, they retain the normal ability to carry out TCR, while being defective in GGR.[22] Retention of this crucial TCR activity renders the cells relatively resistant compared with other XP groups. In contrast, the repair deficiency in the very heterogeneous XP-D group[23] is distributed in both active and inactive genes, and the cells are relatively sensitive. In XP-F cells, repair occurs at a low rate but is fairly prolonged, so that much of the damage is eventually repaired, and the cells are relatively resistant to killing by UV.

MUTABILITY

In vitro mutation experiments measuring UVC-induced resistance to 6-thioguanine, 8-azaguanine or diphtheria toxin reveal that both excision-defective and excision-competent XP fibroblasts are hypermutable when compared with cells from normal individuals.[24–26] The cells are also hypersensitive to the induction of sister chromatid exchanges (SCE)[27] and chromosome aberrations by UVC. They do not, however, have an elevated frequency of spontaneous SCE or chromosome aberrations.[28]

The principal photoproducts produced by UVC irradiation, the cyclobutane pyrimidine dimer (CPD) and the

Table 16.1 *Properties of genes defective in xeroderma pigmentosum, Cockayne syndrome and trichothiodystrophy, and their encoded proteins*

Gene	Chromosome localization	Size of gene (kb)	Size of protein (aa)	Number of exons	Yeast (*S. cerevisiae*) homologue	Protein function
XPA	9q22.3	25	273	6	*RAD14*	DNA binding
XPB	2q21	45	782	14	*RAD25*	Helicase. TFIIH
XPC	3p25.1	24	940	15	*RAD4*	Damage recognition
XPD	19q13.3	15	760	23	*RAD3*	Helicase. TFIIH
XPE	11p11	24	427	10		Damage recognition
XPF	16p13.3	28	916	11	*RAD1*	Nuclease
XPG	13q22	32	1196	15	*RAD2*	Nuclease
XPV	6p21.1	40	713	11	*RAD30*	DNA polymerase
CSA	5q12.1	71	396	12	*RAD28*	WD protein
CSB	10q11	90	1493	21	*RAD26*	DNA-dependent ATPase

pyrimidine (6–4) pyrimidone photodimer, are both produced at sites of adjacent pyrimidines. Mutation spectrum analysis of 6-thioguanine-resistant (hprt⁻) mutants induced by UVC in both untransformed and SV40-immortalized XP (complementation group A) fibroblasts has shown that the sites of the mutations could largely be assigned to such dipyrimidine sequences, on the transcribed strand.[29,30] In contrast, in untransformed normal fibroblasts, although the sites of mutation were again at dipyrimidine sequences, the presumptive damage was largely on the non-transcribed strand of the duplex.[30] This difference may be brought about by preferential repair of damage in the transcribed strand in normal cells. Spectra in XP variant cells were quite different from those in normal and excision-deficient XP cells. Whereas the majority of the latter were G:C to A:T transitions, in the former case, many of the mutations were at thymines, both transitions and transversions.[31] Mutation spectra have also been analysed in a shuttle vector pZ189 passaged in XP or normal cells.[32] A hundred-fold increase in UVC-induced mutant frequency was observed in the marker gene (*supF*) in XP cells, and more G:C to A:T transitions and fewer G:C to T:A transversions were recorded than in normal cells. These spectra are again consistent with damage at dipyrimidine sites.

Measurement of the frequency of 6-thioguanine-resistant mutants amongst circulating T-lymphocytes from peripheral blood revealed an elevated mutant frequency for XP patients as a population, whether they were excision competent or defective.[33] Although most of the mutations occurred at dipyrimidine sites, no strand bias was observed.[34] These data suggested that the enhanced mutant frequency seen in T-lymphocytes of XP patients was not generated by exposure to UVB as cells pass through the skin, although a contribution from this source has not been ruled out.

UNUSUAL RESPONSES

Examples exist of XP patients showing no or little skin cancer. In some cases, this may result from relatively limited exposure to sunlight for particular individuals. In addition, secondary control mechanisms, such as the enhancement of immune surveillance, or the absence of its suppression, may also be important. Two siblings from complementation group B with symptoms of both XP and CS have limited neurological abnormalities, very mild cutaneous symptoms and a complete absence of skin tumours even after 40 years of making no attempt at sun avoidance, even though their levels of NER are very low.[35,36] While T-lymphocytes and fibroblasts from these individuals are hypersensitive to the lethal effects of UVC and UVB, there is no evidence for elevated mutant frequency in blood-derived lymphocytes. There are no data available for UV-induced mutant frequency in these

individuals. Two other XP patients, XP125LO and XP7NE, from complementation groups G and F, respectively, are similarly normal in the mutant frequency amongst circulating T-lymphocytes and are free of skin cancer, despite having low levels of NER (Cole *et al.*[33] and unpublished data). In one fascinating case, an XP patient has been shown to be a mosaic of normal and XP cells.[37]

PARADIGM AND PROSPECTS FOR MANAGEMENT

Taken together, the clinical and cellular features of XP present a convincing conjunction of observation and hypothesis. Thus, the presence of sun sensitivity, leading to skin damage including cancer, is correlated with defects in DNA repair and hypermutability, providing convincing support for the mutational theory of cancer induction. Perhaps the most important lesson to be learnt from the study of this disease is that these unfortunate individuals provide us all with a dramatic model of the consequences of excessive exposure to sunlight.

Several hypotheses have been proposed to account for the neurological abnormalities found in some XP patients (e.g. see Robbins[38]). We do not discuss these further in this chapter.

The defects in repair can be used to confirm clinical diagnoses, which, if achieved early in the life of the individual, can establish a helpful UV light avoidance programme.[39] Successful prenatal diagnosis has also been performed in families with an affected child.[40,41]

As knowledge of XP has progressed, so various routes for its management have become apparent. Clinical observation of skin changes implicates solar irradiation in aetiology of the disease. Thus early diagnosis followed by rigorous protection from sunlight or damaging artificial light can, despite the obvious lifestyle disadvantage, achieve skin and ocular sparing.[39] Significant control of cancer and other skin changes has been achieved with retinoids.[42–44] Here control is based upon tumour suppression and is believed to be a reflection of chemoprophylaxis of skin tumours in both non-XP and XP patients, rather than the correction of any defect in DNA repair. A note of caution should be made with respect to a potential rebound effect as seen in one study,[42] such that, following withdrawal of isotretinoin because of adverse side effects, an increase in tumour incidence was observed.

The endonucleaseV 'dimer endonuclease' from bacteriophage T4 can circumvent the defect in XP cells and restore partial UV resistance when introduced into XP cells in culture.[45] Clinical trials using T4 endonuclease V applied as a liposome cream to the skin of XP individuals gave promising results. The rates of appearance of new actinic keratoses and basal cell carcinomas were significantly reduced in the treatment group as compared with a placebo group.[46]

The possibility that immunosurveillance is perturbed in XP patients has generated a report of a successful outcome of intralesional α-interferon injection of melanoma in one such patient.[9]

Cockayne syndrome

Cockayne syndrome cells are hypersensitive to the lethal effects of UVC, although, in general, this is not as marked as in excision-defective XP cells. Their sensitivities to other DNA-damaging agents are broadly similar to those of XP.[47] They are also hypersensitive to the induction of SCE.[48] Both excision repair and daughter strand repair are normal, but cells from CS patients may be distinguished from normals by the failure of RNA synthesis to recover following UV irradiation.[49] The defect in recovery of post-UV RNA synthesis is used both as a confirmation of clinical diagnosis and for prenatal diagnosis.[12,50] This defect, in combination with normal NER, has allowed the assignment of two complementation groups A and B in this syndrome. Complementation group B is more frequently encountered than A.[51,52]

Although excision repair, as assessed by UDS, is within normal limits in CS cells, transcription-coupled repair is impaired. All genes are repaired at the relatively slow rate at which the bulk of the DNA is repaired in normal cells.[53] This accounts for the lack of recovery of RNA synthesis after UV exposure and is probably responsible for the increased hypersensitivity to the lethal effects of UV.

Considerable efforts have been expended in attempts to determine the mutability of CS cells, but they have been hampered by the tendency of CS fibroblasts to age rapidly on subculture and lose viability. Such data as do exist indicate hypermutability,[54] an observation supported by studies of mutation induction in herpes simplex virus grown in lymphoblastoid cultures of CS.[55]

The measurements of mutant frequencies in circulating T lymphocytes from CS patients are elevated in comparison with normal controls,[56] an observation consistent with the assumption of hypermutability in CS cells.

Trichothiodystrophy

The response of TTD cells to UV-irradiation is very heterogeneous.[57,58] Cells from patients who are not photosensitive are indistinguishable from normal. Cells from photosensitive patients have a wide range of DNA repair capabilities. In nearly all cases, the repair deficiency appears to fall in the XP-D complementation group.[58] One family has, however, been assigned to the XP-B group.[59] Furthermore, cells from one patient, TTD1BR, with a severe repair deficiency, have been shown to complement not only XP complementation group D, but all other XP groups as well. This individual is, therefore, a representative of a new NER complementation group designated TTD-A.[60]

XP GENES AND THEIR PRODUCTS

All of the known genes that are defective in XP and CS have been cloned, and their protein products purified. The roles of the individual XP proteins in NER are now quite well understood. Properties of the XP genes and their products are summarized in Table 16.1. Mutations identified in the XP and CS genes have been recently summarized by Cleaver and coworkers[61] and are presented graphically in Plate 2. A database of mutations identified in XP patients has been established (http://xpmutations.org). The roles of the XP gene products in NER are depicted in Figure 16.1.

XPA

The *XPA* gene encodes a 273 aa zinc-finger protein, which has 33 per cent sequence identity to the yeast *Saccharomyces cerevisiae RAD14* product over a run of 130 aa in the middle of the gene. The XPA protein binds to UV-irradiated DNA better than to unirradiated DNA.[62] It had been hypothesized for many years that *XPA* was responsible for the detection of DNA damage. However, although *XPA* shows an increased affinity to damaged DNA, this increase of only fivefold is much too small for the high lesion specificity observed in NER. In line with this, work by Sugasawa *et al.* and Volker *et al.*, described in the later section on *XPC*, has shown that the XPA protein binds to DNA after the binding of the XPC/HR23B complex, both *in vivo* and *in vitro*.[63,64] This indicates that, although XPA plays a vital role in the early stages of NER (Figure 16.1), it is involved in a function after damage recognition, possibly damage verification or correct positioning of NER proteins. The N-terminal region of the protein is required for nuclear localization, whereas the central part contains a zinc finger DNA-binding domain.[65]

A survey of mutations in XP-A patients has been carried out by Cleaver and colleagues.[61] In Japan, more than 80 per cent of XP-A patients are homozygous for a G→C substitution at the 3′ splice acceptor site of intron 3.[66] This results in two abnormally spliced forms of mRNA and no active protein. Several different mutations were found in the remaining Japanese patients and in Caucasian XP-As[61] (Plate 2). Mutations in the C-terminal exon 6 resulted in relatively less marked UV sensitivity and repair defect, and mild clinical symptoms. The other nonsense and frameshift mutations, the mutations affecting splicing and the missense mutation in the zinc-finger motif in exon 3 all abolished repair activity and resulted in severe clinical symptoms.

Most of the mutations in XP-A patients result in severe truncation of the protein, suggesting that the gene is not essential for life, and this is consistent with the viability

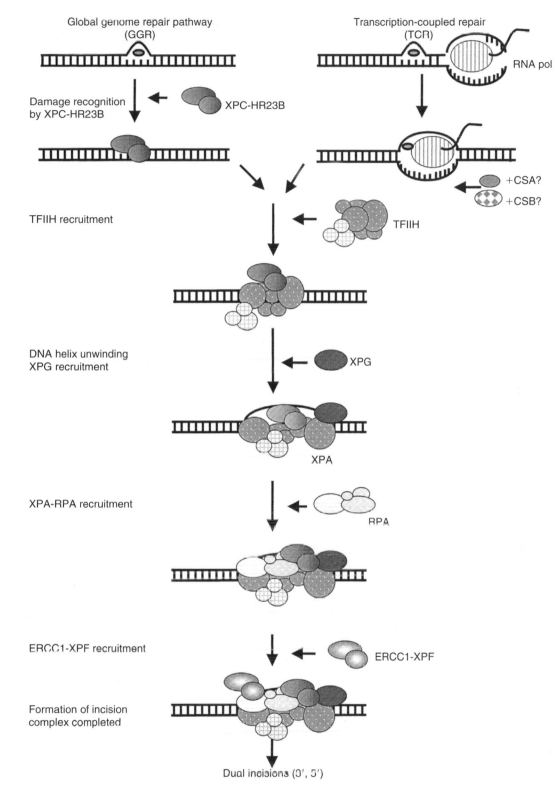

Figure 16.1 *Role of xeroderma pigmentosum and Cockayne syndrome proteins in nucleotide excision repair. For global genome repair, bulky DNA lesions are recognised by the XPC/HR23B heterodimer. The TFIIH complex containing the XPB and XPD proteins is recruited. TFIIH opens out the DNA structure, allowing the XPG nuclease and XPA together with single-strand binding protein to bind and verify the positioning of the proteins relative to the damaged site. The XPF/ERCC1 nuclease is recruited to complete formation of the incision complex. DNA is then cut on both sides of the damage. (The resulting gap is filled in by DNA polymerase ε together with accessory proteins PCNA and RFC, and joining of repaired to pre-existing DNA by a DNA ligase completes the process.) In transcription-coupled repair, RNA polymerase is stalled at the damaged site. By a poorly understood process, the polymerase is displaced from the damaged site, assisted by the CSA and CSB proteins, and TFIIH is recruited. Subsequent steps are the same as for global genome repair. (Modified from Volker et al.[64])*

of XP-A knockout mice. These mice are healthy. They do not show the neurological abnormalities of the human XP-As. Like human XP-A patients, they are extremely sensitive to skin carcinogenesis induced by UVB or dimethylbenzanthracene.[67,68]

XPB

The *XPB* gene encodes a predicted protein of 782 aa. There are only three families described in the literature in the XP-B complementation group.[36,59,69] Two have the combined features of XP and CS (in one case mild, the other severe), the third has TTD. The severely affected XP/CS patient XP11BE has a C→A transversion close to the acceptor site of the C-terminal intron 13 in the only expressed allele.[70] This caused aberrant splicing of the mRNA, resulting in a four-base insertion. The C-terminal 42 aa are, therefore, out of frame. This allele, inherited from the patient's mother is the only one expressed in this cell strain. In two brothers from a second XP-B/CS family, who showed only very mild symptoms (see earlier section on unusual responses), the causative mutation in the only expressed allele was a T→C transition resulting in Phe99Ser.[36] The third patient in the XP-B group has TTD and an A→C transversion, resulting in the amino acid change Thr119Pro.[59]

The first clue to the enigma of mutations in the *XPB* gene (and more dramatically in *XPD*, see below) resulting in different clinical phenotypes came from the unexpected discovery that the XPB protein is the largest subunit of the basal transcription factor TFIIH.[71] This subsequently led to the findings that XPD is also a subunit of TFIIH and that the whole TFIIH complex has a dual role, in NER as well as in initiation of RNA polymerase II-mediated transcription.[72] This is the most striking example of several instances in which DNA repair proteins have multiple functions.[73] Since the transcriptional function of TFIIH is vital for life, *XPB* is an essential gene, and the paucity of XP-B families suggests that the transcriptional function of the *XPB* gene is very intolerant of mutations.

The involvement of TFIIH in both NER and transcription implies that mutations in the TFIIH genes may affect NER, transcription or both. Bootsma and Hoeijmakers proposed that defects in NER alone result in the XP phenotype, whereas subtle defects in transcription result in CS or TTD, thus making XP a repair deficiency syndrome, while CS and TTD are proposed to be transcription deficiency syndromes.[74] In order to resolve the specific roles of TFIIH components in NER and transcription, various experimental systems have been utilized. Like all the *NER* genes, *XPB* is highly conserved, the yeast homologue being designated *RAD25*. The XPB protein has a 3′–5′ helicase[75] and DNA-dependent ATPase activity. The yeast system indicates that the ATPase activity of

XPB is required for both transcription and NER, since a mutation in the ATP binding site of Rad25 results in a defect both in transcription and NER.[76]

More recently, the architecture of the human TFIIH complex has been investigated in detail.[77] The XPB subunit is essential for the transcription reaction.[78] Its role in transcription initiation is the opening of the promoter region.[79] When the transcription substrate contained an artificially open promoter, the XPB protein was no longer required. With regard to its function in NER, *in vivo* and *in vitro* studies showed that the *XPB* mutations described before result in an almost total inhibition (around 95 per cent) of NER, indicating that XPB is indispensable for NER.[70,80,81] Furthermore, an intermediate step in the NER process is the formation of open complexes, prior to incision of the DNA on either side of the damage. XPB is required for this open complex formation (Figure 16.1), suggesting that, within the TFIIH complex, it performs similar roles in NER and transcription. This probably accounts for the rarity of XP-B patients, who must have sufficiently severe mutations to affect repair and give an XP phenotype, yet remain viable by having only a minor effect on transcription.

In summary, XPB is tightly bound in the core of TFIIH and is principally, but not exclusively, involved in generating open structures for both transcription and NER.

XPC

DAMAGE RECOGNITION

The *XPC* gene encodes a protein of 940 aa, and is tightly bound to a smaller subunit, which was found to be one of two human homologues of the *S. cerevisiae RAD23* gene, designated HR23B.[82] The role of the XPC protein in NER had been unclear until Sugasawa *et al.* demonstrated that the affinity of the XPC/HR23B complex for damaged DNA is at least ten times higher than for undamaged DNA and that it is involved in the earliest step of NER, namely the detection of DNA damage (Figure 16.1).[63] This role had been previously ascribed to *XPA*. This early role for *XPC* was confirmed in elegant experiments of Volker *et al.*,[64] who irradiated cells through a membrane filter to introduce damage at localized regions in cell nuclei. They then were able to observe the recruitment of NER proteins to the sites of damage. *XPC* was recruited irrespective of the presence or absence of other XP proteins, whereas recruitment of all other proteins was absolutely dependent on the presence of *XPC*.

Since XPC is involved in GGR but not TCR, it is evident that other proteins must carry out damage recognition in the latter process. It is likely that, in transcribing DNA, the stalling of RNA polymerase at the lesion in some way generates the recognition signal and obviates the need for XPC in this subpathway. The two different repair pathways then come together in the recruitment of TFIIH and, thereafter, NER follows a common pathway. In support of this hypothesis, Mu *et al.* used a model substrate in which a cyclobutane pyrimidine dimer (the major photoproduct produced in DNA on exposure to UV) was present in the middle of a 'bubble' substrate.[83] Repair of the lesion in this conformation did not require the XPC protein, suggesting that this conformation mimicked that of DNA containing a stalled RNA polymerase.

GERMLINE MUTATIONS IN THE *XPC* GENE

Mutations have been identified in several XP-C patients[84,85] and they result in protein truncations in nearly all cases (Plate 2). This demonstrates that *XPC* is not essential for life, which is consistent with the viability of XP-C knockout mice generated in several laboratories.[86–88] These mice are healthy, but sensitive to the carcinogenic effects of UVB irradiation.[86,87,89]

MUTATIONS IN TUMOURS OF XP-C PATIENTS

XP individuals have a 2000-fold increase in the incidence of skin tumours. These are almost exclusively confined to areas exposed to sunlight and are one of the consequences of unrepaired damage. Like other cancers, skin tumours result from a series of mutations and other genetic changes in critical oncogenes or tumour suppressor genes. Mutations induced by UV radiation have a characteristic 'signature', the majority being C:G to T:A transitions, of which a proportion are CC to TT tandem mutations. The latter type of mutation is produced almost exclusively by UV radiation. Sarasin and colleagues have examined the status of the *p53* gene in tumours from several XP patients and found that 80 per cent of them contained mutations in the *p53* gene, 89 per cent of which were C to T transitions and 61 per cent of these were CC to TT tandem mutations. Almost all of the mutations could be attributed to dipyrimidine sites on the non-transcribed strand of the DNA. Most of the patients in this study were in the XP-C group, in which only damage in the transcribed strand of active genes is repaired. These data are consistent with an early stage of tumour formation being a UV radiation-induced mutation resulting from unrepaired damage on the non-transcribed strand of the *p53* gene.[90,91] In subsequent work, the same group also identified a high frequency of mutations in the *patched* (*hptc*) gene in basal cell carcinomas from XP patients.[92]

XPD

The *XPD* gene is highly homologous to the *RAD3* gene of *S. cerevisiae* and the *rad15* gene of *Schizosaccharomyces pombe*.[93,94] The sequence of the 760 aa XPD protein contains seven domains characteristic of DNA helicases, and both the Rad3 and XPD proteins have ATP-dependent 5′–3′ DNA helicase activity.[95,96] Both yeast genes and the human gene have essential functions, which are separable from the repair functions.

GENOTYPE–PHENOTYPE RELATIONSHIPS IN XPD

Like XPB, the XPD protein is a subunit of TFIIH[97] and one might, therefore, anticipate that the effects of *XPB* and *XPD* mutations would be quite similar. In fact, they are quite different. Patients with mutations in the *XPD* gene are relatively frequent.[98,99] This implies that the transcription function of *XPD* is much more tolerant of mutations than *XPB*. XP-D cells are defective in both TCR and GGR, and the *XPD* gene is unique, since mutations in it can lead to different clinical conditions, XP, TTD, COFS, XP with CS or XP with TTD. The transcription syndrome hypothesis leads to the prediction that mutations in *XPD* in TTD patients affect transcription, whereas those in XP patients affect only NER. This further predicts that the sites of the mutations in the *XPD* gene are disease specific. This has proved to be the case[99] consistent with the idea that the site of the mutation in the *XPD* gene determines the distinct clinical phenotypes of XP-D and TTD (see Plate 2).

Further definitive evidence to support this contention has come from the generation of an XP-D mutant mouse. This contained a mutation in the *XPD* gene found in four TTD patients, resulting in Arg722Trp. De Boer *et al.* made the exciting finding that the resulting mouse did indeed have the features of TTD with brittle hair, which went through cyclic periods of loss and re-growth.[100] Furthermore, these mice showed many features of premature ageing,[101] providing strong evidence for a link between defective DNA repair and ageing.

Recent work has shown that cells from the two XP-D patients with the combined features of XP and CS respond to UV-irradiation in a unique way. The DNA damage appears to generate breaks in *trans* in the DNA at sites distant from the damage.[102]

ROLE OF XPD HELICASE IN TFIIH

More insights into the specific role of XPD and its relationship to clinical features has come both from *in vitro* analysis of TFIIH functions and from analysis of patient mutations. The *XPD* gene encodes an ATP-dependent helicase functioning in the 5′–3′ direction. In the yeast homologue Rad3, a mutation in the ATP binding site abolished NER, but did not affect viability[103] and the TFIIH of this mutant was active in transcription.[104] This showed that, in contrast to XPB, the helicase activity of XPD is required only for NER and not for basal transcription. Since many mutations have a drastic effect on NER, but only minor effects on transcription, it is likely that the function of XPD in TFIIH is largely structural. As long as the protein is present in the TFIIH complex, it can tolerate substantial alterations to its structure.

Coin et al. showed that, in the TFIIH complex, the C-terminus of XPD interacts with the p44 subunit, and that this interaction results in a tenfold stimulation of the helicase activity.[105] They then immunopurified TFIIH from normal cells and from XP-D cells with different mutations in the XPD gene. These mutations included the most frequent XP mutation (Arg683Trp), a mutation that gives rise to a combined phenotype of XP with CS (Gly675Arg), a 15 aa deletion (716–730) and (Arg722Trp), which are both associated with TTD. All of these were located at the C-terminal end of the XPD gene. In addition, they constructed a mutation in the ATP binding site of the XPD protein (Lys48Arg). TFIIH from cell extracts from the human disorders all showed 5′–3′ helicase activity, whereas, as expected, the Lys48Arg mutation abolished activity. The co-expression of the patient mutant proteins with p44 showed that these mutations abolished the interaction between XPD and p44, and the helicase activity of XPD was not stimulated by p44. These results explained the effects of mutations in the C-terminal third of the protein on DNA repair activity. However, they did not shed any further light on the disease specificity of these mutations, since they were associated with different disease phenotypes.

The picture emerging from these studies is that it is the helicase activity of XPD within the TFIIH complex that determines the repair capacity of the cell. This is, in turn, determined by the effect of mutations directly on the active site itself, but also on the interaction with the p44 subunit of TFIIH. The effects on transcription are largely determined by the ability of the mutated XPD protein to maintain the integrity of the TFIIH holocomplex.

XPE

The XPE gene encodes the smaller subunit of a heterodimeric DNA binding protein. Chu and Chang reported that a protein that bound specifically to DNA damaged by UV light or cisplatin was absent in an XP-E cell strain.[106] This DNA damage binding activity (UV-DDB) has been purified as a complex with two subunits of 127 and 48 kDa.[107] Sequence analysis of the p48 subunit has shown mutations in the p48 gene of XP-E patients.[108]

Recent work of Hwang and co-workers has shown that the p48/XPE gene is inducible by UV irradiation and that this induction is dependent on p53.[109,110] This work also showed that XPE is specifically involved in the global genome repair of CPDs, but is dispensable for transcription-coupled repair of CPDs and for all repair of the other major UV photoproduct, the 6–4 photodimer. It is likely, therefore, that XPE plays a specific role in recognizing CPDs in non-transcribing DNA.

XPF

The XPF gene encodes the larger (916 aa) subunit of a heterodimeric structure-specific nuclease, XPF/ERCC1. This nuclease incises damaged DNA 5′ to the damaged site. XPF/ERCC1 cuts the DNA 5′ to the damage after XPG (see later) has incised on the 3′-side.[111] Mutations have been identified in several XP-F patients and they are mostly missense mutations[112] (Plate 2). Defects in the partner protein, ERCC1, have not been found in any patients. However, ERCC1 knockout mice have been generated. They are viable but very sick, surviving for only a few weeks. The phenotype of the ERCC1 mice is much more severe than that of XPA mice, even though the XPA mice are completely deficient in NER.[113,114] This implies that ERCC1 and by implication its partner XPF provide a further example of repair proteins having other roles. In the case of ERCC1/XPF, a probable second function is in certain types of recombination. The yeast homologues, Rad1 and Rad10, are known to be required for recombination between short repeats[115] and it is likely that the human proteins have a similar function. It may be that the abolition of this second function is responsible for the more severe phenotype of the ERCC1 mouse, although this remains to be proven.

XPG

XP-G is clinically very heterogeneous. Although nearly all XP-G patients have very low levels of NER, the clinical spectrum ranges from symptoms that are very mild with little sun-sensitivity to severe with associated symptoms of CS. The XPG gene encodes a protein of 1196 aa, which is homologous to the products of the RAD2 gene of S. cerevisiae and the rad13 gene of S. pombe.[116–118] The sequence identity between the three organisms is highest in two regions of about 70 aa close to the termini of the protein. The spacing between these two regions is also conserved between the three organisms, even though there is little similarity in the intervening sequence. These observations suggest that these two domains are crucial for the function of the proteins. The XPG protein is a structure-specific endonuclease with opposite polarity from XPF/ERCC1.[118] It cleaves damaged DNA on the 3′ side of the damaged site (Figure 16.1). This reaction is absolutely dependent on the previous actions of XPA, XPC and TFIIH.[119–121]

Sequence analysis of the XPG gene has shown that patients with the milder symptoms have missense mutations, which abolish nuclease activity. In contrast, the mutations leading to a combined phenotype of XP-G with CS all result in severely truncated XPG proteins[122] (Plate 2). This raised the possibility of a second function of the XPG protein, which was retained in the missense mutants even though nuclease activity was abolished. The viability of XP-G patients with severely truncated XPG protein indicates that XPG does not have an essential role. This is confirmed by the viability of XPG knockout mice, which were, however, very sick with severe growth retardation and death by 23 days post partum.[123]

The increased severity of the abnormalities in XPG mice compared to XPA mice supports the idea of a second function for the XPG protein. This additional function may be a role in the repair of oxidative damage, in addition to its well-characterized role in repair of UV damage. It is possible that a deficiency in this function may be responsible for the features of CS in XP-G patients with the combined features of XP and CS. Cells from XP-G/CS patients are deficient in the transcription coupled repair of thymine glycols (Tg), which, in contrast, is found to be normal in XP-A, XP-F and XP-G cells from patients with XP alone.[124] Recent *in vitro* studies have provided a possible explanation for this specific deficiency.[125] Oxidative damage to DNA is normally removed by base excision repair (BER). Thymines converted into Tg by oxidative damage can be removed by BER, the first step being carried out by the human Nth1 DNA-glycosylase, which simultaneously excises the Tg residue and cleaves the DNA on the 3′-side of the resulting abasic site. hNth1 activity is specifically and strongly stimulated by the XPG protein. XPG appeared to stimulate the binding of hNth1 to DNA. Furthermore, the XPG protein mutated in the nuclease active site maintained its ability to stimulate Nth1.[125,126]

Taken together, there is substantial direct and indirect evidence for the involvement of XPG in the repair of oxidized bases and circumstantial evidence that the loss of oxidative damage repair function may play a causative role in the pathogenesis of CS symptoms in the combined disorder of XP-G/CS (see later section).

XP variants

In about 20 per cent of XP patients, NER is normal, even though the patients exhibit classical XP symptoms[69] and their cells are UV-hypermutable just like those of classical XPs.[177,178] This group, designated XP variants, are not hypersensitive to killing by UV-light.[129] XP-variant cells are defective in a process designated postreplication or daughter-strand repair.[18] This is a mechanism or collection of mechanisms for generating high-molecular-weight daughter-strand DNA after UV irradiation, despite the presence of persisting UV damage in the parental DNA strands. Studies with *E. coli* and lower eukaryotes suggest that there are likely to be different subpathways of postreplication repair. In *E. coli* the major pathway is thought to involve recombination, whereas a minor pathway

involves synthesis past the damage, a process designated translesion synthesis (TLS),[130] whereas in human cells the converse pertains. The precise molecular defect in XP variants remained elusive for a long time. The *XPV* gene was finally cloned in 1999 and found to be a DNA polymerase designated Pol η, which is able to carry out TLS past UV damage.[131–133] Pol η is able to insert adenines opposite a T-T CPD.[131] Abolition of this relatively error-free pathway channels photo-products into more error-prone pathways, resulting in the increased mutability of XP-V cells. It is of interest that the UV mutation spectrum in XP variants is different from that of normal and NER-defective XPs. Whereas the over-riding mutations in the latter are C to T transitions, the XP variant spectrum contains similar numbers of transitions and transversions, at both G:C and A:T sites.[31]

The catalytic activity of Pol η is contained within the highly conserved first 420 amino acids of the protein.[131] The C-terminal 120 amino acids are required to localize the protein in replication factories in the cell nucleus.[134] Many of the mutations found in the Pol η gene in XP variants result in severe protein truncations (see Plate 2), demonstrating that the gene is not essential for life.[131,133,135] A few C-terminal truncation mutations, however, leave the catalytic activity of the polymerase unaffected, but abolish the nuclear localization signals so that the polymerase is unable to gain access to the sites of DNA replication, where it carries out its functions in TLS.[134,135]

CS GENES

As discussed in the earlier section on Cockayne syndrome, CS cells are specifically deficient in TCR, and there are two CS complementation groups (CS-A and CS-B), the latter being the major group.[51] As mentioned before, CS symptoms can also, in rare cases, be associated with mutations in the *XPB*, *XPD* and the *XPG* gene where they coexist with XP symptoms. The defect in TCR indicates a possible role of the *CSA* and *CSB* genes in transcription, and it has been proposed that CS may be a disease that is caused by subtle defects in basal transcription.[136,137] The *CSA* gene encodes a 396 aa WD repeat protein, but there is as yet little information on its specific functions.[138] The CSB protein (chromosome 10q11–21) is a member of the Swi2/Snf2 DNA-dependent ATPase protein family.[139,140] Despite the seven characteristic helicase domains found in all family members, helicase activity has not been demonstrated in any of this family of proteins, including the 1493 aa CSB protein.[141] This protein superfamily is currently thought to be involved in 'chromatin remodelling' by disrupting protein-DNA interactions in chromatin.[142]

CS and transcription

What is the role of the CS proteins in TCR? Initial hypotheses proposed that they were transcription-repair coupling factors, which recruited the NER machinery at sites where RNA polymerase molecules were blocked at lesions. In *E. coli* the product of the *mfd* gene performs such a role,[143] but direct evidence in support of a similar function for the CS proteins is lacking. The failure of CS cells to carry out TCR was proposed as an explanation for the characteristic inability of the cells to restore normal rates of RNA synthesis following UV-irradiation.[49] Van Oosterwijk *et al.* have proposed an alternative model in which, during NER, TFIIH is switched from its transcriptional to its NER role. After repair of damage, the CS proteins are required to switch TFIIH back from repair-mode to transcription-mode, thereby restoring RNA synthesis.[144]

There are several reports of interactions between CS proteins and other repair proteins.[138,145] However, in size fractionation experiments with cell extracts, CSB and CSA ran as separate high-molecular-weight complexes, which did not contain any of the other repair proteins. However, about 10 per cent of RNA polymerase II co-chromatographed and co-immunoprecipitated with CSB.[146] Several other reports have provided evidence for an interaction of CSB with RNA polymerase II.[147–149] These studies suggest a possible role for the CSB protein in assisting RNA polymerase II at positions at which it is stalled.

In another study, UV irradiation was found to result in the ubiquitination of the large subunit of RNA polymerase II in normal cells but not in CS cells. The authors proposed that the function of the CSB proteins is to bring about the ubiquitin-mediated degradation of RNA polymerase II molecules stalled at lesions to enable repair to proceed.[150] There is thus a considerable body of evidence implicating the CS proteins as intermediaries between repair and transcriptional processes, but their precise mode of action is still unclear.

Several studies suggest that neither *CSA* nor *CSB* are essential genes.[138,139,151,152] Many mutations in patients produce drastic truncations of the CS proteins[52] (see Plate 2). Furthermore, the CSB knockout mice are viable and healthy. Although, like CS patients, the mice show hypersensitivity to UV, they have only mild neurological abnormalities in contrast to the severe features of human CS-B individuals.[153] These observations clearly rule out an essential role of the CSB proteins in transcription, but a non-essential accessory role for CS proteins has been proposed.[137]

Oxidative damage

CS cells, like those from XP-G/CS patients discussed above, are defective in transcription-coupled repair of thymine glycols.[154] Work by Le Page *et al.* suggests that CS cells as well as XP/CS cells from the XP-B, XP-C and XP-G groups are also defective in transcription coupled repair of 8-hydroxyguanine,[155] even though this lesion, when on the non-transcribed strand, is repaired efficiently by base excision repair. The relationship of these observations to the stimulation of hNth1 activity by XPG (see earlier section) is unclear. XPG does not affect the activity of hOGG1, the protein responsible for the repair of 8-hydroxyguanine.

TRICHOTHIODYSTROPHY GENES

The majority of cases of TTD (more than 25 reported in the literature) are in the XP-D complementation group. As described in the earlier section on *XPD*, evidence suggests that the site of the mutation in the *XPD* gene determines the phenotype,[99] and these mutations are either found in the very N-terminal or the C-terminal region of the gene (see Plate 2). We have suggested above that the transcriptional role of XPD is maintaining the structure of the TFIIH holocomplex, and that TTD features are largely the result of a transcriptional deficiency. It is likely that each mutation might affect the TFIIH structure to a different extent, and that mutations in which it is more severely disrupted will result in the most severe cases. An extra layer of complexity became apparent from a study of TTD patients in Italy, which revealed a gene dosage effect.[14] The mutation in the majority of these patients was Arg-112→His in the N-terminal region and, although all patients had similarly pronounced defects in NER, their clinical features were very heterogeneous. More detailed examination revealed that the more mildly affected cases were homozygous for this mutation, whereas the severely affected cases were functionally hemizygous, the second allele being null. This suggests that, under conditions in which the XPD protein is partially crippled, its transcriptional role becomes rate-limiting, so that a twofold reduction in its level results in more severe effects. Two studies have shown that the levels of TFIIH are reduced in cells from TTD patients, consistent with the idea that TTD mutations reduce the stability of the TFIIH complex.[156,157]

If, as seems likely, the features of TTD are indeed the result of transcriptional deficiencies, how is the specificity of the features explained? De Boer *et al.* have proposed that the transcriptional deficiency becomes manifest in cells at the end of a differentiation pathway, when there is a high transcriptional load, but the transcription machinery becomes limiting.[100] This would explain the specific deficiency in sulphur-rich matrix proteins of the hair shafts. In support of their ideas, they found that keratinocytes from the TTD mouse were deficient in transcription of the *SPRR2* gene, which encodes a proline-rich protein expressed late in terminal differentiation of inter-follicular keratinocytes. Further support for a transcriptional deficiency in TTD comes from the finding that TTD patients have β-thalassaemia trait, resulting from reduced expression of the β-globin genes.[158]

Although most TTD families are mutated in the *XPD* gene, one family has a point mutation in the *XPB* gene (see earlier section on *XPB*), and three patients have been assigned to a complementation group that has no XP representative (Stefanini[60] and M. Stefanini, N. Jaspers, personal communication). These individuals are, therefore, defective in another gene, designated *TTDA*, which is involved in NER. So far, this gene has not been cloned. Although the defect can be corrected both in cells and cell extracts by microinjection or addition of TFIIH,[80] it does not appear to encode any of the TFIIH subunits. As with other TTD patients, the levels of TFIIH are low in cells from this patient[156] and, indeed, the cellular phenotype can be corrected by microinjecting TFIIH even from the same TTD-A cells. The close association with TFIIH of the three genes in which defects can result in TTD adds further weight to the idea that TTD is a transcription syndrome.

RELATIONSHIP TO CLINICAL SYMPTOMS

In considering the relationship of DNA repair defects to the clinical features of XP, CS and TTD, we need to consider the following questions.

1 What is the relationship of defective DNA repair to the clinical features of XP?
2 How can mutations in *XPB* (in both known families), *XPD* and *XPG* (occasionally) result in the features of XP and CS?
3 How can mutations in *XPD* result in the features of XP alone, XP with CS or TTD?

Cellular and biochemical studies discussed in the earlier section on mutability demonstrated that, in XP cells, defective-excision or daughter-strand repair is associated with UV hypermutability of cultured fibroblasts. This has led to the hypothesis that a high frequency of sunlight-induced mutations in the skin of XP patients is the cause of the freckling and high incidence of skin cancer in these patients. The observations that a large proportion of basal and squamous cell carcinomas in normal individuals contain mutations in the *TP53* gene with a spectrum characteristic of that produced by UV radiation,[159] and that skin tumour cells from many XP patients also contain UV-type mutations in the *TP53* gene[90] are consistent with this hypothesis. A sunlight-induced mutation in *TP53* appears, therefore, to be a crucial event in skin carcinogenesis, and will occur at a greatly elevated frequency in XP patients. This hypothesis is neat, coherent and satisfactorily accounts for the skin abnormalities in XP. Less clear, however, is the explanation for the clinical features of TTD and, in particular, the lack of freckling and skin cancer in TTD patients, even though the cultured fibroblasts have a repair deficiency, and in some cases UV mutability, indistinguishable from that in XP cells.

The brittle hair, ichthyosis and other features of TTD are not related in any obvious way to a DNA repair deficiency. The clue to their possible aetiology comes from the findings discussed in earlier sections that the gene products defective in the three known TTD complementation groups are probably all subunits of or closely involved with the transcription factor TFIIH. It is thus likely that the clinical features of TTD might result from subtle deficiencies in transcription, which are not manifest in cultured fibroblasts but may have more marked effects in specific tissues, e.g. abnormal keratin expression in hair-shaft cells, resulting in trichothiodystrophy.[74,80] In particular, de Boer *et al.* have suggested that the deficiency in TFIIH might be most manifest in tissues that are at the end of differentiation pathways. In such tissue, cells still need to make large amounts of protein, but transcription has been shut off.[100] This is supported by the finding of decreased β-globin expression in erythrocytes from TTD patients.[158]

Mutations in the *XPD* gene can result in the clinical features either of XP or of TTD, but there are only two reported instances of patients with features of both together.[160] There seems to be some consequence of the mutations that result in TTD that inhibits the manifestation of XP skin abnormalities, despite very low levels of NER. Since the clinical features of TTD seem to be unrelated to the repair levels and the latter can range from close to zero up to normal, it seems unlikely that the lack of XP features in TTD has anything to do with differing levels of repair between XP and TTD patients. It is more likely that the subtle transcriptional deficiencies in TTD patients in some way reduce the potential of unrepaired DNA damage to act as a precarcinogenic lesion.[161]

Cockayne syndrome poses further problems. The disorder is associated with a specific deficiency in the ability to carry out TCR. The *CSB* gene is not essential. The features of XP and CS are found in both families in the rare XP-B group, in two families in XP-D and at least seven in XP-G (Hoeijmakers,[21] and S. Clarkson, personal communication). The yeast homologues of the *XPG* gene are not essential, whereas the essential XPB and XPD products are subunits of TFIIH. The latter would suggest that the features of CS may also result from a deficiency in transcription, as suggested for TTD. Indeed, the two disorders do appear to have some features in common, e.g. mental and physical retardation, cataracts, dental caries, abnormal facies. However, the specific hairshaft abnormalities seen in TTD have not been found in CS nor has ichthyosis been reported. The neurological abnormalities in CS are progressive, whereas this does not appear to be the case for TTD. Furthermore, any gene whose product is directly involved in basal transcription must be essential. The features of CS in the CS groups and in XP/CS patients might be related to the deficiencies in repair of oxidative damage described in the sections on *XPG*.[155] Oxidative damage is produced continuously inside cells and they may be particularly prone to the effects of oxidative damage during development.

The rapid progress currently being made in cloning of DNA repair genes and understanding the precise roles of the gene products should help to unravel the complex inter-relationships associated with the disorders discussed in this chapter. These studies are not only contributing to our understanding of the mechanisms of carcinogenesis, but the association of DNA repair proteins with transcription factors may reveal a new category of transcription-related disorders.

SUMMARY

Xeroderma pigmentosum (XP), Cockayne syndrome and trichothiodystrophy are three genetic disorders caused by defects in the ability of cells to remove damage from their DNA. All three disorders are sun sensitive but only XP is cancer prone. XP can result from mutations in any one of eight genes. Seven of these genes encode proteins involved in different steps of nucleotide excision repair of DNA damage. The eighth group is defective in a DNA polymerase, which can replicate past damaged DNA templates. A defect in any of these genes results in a greatly increased incidence of sunlight induced skin cancer. Two of the XP genes encode subunits of the TFIIH basal transcription factor, which has two roles, in basal transcription and in nucleotide excision repair. Trichothiodystrophy is associated with specific mutations in either of these genes and its multisystem clinical phenotype is thought to result from resulting subtle defects in transcription. Cockayne syndrome is also a multisystem disorder with subtle transcriptional deficiencies as well as defects in a subpathway of nucleotide excision repair associated with transcriptionally active genes.

KEY POINTS

- Xeroderma pigmentosum (XP), Cockayne syndrome (CS) and Trichothiodystrophy (TTD) are all due to defects of removal of DNA damage.
- Only XP is cancer prone.
- All three syndromes are sun sensitive.

REFERENCES

1. Bootsma D, Kraemer KH, Cleaver JE, Hoeijmakers JHJ. Nucleotide excision repair syndromes: xeroderma pigmentosum, Cockayne Syndrome, and trichothiodystrophy. In: Vogelstein B, Kinzler KW (eds) *The genetic basis of human cancer.* New York: McGraw-Hill, 1998:245–274.

2. Kraemer KH, Lee MM, Scotto J. Xeroderma pigmentosum. Cutaneous, ocular and neurologic abnormalities in 830 published cases. *Arch Dermatol* 1987; **123**:241–250.

3. Ramsay CA, Giannelli F. The erythemal action spectrum and deoxyribonucleic acid repair synthesis in xeroderma pigmentosum. *Br J Dermatol* 1975; **92**:49–56.

4. Bridges BA (Chairman), Arlett CF, *et al. Solar and ultraviolet radiation.* IARC Monograph. Lyon: IARC, 1992.

5. Kraemer KH, Lee MM, Scotto K. DNA repair protects against cutaneous and internal neoplasia: evidence from xeroderma pigmentosum. *Carcinogenesis* 1984; **5**:511–514.

6. Norris PG, Limb GA, Hamblin AS, *et al.* Immune function, mutant frequency and cancer risk in the DNA repair defective genodermatoses xeroderma pigmentosum, Cockayne's Syndrome and trichothiodystrophy. *J Invest Dermatol* 1990; **94**:94–100.

7. Gaspari AA, Fleisher TA, Kraemer KH. Impaired interferon production and natural killer cell activation in patients with the skin cancer prone disorder, xeroderma pigmentosum. *J Clin Invest* 1993; **92**:1135–1142.

8. Anstey A, Arlett CF, Cole J, *et al.* Long term survival and preservation of natural killer cell activity in a xeroderma pigmentosum patient with spontaneous regression and multiple deposits of malignant melanoma. *Br J Dermatol* 1991; **125**:272–278.

9. Turner ML, Moshell AN, Corbett DW, *et al.* Clearing of melanoma-in-situ with intralesional interferon alpha in a patient with xeroderma pigmentosum. *Arch Dermatol* 1994; **130**:1491–1494.

10. Krutmann J, Bohnert JE, Jung EG. Evidence that DNA damage is a mediate in ultraviolet B radiation-induced inhibition of human gene expression: ultraviolet B radiation effects in intercellular adhesion molecule-1 (ICAM-1) expression. *J Invest Dermatol* 1994; **102**:428–432.

11. Nance MA, Berry SA. Cockayne syndrome: review of 140 cases. *Am J Med Genet* 1992; **42**:68–84.

12. Lehmann AR, Thompson AF, Harcourt SA, *et al.* Cockayne syndrome: correlation of clinical features with cellular sensitivity of RNA synthesis to UV-irradiation. *J Med Genet* 1993; **30**:679–682.

13. Itin PH, Pittelkow MR. Trichothiodystrophy: review of sulfur-deficient brittle hair syndromes and association with the ectodermal dysplasias. *J Am Acad Dermatol* 1990; **20**:705–717.

14. Botta E, Nardo T, Broughton BC, *et al.* Analysis of mutations in the *XPD* gene in Italian patients with trichothiodystrophy: site of mutation correlates with repair deficiency but gene dosage appears to determine clinical severity. *Am J Hum Genet* 1998; **63**:1036–1048.

15. Gartler SM. Inborn errors of metabolism at the cell culture level. In: Fishbein M (ed.) *Second International Conference on Congenital Malformations,* New York: International Medical Congress, 1964:94.

16. Cleaver JE. Deficiency in repair replication of DNA in xeroderma pigmentosum. *Nature* 1968; **218:**652–656.

17. Cleaver JE. Xeroderma pigmentosum: variants with normal DNA repair and normal sensitivity to uv light. *J Invest Dermatol* 1972; **58:**124–128.

18. Lehmann AR, Kirk-Bell S, Arlett CF, *et al.* Xeroderma pigmentosum cells with normal levels of excision repair have a defect in DNA synthesis after UV-irradiation. *Proc Natl Acad Sci USA* 1975; **72:**219–223.

19. Maher VM, McCormick JJ, Grover P, Sims P. Effect of DNA on the cytotoxicity and mutagenicity of polycyclic hydrocarbon derivatives in normal and xeroderma pigmentosum human fibroblasts. *Mutation Res* 1977; **43:**117–138.

20. Arlett CF, Lowe JE, Harcourt SA, *et al.* Hypersensitivity of human lymphocytes to UV-B and solar irradiation. *Cancer Res* 1993; **53:**609–614.

21. Hoeijmakers JHJ. Nucleotide excision repair II: from yeast to mammals. *Trends Genet* 1993; **9:**211–217.

22. van Hoffen A, Venema J, Meschini R, *et al.* Transcription-coupled repair removes both cyclobutane pyrimidine dimers and 6-4 photoproducts with equal efficiency and in a sequential way from transcribed DNA in xeroderma pigmentosum group C fibroblasts. *EMBO J* 1995; **14:**360–367.

23. Johnson RT, Squires S. The XP-D complementation group. Insight into xeroderma pigmentosum, Cockayne syndrome, and trichothiodystrophy. *Mutation Res* 1992; **273:**97–118.

24. Maher VM, McCormick JJ. Effect of DNA repair on the cytotoxicity and mutagenicity of UV irradiation and of chemical carcinogens in normal and xeroderma pigmentosum cells. In: Yuhas JM, Tennant RW, Regan JB(eds) *Biology of radiation carcinogenesis.* New York: Raven Press, 1976:129–145.

25. Arlett CF, Harcourt SA. Variation in response to mutagens amongst normal and repair-defective human cells. In: Lawrence CW (ed.) *Induced mutagenesis. Molecular mechanisms and their implications for environmental protection.* New York: Plenum Press, 1983:240–260.

26. Glover TW, Chang C-C, Trosko JF, Li SS-I. Ultraviolet light induction of diphtheria toxin-resistant mutants in normal and xeroderma pigmentosum human fibroblasts. *Proc Natl Acad Sci USA* 1979; **76:**3982–3986.

27. de Weerd-Kastelein EA, Keijzer W, Rainaldi G, Bootsma D. Induction of sister chromatid exchanges in xeroderma pigmentosum cells after exposure to ultraviolet light. *Mutation Res* 1977; **45:**253–261.

28. Marshall RR, Scott D. The relationship between chromosome damage and cell killing in UV-irradiated normal and xeroderma pigmentosum cells. *Mutation Res* 1976; **36:**397–400.

29. Dorado G, Steingrimsdottir H, Arlett CF, Lehmann AR. Molecular analysis of UV-induced mutations in a xeroderma pigmentosum cell line. *J Mol Biol* 1991; **217:**217–222.

30. McGregor WG, Chen R-H, Lukash L, *et al.* Cell cycle-dependent strand bias for UV-induced mutations in the transcribed strand of excision repair-proficient human fibroblasts but not in repair deficient cells. *Mol Cell Biol* 1991; **11:**1927–1934.

31. Wang YC, Maher VM, Mitchell DL, McCormick JJ. Evidence from mutation spectra that the UV hypermutability of xeroderma pigmentosum variant cells reflects abnormal,

32. Bredberg A, Kraemer KH, Seidman MM. Restricted ultraviolet mutational spectrum in a shuttle vector propagated in xeroderma pigmentosum cells. *Proc Natl Acad Sci USA* 1986; **83:**8273–8277.

33. Cole J, Arlett CF, Norris PG, *et al.* Elevated *hprt* mutant frequency in circulating T-lymphocytes of xeroderma pigmentosum patients. *Mutation Res* 1992; **273:**171–178.

34. Steingrimsdottir H, Rowley G, Waugh A, *et al.* Molecular analysis of mutations in the hprt gene in circulating lymphocytes from normal and DNA-repair-deficient donors. *Mutation Res* 1993; **294:**29–41.

35. Scott RJ, Itui P, Kleijer WJ, *et al.* Xeroderma pigmentosum – Cockayne syndrome complex on two new patients: absence of skin tumors despite severe deficiency of DNA excision repair. *J Am Acad Dermatol* 1993; **29:**883–889.

36. Vermeulen W, Scott RJ, Potger S, *et al.* Clinical heterogeneity within xeroderma pigmentosum associated with mutations in the DNA repair and transcription gene *ERCC3. Am J Hum Genet* 1994; **54:**191–200.

37. Chang HR, Ishizaki K, Sasaki MS, *et al.* Somatic mosaicism for DNA repair capacity in fibroblasts derived from a group A xeroderma pigmentosum patient. *J Invest Dermatol* 1989; **93:**460–465.

38. Robbins JH. Defective DNA repair in xeroderma pigmentosum and other neurologic diseases. *Curr Opin Neurol Neurosurg* 1988; **1:**1077–1083.

39. Kraemer KH. Xeroderma pigmentosum. In: Demis DJ, Dobson RI, McGuire J.(eds) *Clinical dermatology,* Vol. 4, Hagerstown: Harper and Row, 1980:1–33.

40. Ramsay CA, Coltart TM, Blunt S, *et al.* Prenatal diagnosis of xeroderma pigmentosum. *Lancet* 1974; **2:**1109–1112.

41. Holley DJ, Keijzer W, Jaspers NGI, *et al.* Prenatal diagnosis of xeroderma pigmentosum (group C) using assays of unscheduled DNA synthesis and postreplication repair. *Clinic Genet* 1979; **16:**137–146.

42. Kraemer KH, DiGiovanna JJ, Moshell AN, *et al.* Prevention of skin cancer in xeroderma pigmentosum with the use of oral isotretinoin. *N Engl J Med* 1988; **318:**1633–1637.

43. Strong A. Xeroderma pigmentosum variant: prevention of cutaneous neoplasms with etretinate. *Retinoids* 1989; **17:**40–42.

44. Berth-Jones J, Cole J, Lehmann AR, *et al.* Xeroderma pigmentosum variant: 5 years of tumor suppression by etretinate. *J Roy Soc Med* 1993; **86:**355–356.

45. Tanaka K, Hayakawa H, Sekiguchi M, Okada Y. Specific action of T4 endonuclease V on damaged DNA in xeroderma pigmentosum cells *in vivo. Proc Natl Acad Sci USA* 1977; **74:**2958–2962.

46. Yarosh D, Klein J, O'Connor A, *et al.* Effect of topically applied T4 endonuclease V in liposomes on skin cancer in xeroderma pigmentosum: a randomised study. Xeroderma Pigmentosum Study Group. *Lancet* 2001; **357:**926–929.

47. Wade MH, Chu EHY. Effects of DNA damaging agents on cultured fibroblasts derived from patients with Cockayne syndrome. *Mutation Res* 1979; **59:**49–60.

48. Marshall RR, Arlett CF, Harcourt SA, Broughton BC. Increased sensitivity of cell strains from Cockayne syndrome to sister-chromatid-exchange induction and cell killing by UV light. *Mutation Res* 1980; **69:**107–112.

49. Mayne LV, Lehmann AR. Failure of RNA synthesis to recover after UV-irradiation: an early defect in cells from individuals with Cockayne syndrome and xeroderma pigmentosum. *Cancer Res* 1982; **42**:1473–1478.

50. Lehmann AR, Francis AJ, Giannelli F. Prenatal diagnosis of Cockayne syndrome. *Lancet* 1985; **i**:486–488.

51. Stefanini M, Fawcett H, Botta E, *et al.* Genetic analysis of twenty-two patients with Cockayne syndrome. *Hum Genet* 1996; **97**:418–423.

52. Mallery DL, Tanganelli B, Colella S, *et al.* Molecular analysis of mutations in the *CSB(ERCC6)* gene in patients with Cockayne syndrome. *Am J Hum Genet* 1998; **62**:77–85.

53. van Hoffen A, Natarajan AT, Mayne LV, *et al.* Deficient repair of the transcribed strand of active genes in Cockayne syndrome cells. *Nucl Acids Res* 1993; **21**:5890–5895.

54. Arlett CF, Cole J. Photosensitive human syndromes and cellular defects in DNA repair. In: Jones RR, Wigley T (eds) *Ozone depletion: health and environmental consequences.* Chichester: Wiley and Sons Ltd, 1989:147–160.

55. Henderson EE, Long WK. Host cell reactivation of UV- and X-ray-damaged herpes simplex virus by Epstein-Barr Virus (EBV)-transformed lymphoblastoid cell lines. *Virology* 1981; **115**:237–248.

56. Norris PG, Lehmann AR, Cole J, *et al.* Photosensitivity and lymphocyte hypermutability in Cockayne syndrome. *Br J Dermatol* 1991; **124**:453–460.

57. Broughton BC, Lehmann AR, Harcourt SA, *et al.* Relationship between pyrimidine dimers, 6-4 photoproducts, repair synthesis and cell survival: studies using cells from patients with trichothiodystrophy. *Mutation Res* 1990; **235**:33–40.

58. Stefanini M, Lagomarsini P, Giliani S, *et al.* Genetic heterogeneity of the excision repair defect associated with trichothiodystrophy. *Carcinogenesis* 1993; **14**:1101–1105.

59. Weeda G, Eveno E, Donker I, *et al.* A mutation in the *XPB/ERCC3* DNA repair transcription gene, associated with trichothiodystrophy. *Am J Hum Genet* 1997; **60**:320–329.

60. Stefanini M, Vermeulen W, Weeda G, *et al.* A new nucleotide excision repair gene associated with the genetic disorder trichothiodystrophy. *Am J Hum Genet* 1993; **53**:817–821.

61. Cleaver JE, Thompson LH, Richardson AS, States JC. A summary of mutations in the UV-sensitive disorders: xeroderma pigmentosum, Cockayne syndrome, and trichothiodystrophy. *Hum Mutat* 1999; **14**:9–22.

62. Robins P, Jones CJ, Biggerstaff M, *et al.* Complementation of DNA repair in xeroderma pigmentosum group A cell extracts by a protein with affinity for damaged DNA. *EMBO J* 1991; **10**:3913–3921.

63. Sugasawa K, Ng JM, Masutani C, *et al.* Xeroderma pigmentosum group C protein complex is the initiator of global genome nucleotide excision repair. *Mol Cell* 1998; **2**:223–232.

64. Volker M, Mone MJ, Karmakar P, *et al.* Sequential assembly of the nucleotide excision repair factors *in vivo. Mol Cell* 2001; **8**:213–224.

65. Miyamoto I, Miura N, Niwa H, *et al.* Mutational analysis of the structure and function of the xeroderma pigmantosum group A complementing protein. *J Biol Chem* 1992; **267**:12182–12187.

66. Nishigori C, Moriwaki S-I, Takebe H, *et al.* Gene alterations and clinical characteristics of xeroderma pigmentosum group A patients in Japan. *Arch Dermatol* 1994; **130**:191–197.

67. de Vries A, van Oostrom CT, Hofhuis FM, *et al.* Increased susceptibility to ultraviolet-B and carcinogens of mice lacking the DNA excision repair gene *XPA. Nature* 1995; **377**:169–173.

68. Nakane H, Takeuchi S, Yuba S, *et al.* High incidence of ultraviolet-B- or chemical-carcinogen-induced skin tumours in mice lacking the xeroderma pigmentosum group A gene. *Nature* 1995; **377**:165–168.

69. Robbins JH, Kraemer KH, Lutzner MA, *et al.* Xeroderma pigmentosum: an inherited disease with sun-sensitivity, multiple cutaneous neoplasms, and abnormal DNA repair. *Ann Intern Med* 1974; **80**:221–248.

70. Weeda G, van Ham RCA, Vermeulen W, *et al.* A presumed DNA helicase encoded by *ERCC-3* is involved in the human repair disorders xeroderma pigmentosum and Cockayne syndrome. *Cell* 1990; **62**:777–791.

71. Schaeffer L, Roy R, Humbert S, *et al.* DNA repair helicase: a component of BTF2 (TFIIH) basic transcription factor. *Science* 1993; **260**:58–63.

72. Hoeijmakers JHJ, Egly J-M, Vermeulen W. TFIIH: a key component in multiple DNA transactions. *Curr Opin Gen Dev* 1996; **6**:26–33.

73. Lehmann AR. Dual functions of DNA repair genes: molecular, cellular, and clinical implications. *BioEssays* 1998; **20**:146–155.

74. Bootsma D, Hoeijmakers JHJ. Engagement with transcription. *Nature* 1993; **363**:114–115.

75. Ma L, Siemssen ED, Noteborn M, Van der Eb AJ. The xeroderma pigmentosum group B protein ERCC3 produced in the baculovirus system exhibits DNA helicase activity. *Nucl Acids Res* 1994; **22**:4095–4102.

76. Park E, Guzder SN, Koken MHM, *et al. RAD25 (SSL2),* the yeast homolog of the human xeroderma pigmentosum group B DNA repair gene, is essential for viability. *Proc Natl Acad Sci USA* 1992; **89**:11416–11420.

77. Schultz P, Fribourg S, Poterszman A, *et al.* Molecular structure of human TFIIH. *Cell* 2000; **102**:599–607.

78. Tirode F, Busso D, Coin F, Egly JM. Reconstitution of the transcription factor TFIIH: assignment of functions for the three enzymatic subunits, XPB, XPD, and cdk7. *Mol Cell* 1999; **3**:87–95.

79. Coin F, Bergmann E, Tremeau-Bravard A, Egly JM. Mutations in XPB and XPD helicases found in xeroderma pigmentosum patients impair the transcription function of TFIIH. *EMBO J* 1999; **18**:1357–1366.

80. Vermeulen W, van Vuuren AJ, Chipoulet M, *et al.* Three unusual repair deficiencies associated with transcription factor BTF2(TFIIH): evidence for the existence of a transcription syndrome. *Cold Spring Harb Symp Quant Biol* 1994; **59**:317–329.

81. Evans E, Moggs JG, Hwang JR, *et al.* Mechanism of open complex and dual incision formation by human nucleotide excision repair factors. *EMBO J* 1997; **16**:6559–6573.

82. Masutani C, Sugasawa K, Yanagisawa J, *et al.* Purification and cloning of a nucleotide excision-repair complex involving the xeroderma-pigmentosum group-C protein and a human homolog of yeast RAD23. *EMBO J* 1994; **13**:1831–1843.

83. Mu D, Sancar A. Model for XPC-independent transcription-coupled repair of pyrimidine dimers in humans. *J Biol Chem* 1997; **272**:7570–7573.

84. Li L, Bales ES, Peterson CA, Legerski RJ. Characterization of molecular defects in xeroderma pigmentosum group C. *Nature Genet* 1993; **5**:413–417.

85. Chavanne F, Broughton BC, Pietra D, *et al*. Mutations in the *XPC* gene in families with xeroderma pigmentosum and consequences at the cell, protein and transcript levels. *Cancer Res*. 2000; **60**:1974–1982.

86. Sands AT, Abuin A, Sanchez A, *et al*. High susceptibility to ultraviolet-induced carcinogenesis in mice lacking XPC. *Nature* 1995; **377**:162–165.

87. Berg RJ, Ruven HJ, Sands AT, *et al*. Defective global genome repair in XPC mice is associated with skin cancer susceptibility but not with sensitivity to UVB induced erythema and edema. *J Invest Dermatol* 1998; **110**:405–409.

88. Cheo DL, Ruven HJ, Meira LB, *et al*. Characterization of defective nucleotide excision repair in XPC mutant mice. *Mutat Res* 1997; **374**:1–9.

89. Cheo DL, Meira LB, Hammer RE, *et al*. Synergistic interactions between *xpc* and *p53* mutations in double-mutant mice: neural tube abnormalities and accelerated UV radiation-induced skin cancer. *Curr Biol* 1996; **6**:1691–1694.

90. Dumaz N, Drougar C, Sarasin A, Daya-Grosjean L. Specific UV-induced mutation spectrum in the *p53* gene of skin tumors from DNA repair deficient xeroderma pigmentosum patients. *Proc Natl Acad Sci USA* 1993; **90**:10529–10533.

91. Giglia G, Dumaz N, Drougard C, *et al*. *p53* mutations in skin and internal tumors of xeroderma pigmentosum patients belonging to the complementation group C. *Cancer Res* 1998; **58**:4402–4409.

92. Bodak N, Queille S, Avril MF, *et al*. High levels of *patched* gene mutations in basal-cell carcinomas from patients with xeroderma pigmentosum. *Proc Natl Acad Sci USA* 1999; **96**:5117–5122.

93. Weber CA, Salazar EP, Stewart SA, Thompson LH. *ERCC-2*: cDNA cloning and molecular characterization of a human nucleotide excision repair gene with high homology to yeast RAD3. *EMBO J* 1990; **9**:1437–1448.

94. Murray JM, Doe C, Schenk P, *et al*. Cloning and characterisation of the *S. pombe rad15* gene, a homologue to the *S. cerevisiae RAD3* and human *ERCC2* genes. *Nucl Acids Res* 1992; **20**:2673–2678.

95. Sung P, Prakash L, Matson SW, Prakash S. RAD3 protein of *Saccharomyces cerevisiae* is a DNA helicase. *Proc Natl Acad Sci USA* 1987; **84**:8951–8955.

96. Sung P, Bailly V, Weber C, *et al*. Human xeroderma pigmentosum group D gene encodes a DNA helicase. *Nature* 1993; **365**:852–855.

97. Schaeffer L, Monocollin V, Roy R, *et al*. The ERCC2/DNA repair protein is associated with the class II BTF2/TFIIH transcription factor. *EMBO J* 1994; **13**:2388–2392.

98. Lehmann AR. Nucleotide excision repair and the link with transcription. *Trends Biochem Sci* 1995; **20**:402–405.

99. Taylor EM, Broughton BC, Botta E, *et al*. Xeroderma pigmentosum and trichothiodystrophy are associated with different mutations in the *XPD* (*ERCC2*) repair/transcription gene. *Proc Natl Acad Sci USA* 1997; **94**:8658–8663.

100. de Boer J, de Wit J, van Steeg H, *et al*. A mouse model for the basal transcription/DNA repair syndrome trichothiodystrophy. *Mol Cell* 1998; **1**:981–990.

101. de Boer J, Andressoo JO, de Wit J, *et al*. Premature ageing in mice deficient in DNA repair and transcription. *Science* 2002; **296**:1276–1279.

102. Berneburg M, Lowe JE, Nardo T, *et al*. UV damage causes uncontrolled DNA breakage in cells from patients with combined features of XP-D and Cockayne syndrome. *EMBO J* 2000; **19**:1157–1166.

103. Sung P, Higgins D, Prakash L, Prakash S. Mutation of lysine-48 to arginine in the yeast RAD3 protein abolishes its ATPase and DNA helicase activities but not the ability to bind ATP. *EMBO J* 1988; **7**:3263–3269.

104. Feaver WJ, Svejstrup JQ, Bardwell L, *et al*. Dual roles of a multiprotein complex from *S. cerevisiae* in transcription and DNA repair. *Cell* 1993; **75**:1379–1387.

105. Coin F, Marinoni JC, Rodolfo C, *et al*. Mutations in the *XPD* helicase gene result in XP and TTD phenotypes, preventing interaction between *XPD* and the p44 subunit of TFIIH. *Nature Genet* 1998; **20**:184–188.

106. Chu G, Chang E. Xeroderma pigmentosum group E cells lack a nuclear factor that binds to damaged DNA. *Science* 1988; **242**:564–567.

107. Keeney S, Chang GJ, Linn S. Characterization of a human DNA damage binding protein implicated in xeroderma pigmentosum E. *J Biol Chem* 1993; **268**:21293–21300.

108. Nichols AF, Ong P, Linn S. Mutations specific to the xeroderma pigmentosum group E Ddb-phenotype. *J Biol Chem* 1996; **40**:24317–24320.

109. Hwang BJ, Toering S, Francke U, Chu G. p48 Activates a UV-damaged-DNA binding factor and is defective in xeroderma pigmentosum group E cells that lack binding activity. *Mol Cell Biol* 1998; **18**:4391–4399.

110. Hwang BJ, Ford JM, Hanawalt PC, Chu G. Expression of the p48 xeroderma pigmentosum gene is p53-dependent and is involved in global genomic repair. *Proc Natl Acad Sci USA* 1999; **96**:424–428.

111. Sijbers AM, de Laat WL, Ariza RR, *et al*. Xerderma pigmentosum group F caused by a defect in a structure-specific DNA repair endonuclease. *Cell* 1996; **86**:811–822.

112. Matsumura Y, Nishigori C, Yagi T, *et al*. Characterization of molecular defects in xeroderma pigmentosum group F in relation to its clinically mild symptoms. *Hum Mol Genet* 1998; **7**:969–974.

113. McWhir J, Selfridge J, Harrison DJ, *et al*. Mice with DNA repair gene (*ercc-1*) deficiency have elevated levels of p53, liver nuclear abnormalities and die before weaning. *Nature Genet* 1993; **5**:217–223.

114. Weeda G, Donker I, de Wit J, *et al*. Disruption of mouse *ERCC1* results in a novel repair syndrome with growth failure, nuclear abnormalities and senescence. *Curr Biol* 1997; **7**:427–439.

115. Fishman-Lobell J, Haber JE. Removal of nonhomologous DNA ends in double-strand break recombination: the role of the yeast ultraviolet repair gene *RAD1*. *Science* 1992; **258**:480–484.

116. Scherly D, Nouspikel T, Corlet J, *et al*. Complementation of the DNA repair defect in xeroderma pigmentosum group G cells by a human cDNA related to yeast *RAD2*. *Nature* 1993; **363**:182–185.

117. MacInnes MA, Dickson JA, Hernandez RR, *et al*. Human ERCC5 cDNA-cosmid complementation for excision repair and bipartite amino acid domains conserved with RAD proteins of *Saccharomyces cerevisiae* and *Schizosaccharomyces pombe*. *Mol Cell Biol* 1993; **13**:6393–6402.

118. O'Donovan A, Scherly D, Clarkson SG, Wood RD. Isolation of active recombinant XPG protein, a human DNA repair endonuclease. *J Biol Chem* 1994; **269**:15965–15968.

119. O'Donovan A, Davies AA, Moggs JG, *et al*. XPG endonuclease makes the 3' incision in human DNA nucleotide excision repair. *Nature* 1994; **371**:432–435.

120. Cloud KG, Shen B, Strniste GF, Park MS. XPG protein has a structure-specific endonuclease activity. *Mutat Res* 1995; **347**:55–60.

121. Evans E, Fellows J, Coffer A, Wood RD. Open complex formation around a lesion during nucleotide excision repair provides a structure for cleavage by human XPG protein. *EMBO J* 1997; **16**:625–638.

122. Nouspikel T, Lalle P, Leadon SA, *et al*. A common mutational pattern in Cockayne syndrome patients from xeroderma pigmentosum group G: implications for a second XPG function. *Proc Natl Acad Sci USA* 1997; **94**:3116–3121.

123. Harada YN, Shiomi N, Koike M, *et al*. Postnatal growth failure, short life span, and early onset of cellular senescence and subsequent immortalization in mice lacking the xeroderma pigmentosum group G gene. *Mol Cell Biol* 1999; **19**:2366–2372.

124. Cooper PK, Nouspikel T, Clarkson SG, Leadon SA. Defective transcription-coupled repair of oxidative base damage in Cockayne syndrome patients from XP group G. *Science* 1997; **275**:990–993.

125. Klungland A, Hoss M, Gunz D, *et al*. Base excision repair of oxidative DNA damage activated by XPG protein. *Mol Cell* 1999; **3**:33–42.

126. Bessho T. Nucleotide excision repair 3' endonuclease XPG stimulates the activity of base excision repair enzyme thymine glycol DNA glycosylase. *Nucl Acids Res* 1999; **27**:979–983.

127. Maher VM, Ouellette LM, Curren RD, McCormick JJ. Frequency of ultraviolet light-induced mutations is higher in xeroderma pigmentosum variant cells than in normal human cells. *Nature* 1976; **261**:593–595.

128. Myhr BC, Turnbull D, DiPaolo JA. Ultraviolet mutagenesis of normal and xeroderma pigmentosum variant human fibroblasts. *Mutation Res* 1979; **62**:341–353.

129. Arlett CF, Harcourt SA, Broughton BC. The influence of caffeine on cell survival in excision-proficient and excision-deficient xeroderma pigmentosum and normal human cell strains following ultraviolet light irradiation. *Mutation Res* 1975; **33**:341–346.

130. Lawrence CW, Hinkle DC. DNA polymerase zeta and the control of DNA damage induced mutagenesis in eukaryotes. *Cancer Surv* 1996; **28**:21–31.

131. Masutani C, Kusumoto R, Yamada A, *et al*. The human *XPV* (xeroderma pigmentosum variant) gene encodes human polymerase h. *Nature* 1999; **399**:700–704.

132. Masutani C, Araki M, Yamada A, *et al*. Xeroderma pigmentosum variant (XP-V) correcting protein from HeLa cells has a thymine dimer bypass DNA polymerase activity. *EMBO J* 1999; **18**:3491–3501.

133. Johnson RE, Kondratick CM, Prakash S, Prakash L. *RAD30* mutations in the variant form of xeroderma pigmentosum. *Science* 1999; **285**:263–265.

134. Kannouche P, Broughton BC, Volker M, *et al*. Domain structure, localization and function of DNA polymerase h, defective in xeroderma pigmentosum variant cells. *Genes Dev* 2001; **15**:158–172.

135. Broughton BC, Cordonnier A, Kleijer WJ, *et al*. Molecular analysis of mutations in DNA polymerase eta in xeroderma pigmentosum-variant patients. *Proc Natl Acad Sci USA* 2002; **99**:815–820.

136. Friedberg EC. Cockayne syndrome – a primary defect in DNA repair, transcription, both or neither? *BioEssays* 1996; **18**:731–738.

137. van Gool AJ, van der Horst GTJ, Citterio E, Hoeijmakers JHJ. Cockayne syndrome: defective repair of transcription. *EMBO J* 1997; **16**:4155–4162.

138. Henning KA, Li L, Iyer N, *et al*. The Cockayne-syndrome group-A gene encodes a WD repeat protein that interacts with CSB protein and a subunit of RNA-polymerase-II TFIIH. *Cell* 1995; **82**:555–564.

139. Troelstra C, van Gool A, de Wit J, *et al*. ERCC6, a member of a subfamily of putative helicases, is involved in Cockayne syndrome and preferential repair of active genes. *Cell* 1992; **71**:939–953.

140. Eisen JA, Sweder KS, Hanawalt PC. Evolution of the SNF2 family of proteins – subfamilies with distinct sequences and functions. *Nucl Acids Res* 1995; **23**:2715–2723.

141. Selby CP, Sancar A. Human transcription-repair coupling factor CSB/ERCC6 is a DNA-stimulated ATPase but is not a helicase and does not disrupt the ternary transcription complex of stalled RNA polymerase II. *J Biol Chem* 1997; **272**:1885–1890.

142. Pazin MJ, Kadonaga JT. SWI2/SNF2 and related proteins: ATP-driven motors that disrupt protein-DNA interactions. *Cell* 1997; **88**:737–740.

143. Selby CP, Sancar A. Mechanisms of transcription-repair coupling and mutation frequency decline. *Microbiol Rev* 1994; **58**:317–329.

144. van Oosterwijk MF, Versteeg A, Filon R, *et al*. The sensitivity of Cockayne's Syndrome cells to DNA-damaging agents is not due to defective transcription-coupled repair of active genes. *Mol Cell Biol* 1996; **16**:4436–4444.

145. Iyer N, Reagan MS, Wu KJ, *et al*. Interactions involving the human RNA polymerase II transcription/nucleotide excision repair complex TFIIH, the nucleotide excision repair protein XPG, and Cockayne syndrome group B (CSB) protein. *Biochemistry* 1996; **35**:2157–2167.

146. van Gool AJ, Citterio E, Rademakers S, *et al*. The Cockayne syndrome B protein, involved in transcription-coupled DNA repair, resides in a RNA polymerase II containing complex. *EMBO J* 1997; **16**:5955–5965.

147. Selby CP, Sancar A. Cockayne syndrome group B protein enhances elongation by RNA polymerase II. *Proc Natl Acad Sci USA* 1997; **95**:11205–11209.

148. Tantin D, Kansal A, Carey M. Recruitment of the putative transcription-repair coupling factor CSB/ERCC6 to RNA polymerase II elongation complexes. *Mol Cell Biol* 1997; **17**:6803–6814.

149. Tantin D. RNA polymerase II elongation complexes containing the Cockayne syndrome group B protein interact with a molecular complex containing the transcription factor IIH components xeroderma pigmentosum B and p62. *J Biol Chem* 1998; **273**:27794–27799.

150. Bregman DB, Halaban R, van Gool AJ, *et al*. UV-induced ubiquitination of RNA polymerase II: a novel modification deficient in Cockayne syndrome cells. *Proc Natl Acad Sci USA* 1996; **93**:11586–11590.

151. van Gool AJ, Verhage R, Swagemakers SMA, *et al*. RAD26, the functional *S. cerevisiae* homolog of the cockayne syndrome B gene *ERCC6. EMBO J* 1994; **13**:5361–5369.

152. Bhatia PK, Verhage RA, Brouwer J, Friedberg EC. Molecular cloning and characterization of *Saccharomyces cerevisiae RAD28*, the yeast homolog of the human Cockayne Syndrome A (*CSA*) gene. *J Bacteriol* 1996; **178**:5977–5988.

153. van der Horst GTJ, van Steeg H, Berg RJW, *et al*. Defective transcription-coupled repair in Cockayne syndrome B mice is associated with skin cancer predisposition. *Cell* 1997; **89**:425–435.

154. Leadon SA, Cooper PK. Preferential repair of ionizing radiation-induced damage in the transcribed strand of an active human gene is defective in Cockayne syndrome. *Proc Natl Acad Sci USA* 1993; **90**:10499–10503.

155. Le Page F, Kwoh EE, Avrutskaya A, *et al*. Transcription-coupled repair of 8-oxoguanine:requirement for XPG, TFIIH, and CSB and implications for Cockayne syndrome. *Cell* 2000; **101**:159–171.

156. Vermeulen W, Bergmann E, Auriol J, *et al*. Sublimiting concentration of TFIIH transcription/DNA repair factor causes TTD-A trichothiodystrophy disorder. *Nature Genet* 2000; **26**:307–313.

157. Botta E, Nardo T, Lehmann AR, *et al*. Reduced level of the repair/transcription factor TFIIH in trichothiodystrophy. *Hum Mol Genet* 2002; **11**:2919–2928.

158. Viprakasit V, Gibbons RJ, Broughton BC, *et al*. Mutations in the general transcription factor TFIIH result in beta-thalassaemia in individuals with trichothiodystrophy. *Hum Mol Genet* 2001; **10**:2797–2802.

159. Ziegler A, Leffell DJ, Kunala S, *et al*. Mutation hotspots due to sunlight in the p53 gene of nonmelanoma skin cancers. *Proc Natl Acad Sci USA* 1993; **90**:4216–4220.

160. Broughton BC, Berneburg M, Fawcett H, *et al*. Two individuals with features of both xeroderma pigmentosum and trichothiodystrophy highlight the complexity of the clinical outcomes of mutations in the *XPD* gene. *Hum Mol Genet* 2001; **10**:2539–2547.

161. Berneburg M, Clingen PH, Harcourt SA, *et al*. The cancer-free phenotype in trichothiodystrophy is unrelated to its repair defect. *Cancer Res* 2000; **60**:431–438.

PART 4

The common cancers

17

Genetics and the common cancers

RICHARD S. HOULSTON AND JULIAN PETO

INTRODUCTION

The importance of inherited predisposition is now well established for a number of common cancers and the mechanisms by which mutation in some genes leads to cancer are at least partially understood. The ability to identify susceptible individuals among cancer patients and in the general population provides a basis for estimating the contribution of each such gene to overall cancer incidence. These powerful strategies will continue to dominate cancer research for many years, and not only in the field of genetic susceptibility. The same genes are often lost or mutated somatically in the multistep evolution of cancer in non-susceptible individuals and may, therefore, be targets for novel screening and treatment methods. Most cancer susceptibility genes so far discovered are highly penetrant but too rare to account for more than a few per cent of most types of cancer. There is increasing evidence that a greater proportion of cancers are attributable to genetic susceptibility, but the relevant genes or gene combinations do not confer high enough risks to produce large multiple-case families and, therefore, may be difficult to identify by conventional linkage analysis. If a small number of common susceptibility genes account for these moderate cancer risks, many of them will probably be identified rapidly through methods discussed below. However, if large numbers of rare susceptibility genes are involved, whether acting independently or synergistically, they may be discoverable only through advances in cell and molecular biology.

In this chapter, we review the evidence on the role of genes of high and low penetrance in the aetiology of the common cancers, and discuss the implications of this knowledge.

FAMILIAL CLUSTERING OF COMMON CANCERS

Risks in first-degree relatives

For many common cancers, first-degree relatives (i.e. parents, siblings, offspring) of patients are at increased risk for cancer at the same site.[1–34] This has been recognized for many years but, for most cancers, there are still too few systematic studies to provide precise estimates of these familial risks, particularly for relatives of younger patients. Some cohort studies have been conducted but most estimates of familial cancer risks have been based on case-control studies. Table 17.1 provides summary estimates of risks to relatives of affected cases for a number of common cancers. Estimates from early case-control studies may be somewhat inflated by under-reporting of affected relatives by controls but, in most recent studies, this bias is minimized by systematic questioning about each relative. For first degree relatives of patients with most common cancers, the risk of developing cancer at the same site is generally increased by 2–5-fold above that in the general population. Such apparently moderate increases in risk could be due to a shared environment or a polygenic mechanism, but Table 17.2 shows that, if they are caused by single genes, the genetic effect must be substantial. For a dominant gene to cause a relative risk of two in patients' siblings, the risk in susceptible

Table 17.1 *Summary estimates of the relative risk for the same type of cancer in patients' first-degree relatives. Where single references are given, estimates are abstracted from published pooled estimates, otherwise estimates are based on a meta-analysis of published studies*

Site	Type of relative	Relative risk	95% confidence interval	Reference
Breast	All	2.1	2.0–2.2	1
	Age < 50	2.3	2.2–2.5	
	Age > 50	1.8	1.6–2.0	
	Sister	2.3	2.1–2.4	
	Mother	2.0	1.8–2.1	
	Daughter	1.8	1.6–2.0	
	Mother and sister	3.6	2.5–5.0	
Ovary	All	3.1	2.6–3.7	2
	Mother	1.1	0.8–1.6	
	Sister	3.8	2.9–5.1	
	Daughter	6.0	3.0–11.9	
Uterus	All	2.1	1.3–3.4	3–6
Stomach	All	2.5	2.0–3.0	6–9
Colorectal	All	2.3	2.0–2.5	10
	<45	3.9	2.4–6.2	
	2+ relatives	4.3	3.0–6.1	
Prostate	All	2.2	1.1–2.4	6,9,11–17
Renal	All	4.4	2.0–9.7	6,18
Testicular	Father	2.3	1.5–3.6	6,19–24
	Brother	9.8	7.1–13.7	
Bladder	All	1.4	1.2–1.6	6,25–27
Melanoma	All	2.5	2.1–3.0	6,9,28–32
Thyroid	All	8.6	6.3–11.8	6,9,33,34

Table 17.2 *Dominant and recessive gene models causing specific relative risk in siblings of affected cases.[a] Tabulated values are the ratios of risks in susceptible to non-susceptible individuals*

	Gene frequency	Relative risk to sibling			
		1.5	2	3	5
Dominant gene model	0.001	25	35	50	74
	0.01	10	14	21	35
	0.05	6	10	21	35
	0.1	6	13	280	–
	0.2	10	–	–	–
Recessive gene model	0.01	143	203	289	414
	0.05	30	44	64	96
	0.1	16	24	36	60
	0.5	8	35	–	–

individuals has to be at least ten times greater than in non-susceptible individuals, and, for a recessive gene, the risk ratio must be over 20. Table 17.2 also shows that a moderate familial risk is consistent with a wide range of gene frequencies and genetic mechanisms, so the underlying genetic model cannot be reliably inferred from relative risks in first-degree relatives.

Age-specific familial risks

If cancers develop earlier in susceptible persons, the relative risk in patients' relatives will be greatest in young relatives of young cases. This pattern of risk is displayed by most common cancers, including breast, colon, prostate and melanoma (Table 17.1). The distribution of age at diagnosis in susceptible individuals can differ from that in non-susceptible persons for two reasons. First, those susceptible may have a different underlying disease process. Over 30 years ago, Ashley proposed that familial adenomatous polyposis (FAP) patients have inherited one of a series of

carcinogenic 'hits' that occur somatically in the development of sporadic colon cancer, based on the observation that the susceptible to non-susceptible incidence ratio declines with increasing age.[35] In the same year, DeMars suggested that apparently autosomal dominant syndromes, such as FAP and familial retinoblastoma, should be viewed as autosomal recessives at the cellular level, because the cancers 'appear as a result of subsequent somatic mutations in which individuals cells become homozygous for a recessive neoplasm causing gene'.[36] Confirmation of this hypothesis has been one of the key achievements of the last two decades of cancer research, and it is now established that susceptibility to these and several other dominant cancer syndromes is caused by germline mutation in one allele of a tumour suppressor gene, both alleles of which are frequently damaged or deleted somatically in the development of non-hereditary cancers of the same type. In a plausible extension to this model, inherited mutation in a DNA repair gene followed by somatic loss of the wild-type allele may cause genetic instability that generally kills the cell, but occasionally causes multiple damage leading immediately to cancer, so these subsequent events in carcinogenesis are no longer rate-limiting. This mechanism has been proposed for hereditary non-polyposis colon cancer (HNPCC) to explain the flat age-incidence curve in susceptible adults.[37]

Progressive elimination of susceptible individuals would lead to an earlier age at first cancer in susceptibles even if the susceptible to non-susceptible incidence ratio were identical at each age. Incidence rates of second and subsequent skin cancers in mice treated with benzo(a)pyrene are consistent with such a model.[38] The marked difference between the age distribution at diagnosis of the patients' first tumours for hereditary and sporadic retinoblastomas is almost all due to the effect of elimination. In contrast to FAP, where the majority of somatic events occur later in life, the susceptible to non-susceptible incidence ratio will be virtually

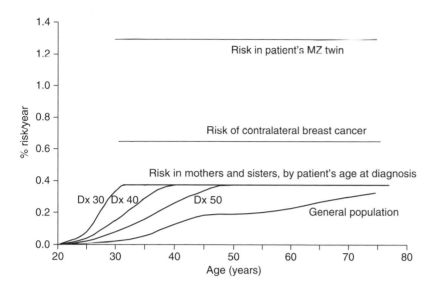

Figure 17.1 *Incidence of breast cancer in the general population and in patient's relatives. Dx, age at diagnosis of breast cancer.*

independent of age for embryological tumours where sporadic cases involve an additional mutation in a tumour suppressor gene that arises in the rapidly developing target organ.

DeMar's hypothesis of germline mutation among susceptible individuals in one allele of a tumour suppressor gene has proved to be the correct explanation of the 100 000-fold difference in incidence between hereditary and sporadic retinoblastomas. However, as Hethcote and Knudson[39] noted, their data were also consistent with a model in which the number of somatic mutations, and hence the distribution of ages at diagnosis for all tumours – not first tumours, as most susceptible individuals develop multiple tumours – are the same for hereditary as for sporadic retinoblastoma.

Models of inherited cancer susceptibility based on age-specific rates have occasionally suggested unexpected mechanisms. An example is the novel hypothesis concerning breast cancer susceptibility proposed by Peto and Mack.[40] Figure 17.1 shows the pattern of incidence in patients' contralateral breasts, and in their monozygotic (MZ) twins, sisters and mothers. The high contralateral and MZ twin rates imply that a high proportion, and perhaps most, of all breast cancers arise in a susceptible minority of women; but the most surprising aspect of these data is the approximately constant breast cancer incidence in patients' mothers and sisters, and in their contralateral breast which suggests that the incidence rate abruptly rises to a constant level at different ages in different families. Such an effect is difficult to reconcile with established mechanisms of carcinogenesis and susceptibility, but no equally simple model seems to fit the pattern shown in Figure 17.1. Data on familial age-specific incidence rates for breast cancer are still relatively imprecise however, especially for twins and young relatives.

Familial associations between common cancers

A number of dominantly inherited susceptibility genes cause cancer at several sites. These include clustering of adenocarcinomas of the colorectum and endometrium in HNPCC families,[41] soft tissue sarcomas, brain and breast tumours in the Li–Fraumeni syndrome,[42] and cancers of the breast and ovary, with smaller risks for colon and prostate cancer in *BRCA1* and *BRCA2* families.[43,44]

A large number of epidemiological studies have examined the risk to relatives for cancer at the same site as the proband, but few have systematically examined the risk of cancer at other sites. Tables 17.3 and 17.4 detail the results of Goldgar *et al.*[6] who carried out a systematic study of the clustering of cancer at 28 distinct sites using the Utah Population Database. Strong familial relationships were seen between a number of sites. Some of these are caused by rare penetrant genes. *BRCA1* and *BRCA2* presumably contribute to the associations between breast, colon and prostate, and between ovary and pancreas, and the increased risk of soft tissue cancers among relatives of breast cancer cases must be due in part to the Li–Fraumeni syndrome.

Environmental and behavioural risk factors that are similar within families may account for some associations, such as the familial clustering seen for cancers at smoking-related sites (lung, lip, cervix). Clustering of cancers of the female genitalia, lip and oral cavity may reflect a common viral aetiology. In addition to these previously reported associations between cancer sites, highly significant excesses of thyroid cancer and non-Hodgkin's lymphoma were seen in relatives of breast cancer probands, suggesting a hitherto unrecognized inherited association. Relationships were also identified between ovarian and pancreatic cancer, and between colorectal cancer and leukaemias.

Table 17.3 *Familial relative risks in first degree relatives of cancer probands with gastrointestinal, urogenital and haemopoietic soft-tissue tumours and melanoma*[6]

Proband site	Second site	Risk
Gastrointestinal cancers		
Rectum	Colon	2.0[c]
Early rectum	Colon	3.5[c]
Colon	Prostate	1.3[c]
Colon	Breast	1.2[c]
Rectum	Prostate	1.3[c]
Early colon	Lung	1.7[b]
Colon	Leukaemia	1.7[b]
Early colon	Breast	1.4[b]
Colon	Anus	1.8[b]
Colon	Lung	1.3[b]
Early colon	Melanoma	1.8[b]
Rectum	Lymphatic leukaemia	2.0[b]
Early colon	Granulocytic leukaemia	2.2[a]
Pancreas	Gall bladder	2.5[a]
Stomach	Female genitals	2.4[a]
Urogenital tract cancers		
Prostate	Colon	1.3[c]
Prostate	Non-Hodgkin's	1.2[b]
Prostate	Rectum	1.3[b]
Early prostate	Rectum	2.0[b]
Prostate	Brain/CNS	1.3[a]
Early bladder	Lymphatic leukaemia	3.6[a]
Early badder	Cervix	2.3[a]
Testis	Myeloma	3.7[a]
Testis	Bladder	2.4[a]
Haemopoietic soft-tissue tumours and melanoma		
Early NHL	Prostate	1.6[c]
Non-Hodgkin's	Prostate	1.3[b]
Melanoma	Brain/CNS	1.7[b]
Granulocytic leukaemia	Colon	1.7[b]
Lymphatic leukaemia	Rectum	2.0[b]
Soft tissue	Granulocytic leukaemia	3.2[a]
Lymph	Thyroid	2.4[a]
Soft tissue	Thyroid	2.8[a]

[a] $p < 0.05$; [b] $p < 0.01$; [c] $p < 0.001$.
CNS, central nervous system.

Table 17.4 *Familial relative risks in first-degree relatives of cancer probands with female reproductive cancers and other cancers*[6]

Proband site	Second site	Risk
Female reproductive sites		
Breast	Colon	1.2[a]
Breast	Thyroid	1.7[a]
Early breast	Colon	1.7[a]
Breast	Non-Hodgkin's	1.4[a]
Early breast	Non-Hodgkin's	1.9[a]
Ovary	Lip	2.2[b]
Cervix	Lung	1.6[b]
Early breast	Prostate	1.4[b]
Ovary	Pancreas	2.1[b]
Cervix	Colon	1.5[b]
Early uterine	Colon	1.6[b]
Early uterine	Female genitals	2.9[a]
Female genitals	Oral cavity	3.0[a]
Female genitals	Stomach	2.6[a]
Female genitals	Lip	2.5[a]
Ovary	Soft-tissue cancers	2.2[a]
Cancers at other sites		
Thyroid	Breast	1.7[a]
Larynx	Lip	3.5[a]
Lung	Lip	1.7[a]
Early brain/CNS	Pancreas	4.7[a]
Brain/CNS	Prostate	1.3[b]
Lung	Cervix	1.6[b]
Larynx	Lung	2.1[b]
Brain	Stomach	1.9[b]
Brain	Melanoma	1.6[b]
Early brain	Stomach	3.6[b]
Lip	Ovary	1.9[b]
Thyroid	Prostate	1.4[b]
Lung	Colon	1.3[b]
Oral cavity	Female genitals	3.0[a]
Thyroid	Lymphatic leukaemia	2.7[a]
Thyroid	Soft tissue	2.9[a]
Lip	Female genitals	2.3[a]
Larynx	Thyroid	3.0[a]

[a] $p < 0.05$; [b] $p < 0.01$; [c] $p < 0.001$.
CNS, central nervous system.

Benign lesions

A number of benign lesions are associated with an increased risk of cancer, and many of these have an inherited basis (Table 17.5). In addition to the classical highly penetrant syndromes, such as FAP and xeroderma pigmentosum (XP), several such lesions are associated with moderate site-specific cancer risks. Melanoma risk is strongly correlated with numbers of melanocytic naevi.[46] Numbers of naevi have been shown to be highly correlated in MZ twins, but not in dizygotic twins, suggesting a major genetic component in the prevalence of naevi and presumably melanoma risk.[47] Further evidence of genetic susceptibility to naevi was found by Goldgar *et al.* in studies of families of melanoma cases.[48]

Palmar keratoses, which are strongly associated with bladder cancer,[49] are more frequent in first-degree relatives of bladder cancer cases, especially if the individual also had keratoses. Spouses of cases also had an increased, but smaller, risk of bladder cancer, especially if the case had keratoses.[49] These results implicate genetic as well as environmental – possibly viral – factors in the aetiology of keratoses. Other examples in this class of cancer susceptibility genes are those predisposing to

Table 17.5 *Diseases and phenotypes associated with cancer susceptibility*[45]

Disease or phenotype	Population prevalence (%)	Sibling risk (%)	Cancer risk
Cryptorchidism	1	6	Testicular (6-fold)
Palmar keratoses	23	–	Bladder (12-fold), lung (4-fold)
Supernumerary nipples	1	–	Urogenital (8-fold)
Paget's disease of bone	2	12	Osteosarcoma (100-fold)
Multinodular goitre	1	4	Thyroid (4-fold; 20% of cases), breast (4-fold)
Coeliac disease	0.3	10	Lymphoproliferative disease (30–40-fold), oesophagus (8–12-fold), mouth and pharynx (10-fold)
Inflammatory bowel disease	0.3	8	Colorectal (6-fold)
Endometriosis	10	70	Breast (1.3-fold), ovary (1.9-fold)
Naevi	NA	$h^2 = 84$	Melanoma
Radiosensitivity	9	18	Breast (9-fold), lung (14-fold)

NA, not applicable; h^2, heritability.

cryptorchidism, supernumerary nipples, inflammatory bowel disease, Paget's disease and endometriosis.[45]

Genetic models of predisposition to common cancer

Genetic models of familial cancer can be formally tested using segregation analysis. This involves comparing the observed pattern of disease incidence in each pedigree with that predicted by different models. The major segregation analyses of breast, colorectal, lung, ovarian and testicular cancer are summarized in Table 17.6. The majority of these studies have found evidence for dominant genes predisposing to these cancers.[50–65]

In principle, risks to second-degree and more distant relatives provide useful additional evidence on the mode of inheritance because, for a simple dominant gene, the excess relative risk (R-1) reduces by a factor of two for each degree of relationship.[66] However, in practice, this approach is unlikely to be helpful even for common cancers, since complete unbiased data on second- and third-degree relatives are rarely available.

If a single gene accounts for the familial risk, segregation analysis of cancer families ascertained within population-based studies can, in principle, provide estimates of both gene frequency and age-specific cancer incidence for susceptibles and non-susceptibles. For the majority of cancers, however, it is likely that several genes with varying penetrances contribute to the risk in relatives. For example, in the CASH study of breast cancer, a dominant gene with a frequency of 0.0033 provided the most parsimonious model, conferring a risk of 14 per cent by age 40, 38 per cent by age 50 and 67 per cent by age 70.[52] It is, however, now known that the two major breast cancer susceptibility genes (*BRCA1* and *BRCA2*),

the rare Li–Fraumeni (*TP53*) syndrome, CHEK2 and ataxia telangiectasia (A-T) heterozygotes all contribute to the familial risk. Segregation analysis can be particularly misleading when there are several genes with different modes of inheritance. This is illustrated by testicular cancer, in which segregation analysis predicted an autosomal recessive gene.[65] The recently identified testicular cancer locus *TCG1* on the X-chromosome[67] accounts for many fraternal pairs but none of the father–son associations.

In addition to the highly penetrant genes causing colorectal cancer that have been identified by linkage, such as the APC and HNPCC genes, segregation studies have suggested the presence of more common genes with lower penetrance predisposing to colorectal cancer in the general population.[57,58] Cannon-Albright *et al.* fitted a dominant model with a gene frequency of 19 per cent and a lifetime penetrance of 40 per cent for adenomas or colorectal cancer in susceptible individuals. This model implies that most, and perhaps all, adenomas arise through inherited predisposition, although the confidence limits were wide.[57]

One feature of familial breast cancer risk which is not readily explained by a dominant model is the higher risk reported in sisters of breast cancer cases than in their mothers in some studies (e.g. Peto *et al.*[68]). If real, this could be due to shared lifestyle factors among sisters, anticipation, reduced fertility in female carriers, or the presence of co-dominant or recessive susceptibility genes. Few segregation analyses of familial cancer have incorporated data on environmental risk factors. In an analysis of lung cancer Sellers *et al.* fitted a model in which lung cancer risk is increased both by genetic susceptibility and by smoking.[64] The observed pattern of familial aggregation was compatible with the inheritance of a co-dominant gene conferring an increased susceptibility to lung cancer.[64]

Table 17.6 *Segregation analyses of breast, colorectal, ovarian, prostate, lung and testicular cancers*

Site of cancer	Number of families	Genetic model			Comments
		Mode of inheritance	Gene frequency	Penetrance	
Breast cancer					
Williams and Anderson (1984)[50]	200	AD	0.0076	0.57	Analysis of Jacobsen pedigrees: possible enrichment of premenopausal cases; specific mortality neglected
Goldstein et al. (1987)[52]	286	AD	0.00140	?	Bilateral cases
	252		0.00092	?	All cases
Claus et al. (1991)[51]	4730	AD	0.003	0.95	Premenopausal: evidence of non-Mendelian transmission
Chen et al. (1995)[53]	251	CD		–	Analysis of CASH study: probands aged <55
Grabrick et al. (1999)[54]	426				
Baffoe-Bonnie et al. (2000)[55]	389	CD	0.026	0.16/0.32	Enrichment of premenopausal cases
Cui et al. (2000)[56]	858	AD/AR			Cases aged <40; exclusion of BRCA1/2 cases; evidence for a recessive component
Colorectal cancer					
Cannon-Albright et al. (1988)[57]	34	AD	0.19	0.4	Large extended families
Houlston et al. (1992)[58]	209	AD	0.006	0.64	
Houlston et al. (1995)[59]	305	AD			
Ovarian					
Eccles et al. (1997)[60]		AD		0.50	
Auranen and Iselius (1998)[61]	663	AR			
Prostate					
Carter et al. (1992)[62]	691	AD	0.003	0.88	Enrichment for younger cases
Gronberg et al. (1997)[63]	2857	AD	0.017	0.63	
Lung					
Sellers et al. (1990)[64]	337	CD	0.052		
Testicular					
Heimdal et al. (1997)[65]	978	AR	0.038	0.076	

AD, autosomal dominant; AR, autosomal recessive; CD, co-dominant.

HIGHLY PENETRANT GENES

Linkage analysis

A large number of rare hereditary syndromes in which carriers have a characteristic phenotype and are at high risk of developing cancer have been recognized for many years. Online Mendelian Inheritance in Man (OMIM) lists several hundred inherited disorders for which neoplasia is a major feature or complication, but the majority are rare[69] and, in total, they are unlikely to be responsible for more than 1 per cent of all cancers. There are also several hereditary syndromes with no associated phenotype that produce multiple-case families with one or more common types of cancer. Genetic linkage analysis of multiple-case families has been instrumental in the localization of most of these highly penetrant rare genes. Examples of common cancers for which susceptibility genes have been identified include breast and ovarian cancers (*BRCA1* and *BRCA2* on chromosomes 17 and 13),[70,71] colon cancer with adenomatous polyposis coli (*APC* on chromosome 5),[72] HNPCC (the mismatch repair genes *MSH2*, *MLH1*, *MSH6*, *PMS1* and *PMS2* on chromosomes 2, 3 and 7),[73,74] melanoma (*CDNK2A* on chromosome 9),[75,76] testicular cancer (*TCG1* on the X chromosome)[67] and the Li–Fraumeni syndrome (*TP53* on chromosome 17).[42]

Gene frequency and penetrance

Once a susceptibility gene has been identified, its frequency and penetrance can only be estimated reliably from extremely large population-based studies of unaffected individuals as well as cancer cases. Such studies have not been performed to date. Families used for linkage analyses cannot be utilized to estimate gene frequency because they have been selected for the occurrence of multiple cases. Penetrance estimates based on such families may be misleading. For example, penetrance estimates for mutant *BRCA1* and *BRCA2*, based on risks to relatives of unselected breast cancer cases in whom these genes were sequenced,[77] were substantially lower than those obtained from analysis of multiple case families.[78] Both genetic and shared environmental factors may contribute to such differences.

LOW-PENETRANCE GENES

Highly penetrant genes that underlie multiple case families are too rare to account for a substantial proportion of common cancers. There may also be predisposing genes of lower penetrance, which account for a larger proportion of cancers. The relative risk for most common cancers in first-degree relatives of cases is of the order of two at older ages. The range of dominant and recessive models consistent with a relative risk of between 1.5 and 2 is shown in Table 17.2. If the relative risk were two, for example, a dominantly acting predisposition gene carried by 25 per cent of the population would cause a risk in carriers about ten times that in the general population. This would rarely produce striking multiple-case families. Even for lung cancer a ten-fold increase in risk would correspond to a penetrance by age 70 years of less than 50 per cent, and for colon cancer a tenfold relative risk in susceptibles would correspond to a penetrance of only 10 per cent by age 70 years. Such a gene might be detectable by linkage analysis of affected sibling pairs, haplotypes in linkage disequilibrium with founder mutations, or an associated phenotype. Direct sequencing of candidate genes in cases and controls probably represents the most promising approach, although so far it has proved unproductive. If low-penetrance genes cause a substantial proportion of all cancers, their identification will be of great practical importance. There may also be susceptibility genes which are carried by the majority of the population, but these could not cause a detectable risk in relatives and their identification will be of scientific rather than clinical value. In the extreme case of the polymorphic *CYP2D6* locus, where more than 90 per cent of the population are at high risk, even if poor metabolizers were totally immune from lung cancer, the resulting relative risk in first-degree relatives would be only around 1.02.

Genetic polymorphisms

The only viable strategy for identifying low-penetrance cancer susceptibility genes to date has been through the analysis of polymorphisms at candidate loci. There have been many studies comparing the prevalence in cancer cases and unaffected controls of polymorphisms in the genes involved in metabolism of exogenous or endogenous mutagens or in the production or processing of sex hormones or their analogues.[45] Common sequence variants reported to act as low-penetrance genes in more than one study are detailed in Table 17.7. A few polymorphisms in such genes appear to alter the risk substantially, such as the N-acetyltransferase 2 (NAT-2) slow acetylator phenotype, which increases the risk of bladder cancer,[79] especially in workers heavily exposed to certain aromatic amines. Systematic meta-analysis reveals little or no effect for most of these polymorphisms, and the pooled data for the minority that are statistically significant usually suggest odds ratios of less than two, and often much less.[80–85] Thus, for example, early reports suggested that glutathione-S-transferase μ1 (GSTM1) deficiency more than

Table 17.7 *Genes reported to act as low-penetrance susceptibility loci[45]*

Class/locus	Cancer	Putative mechanism
Metabolic polymorphisms		
CYP1A1	Lung, breast, colorectal, uterine, BCC	Altered metabolism (procarcinogen activation: polycyclic aromatic hydrocarbons)
CYP1A2	Bladder, colorectal	Altered metabolism (procarcinogen activation: nitrosamines and arylamines)
CYP2D6	Lung, liver	Altered metabolism (procarcinogen activation: nitrosamines)
GSTM1	Lung, bladder, breast, gastric, colon, head and neck, uterine	Altered metabolism (carcinogen detoxification: electrophilic compounds)
GSTT1	Colorectal, larynx, BCC, brain	Altered metabolism (carcinogen: electrophilic compounds)
NAT2	Bladder, colon, liver	Altered metabolism (carcinogen detoxification: aromatic amines, hydazines)
Androgen receptor	Prostate	Altered metabolism (testosterone and dihyrotestosterone transactivation)
MTHFR	Colorectal, uterine	Methylation status
Tumour suppressor genes		
APC -I1307K	Colorectal	Hypermutability
DNA repair genes		
ATM	Breast	Genomic instability
Proto-oncogene polymorphisms		
H-ras-VNTR	Colorectal, breast, lung, bladder, leukaemia	Altered transcription/linkage disequilibrium

BCC, basal cell carcinoma.

doubled the risk of lung cancer; however, pooled results of subsequent typing studies give an odds ratio of only 1.14 (95 per cent confidence interval (CI) 1.03–1.25).[80]

Polymorphisms in tumour suppressor genes or oncogenes may also confer a moderate increase in cancer risk. An example of a sequence variant in this class is the I1307K single nucleotide polymorphism (SNP) in *APC*, which is carried by around 6 per cent of Ashkenazi Jews and appears to almost double their risk of colorectal cancer.[86] To estimate the individual effects of rare polymorphisms will generally require very large studies, although enhanced power can be achieved by analysis of cases with a family history of the disease.

The increased cancer risk associated with rare alleles of the *HRAS1*-associated minisatellite was among the first such associations to be reported. Such alleles, which are carried by around 5 per cent of the population, appear to increase the risk of several common cancers by 1.5–2-fold.[87] More recent studies, however, have found no effect.

There have been various reports of statistically significant gene–environment interactions, such as much larger lung cancer risks due to passive smoking in women who were GSTM1-deficient,[88] or an increased breast cancer risk due to smoking in postmenopausal women confined to NAT2 slow acetylators.[89] In these examples, however, the estimates of the risk in susceptibles (although not their lower confidence limits) were inconsistent with the much lower overall effect of passive smoking on lung cancer,[90] or of smoking on breast cancer (which is nil) in larger studies.[91] Many apparently significant gene–gene or gene–exposure interactions will arise by chance, but some will be real. The effects of such polymorphisms in combination with each other and with environmental risk factors could be substantial, but their contribution to cancer incidence will not be known until data on risk factors and extensive genotyping are available for very large numbers of patients and controls. Molecular epidemiology is increasingly focusing on genes that may modify endogenous carcinogenic processes rather than those that affect susceptibility to environmental carcinogens.[92]

DNA replication and repair genes

Some classical inherited diseases such as Fanconi anaemia, ataxia telangectasia, xeroderma pigmentosum and Bloom's syndrome, which are associated with increased cancer risk, involve chromosome instability or DNA replication or repair defects. Other important cancer susceptibility genes are also of this type. A normal function of the *TP53* gene is either to cause cell-cycle arrest or to induce apoptosis in response to DNA damage, and inactivation of the

HNPCC genes on chromosomes 2, 3 and 7 is associated with somatic instability of dinucleotide and trinucleotide repeats. The *p16* cell-cycle regulator gene (*CDKN2A*) on chromosome 9, originally located by linkage in familial melanoma, is deleted or mutated in a high proportion of cancers at many sites.[76] If *p16* inactivation leads to uncontrolled cell division it is also likely to increase the risk of other mutations. The possibility that other 'mutator' genes of this general class might be detectable phenotypically is suggested by the observation that more than a third of breast cancer patients exhibit lymphocyte radiation sensitivity, while only 10 per cent of the population have this phenotype.[93] Formal modelling of radiation sensitivity in breast cancer families is compatible with a dominant mechanism[94] that causes a relative risk of 1.5–2 in first-degree relatives of breast cancer patients and approximately 3 in their monozygotic twins. These figures are in the range of the risks seen in relatives of breast cancer patients above the age of 50 (Figure 17.1). This effect, if real, is not due to a single gene. While A-T heterozygotes have been shown to exhibit high radiation sensitivity in the test, they do not constitute 10 per cent of the population.

Linkage analysis of low–penetrance genes

Highly penetrant genes do not cause a high proportion of most cancers, but the preceding example shows that less penetrant genes carried by up to 20 per cent of the population (Table 17.2) could well do so. If such genes cause a high proportion of cancers of a particular type, they may be detectable by linkage analysis of affected pairs of siblings, particularly if the mode of inheritance is recessive, as the examples of Hodgkin's disease[95] and nasopharyngeal carcinoma[96] have demonstrated. For low-penetrance genes that cause a small proportion of cancers, the number of affected relative pairs required will be prohibitively large[97,98] but the sample size for a test based on allelic association can be very much smaller, even allowing for multiple comparisons.

The observation that linkage disequilibrium can extend up to 100 kb or more among populations of European origin[99] lends some support to the idea that susceptibility genes might be found by discovering ancient DNA sequences that are commoner in cancer patients than in controls. Such disequilibrium studies are now feasible using the dense genome-wide map of over a million SNPs together with the human genome sequence.[99] This approach could detect any founder mutation that causes a substantial fraction of cancers of a particular type. *BRCA2* might, for example, have been discoverable through the higher prevalence among breast cancer patients of the sequences flanking the 6174delT mutation among Ashkenazi Jews or the 999del5 mutation in Icelanders. Less penetrant mutations would be more difficult to detect, however, particularly in genetically heterogeneous populations in which founder mutations are rarer. A similar idea underlies admixture analysis.[100] Most international differences in cancer rates are due to environmental or lifestyle rather than genetic effects, but some, such as the higher prostate cancer risk among African Americans than among White Americans, could be due to racial differences in the allelic spectrum of a particular gene. If so, in a population of mixed descent the high-risk African alleles would remain within long DNA sequences of African origin for many generations, and these sequences would be commoner in cancer patients of mixed race than in their siblings.

Another strategy by which such genes might be detected is linkage analysis in large families of an associated phenotypic or molecular marker of susceptibility, such as the lymphocyte sensitivity in breast cancer patients described above or the susceptibility to adenomas in colon cancer modelled by Cannon-Albright and colleagues.[57] Other established or suspected susceptibility markers include clinically detectable lesions such as naevi, benign fibrocystic breast disease or palmar keratoses, metabolic markers, such as slow acetylation, and various markers of DNA repair efficiency or chromosomal instability detectable by cellular assay or DNA analysis.[45]

CONCLUSIONS

Studies of multiple case families have led to the identification of highly penetrant genes predisposing to colon, breast, ovarian and testicular cancers, and melanoma. Such genes account for most striking multiple-case families and a substantial proportion of cancers diagnosed below age 40 years, although they cause a much smaller proportion of older cases. The large risks observed in relatives of young patients suggest the existence of such genes predisposing to other common cancers. With the possible exception of ovarian cancer, however, most of the familial risk in first-degree relatives of older cancer patients is probably not due to highly penetrant genes. A major unanswered question in cancer genetics is whether a substantial proportion of all cancers arise in susceptible individuals as a result of genes of lower penetrance. If so, some of these genes may be detectable by the various linkage approaches discussed above. Novel candidate genes will continue to be discovered through research on growth control and DNA repair pathways, and somatic mutations in oncogenes and tumour suppressor genes, some of which can also be inherited, will be discovered by powerful new methods, such as the detection of all sequence differences between tumour DNA and normal DNA from the same patient.

The ability to identify a large number of individuals with a lifetime risk for a particular cancer of the order of 20–50 per cent would present a number of practical opportunities and ethical difficulties. Phenotypic or genetic tests might be offered routinely as an adjunct to screening for cancers such as breast, colon and prostate, extending the ethical difficulties of obtaining fully informed consent for genetic testing to the general population. There would also be important implications for industrial and environmental exposure to carcinogens. Susceptible individuals can perhaps be excluded from certain occupations or persuaded to give up smoking, but if identified individuals in the general population suffer much higher than average risks from carcinogenic agents such as ionizing radiation, it could be argued that much more stringent environmental limits must be introduced. The discovery of mutant genes such as those predisposing to HNPCC has already raised these ethical quandaries.

The study of cancer genetics has given rise to a succession of statistical fallacies during the 70 years since Cramer noted that the overall cancer rate varies much less than the rates for individual sites between different countries.[101] The correct explanation is found in the statistical formula for adding variances, but Cramer inferred that a certain fixed proportion of all populations must be 'cancer prone'. The low relative risks seen in relatives of cancer patients were mistakenly believed to be inconsistent with the large effects due to mendelian genes. Familial clusters of common cancers that could not possibly have arisen by chance were often ascribed to ascertainment bias by those sceptical of the importance of genetic susceptibility in carcinogenesis. For example, a family in which four sisters develop breast cancer before 45 years would be expected to occur by chance less than once every 1000 years in the whole of Britain. The probability that one of the trillions of cells in a smoker's bronchus will become fully cancerous after 60 years of smoking is approximately one in four, yet the illogical argument that genetics must play a dominant role because heavy smokers do not all develop lung cancer remains as popular as ever.

The contribution of early multistage models to subsequent discoveries of molecular mechanisms in carcinogenesis is also widely misunderstood. The most cited example, the hypothesis that hereditary retinoblastoma is due to an inherited or germline mutation in a tumour suppressor gene, provided a biologically plausible explanation both of the apparently dominant pattern of inheritance and of the 100 000-fold higher risk in susceptibles. This has proved to be correct, but the persistent belief[102] that differences between the distributions of age at diagnosis of hereditary and sporadic cases constituted an important part of the evidence for an extra rate-limiting step in sporadic retinoblastoma is wrong.

These statistical misconceptions are not merely footnotes in the history of cancer research. Statisticians were right when they predicted more than 20 years ago that the discovery of penetrant susceptibility genes would also elucidate some of the fundamental processes of spontaneous carcinogenesis. There is now a consensus among statisticians, again largely unsupported by laboratory evidence, that a substantial proportion of human cancers arise in carriers of less penetrant susceptibility genes. Modelling the relationship between the kinetics of specific genetic and cellular processes and age-specific cancer incidence rates may play a role in the discovery of these genes, and will certainly be an important goal once they have been identified. The predictions of even the simplest genetic models are often counterintuitive, and cancer researchers should be aware of familial incidence patterns and the range of biological mechanisms that are consistent with them, if this ultimate synthesis of cancer epidemiology and molecular biology is to be achieved.

KEY POINTS

- Many cancer sites are associated with an increased relative risk of the same cancer in first-degree relatives.
- It is possible that a substantial proportion of cancers could be due to genetic predisposition if lower penetrance genes (which are more common than the rarer, highly penetrant genes) are found to confer an increase in cancer risk.

REFERENCES

1. Stratton JF, Pharoah P, Smith SK, et al. A systematic review and meta-anlysis of family history and risk of ovarian cancer. Br J Obstet Gynaecol 1998; 105:493–499.
2. Pharoah PDP, Day NE, Duffy A, et al. Family history and risk of breast cancer: a systematic review and meta-analysis. Int J Cancer 1997; 71:800–809.
3. Schildkraut JM, Risch N, Thompson WD. Evaluating genetic association among ovarian, breast, and endometrial cancer: evidence for a breast/ovarian cancer relationship. Am J Hum Genet 1989; 45:521–529.
4. Parazzini F, La Vecchia C, Moroni S, et al. Family history and the risk of endometrial cancer. Int J Cancer 1994; 59:460–462.
5. Hemminki K, Vaittinen P, Dong C. Endometrial cancer in the family-cancer database. Cancer Epidemiol Biomarkers Prev 1999; 8:1005–1010.
6. Goldgar DE, Easton DF, Cannon-Albright LA, Skolnick MH. Systematic population-based assessment of cancer risk in first-degree relatives of cancer probands. J Natl Cancer Inst 1994; 86:1600–1608.

7. Macklin MT. Inheritance of cancer of the stomach and large intestine in man. *J Natl Cancer Inst* 1960; **24**:551–571.

8. La Vecchia C, Negri E, Franceschi S, Gentile A. Family history and the risk of stomach and colorectal cancer. *Cancer* 1992; **70**:50–55.

9. Hemminki K, Vaittinen P, Kyyronen P. Age-specific familial risks in common cancers of the offspring. *Int J Cancer* 1998; **78**:172–175.

10. Johns LE, Houlston RS. A systematic review and meta-analysis of familial colorectal cancer risk. *Am J Gastroenterol* 2001; **96**:2992–3003.

11. Steinberg GD, Carter BS, Beaty TH, *et al.* Family history and the risk of prostate cancer. *Prostate* 1990; **17**:337–347.

12. Ghadrain P, Cadotte M, Perret C. Familial aggregation of cancer of the prostate in Quebec: the tip of the iceberg. *Prostate* 1991; **19**:43–52.

13. Spitz MR, Currier RD, Fueger JJ, *et al.* Familial patterns of prostate cancer: a case control analysis. *J Urol* 1991; **146**:1305–1307.

14. Isaacs SD, Kiemeney LA, Baffoe-Bonnie A, *et al.* Risk of cancer in relatives of prostate cancer probands. *J Natl Cancer Inst* 1995; **87**:991–996.

15. Lesko SM, Rosenberg L, Shapiro S. Family history and prostate cancer risk. *Am J Epidemiol* 1996; **144**:1041–1047.

16. Bratt O, Kristoffersson U, Lundgren R, Olsson H. Familial and hereditary prostate cancer in southern Sweden. A population-based case-control study. *Eur J Cancer* 1999; **35**:272–277.

17. Ghadirian P, Howe GR, Hislop TG, Maisonneuve P. Family history of prostate cancer: a multi-center case-control study in Canada. *Int J Cancer* 1997; **70**:679–681.

18. Mellemgaard A, Niwa S, Mehl ES, *et al.* Risk factors for renal cell carcinoma in Denmark: role of medication and medical history. *Int J Epidemiol* 1994; **23**:923–930.

19. Westergaard T, Olsen JH, Frisch M, *et al.* Cancer risk in fathers and brothers of testicular cancer patients in Denmark. A population-based study. *Int J Cancer* 1996; **66**:627–631.

20. Tollerud DJ, Blattner WA, Fraser MC, *et al.* Familial testicular cancer and urogenital developmental anomalies. *Cancer* 1985; **55**:1849–1854.

21. Heimdal K, Olsson H, Tretli S, *et al.* Familial testicular cancer in Norway and southern Sweden. *J Cancer* 1996; **73**:964–969.

22. Forman D, Oliver RT, Brett AR, *et al.* Familial testicular cancer: a report of the UK family register, estimation of risk and an HLA class 1 sib-pair analysis. *Br J Cancer* 1992; **65**:255–262.

23. Dieckmann KP, Pichlmeier U. The prevalence of familial testicular cancer: an analysis of two patient populations and a review of the literature. *Cancer* 1997; **80**:1954–1960.

24. Sonneveld DJ, Sleijfer DT, Schrafford Koops H, *et al.* Familial testicular cancer in a single-centre population. *Eur J Cancer* 1999; **35**:1368–1373.

25. Kantor AF, Hartge P, Hoover RN, Fraumeni JF. Familial and environmental interactions in bladder cancer risk. *Int J Cancer* 1985; **35**:703–706.

26. Kunze E, Chang-Claude J, Frentzel-Beyme R. Life style and occupational risk factors for bladder cancer in Germany. A case-control study. *Cancer* 1992; **69**:1776–1790.

27. Kiemeney LA, Moret NC, Witjes JA, Schoenberg MP, Tulinius H. Familial transitional cell carcinoma among the population of Iceland. *J Urol* 1997; **157**:1649–1651.

28. Holman CD, Armstrong BK. Pigmentary traits, ethnic origin, benign nevi, and family. *J Natl Cancer Inst* 1984; **72**:257–266.

29. Green A, Battistutta D. Incidence and determinants of skin cancer in a high-risk Australian population. *Int J Cancer* 1990; **46**:356–361.

30. Cristofolini M, Franceschi S, Tasin L, *et al.* Risk factors for cutaneous malignant melanoma in a northern Italian population. *Int J Cancer* 1987; **39**:150–154.

31. Holly EA, Kelly JW, Shpall SN, Chiu SH. Number of melanocytic nevi as a major risk factor for malignant melanoma. *J Am Acad Dermatol* 1987; **17**:459–468.

32. Osterlind A, Tucker MA, Hou-Jensen K, *et al.* The Danish case-control study of cutaneous malignant melanoma. I. Importance of host factors. *Int J Cancer* 1988; **42**:200–206.

33. Stoffer SS, Van Dyke DL, Bach JV, *et al.* Familial papillary carcinoma of the thyroid. *Am J Med Genet* 1986; **25**:775–782.

34. Ron E, Kleinerman RA, Boice JD Jr, *et al.* A population-based case-control study of thyroid cancer. *J Natl Cancer Inst* 1987; **79**:1.

35. Ashley DJB. Colonic cancer arising in polyposis coli. *J Med Genet* 1969; **6**:276–378.

36. DeMars R. Contributation to discussion. In: *Genetic Concepts and Neoplasia. Twenty-third Annual Symposium on Fundamental Cancer Research 1969* (University of Texas M.D. Anderson Hospital). Baltimore: Williams and Wilkins, 1970;105–106.

37. Janin N. A simple model for carcinogenesis of colorectal cancers with microsatellite instability. *Adv Cancer Res* 2000; **77**:189–221.

38. Peto R, Parish SE, Gray RG. There is no such thing as ageing, and cancer is not related to it. In: Likhachev A, Anisimov V, Montesano R (eds) *Age-related factors in carcinogenesis.* IARC Scientific Publications no. 58. Lyon: IARC, 1986.

39. Hethcote HW, Knudson AG Jr. Model for the incidence of embryonal cancers: application to retinoblastoma. *Proc Natl Acad Sci USA* 1978; **75**:2453–2457.

40. Peto J, Mack TM. High constant incidence in twins and other relatives of women with breast cancer. *Nature Genet* 2000; **26**:411–414.

41. Olschwang S. Germline mutation and genome instability. *Eur J Cancer Prev* 1999; **8**(Suppl. 1):S33–S37.

42. Varley JM, Evans DG, Birch JM. Li-Fraumeni syndrome – a molecular and clinical review. *Br J Cancer* 1997; **76**:1–14.

43. Ford D, Easton DF, Bishop DT, *et al.* and the Breast Cancer Linkage Consortium. Risks of cancer in *BRCA1*-mutation carriers. *Lancet* 1994; **343**:692–695.

44. Cancer risks in BRCA2 mutation carriers. The Breast Cancer Linkage Consortium. *J Natl Cancer Inst* 1999; **91**:1310–1316.

45. Houlston RS, Tomlinson IP. Detecting low penetrance genes in cancer: the way ahead. *J Med Genet* 2000; **37**:161–167.

46. Swerdlow AJ, Green A. Melanocytic naevi and melanoma: an epidemiological perspective. *Br J Dermatol* 1987; **117**:137–146.

47. Easton DF, Cox GM, Macdonald AM, Ponder BAJ. Genetic susceptibility to naevi – a twin study. *Br J Cancer* 1991; **64**:1164–1167.

48. Goldgar DE, Cannon-Albright LA, Meyer LJ, *et al.* Inheritance of nevus number and size in melanoma/DNS kindreds. *Cytogenet Cell Genet* 1992; **59**:200–202.

49. Cuzick J, Babiker A, de Stovola BL, *et al.* Palmar keratoses in family members with bladder cancer. *J Clin Epidemiol* 1990; **43**:1421–1426.

50. Williams WR, Anderson DE. Genetic epidemiology of breast cancer: segregation analysis of 200 Danish pedigrees. *Genet Epidemiol* 1984; **1**:7–20.

51. Claus EB, Risch N, Thompson WD. Genetic analysis of breast cancer in the cancer and steroid hormone study. *Am J Hum Genet* 1991; **48**:232–241.

52. Goldstein AM, Haile RWC, Marazita ML, Paganni-Hill AA. Genetic epidemiologic investigation of breast cancer in families with bilateral breast cancer, I: segregation analysis. *J Natl Cancer Inst* 1987; **78**:911–918.

53. Chen PL, Sellers TA, Rich SS, *et al.* Segregation analysis of breast cancer in a population-based sample of postmenopausal probands: The Iowa Women's Health Study. *Genet Epidemiol* 1995; **12**:401–415.

54. Grabrick DM, Anderson VE, King RA, *et al.* Inclusion of risk factor covariates in a segregation analysis of a population-based sample of 426 breast cancer families. *Genet Epidemiol* 1999; **16**:150–164.

55. Baffoe-Bonnie AB, Beaty TH, Bailey-Wilson JE, *et al.* Genetic epidemiology of breast cancer: segregation analysis of 389 Icelandic pedigrees. *Genet Epidemiol* 2000; **18**:81–94.

56. Cui J, Antoniou AC, Dite GS, *et al.* After *BRCA1* and *BRCA2* – what next? Multifactorial segregation analyses of three-generation, population-based Australian families affected by female breast cancer. *Am J Hum Genet* 2001; **68**:420–431.

57. Cannon-Albright LA, Skolnick MH, Bishop DT, *et al.* Common inheritance of susceptibility to colonic adenomatous polyps and associated colorectal cancers. *N Engl J Med* 1988; **319**:533–537.

58. Houlston RS, Collins A, Slack J, Morton NE. Dominant genes for colorectal cancer are not rare. *Ann Human Genet* 1992; **56**:99–103.

59. Houlston RS, Collins A, Kee F, *et al.* Segregation analysis of colorectal cancer in Northern Ireland. *Hum Hered* 1995; **45**:41–48.

60. Eccles DM, Forabosco P, Williams A, *et al.* Segregation analysis of ovarian cancer using diathesis to include other cancers. *Ann Hum Genet* 1997; **61**:243–252.

61. Auranen A, Iselius L. Segregation analysis of epithelial ovarian cancer in Finland. *Br J Cancer* 1998; **77**:1537–1541.

62. Carter BS, Beaty TH, Steinberg GD, *et al.* Mendelian inheritance of prostate cancer. *Proc Natl Acad Sci USA* 1992; **89**:3367–3371.

63. Gronberg H, Damber L, Damber JE, Iselius L. Segregation analysis of prostate cancer in Sweden: support for dominant inheritance. *Am J Epidemiol* 1997; **146**:552–557.

64. Sellers TA, Bailey-Wilson JE, Elston RC, *et al.* Evidence for mendelian inheritance in the pathogenesis of lung cancer. *J Natl Cancer Inst* 1990; **82**:1272–1279.

65. Heimdal K, Olsson H, Tretli S, *et al.* A segregation analysis of testicular cancer based on Norwegian and Swedish families. *Br J Cancer* 1997; **75**:1084–1087.

66. Risch N. Linkage strategies for genetically complex multilocus traits, I: multilocus models. *Am J Hum Genet* 1990; **46**:222–228.

67. Rapley EA, Crockford GP, Teare D, *et al.* Localization to Xq27 of a susceptibility gene for testicular germ-cell tumours. *Nature Genet* 2000; **24**:197–200.

68. Peto J, Easton DF, Matthews FE, *et al.* Cancer mortality in relatives of women with breast cancer: the OPCS Study. Office of Population Censuses and Surveys. *Int J Cancer* 1996; **65**:275–283.

69. Online Mendelian Inheritance in Man: http://www.ncbi.nlm.nih.gov/entrez/query.fcgi?db=OMIM.

70. Hall JM, Lee MK, Morrow J, *et al.* Linkage analysis of early onset familial breast cancer to chromosome 17q21. *Science* 1990; **250**:1684–1689.

71. Wooster R, Neuhausen SL, Mangion J, *et al.* Localization of a breast cancer susceptibility gene, *BRCA2*, to chromosome 13q12–13. *Science* 1994; **265**:2088–2090.

72. Bodmer W. Familial adenomatous polyposis (FAP) and its gene, APC. *Cytogenet Cell Genet* 1999; **88**:99–104.

73. Lindbolm A, Tannergaard P, Werelius B, Nordenskjoid B. Genetic mapping of a second locus predisposing to hereditary non-polyposis colon cancer. *Nature Genet* 1993; **5**:279–282.

74. Peltomaki P, Aaltonen LA, Sistonen P, *et al.* Genetic mapping of a locus predisposing to human colorectal cancer. *Science* 1993; **260**:810–812.

75. Cannon-Albright LA, Goldgar DE, Meyer LJ, *et al.* Assignment of a locus for familial melanoma, MLM, to chromosome 9p13–p22. *Science* 1992; **258**:1148–1152.

76. Piepkorn M. Melanoma genetics: an update with focus on the *CDKN2A(p16)/ARF* tumor suppressors. *J Am Acad Dermatol* 2000; **42**:705–722.

77. Peto J, Collins N, Barfoot R, *et al.* Prevalence of *BRCA1* and *BRCA2* gene mutations in patients with early-onset breast cancer. *J Natl Cancer Inst* 1999; **91**:943–949.

78. Ford D, Easton DF, Peto J. Estimates of the gene frequency of *BRCA1* and its contribution to breast and ovarian cancer incidence. *Am J Hum Genet* 1995; **57**:1457–1462.

79. Hein DW, Doll MA, Fretland AJ, *et al.* Molecular genetics and epidemiology of the NAT1 and NAT2 acetylation polymorphisms. *Cancer Epidemiol Biomarkers Prev* 2000; **9**:29–42.

80. Houlston RS. Glutathione S-transferase M1 status and lung cancer risk: a meta-analysis. *Cancer Epidemiol Biomarkers Prev* 1999; **8**:675–682.

81. Johns LE, Houlston RS. Glutathione S-transferase μ1 (GSTM1) status and bladder cancer risk: a meta-analysis. *Mutagenesis* 2000; **15**:399–404.

82. Dunning AM, Healey CS, Pharoah PD, *et al.* A systematic review of genetic polymorphisms and breast cancer risk. *Cancer Epidemiol Biomarkers Prev* 1999; **8**:843–854.

83. Johns LE, Houlston RS. N-acetyl transferase-2 and bladder cancer risk: a meta-analysis. *Environ Mol Mutagen* 2000; **36**:221–227.

84. Houlston RS, Tomlinson IP. Polymorphisms and colorectal tumor risk. *Gastroenterology* 2001; **121**:282–301.

85. Houlston RS. CYP1A1 polymorphisms and lung cancer risk: a meta-analysis. *Pharmacogenetics* 2000; **10**:105–114.

86. Laken SJ, Petersen GM, Gruber SB, *et al.* Familial colorectal cancer in Ashkenazim due to a hypermutable tract in APC. *Nature Genet* 1997; **17**:79–83.

87. Krontiris TG, Devlin B, Karp DD, *et al.* An association between the risk of cancer and mutations in the *HRAS1* minisatellite locus. *N Engl J Med* 1993; **329**:517–523.

88. Bennett WP, Alavanja MC, Blomeke B, *et al.* Environmental tobacco smoke, genetic susceptibility, and risk of lung cancer in never-smoking women. *J Natl Cancer Inst* 1999; **91**:2009–2014.

89. Ambrosone CB, Freudenheim JL, Graham S, *et al.* Cigarette smoking, N-acetyltransferase 2 genetic polymorphisms, and breast cancer risk. *JAMA* 1996; **276**:1494–1501.

90. Weinberg CR, Sandler DP. Gene-by-environment interaction for passive smoking and glutathione S-transferase M1? *Natl Cancer Inst* 1999; **91**:1985–1986.

91. IARC. *Tobacco smoking.* IARC Monographs on the Evaluation of Carcinogenic Risks to Humans, no. 38. Lyon: IARC, 1986.

92. Perera FP, Weinstein IB. Molecular epidemiology: recent advances and future directions. *Carcinogenesis* 2000; **21**:517–524.

93. Scott D, Barber JB, Levine EL, *et al.* Radiation-induced micronucleus induction in lymphocytes identifies a high frequency of radiosensitive cases among breast cancer patients: a test for predisposition? *Br J Cancer* 1998; **77**:614–620.

94. Roberts SA, Spreadborough AR, Bulman B, *et al.* Heritability of cellular radiosensitivity: a marker of low-penetrance predisposition genes in breast cancer? *Am J Hum Genet* 1999; **65**:784–794.

95. Risch N. Assessing the role of HLA-linked and unlinked determinants of disease. *Am J Hum Genet* 1987; **40**:1–14.

96. Lu S, Day NE, Degos L, *et al.* Linkage of a nasopharyngeal carcinoma susceptibility locus to the HLA region. *Nature* 1990; **346**:470–471.

97. Risch N, Merikangas K. The future of genetic studies of complex human disease. *Science* 1996; **273**:1516–1517.

98. Camp NJ. Genomewide transmission/disequilibrium testing-consideration of the genotypic relative risks at disease loci. *Am J Hum Genet* 1997; **61**:1424–1430.

99. Reich DE, Cargill M, Bolk S, *et al.* Linkage disequilibrium in the human genome. *Nature* 2001; **411**:199–204.

100. McKeigue PM. Mapping genes underlying ethnic differences in disease risk by linkage disequilibrium in recently admixed populations. *Am J Hum Genet* 1997; **60**:188–196.

101. Cramer W. The prevention of cancer. *Lancet* 1934; **1**:1–5.

102. Ponder BA. Cancer genetics. *Nature* 2001; **411**:336–341.

18

Familial breast cancer

ASHER Y. SALMON AND ROSALIND A. EELES

INTRODUCTION

Breast cancer has been recognized for over 100 years as having a familial component.[1] More recently, a number of epidemiological investigations have attempted to quantify the risks of breast cancer associated with a positive family history. Attempts have also been made to examine whether the pattern of related individuals with breast cancer are consistent with the effects of a single gene of large effect, shared environmental effects, many genes acting in an additive manner or, more likely, a combination of two or more of these effects. In addition to this statistical and observational evidence for the role of genes in the development of breast cancer, a number of specific genes have been identified as playing a role. Perhaps the most notable of these genes are *BRCA1* and *BRCA2*, which were identified through genetic linkage studies and localized to the long arms of chromosomes 17 and 13, respectively.[2,3] Because *BRCA1* and *BRCA2* have been extensively studied, they are the subjects of a separate chapter (Chapter 19) in this book. However, the *BRCA1* and *BRCA2* genes account for less than half of all familial breast cancer.[4]

In this chapter, we will begin by examining the epidemiological evidence for familial risks in breast cancer, then discuss the results of statistical analyses of breast cancer families for the presence of major genetic effects, and describe specific genes other than *BRCA1* and *BRCA 2* that influence breast cancer risk. We will also discuss additional genetic syndromes, which account for a proportion of familial breast cancer.

FAMILIAL RISK OF BREAST CANCER

Evidence that women with a positive family history of breast cancer are at increased risk for developing the disease has been accumulating for over 50 years; virtually every study in which this question has been examined has found significantly elevated relative risks to female relatives of breast cancer patients. However, the magnitude of these risks has varied considerably according to the number and type of affected relatives, age at diagnosis of the proband(s), laterality, relatives suffering from ovarian cancer and the overall study design. There are over 50 epidemiological studies examining risks to close relatives of breast cancer patients. Most studies have found relative risks of between 2 and 3 for first-degree relatives of breast cancer patients selected without regard to age at diagnosis or laterality. In one of the first studies of familial breast cancer in a population-based series,[5] sisters of unilateral breast cancer cases diagnosed at age 50 or younger did not show significantly increased risk; however, sisters of bilateral patients diagnosed at age 40 or younger did appear to have increased risk (relative risk (RR) = 2.4).

In a comprehensive population-based study of familial cancer using the Utah Population Database, Goldgar *et al.* studied the incidence of breast and other cancers among

49 202 first-degree relatives of 5559 breast cancer probands diagnosed before age 80.[6] This study estimated a relative risk of 1.8 in relatives of these breast cancer probands. When the age criterion was restricted to early-onset cancer (diagnosed before age 50), the relative risk of breast cancer among first-degree relatives increased to 2.6 and the risk for early-onset breast cancer among these relatives was 3.7 (95 per cent confidence interval (CI) 2.8–4.6). Similarly, when the risk to subsequent relatives in families with two affected sisters was considered, the risk increased to 2.7 with a particularly high risk of 4.9 for breast cancers diagnosed before age 50. When the study was extended to examine only second-degree relatives of early-onset probands, the relative risk estimate decreased to 1.4 (CI 1.1–1.8) for all breast cancer, and 1.7 (CI 0.9–2.8) for early-onset breast cancer. Similarly, when cousins of early-onset probands were considered, the overall familial relative risks were 1.2 for all breast cancer cases and 1.5 (CI 1.1–2.0) for those diagnosed before the age of 50.

Although most studies have shown the risk to relatives of early-onset probands to be higher than that for probands diagnosed after age 50 or for relatives of all probands, one study found a higher relative risk (1.8) among probands diagnosed over the age of 55 than that for probands diagnosed at an earlier age.[7]

Perhaps the largest population-based study of familial breast cancer is the one done as part of the Cancer and Steroid Hormone (CASH) case-control study of 4730 probands with breast cancer diagnosed between the ages of 20 and 54. The risk of breast cancer in the first-degree relatives of these women compared with controls was 2.1.[8] From this large data set, Claus et al. estimated age-specific risks as a function of the age at diagnosis of the proband and the number of affected relatives.[9] Some of these data (reproduced from Claus et al.[10]) are shown in Figure 18.1. The RR increases as the number of affected relatives increases. For example, a woman with a sister affected at age 50 has an estimated lifetime risk of 3.6 (CI 2.1–6.1), while a woman at age 50 with a mother and a sister affected has an estimated lifetime risk of 17.1 (CI 9.4–31.3). A recent study performed a reanalysis of data from 52 epidemiological studies including 58 209 women with breast cancer and 101 986 women without the disease.[11] The authors found that the risk ratios for breast cancer increased with increasing numbers of affected first-degree relatives: compared with women who had no affected relative, the ratios were 1.80, 2.93 and 3.90, respectively, for one, two and three or more affected first-degree relatives. The risk ratios were greatest at young ages and, for women of a given age, were greater the younger the relative was when diagnosed. The results did not differ substantially between women reporting an affected mother or sister.

In addition to the relationship between age at diagnosis and the magnitude of the familial component of

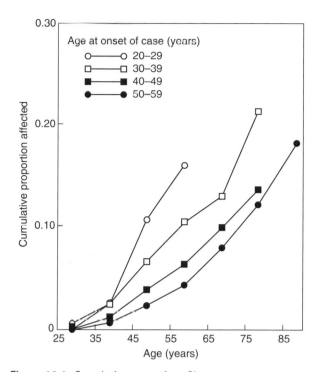

Figure 18.1 *Cumulative proportion of breast cancer cases occurring in first-degree relatives of cases by age of case. (Reproduced from Claus EB, Risch N, Thompson WD. Age of onset as an indicator of familial risk of breast cancer. Am J Epidemiol 1990; 131:961–972 by permission of Oxford University Press.)*

breast cancer (as discussed above), other investigators have examined the role of other factors with respect to family history. Ottman et al. found larger familial effects among relatives of young bilateral probands compared with young probands with unilateral breast cancer.[5] Similar findings have been reported by Anderson.[12]

The issue of relationship of histology to familial breast cancer is less clear. Some studies have found that lobular carcinoma is more often associated with a positive family history.[13] However, Lagios et al. found that cases with tubular carcinoma more frequently reported a positive family history than other histological subtypes.[14] Multicentricity was also found to be positively associated with family history.[15] Other studies have shown conflicting reports of correlation between family history and subtypes or found no differences.[16–18] In the CASH study, Claus et al. found that cases with lobular carcinoma *in situ* were significantly more likely to have a mother or sister affected with breast cancer.[19] The pattern that is emerging is that, within the *BRCA1* subset of genetically-predisposed breast cancer, there is a higher likelihood of grade 3, oestrogen receptor-negative tumours without an *in situ* component (see Chapter 19).

Another feature that conveys strong familial risk of breast cancer is the occurrence of breast cancer in a male. It has been estimated that female relatives of probands with male breast cancer have a 2–3-fold increased risk of breast cancer.[20,21] Male breast cancer has been found to be associated particularly with *BRCA2* families.[22]

FAMILIAL ASSOCIATIONS OF BREAST AND OTHER CANCERS

A number of studies, including those described earlier, have found increased risks for other cancers among relatives of breast cancer probands. The most commonly reported sites have been ovarian, uterine, prostate and colon cancer. However, most of these studies have only examined risks at selected sites in relatives.

The most prominent association is with ovarian cancer in *BRCA1* and *BRCA2* families, where a carrier risk of developing ovarian cancer is between 10 and 60 per cent (RR of 10–60 fold lifetime).[23,24] In families with a significant history of breast cancer and wild-type *BRCA1* or *BRCA2* profiles, the association with ovarian cancer is less prominent.[25] A study by Goldgar *et al.* examined risks to all other sites among such probands.[6] Statistically significant familial associations were found between breast cancer and cancers of the prostate ($RR = 1.2$, $p < 0.0001$), colon ($RR = 1.35$, $p < 0.0001$), thyroid ($RR = 1.7$, $p < 0.001$) and non-Hodgkin's lymphoma ($RR = 1.4$, $p < 0.001$). When the analysis was confined to relatives of the 1145 probands diagnosed before age 50, the risks for colon cancer and non-Hodgkin's lymphoma were increased, with familial RR of 1.7 ($p < 0.00l$) and 1.9 ($p < 0.00l$), respectively. In this study, there did not appear to be an increased risk of ovarian cancer among the relatives of breast cancer probands (70 observed vs. 68 expected). There was a slightly increased frequency of ovarian cancer among relatives of the early onset breast cancer cases (17 observed, 11.3 expected, RR = 1.5) but this difference was *not* statistically significant.

Another consistently identified familial association of other cancers with breast cancer is prostate cancer. In addition to the comprehensive study of familial cancer association described previously, a number of other investigators have also observed significant associations between breast cancer and prostate cancer. Using the Utah Genealogy, Cannon *et al.* found that, among all pairs of individuals in which one member of the pair had prostate cancer and the other breast cancer, there was a significantly higher average degree of relatedness between the affected pair than among cohort-matched control pairs.[26] Tulinius *et al.*, in a similar population-based study of the Iceland genealogies and cancer registry, found a significantly increased risk of prostate cancer in all relatives of women with breast cancer; a relative risk of 1.5 in first-degree relatives, and 1.3 in second-degree relatives.[27] Anderson and Badzioch reported a greater than twofold

risk of familial breast cancer when prostate cancer is also in the family history.[21] Analysis of a subset of the Breast Cancer Linkage Consortium (BCLC) families suggests that particularly the *BRCA2* locus confers an increased risk of prostate cancer.[28]

Other studies have also shown relationships between breast cancer, and colon and uterine cancers, although the results have not been consistent across studies. Some of these families may be modified Lynch type II families (see Chapter 24), although classically, breast cancer is not thought to be increased in frequency in Lynch syndrome. Until the underlying genetic basis for such families is elucidated, this debate will continue.

IMPLICATIONS OF MAJOR GENES IN BREAST CANCER AETIOLOGY

Because of the increased risk of breast cancer in relatives of breast cancer cases and the existence of families with unusual clusters of breast cancer cases, genes have been recognized to play an important role in breast cancer aetiology.[29] Numerous investigators have examined the evidence for genetic inheritance[9,30] in breast cancer families ascertained from a variety of population and non-population-based sources and concluded that the data were most consistent with autosomal dominant inheritance for a major susceptibility locus/loci with high, but incomplete, lifetime penetrance in genetically susceptible women. The genetic models arising from these studies also implied that there was a non-negligible risk of breast cancer among women who did not carry this genetic susceptibility, and that, because the risks to gene carriers was not 100 per cent, there must be other genetic or environmental effects that influence risk.

In 1986, the fourth Genetic Analysis Workshop examined segregation and linkage analysis in several large data sets of breast cancer families. These workshops were conceived as a way of bringing together many different genetic epidemiologists with a variety of approaches to tackle a common problem. The group analysed data consisting of 200 families of sequential breast cancer probands in the Danish Cancer Registry from 1942 to 1945 collected by Jacobson *et al.* 18 Nebraskan families ascertained in a variety of ways by Henry Lynch *et al.*, 16 2–5-generation pedigrees collected in the Netherlands by Cleton *et al.* and nine families ascertained from the Utah Genealogy by Skolnick *et al.* (families and data are described by Bailey-Wilson *et al.*[31]) were analysed,[32,33] and they confirmed the presence of an autosomal dominant susceptibility locus or loci acting to increase breast cancer susceptibility, at least in a subset of familial breast cancer.

Claus *et al.* analysed a large data set collected as part of the CASH study and demonstrated a rare dominant susceptibility allele for breast cancer.[9] The estimated frequency of the allele that conferred increased susceptibility to breast cancer was 0.003, implying a carrier rate in the general population of 6/1000. The estimated increased risk due to this susceptibility allele ranged from almost 100-fold in women in their 20s to a modest twofold increase in women in their 80s. However, it must be recognized that the results of any segregation analysis of breast cancer families is likely to reflect the effects of a number of different susceptibility loci, given that we now know that familial breast cancer is not all due to a single locus. Thus, the estimates of a gene frequency derived from such analyses would represent the sum of the allele frequencies of a number of specific susceptibility loci. Similarly, the penetrance estimates are an average of the effects of each individual susceptibility locus. Confirmation of the existence of one or more loci that contribute to familial breast cancer and elucidation of the effects of individual loci can come only through localization of such genes to specific chromosomal regions by linkage analysis of breast cancer families, or through identification of germline mutations of specific candidate loci in familial breast cancer patients, such as has occurred for BRCA1 and BRCA2 (see Chapter 19).

GENE MAPPING STUDIES IN FAMILIAL BREAST CANCER

A number of possible linkages between genetic markers and familial breast cancer have been reported in the past. The first such linkage was found between a polymorphism at the glutamate–pyruvate transaminase (GPT) locus on chromosome 10.[34] Later, Skolnick et al. reported an initial linkage of a single kindred to the ABO blood group locus on chromosome 9q.[35] The LOD score reached a maximum value of 3.0 before subsequent observations in new cases of breast cancer in the family reduced the strength of this evidence. These findings illustrate the difficulty in linkage analysis of complex traits, and demonstrate the need for confirmation in multiple families by different investigators. In spite of these difficulties, the existence of a specific gene, denoted BRCA1, conferring increased susceptibility to breast cancer, was confirmed in late 1990 with the finding of linkage between early-onset breast cancer and a specific marker (DI7S74) on the long arm of chromosome 17[2] (see also Chapter 19). The discovery of linkage to BRCA2 illustrated the use of phenotypic classification to aid grouping of families for linkage studies. Families were selected on the presence of male breast cancer in addition to early-onset ovarian cancer and this was found to select against the presence of BRCA1[22,36] (see also Chapter 19).

OTHER GENES CONFERRING INCREASED RISK OF BREAST CANCER

Aside from BRCA1 and BRCA2, there are a number of specific genes that have been associated with an increased risk of breast cancer (Table 18.1). The most striking of these genes is the TP53 tumour suppressor locus (on chromosome 17p, see Chapter 11). Although mutations

Table 18.1 *Genes associated with hereditary breast cancer*

Gene	Clinical syndrome	Location	Other familial cancers associated	Breast cancer lifetime penetrance	Protein function
BRCA1	Familial breast–ovarian cancer	17q21	Ovarian, others?	Up to 85%	DNA repair complex
BRCA2	Familial breast–ovarian cancer	13q12	Ovarian, prostate, pancreas, bile duct, fallopian tube, male breast	Up to 80%	DNA repair complex
TP53	Li–Fraumeni	17p13.1	Sarcoma, CNS, adrenocortical leukaemia	~90%	Cell-cycle and apoptosis regulation
ATM	Ataxia telangiectasia	11q22	Leukaemia, lymphoma (in homozygotes)	Up to 60% in homozygote (short lifespan) 24% in heterozygotes	DNA damage signalling
PTEN	Cowden syndrome	10q23.3	Thyroid (follicular)	20–50%	Lipid and protein phosphatase upstream of protein kinase B
MLH1α MSH2	Hereditary non-polyposis colorectal cancer/Lynch	3p21 2p27	Colorectal, ovarian endometrial, other gastrointestinal	?16% (debated)	DNA mismatch repair
CHEK2		22q		RR ~2.2	Cell-cycle checkpoint kinase
H-RAS		11p15.5		RR ~2.3	GTP-binding protein (proto-oncogene)

in this gene are commonly found in many types of tumours, germline *TP53* mutations are most often associated with the Li–Fraumeni syndrome (LFS) in which families typically exhibit multiple affected members with childhood cancers, primarily sarcomas and brain tumours,[37] in addition to very early-onset breast cancer, often diagnosed before age 30. It has been estimated that 50–75 per cent of Li–Fraumeni families are due to germline *TP53* mutations in the coding region of the gene.[38] However, in families that have some of these characteristics but do not fulfill the classical definition of LFS, only 10–27 per cent are attributable to germline *TP53* mutations.[38] Loss of heterozygosity (LOH) in the *TP53* gene has been shown to be a common event in primary breast carcinomas and this is accompanied by mutation of the residual allele in some cases. It is important to emphasize that, overall, germline *TP53* mutations account for only a small (<1 per cent) proportion of early-onset breast cancers and a negligible fraction of familial breast cancer in general. For example, Borreson *et al.*[39] screened 237 women with early-onset breast cancer and found only two germline *TP53* mutations; both cases belonged to families with features seen in the Li–Fraumeni or LFS-like syndrome. Sidransky *et al.* examined 126 cases and found only one patient with breast cancer diagnosed before age 40 to have a germline *TP53* mutation;[40] again, this case came from a Li–Fraumeni-like family (see also Chapter 11). However, individuals who carry a germline *TP53* mutation have a very high penetrance of breast cancer, which is of particularly early onset (90 per cent by age 60).[41]

Ataxia telangiectasia (A-T) is an autosomal recessive disorder associated with a high incidence of cancer (61–184-fold), particularly lymphomas and leukaemias, but also primary carcinomas of other organs, including the breast.[42] It has been reported that individuals who carry one copy of the abnormal *ATM* gene are also at an increased risk (RR = 3) for breast cancer.[43] If this result is true and the *ATM* gene frequency is as high as some estimates have indicated, the *ATM* locus could account for a substantial proportion of the observed familial relative risk (see Chapter 13). In a study of a number of early-onset breast cancer families that were not linked to *BRCA1*, no evidence of linkage to the *ATM* region of chromosome 11 was found.[44] However, if the *ATM* gene has a moderate penetrance, it may not cause the dramatic familial clusters needed for linkage analysis, but may still make an important contribution to genetic breast cancer. Further studies have tried to address these questions, both by trying to estimate the incidence of breast cancer among known *ATM* heterozygotes in A-T families[45,46] and by linkage and *ATM*-mutation screening among affected individuals in breast cancer families.[44,47] These studies report contrasting conclusions about the degree of risk of developing breast cancer among *ATM* heterozygotes.

While some studies showed an association, others did not. Gatti suggested a model in which hetrozygotes of *ATM* mutations that result in a truncated non-functional protein (such as are found in the A-T syndrome) would not predispose to a high cancer risk, while a missense mutation that will alter the activity of the protein would be associated with a high risk of cancer.[48] This model has not yet been confirmed, although mouse models of a mutant *atm* polypeptide lacking the PI3-kinase domain have been shown to increase genetic instability and have a negative dominant effect. A recent study has shown that two *ATM* mutations (T7271G and IVS10–6t → g) are associated with a significantly high risk of breast cancer, which has been found in multiple-case breast cancer families. The investigators estimated that penetrance of the mutations could be as high as 60 per cent at age 70 years, equivalent to a 15.7-fold increased relative risk compared with that of the general population.[49] As they found no evidence of LOH for either the wild-type or mutant allele, they concluded that the high penetrance observed was related to the dominant negative nature of these mutations.

Recently, a few mutations have been described in the *CHEK2* gene that were shown to be involved in low-penetrance breast cancer susceptibility. The *CHEK2* gene is located on chromosome 22q. The CHEK2 protein functions downstream of the ATM protein in response to DNA damage to phosphorylate TP53 and BRCA1.[50] Activation of these proteins in response to DNA damage prevents cellular entry into mitosis in mammalian cells, therefore, regulating the tumour suppressor functions of these proteins. *CHEK2* 1100delC, a truncating variant that abrogates the kinase activity, has a frequency of 1.1 per cent in healthy individuals. However, this variant is present in 5.1 per cent of individuals with breast cancer from 718 families that do not carry mutations in *BRCA1* or *BRCA2*, including 13.5 per cent of individuals from families with male breast cancer. It was estimated that the *CHEK2**1100delC variant results in an approximately twofold increase of breast cancer risk in women and a tenfold increase of risk in men.[51] Similar results were reported by another group.[52] Other mutations, Arg180His, Arg117Gly and Arg137Gln, were also found in breast cancer families, but their overall contribution to breast cancer risk may be small.[53,54]

Other previously identified genes, which might be biologically plausible candidates for breast cancer, include the oestrogen receptor (*ESR*) and the *HRAS1* locus. The *ESR* locus on chromosome 6q is a biological candidate in a region frequently lost in tumours,[55] for which possible genetic linkage in a single postmenopausal breast cancer family has been reported.[56] The LOD score for this family with *ESR* was only 1.85, indicating a suggestive but not conclusive evidence of linkage in this family. In a test of candidate gene loci in a set of *BRCA1*-unlinked breast cancer and breast–ovarian cancer families, no evidence of linkage to the *ESR* locus was found; however, it should be noted that these families were selected primarily for premenopausal breast cancer.

One study showed a small but significant elevated risk of 2.29 for breast cancer associated with certain rare variants at a minisatellite locus located in the three prime untranslated region of the *HRAS1* oncogene locus on the distal short arm of chromosome 11.[57] The authors of this study hypothesize that *HRAS1* minisatellite mutations interfere with regulatory mechanisms governing the control of gene expression. A more recent study did not show a susceptibility to early-onset breast cancer among individuals with the higher risk genotype described in earlier studies.[58]

Cowden syndrome (see Chapter 12) is an autosomal dominant disorder characterized by multiple hamartomas and breast cancer.[59] Mutations of the *PTEN* gene, a tumour suppressor gene on 10q23.3,[60,61] which encodes a lipid and protein phosphatase that lies upstream of protein kinase B, was found to be associated with the syndrome. The real incidence of breast cancer among *PTEN* mutation carriers is not well defined, although several authors have suggested that it is as high as 25–50 per cent of all female carriers by the age of 50 years.[59] This syndrome is also now known to be associated with male breast cancer.[62]

THE SEARCH FOR ADDITIONAL BREAST CANCER SUSCEPTIBILITY GENES – THE *BRCA3* STORY

At least 20 per cent of large familial breast cancer clusters are not related to the *BRCA1* or *BRCA2* genes.[63] In fact, the majority of families with less than six cases of breast cancer and no ovarian cancer are not linked to either *BRCA1* or *BRCA2*.[36] Linkage at a few chromosomal loci has been reported in these families. A locus on chromosome 8p12–22 has been reported to account for some of these families.[64] Further studies did not confirm this locus in other non *BRCA1/2*-linked high risk breast cancer families.[65]

A study of 77 multiple case breast cancer families from Scandinavia found evidence of linkage between the disease and polymorphic markers on chromosome 13q21. A recent study has evaluated the contribution of this candidate 'BRCA3' locus to breast cancer susceptibility in 128 high-risk breast cancer families of Western European ancestry with no identified *BRCA1* or *BRCA2* mutations. No evidence of linkage was found.[66]

Owing to the fact that *BRCA1* and *BRCA2* cannot explain all the observed familial breast cancer clustering, the search for a third hypothetical gene, 'BRCA3', is in progress. The dilemma is whether another highly penetrant gene such as *BRCA1* or *BRCA2* really exists. It is

possible that this is so, but that only a very small fraction of families are due to such a gene and the remainder are due to more moderate risk genes together with a proportion of clusters that have occurred due to chance. The discovery of *CHEK2* was the first more moderate risk breast cancer gene to be reported. It has an overall relative risk of 2.4-fold on a meta-analysis of about 11000 breast cancer cases.[67] This discovery illustrates the need for very large numbers of cases in such experiments to find effects of this more modest magnitude.

KEY POINTS

- It is well established that a positive family history is the strongest epidemiological risk factor known for breast cancer, stronger than any known reproductive, hormonal or dietary factors.
- Although a common family environment could account for a proportion of the observed familiarity, there is substantial evidence that the majority of this familial effect is due to the action of a number of specific genes. This evidence comes from several sources: the observation that there is an increased risk to more distant relatives of breast cancer probands who do not share common environments; the results of segregation analyses, which show that the pattern of familiarity is consistent with the actions of dominant high penetrant susceptibility loci; and, most convincingly, the cloning of two such susceptibility genes, *BRCA1* and *BRCA2*, and the identification by candidate gene analysis of *TP53*, *PTEN* and *CHEK2*.
- The role of mutations in other known genes, such as *ATM* and *HRAS*, remains to be clarified.

REFERENCES

1. Broca PP. *Traites des Tumeurs.* Paris: Asselin, 1866.
2. Hall MJ, Lee MK, Newman B, *et al.* Linkage of early-onset familial breast cancer to chromosome 17q21. *Science* 1991; **250**:1684–1689.
3. Wooster R, Neuhausen S, Mangion J, *et al.* Localization of a breast cancer susceptibility gene, *BRCA2*, to chromosome 13q?,12-13. *Science* 1994; **265**:2088–2090
4. Peto J, Collins N, Barfoot R, *et al.* Prevalence of *BRCA1* and *BRCA2* gene mutations in patients with early-onset breast cancer. *J Natl Cancer Inst.* 1999; **91**:943–949.
5. Ottman R, Pike MC, King M-C, *et al.* Familial breast cancer in a population based series. *Am J Epidemiol* 1986; **123**:15–21.
6. Goldgar DE, Easton DF, Cannon Albright LA, Skolnick MH. Systematic population-based assessment of cancer risk in first degree relatives of cancer probands. *J Natl Cancer Inst* 1994; **86**:1600–1607.

7. Mettlin C, Croghan I, Natarajan N, Lane W. The association of age and familial risk in a case-control study of breast cancer. *Am J Epidemiol* 1990; **131**:973–983.

8. Schildkraut JM, Risch N, Thompson WD. Evaluating genetic association among ovarian, breast, and endometrial cancer: evidence for a breast/ovarian cancer relationship. *Am J Hum Genet* 1989; **45**:521–529.

9. Claus EB, Risch N, Thompson W. Genetic analysis of breast cancer in the cancer and steroid hormone study. *Am J Hum Genet* 1991; **48**:232–242.

10. Claus EB, Risch N, Thompson WD. Age of onset as an indicator of familial risk of breast cancer. *Am J Epidemiol* 1990; **131**:961–972.

11. Familial breast cancer: collaborative reanalysis of individual data from 52 epidemiological studies including 58 209 women with breast cancer and 101 986 women without the disease. *Lancet* 2001; **358**:89–99.

12. Anderson DE. Genetic study of breast cancer: identification of a high risk group. *Cancer* 1974; **34**:1090–1097.

13. Erdreich LS, Asal NR, Hoge AF. Morphologic types of breast cancer: age, bilaterality, and family history. *South Med J* 1980; **73**:28–32.

14. Lagios MD, Rose ME, Margolin FR. Tubular carcinoma of the breast: association with multicentricity, bilaterality and family history. *Am J Clin Pathol* 1980; **73**:25–30.

15. Lagios MD. Multicentricity of breast carcinoma demonstrated by routine correlated serial subgross and radiographic examination. *Cancer* 1977; **40**:1726–1734.

16. Lynch HT, Albano WA, Heieck JJ, *et al.* Genetics, biomarkers, and control of breast cancer: a review. *Cancer Genet Cytogenet* 1984; **13**:43–92.

17. Rosen PP, Lesser ML, Senie RT, Kinne DW. Epidemiology of breast carcinoma. III. Relationship of family history to tumor type. *Cancer* 1982; **50**:171–179.

18. Burki N, Buser M, Fmmons ER, *et al.* Malignancies in families of women with medullary, tubular, and invasive ductal breast cancer. *Eur J Cancer Clinc Oncol* 1990; **26**:295–303.

19. Claus EB, Risch N, Thompson WD. Relationship between breast histopathology and family history of breast cancer. *Cancer* 1993: **71**:147–153.

20. Rosenblatt KA, Thomas DB, McTiernan A, *et al.* Breast cancer in men: aspects of familial aggregation. *J Natl Cancer Inst* 1991; **83**:849–853.

21. Anderson DL. Badzioch MD. Familial breast cancer risks: effects of prostate and other cancers. *Cancer* 1993; **7**:114–119.

22. Stratton MR, Ford D, Seal S. Familial male breast cancer is not linked to the *BRCA1* locus on chromosome 17q. *Nature Genet* 1994; **7**:103–107.

23. Struewing JP, Hartge P, Wacholder S, *et al.* The risk of cancer associated with specific mutations of *BRCA1* and *BRCA2* among Ashkenazi Jews. *N Engl J Med* 1997; **336**:1401–1408.

24. Ford D, Easton DF, Stratton M, *et al.* (1998) Genetic heterogeneity and penetrance analysis of the *BRCA1* and *BRCA2* genes in breast cancer families. The Breast Cancer Linkage Consortium. *Am J Hum Genet* **62**:676–689.

25. Antoniou AC, Pharoah PD, McMullan G, *et al.* Evidence for further breast cancer susceptibility genes in addition to *BRCA1* and *BRCA2* in a population-based study. *Genet Epidemiol* 2001; **1**:1–18.

26. Cannon I, Bishop DT, Skolnick MH, *et al.* Genetic epidemiology of prostate cancer in the Utah Mormon genealogy. *Cancer Surv* 1982; **1**:1–12.

27. Tulinius H, Egilsson V, Olafsdottir GH, Sigvaldsson H. Risk of prostate, ovarian and endometrial cancer among relatives of women with breast cancer. *Br Med J* 1992; **305**:855–857.

28. The Breast Cancer Linkage Consortium. Cancer Risks in *BRCA2* Mutation Carriers. *J Natl Cancer Inst* 1999; **91**:1310–1316.

29. Lynch HI, Guirgis HA, Albert S, *et al.* Familial association of carcinoma of the breast and ovary. *Surgery* 1974; **138**:717–724.

30. Bishop DT, Albright EG, McClellan T, *et al.* Segregation and linkage analysis of nine Utah breast cancer pedigrees. *Genet Epidemiol* 1988; **5**:151–169.

31. Bailey-Wilson JE, Cannon LA, King M.-C. Genetic analysis of human breast cancer: a synthesis of contributions to GAW IV. *Genet Epidemiol (Suppl.)* 1986; **1**:15–35.

32. King M-C, Cannon LA, Bailey-Wilson JE, *et al.* Genetic analysis of human breast cancer: literature review and description of family data in workshop. *Genet Epidemiol (Suppl.)* 1986; **1**:3–13.

33. Cannon LA, Bishop DT, Skolnick MH. Segregation and linkage analysis of breast cancer in the Dutch and Utah families. *Genet Epidemiol* 1986; **3**:43–46.

34. King M-C, Go RCP, Elsten RC, *et al.* Allele increasing susceptibility to human breast cancer may be linked to the glutamate–pyruvate transaminase locus. *Science* 1980; **208**:406–408.

35. Skolnick MH, Thompson LA, Bishop DT, Cannon LA. Possible linkage of a breast cancer susceptibility locus to the ABO locus: sensitivity of LOD scores to a single new recombinant observation. *Genet Epidemiol* 1984; **1**:363–373.

36. Stratton MR. Recent advances in understanding of genetic susceptibility to breast cancer. *Hum Mol Genet* 1996; **5**:1515–1519.

37. Li FP, Fraumeni JF. Soft tissue sarcomas, breast cancer and other neoplasms: a familial syndrome? *Ann Intern Med* 1969; **71**:747–760.

38. Birch JM, Hartley AL, Tricker KJ, *et al.* Prevalence and diversity of constitutional mutations in the *p53* gene among 21 Li–Fraumeni families. *Cancer Res* 1994; **54**:1298–1304.

39. Borreson AL, Anderson LL, Garber J, *et al.* Screening for germ line *TP53* mutations in breast cancer patients. *Cancer Res* 1992; **52**:3234–3236.

40. Sidransky D, Tokino T, Helzlsouer K, *et al.* Inherited *p53* mutations in breast cancer. *Cancer Res* 1992; **52**:2984–2986.

41. La Bihan C, Bonati-Pellie C. A method for estimating cancer risk in *p53* mutation carriers. *Cancer Detect Prev* 1994; **18**:171–178.

42. Swift M, Reitnauer PJ, Morrell D, Chase CL. Incidence of cancer in 161 families affected by ataxia telangiectasia. *N Engl J. Med* 1991; **325**:1831–1836.

43. Olsen JH, Hahnemann JM, Borresen-Dale AL. Cancer in patients with ataxia-telangiectasia and in their relatives in the nordic countries. *J Natl Cancer Ins.* 2001; **93**:121–127.

44. Wooster R, Ford D, Mangion J, *et al.* Absence of linkage to the ataxia-telangiectasia locus in familial breast cancer. *Hum Genet* 1993; **92**:91–94.

45. Easton DF. Cancer risks in A-T heterozygotes. *Int J Radiat Biol* 1994; **66**:S177–182.

46. Janin N, Andrieu K, Ossian A, et al. Breast cancer risk in ataxia telangiectasia (AT) heterozygotes: haplotype study in French AT families. Br J Cancer 1999; 80:1042–1045.

47. Vorechovsky I, Luo L, Lindblom A, et al. ATM mutations in cancer families. Cancer Res 1996; 56:4130–4133.

48. Gatti RA, Tward A, Concannon P, et al. Cancer risk in ATM heterozygotes: a model of phenotypic and mechanistic differences between missense and truncating mutations. Mol Genet Metab 1999; 68:419–423.

49. Chenevix-Trench G, Spurdle AB, Gatei M, et al. Dominant negative ATM mutations in breast cancer families. J Natl Cancer Inst 2002; 94:205–215.

50. Falck J, Mailand N, Syljuasen RG, et al. The ATM-Chk2-Cdc25A checkpoint pathway guards against radioresistant DNA synthesis. Nature 2001; 41:842–847.

51. Meijers-Heijboer H, van den Ouweland A, Klijn J, et al. The CHEK2-Breast Cancer Consortium. Low-penetrance susceptibility to breast cancer due to CHEK2(*)1100delC in noncarriers of BRCA1 or BRCA2 mutations. Nature Genet 2002; 31:55–59.

52. Vahteristo P, Bartkova J, Eerola H, et al. A CHEK2 genetic variant contributing to a substantial fraction of familial breast cancer. Am J Hum Genet 2002; 71:432–438.

53. Schutte M, Seal S, Barfoot R, et al. Variants in CHEK2 other than 1100delC do not make a major contribution to breast cancer susceptibility. Am J Hum Genet 2003; 73(4): 1023–1028.

54. Sodha N, Bullock S, Taylor R, et al. CHEK2 variants in susceptibility to breast cancer and evidence of retention of the wild type allele in tumours. Br J Cancer 2002; 87:1445–1448.

55. Fuqua SA, Chamness GC, McGuire WL. Estrogen receptor mutations in breast cancer. J Cell Biochem 1993; 51:135–139.

56. Zuppan P, Hall JM, Lee MK, et al. Possible linkage of the estrogen receptor gene to breast cancer in a family with late-onset disease. Am J Hum Genet 1991; 48:1065–1068.

57. Krontiris TG, Devlin B, Karp DD, et al. An association between the risk of cancer and mutations in the HRAS1 minisatellite locus. N Engl J Med 1993; 329:517–523.

58. Firgaira FA, Seshadri R, McEvoy CR, et al. HRAS1 rare minisatellite alleles and breast cancer in Australian women under age forty years. J Natl Cancer Inst 1999; 91:2107–2111.

59. Eng C. Genetics of Cowden syndrome: through the looking glass of oncology. Int J Oncol 1998; 12:701–710.

60. Nelen MR, Padberg GW, Peeters EA, et al. Localization of the gene for Cowden disease to chromosome 10q22–23. Nature Genet 1996; 13:114–116.

61. Liaw D, Marsh DJ, Li J, et al. Germline mutations of the PTEN gene in Cowden disease, an inherited breast and thyroid cancer syndrome. Nature Genet 1997; 16:64–67.

62. Fackenthal JD, Marsh DJ, Richardson AL, et al. Male breast cancer in Cowden syndrome patients with germline PTEN mutations. J Med Genet 2001; 38:159–164.

63. Antoniou AC, Pharoah PD, McMullan G, et al. Evidence for further breast cancer susceptibility genes in addition to BRCA1 and BRCA2 in a population-based study. Genet Epidemiol 2001; 1:1–18.

64. Imbert A, Chaffanet M, Essioux L, et al. Integrated map of the chromosome 8p12–p21 region, a region involved in human cancers and Werner syndrome. Genomics 1996; 32:29–38.

65. Rahman N, Teare MD, Seal S, et al. Absence of evidence for a familial breast cancer susceptibility gene at chromosome 8p12–p22. Oncogene 2000; 19:4170–4173.

66. Thompson D, Szabo CI, Mangion J, et al. Evaluation of linkage of breast cancer to the putative BRCA3 locus on chromosome 13q21 in 128 multiple case families from the Breast Cancer Linkage Consortium. Proc Natl Acad Sci USA 2002; 99:827–831.

67. The CHEK2 Breast Cancer Case Control Consortium (2004). CHEK2 1100 delc and susceptibility to breast cancer: a collaborative analysis involving 10860 breast cancer cases and 9065 controls from 10 studies. Amer J Hum Genet 2004; 74:1175–1182.

19

The *BRCA1* and *BRCA2* genes

DEBORAH THOMPSON AND DOUGLAS F. EASTON

INTRODUCTION

Germline mutations in the *BRCA1* and *BRCA2* genes are the most important known causes of inherited susceptibility to breast and ovarian cancer. In this chapter, we outline the research leading to the identification of these genes. We discuss the risks of breast, ovarian and other cancers conferred by mutations in these genes; their contribution to breast and ovarian cancer incidence; and the pathology and clinical outcome of these tumours. We also discuss the role of genetic and lifestyle modifiers of risk in mutation carriers and, briefly, the function of these genes. Management of *BRCA1* and *BRCA2* mutation carriers is discussed in more detail in Chapters 21–23.

Family history is an important risk factor for both breast cancer, particularly at young ages, and ovarian cancer. A recent meta-analysis found that the risk of breast cancer in women with an affected mother or sister is increased by approximately fivefold below age 40, falling to approximately 1.4-fold above age 60.[1] The higher risks of breast cancer in monozygotic twins of cases indicate that much of this familial aggregation is likely to have a genetic basis.[2,3] Some, but not all, formal segregation analyses[4] have suggested that rare autosomal alleles conferring a high lifetime risk of the disease may explain this familial aggregation. This hypothesis has been supported by many anecdotal examples of high-risk families consistent with the inheritance of an autosomal dominant gene.

Ovarian cancer also exhibits familial aggregation, the disease being 2–3-fold more common in the first-degree relatives of cases (see Chapter 23). Moreover, several studies have shown that breast cancer is 30–60 per cent more common in the first-degree relatives of ovarian cancer cases and vice versa (e.g. Schildkraut *et al.*[5] and Easton *et al.*[6]), suggesting the existence of genes predisposing to both cancers. This hypothesis is supported by numerous reports of families displaying striking aggregations of both breast and ovarian cancer, including individual women with primary tumours at both sites.[5,7,8] Such families formed the basis for genetic linkage studies to map breast–ovarian cancer susceptibility genes.

IDENTIFICATION OF *BRCA1*

The *BRCA1* gene was initially localized by Hall *et al.* using 23 families with multiple cases of breast cancer.[9] It was the first breast cancer locus and one of the first for any common disease to be mapped in this manner. The disease in this set of families showed evidence of linkage to the marker D17S74 on chromosome 17q21, with a heterogeneity LOD score of 3.28 and an estimated 40 per cent of the families being linked to this locus[9] (see also Chapter 3). These findings were confirmed, and the phenotypic definition extended to include ovarian cancer, by a study of five large US families segregating both breast and ovarian cancer.[8] An analysis of 214 families assembled by the Breast Cancer Linkage Consortium (BCLC) provided overwhelming evidence of 17q linkage (LOD score 27), with an estimated 45 per cent of the 153 families with breast cancer alone, and 100 per cent of the 57 families that contained both breast and ovarian cancer cases being linked to this locus.[10] This analysis localized *BRCA1* to the interval bounded by the markers D17S250 and D17S588.

After further narrowing of the region by several groups using multipoint linkage, *BRCA1* (MIM 113705)[11] was finally identified in 1994 by positional cloning, using individuals from eight families with evidence of linkage to *BRCA1*.[12] Mutations segregating with disease were detected in five families, but were not seen in a panel of controls. The gene contains 22 exons, spans approximately 100 kb of genomic DNA and encodes a protein of 1863 amino acids. The presence of mutations in *BRCA1* in breast–ovarian cancer families linked to 17q has been confirmed in many studies (e.g. Friedman *et al.*[13] and Simard *et al.*[14]).

IDENTIFICATION OF *BRCA2*

Evidence for a second breast cancer susceptibility locus, '*BRCA2*' (MIM 600185)[15] on chromosome 13q12–13, was found by Wooster *et al.*,[16] by genetic linkage analysis in 15 families showing strong evidence against linkage to *BRCA1*. The gene was localized to a 6 cM interval around D13S260 (maximum heterogeneity LOD score 11.65). The gene itself was identified 15 months later by positional cloning, with identification of protein truncating mutations in *BRCA2* among 46 families with evidence of linkage to the region.[17] Wooster *et al.*[17] identified and screened approximately two-thirds of the *BRCA2* coding sequence; the remaining information was provided by Tavtigian *et al.*, who identified a further ten distinct mutations in 18 putative *BRCA2*-linked families.[18]

The *BRCA2* gene consists of 27 exons, spans approximately 70 kb of genomic DNA and encodes a protein of 3418 amino acids (i.e. approximately twice the size of *BRCA1*). Like *BRCA1*, it has no apparent close homologue in the human genome.

MUTATIONS IN *BRCA1* AND *BRCA2*

By February 2003, the Breast Cancer Information Core (BIC) database[19] had recorded 1237 distinct *BRCA1* mutations and 1381 *BRCA2* mutations. Of these, 711 and 872 respectively have been reported just once (i.e. over 60 per cent of reported mutations are unique). Mutations appear to be reasonably evenly distributed across the coding sequences, with no obvious 'mutation hot spots'.

The majority of mutations found in individuals in breast–ovarian families linked to 17q or 13q (and hence believed to be deleterious) are mutations leading to a truncated protein. These include small insertions or deletions resulting in a frameshift, nonsense mutations, mutations in splice-sites leading to aberrant splicing and large-scale rearrangements (insertions, deletions or duplications). Such alterations are generally regarded as disease associated and would be utilized in clinical genetic testing. There is some uncertainty in the case of splice-site alterations that are not at a strongly conserved site since RNA is often not available to confirm aberrant splicing directly. The other major exception is the nonsense mutation 3326 Ter near the 3′ end of *BRCA2*.[20] This mutation has been shown to occur with a frequency of approximately 2 per cent in the normal population, and is not associated with any marked breast or ovarian cancer risk. A smaller number of in-frame deletions have been identified in high-risk individuals; their association with disease is less clear than for truncating alterations.

In addition to the protein-truncating mutations reported above, a large number of amino-acid substitutions have been identified in both genes. A few of these occur at significant population frequencies (see later) but the majority are rare. A small number of these, principally those involving cysteine residues in the *BRCA1* RING domain (e.g. Cys61Gly), have occurred consistently in high-risk families and are regarded as deleterious, but the status of the majority of these 'rare variants' is uncertain. Given their frequency (they account for approximately 30 per cent of all mutations on BIC) and the fact that many occur in patients with another deleterious mutation, it is clear that the large majority of these variants cannot be strongly associated with disease. At the present time, no reliable functional assay exists to determine whether such a variant is likely to be deleterious, and only the epidemiological evidence on the frequency of the variant in breast cancer cases or families and in controls, and on the co-segregation of the variant with disease in families, can be regarded as definitive. Unfortunately, this evidence is lacking for most variants. Only six variants outside the RING domain of *BRCA1* are classified as missense mutations by BIC – R1347G, S1448T, A1708E, M1775R, R1699Q and R1699W, and, for some of these, the evidence that they are pathogenic is not totally convincing. No clearly deleterious missense *BRCA2* mutations have yet been defined.

It is important to note that the frequency of reported mutation types does not necessarily reflect their overall population frequency. Many laboratories use mutation-screening techniques (e.g. single-stranded conformation polymorphism, SSCP; or conformational strand-gel electrophoresis, CSGE) that have better sensitivity for detecting small deletions and insertions than for detecting point mutations.

Large insertions, deletions and rearrangements

Screening for germline mutations in *BRCA1* and *BRCA2* is usually performed by sequencing of the coding sequence and splice sites, or by screening techniques, such as single stranded conformational polymorphism (SSCP), denaturing gradient gel electrophoresis (DGGE), conformational sequence gel electrophoresis (CSGE), denaturing high performance liquid chromatography (DHPLC) or protein truncation test (PTT). A comparative study has suggested that these latter techniques have sensitivities ranging from 60 to 100 per cent, relative to sequencing.[21] Even sequencing does not, however, detect mutations in all linked families. By examination of the mutation detection rate among families likely to be linked to *BRCA1*, the sensitivity of these techniques, including sequencing, for *BRCA1* mutation detection has been estimated to be around 63 per cent.[21,22] This incomplete sensitivity is due, at least in part, to the existence of large-scale insertions and deletions that are not detectable using conventional screening techniques. To date there have been reports of around 16 distinct large genomic rearrangements in *BRCA1* (all associated with breast or ovarian cancer), generally identified using protein-truncation analyses or Southern blots. The majority are deletions of one or more exons.[23–30] For example, a 6 kb *BRCA1* duplication of exon 13 has been identified in 15 unrelated families (all compatible with a common haplotype), suggesting a common origin for the mutation, possibly in the North of England.[31] By 1997, 36 per cent of all *BRCA1* mutations found in Dutch families were large-scale deletions.[25] The high density of Alu repetitive sequences in the *BRCA1* gene (41.5 per cent)[32] is thought to contribute to the number of large deletions and duplications observed; all but one of the reported rearrangements has involved a non-homologous recombination between two similar Alu sequences at different locations. To date, there have been just two reports of large rearrangements in *BRCA2*.[33,34] *BRCA2* has a lower density of Alu repeat sequences than *BRCA1* (20 per cent), although it has a higher density of other types of repetitive DNA sequences.[35] It is not yet clear whether the difference in the frequency of large rearrangements between *BRCA1* and *BRCA2* is genuine, or the result of bias in the studies performed. A lower frequency of large rearrangements in *BRCA2* would be consistent with the higher mutation detection sensitivity that has been observed for *BRCA2* (approximately 78 per cent based on BCLC data; D.F. Easton, personal communication).

Polymorphisms

The BIC database lists 164 neutral polymorphisms in *BRCA1* and *BRCA2*. Most of these are quite rare, but five polymorphisms in *BRCA1* (Pro871Leu, Glu1038Gly, Lys1183Arg, Ser1613Gly, and Gln356Arg) and three in *BRCA2* (Asn289His, His372Asn, Asn991Asp) have population frequencies in excess of 5 per cent.[36–38] Remarkably, the first four listed polymorphisms in *BRCA1* are in virtually complete linkage disequilibrium and hence define just two common haplotypes, Pro871Glu1038Lys1183Ser1613 and Leu871Gly1038Arg1183Gly1613, with frequencies (at least in the Caucasian populations studied) of approximately 63 per cent and 32 per cent, respectively. The Arg356 allele occurs only on the Pro871Glu1038Lys1183Ser1613 background, and has a frequency of ~6 per cent. It is clear that these polymorphisms cannot be associated with the high cancer risks conferred by the truncating mutations. Several studies have examined whether these polymorphisms might be associated with moderate risks of breast or ovarian cancer by comparing polymorphism frequencies in cases and controls. To date, there is no consistent evidence that any of the *BRCA1* polymorphisms tested so far confers an increased risk of breast cancer.[36,38] The *BRCA2* variant N372H has, however, been shown to be associated with a moderately increased risk of breast cancer in two studies.[39,40] Homozygotes for the His allele were associated with a relative risk of about 1.3-fold in both studies. Intriguingly, among female controls, including newborns, the frequency of homozygous carriers of this variant was significantly lower than that expected under Hardy–Weinberg equilibrium whereas, among newborn males, a deficit of heterozygotes was identified. This suggests that *BRCA2* may have different roles in the fetal development of males and females, leading to differential selection.

Founder mutations

While the majority of *BRCA1* and *BRCA2* mutations have only been observed once or at most a few times, certain mutations in *BRCA1* and *BRCA2* have been observed multiple times. Haplotype analysis using markers flanking the genes has demonstrated that, in most cases, these recurrent mutations occur on a common haplotype background and hence are descended from a single founder. Consistent with this, such mutations tend to be common in specific populations, so that mutations common in, for example, The Netherlands, are rare in other populations. This indicates that most mutations observed now have arisen over the past few hundred years.

Although *BRCA1* and *BRCA2* mutations are rare in most populations (see later), mutations can be more frequent if the population has arisen from a relatively recent small founder population. The best characterized examples occur in the Icelandic and the Ashkenazi Jewish populations.

ASHKENAZI JEWISH FOUNDER MUTATIONS

Around 90 per cent of the 6 million Jews living in North America are described as being Ashkenazi, a distinct group originating from Central and Eastern Europe. Three mutations are commonly found in this population: 185delAG and 5382insC in *BRCA1*[14,41–43] and 6174delT in *BRCA2*.[18] These three mutations account for almost all the *BRCA1* and *BRCA2* mutations found in this population,[44] facilitating quicker, cheaper and more complete mutation testing. The 185delAG mutation is one of the most commonly reported mutations. Although the large majority of carrier families are Ashkenazi, the mutation has also been reported in other Jewish groups, indicating an older origin.[45] The 6174delT mutation appears to be virtually restricted to the Ashkenazim, and has only once been reported in anyone of proven non-Ashkenazi Jewish heritage.[46] The 5382insC mutation is, however, more widespread, being common in Poland, Russia and other parts of Eastern Europe, and occurring in most European populations.

The frequencies of these mutations are much higher than the frequencies of *BRCA1* and *BRCA2* mutations in other populations and, in consequence, they are found in a high proportion of breast and ovarian cancer patients and families in this population. Based on a pooled analysis of five population studies, the frequencies of the 185delAG and 6174delT mutations in the Ashkenazim are both about 1 in 100, with the frequency of 5382insC being about 1 in 400.[47] This is in agreement with a study of volunteers in Washington DC, which found a combined carrier frequency of 2.3 per cent.[48] These mutations are found in approximately 30 per cent of breast cancer cases diagnosed below age 40 years[49–53] and approximately 40–60 per cent of ovarian cancer cases.[54,55]

THE ICELANDIC *BRCA2* FOUNDER MUTATION

One predominant *BRCA2* mutation, 999del5, has been identified in the geographically isolated population of Iceland. This mutation is present in the majority of multiple case breast cancer families in this population.[56,57] This is the only *BRCA2* mutation found so far in Iceland and appears to be considerably more frequent than *BRCA1* mutations in this population. The 999del5 mutation is estimated to account for 8 per cent of ovarian cancers and 8–10 per cent of female breast cancers, rising to 24 per cent of female breast cancers diagnosed before age 40 years.[58] The mutation is also present in 38 per cent of the 34 cases of male breast cancer diagnosed in Iceland in the period 1955–96.[57] About 1 in 200 Icelanders are thought to carry a 999del5 mutation, a much higher frequency than that of all mutations in larger more heterogeneous populations.[58–61] The mutation is also present, at a lower frequency, in Finland[62] and other northern European populations.

Homozygous mutations

To date, there is only a single report of an individual inheriting a germline *BRCA1* mutation from both parents.[63] It describes a Scottish woman diagnosed with breast cancer at age 32 years, who was homozygous for the *BRCA1* protein-truncating mutation 2800delAA. However, in a report of a second woman, apparently homozygous for the same mutation, it was shown that the homozygosity was an artefact resulting from non-amplification of the wild-type allele.[64]

Individuals homozygous for *BRCA1* or *BRCA2* mutations, if they exist, would be expected to be most common in populations with common founder mutations, particularly the Ashkenazi and Icelandic populations. However, no such individuals have been reported. An investigation of around 1500 Ashkenazim with breast or ovarian cancer, or a family history of breast or ovarian cancer revealed no carriers homozygous for any of the three Ashkenazi founder mutations.[65] Given that several hundred carriers of the *BRCA1* 185delAG and *BRCA2* 6174delT mutations have been identified, and that the frequencies of these mutations are 1 per cent or more in Ashkenazi Jews, these results suggest reduced homozygote viability in humans, consistent with reports of embryonic lethality or severe developmental abnormalities in mice homozygous for various *brca1* or *brca2* mutations.[66–69] Similar arguments apply to the Icelandic *BRCA2* 999del5 mutation.

However, a recent study has found that certain individuals with Fanconi anaemia complementation groups D1 (and perhaps also B; see Chapter 14) carried two distinct germline *BRCA2* mutations.[70] This phenotype is consistent with the hypothesized functions of *BRCA2* (see later). Interestingly, in all cases, at least one of the two mutations was towards the 3′ end of *BRCA2*, so that, for example, the RAD51 binding domain was retained. This may explain the apparent viability of these double mutations as compared with homozygotes for the 999del5 or 6174delT mutations.

In contrast to *BRCA1* or *BRCA2* homozygotes, individuals heterozygous for both *BRCA1* and *BRCA2* have been found in several breast–ovarian cancer families, and their phenotype appears similar to that of carriers of either mutation alone (e.g. Friedman et al.,[65] Liede et al.[71] and Ramus et al.[72]).

PENETRANCE OF *BRCA1* AND *BRCA2* MUTATIONS

Knowledge of the age-specific cancer risks (or penetrance) associated with *BRCA1* and *BRCA2* mutations is central to the genetic counselling of mutation carriers. To this end, there have been several attempts to estimate these risks. Ultimately, estimates of penetrance based on prospective follow-up of unaffected carriers will be available but, at the present time, estimates must be derived from retrospective data. Several techniques have been used, each with advantages and disadvantages.

1 The maximum LOD score (or linkage) method. Estimates are based on cancer incidence and mutation carrier status in families, often ascertained on the basis of a large number of cancer cases. The LOD score (see Chapter 2) is maximized with respect to a range of penetrance models with different age-specific risks; this is equivalent to conditioning the observed pattern of carrier status data on all available phenotypic information.[73,74] In general, estimates based on high-risk families have the benefit of being directly relevant to that type of family. However, the high cancer incidence within these families may, in part, be attributable to other modifying factors shared within the family, either genetic or environmental. The failure of this technique to account for any other form of familial shared risk is likely to result in an overestimate of the penetrance, in the sense that it would not be applicable to a randomly selected carrier in the population.

2 Population studies (the 'kin-cohort' design). These studies are based on the incidence of cancer in the first-degree relatives of carriers identified in a population-based series of cases, unselected for family history. This has the advantage of removing some of the bias due to modifiers, which may be present in high-risk families, and gives results that are more closely related to the experience of the majority of mutation carriers. However, a degree of selection remains since the cohort are all, by definition, relatives of cancer patients. Unfortunately, the low frequency of *BRCA1* and *BRCA2* mutations means that even large studies often detect only a small number of mutation carriers, resulting in imprecise estimates and very large confidence intervals. This difficulty has been circumvented to some extent by a recent meta-analysis (see later).

3 Case-control studies, that is, a direct estimate of mutation frequency in cases and controls. This approach does avoid completely the potential selection owing to other familial factors. However, it is severely limited by the low population frequency of mutations. It is only possible in populations with founder mutations, and even then the estimates lack precision.

The *BRCA1* penetrance estimates from the recent meta-analysis of population studies by Antoniou *et al.*[75] are shown in Figure 19.1. The cumulative risks of both breast and ovarian cancer are higher in *BRCA1* carriers than *BRCA2* carriers, but the difference is more marked for ovarian cancer (39 per cent vs. 11 per cent by age 70). The difference is also more marked for breast cancer at younger ages (38 per cent vs. 16 per cent by age 50) than at older ages (65 per cent vs. 45 per cent by age 70). This is a consequence of the fact that *BRCA1* breast cancer incidence rates rise steeply to approximately 3–4 per cent per annum in the 40–49 age group, and are roughly constant thereafter, whereas the *BRCA2* rates show a pattern similar to that in the general population (though approximately tenfold higher), rising steeply up to age 50 and more slowly thereafter. Ovarian cancer risks in *BRCA1* carriers are very low (in absolute terms) below age 40, rising thereafter to 1–2 per cent per annum. Ovarian cancer risks in *BRCA2* carriers are in contrast very low below age 50 but then increase sharply.

Figure 19.2 shows the corresponding penetrance estimates derived from the BCLC studies of high-risk families for comparison.[22,76] It is notable that the risks are somewhat higher than those in Figure 19.1, especially the breast cancer risks for *BRCA2* carriers. These differences in risk suggest the existence of additional familial factors modifying the cancer risk in carriers.

Risks of second cancers

The risks of second cancers in carriers affected with breast cancer have been estimated by constructing cohorts of affected carriers identified in the BCLC families.[77,78] (There is some potential bias in these studies, since families containing cases with two cancers may be more likely to be ascertained, but the bias is probably fairly small given that most of the families contained four or more breast cancer cases.) Estimates of the incidence rates and cumulative risks of a contralateral breast cancer or of an ovarian cancer following a breast cancer are given in Table 19.1. The incidence of contralateral breast

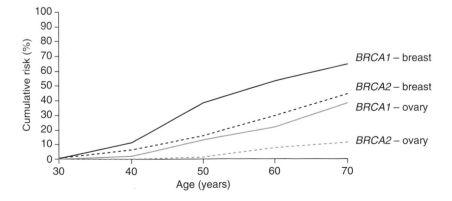

Figure 19.1 *Cumulative risks of breast and ovarian cancer in* BRCA1 *and* BRCA2 *carriers, based on relatives of unselected cancer cases.*

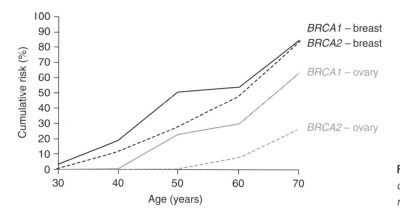

Figure 19.2 *Cumulative risks of breast and ovarian cancer in* BRCA1 *and* BRCA2 *carriers, based on high risk families.*[22,76]

Table 19.1 *Incidence rates for second cancers in* BRCA1 *and* BRCA2 *carriers affected with breast cancer. Estimates derived from BCLC studies.*[77,78]

Age group (years)	Contralateral breast cancer		Ovarian cancer	
	BRCA1	*BRCA2*	*BRCA1*	*BRCA2*
30–39	4.0% (7)	1.7% (9)	1.4% (4)	–
40–49	2.8% (9)	2.6% (28)	2.4% (12)	0.2% (3)
50–59	2.3% (7)	1.9% (20)	1.3% (5)	0.7% (8)
60–69	1.5% (3)	0.8% (6)	1.0% (2)	0.8% (7)

cancer in *BRCA1* carriers reaches a maximum of approximately 4 per cent per annum in women aged 30–39 years before declining at later ages, while the incidence rates in *BRCA2* carriers are approximately 2 per cent across the age range 30–60 years. These rates contrast with a rate of approximately 0.7 per cent in unselected breast cancer cases. While these estimates remain imprecise owing to small numbers, it is notable that observed rates of contralateral breast cancer are markedly higher than one would predict from simply halving the incidence rates in unaffected carriers to allow for only one breast being at risk. This higher risk presumably reflects additional genetic, lifestyle or stochastic factors that can increase individual risk. The incidence rates of ovarian cancer following a breast cancer are generally comparable to the estimated incidence rates for a first ovarian cancer.

Genotype–phenotype correlations

The estimates of penetrance described above assume that all mutations confer the same cancer risks. Although most reported deleterious mutations are protein-truncating, some expression is still present in the majority of cases and it is plausible that gene-products truncated to differing degrees may confer different cancer risks.

Given the large number of distinct mutations already discovered, establishing the risks associated with each individual mutation is impractical. This difficulty can be avoided by grouping mutations by their location within the gene. Gayther *et al.*[79] reported that *BRCA1* families with mutations 5′ to exon 13 had a higher proportion of ovarian cancer cases than families with mutations within and 3′ to exon 13. A more recent analysis, based on 356 families with protein-truncating *BRCA1* mutations, found that the risk of breast cancer was 29 per cent lower in carriers of mutations between nucleotides 2401 and 4191 (exon 11) than for mutations outside this central region.[80] The risk of ovarian cancer was found to be 19 per cent lower for mutations 3′ to this region, although this result was statistically less significant. Missense mutations in the ring finger domain appeared to be associated with similar cancer risks to truncating mutations at the 3′ end of the gene.

For *BRCA2*, the mutations in the region between nucleotides 3035 and 6629 on exon 11, referred to as the 'ovarian cancer cluster region' (OCCR), appear to be associated with a higher proportion of ovarian cancer than those located elsewhere.[81] This region is coincident with a domain containing eight BRC repeats that are responsible for binding to RAD51 (see later). A study of 164 families with protein-truncating *BRCA2* mutations found that mutations in the OCCR were associated with a 37 per cent lower breast cancer risk, but an 88 per cent higher ovarian cancer risk.[82] This effect is consistent with the observation that the prevalence of the 6174delT mutation (that lies within the OCCR) in the Ashkenazim is higher in ovarian cancer patients than breast cancer patients, whereas the prevalence of the 999del5 mutation in Icelandic ovarian cancer patients and breast cancer patients is similar. There is also some evidence that the *BRCA2* prostate cancer risk is lower for OCCR than for non-OCCR mutations.[82]

BRCA1 AND *BRCA2* MUTATION PREVALENCE

Contribution of *BRCA1* and *BRCA2* to familial breast and ovarian cancer

The earliest studies of *BRCA1* and *BRCA2* were based on multiple-case breast or breast–ovarian families informative for genetic linkage studies. The largest such study was based on 237 families with four or more cases of breast cancer diagnosed below age 60 years.[22] Genetic linkage analysis estimated that, overall, 52 per cent of such families were linked to *BRCA1*, 32 per cent to *BRCA2* and 16 per cent were unlinked to either loci. However, these proportions were strongly dependent on the family type; among families with one or more additional cases of ovarian cancer, 81 per cent were linked to *BRCA1* and 14 per cent to *BRCA2*. This is consistent with the notion that *BRCA1* mutations predispose more strongly than *BRCA2* mutations to ovarian cancer. Conversely, among families with one or more cases of male breast cancer, 16 per cent were linked to *BRCA1* and 76 per cent to *BRCA2*, indicating a higher risk of male breast cancer in *BRCA2* carriers. Among families without ovarian or male breast cancer, the contribution of these genes was more modest, with 42 per cent not linked to either gene. This was particularly true among families with less than six cases of breast cancer, where 67 per cent were unlinked.

While *BRCA1* and *BRCA2* mutations are common among families with four or more cases of breast cancer, the prevalence in the more common types of family with fewer cases is markedly lower.[83,84] Two studies have estimated the overall contribution of *BRCA1* and *BRCA2* to familial breast cancer by examining the familial risks in carriers and non-carriers in population studies; both studies estimated that approximately 15 per cent of the excess familial risk of breast cancer is due to mutations in these genes.[85,86] The most likely explanation for these observations is that, while *BRCA1* and *BRCA2* are the most important high-penetrance breast cancer susceptibility genes, other genes conferring lower risks explain the majority of the familial aggregation.

The prevalence of mutations in families with two or more cases of ovarian cancer is markedly higher than for breast cancer; Gayther *et al.* found *BRCA1* or *BRCA2* mutations in 42 per cent of 112 families with two or more cases of ovarian cancer.[87] Antoniou *et al.* estimated that over 50 per cent, and possibly close to 100 per cent, of the familial aggregation of ovarian cancer may be due to these two genes.[88]

Contribution of *BRCA1* and *BRCA2* to breast and ovarian cancer incidence

The prevalences of *BRCA1* and *BRCA2* mutations in breast and ovarian cancer cases overall (as opposed to cases with a family history) have been estimated in various studies (summarized in Tables 19.2 and 19.3). Most studies have focused on cases diagnosed at a young age, although some have compared the mutation prevalence among cases diagnosed at different ages. As anticipated, mutations in both genes account for a higher proportion of breast cancer cases in the younger age groups.

Pooling the applicable results in Table 19.2 gives crude estimates of the prevalence of mutations in *BRCA1* and *BRCA2* among breast cancer patients diagnosed below their mid-thirties of approximately 4.6 per cent and 3.5 per cent, respectively. In contrast, the Anglian Breast Cancer Study (the largest population-based study to date) found the prevalences among cases diagnosed between 45 and 54 years of age to be just 0.3 per cent and 1.0 per cent, respectively.[86] The values given in the tables clearly underestimate the true prevalence, owing to the insensitivity of the mutation detection techniques used. Assuming an overall sensitivity of 63 per cent,[22] the 'true' prevalences would, on average, be 59 per cent higher. More accurate estimates would require knowledge of the sensitivities of the techniques used in each study. Nevertheless, the overall fraction of breast cancer patients in outbred populations carrying *BRCA1* and *BRCA2* mutations is probably close to 1–2 per cent for each gene.

The estimated prevalence of *BRCA1* mutations in ovarian cancer patients varies from 3.5 per cent in a UK study to 6 per cent in Canadian and US studies, while the *BRCA2* prevalence is approximately 3 per cent in both the North American studies (Table 19.3[89–92]). Some of the difference in rates may be explained by the higher prevalence of the Ashkenazi Jewish mutation 6174delT in the North American series. The prevalence rates vary with age in a manner consistent with the penetrance estimates: that is, for *BRCA1*, a low rate below age 40 rising to a peak in the 40–49 age group followed by a decline; and, for *BRCA2*, a later peak.[54,89]

The frequency of *BRCA1* and *BRCA2* mutations within large outbred populations (as distinct from the Ashkenazi Jewish and Icelandic populations, which have a limited number of founder mutations) have not been estimated directly, but can be inferred indirectly. Ford *et al.*[59] estimated the *BRCA1* mutation frequency by assuming that the overall excess risk of ovarian cancer in first-degree relatives of breast cancer patients (and vice versa) was due to mutations in *BRCA1*. Based on the *BRCA1* penetrance model of Easton *et al.*,[76] they estimated a mutation frequency of 0.0006, i.e. approximately one heterozygous carrier per 800 individuals. Alternative estimates have been calculated from the prevalence of *BRCA1/2* mutations

Table 19.2 *Published prevalences for* BRCA1 *and* BRCA2 *among breast cancer patients unselected for cancer family history*

Study	Country	Age group (years)	Sample size	BRCA1 mutations Count	BRCA1 mutations %	BRCA2 mutations Count	BRCA2 mutations %	Mutation detection technique
Krainer *et al.* (1997)[207] [a]	USA	<33	73	9	12.3	2	2.7	Protein-truncation assays + sequencing
Eccles *et al.* (1998)[208]	UK	<40	155	10	6.5			HD/SSCP for all coding regions
Malone *et al.* (1998)[209] [b]	USA	20–29	44	5	11.4			SSCP; entire coding + intron–exon boundaries
		30–34	149	7	4.7%			
Newman *et al.* (1998)[210]	USA	20–74	211	3	1.4			SSCP; coding region + intron–exon boundaries; PTT exon 11
Hopper *et al.* (1999)[211]	Australia	<40	388	9	2.3	9	2.3	HD of *BRCA1* exons 2, 11, 20 and *BRCA2* exons 10, 11
Peto *et al.* (1999)[85]	UK	<36	254	9	3.5	6	2.4	Full coding sequence and splice junctions using CSGE
		36–45	363	7	1.9	8	2.2	
Anglian Breast Study Group (2000)[86]	UK	<35	57	2	4.1[c]	4	8.3[c]	Entire coding sequence and intron–exon boundaries by multiplex HD analysis
		35–44	341	3	1.0[c]	4	1.4[c]	
		45–54	917	3	0.3[c]	8	1.0[c]	
Loman *et al.* (2001)[212]	Sweden	<41	234	16	6.8	5	2.1	PTT, SSCP, dHPLC, sequencing

[a] Subset first published by Fitzgerald *et al.*[49]
[b] Subset first published by Langston *et al.*[213]
[c] Percentage prevalences are adjusted for 15% failure rate in DNA amplification by the polymerase chain reaction.
CSGE, confirmation-sensitive gel electrophoresis; dHPLC, denaturing high-performance liquid chromatography; HD, heteroduplex analysis; PTT, protein truncation test; SSCP, single-strand conformation polymorphism analysis.

Table 19.3 *Published prevalences for* BRCA1 *and* BRCA2 *among ovarian cancer patients unselected for cancer family history*

Study	Country	Age group (years)	Sample size	BRCA1 mutations Count	BRCA1 mutations %	BRCA2 mutations Count	BRCA2 mutations %	Mutation detection technique
Takahashi *et al* (1995)[90]	USA	Unspecified	115	7	6.1			SSCP; entire coding region
Takahashi *et al.* (1996)[92]	USA	Unspecified	130			4	3.1	SSCP; entire coding region
Stratton *et al.* (1997)[91]	UK	<70	374	13	3.5			HD; entire coding region and intron–exon boundaries
Risch *et al* (2001)[89]	Canada	<41	96	3	3.1	1	1.0	Rapid multiplex, DGGE, PTT
		41–50	136	21	15.4	4	2.9	
		51–60	165	9	5.5	7	4.2	
		>60	252	6	6.0	9	3.6	

DGGE, denaturing gradient gel electrophoresis; HD, heteroduplex analysis; PTT, protein truncation test; SSCP, single-strand conformation polymorphism analysis.

in population-based studies of breast cancer patients or from segregation analyses.[85,93] These studies gave similar estimated frequencies in the UK: 0.05–0.11 per cent for *BRCA1*, and 0.08–0.12 per cent for *BRCA2*. Larger estimates (0.26 per cent for *BRCA1*, 0.34 per cent for *BRCA2*) were obtained in a segregation analysis based on ovarian cancer patients; these may be overestimates, as the analysis did not allow for other familial risk factors.[88]

Male breast cancer

Male cases account for approximately 1 per cent of all breast cancers.[94] A family history of breast cancer in either sex is a known risk factor for male breast cancer, and the discoveries of *BRCA1* and *BRCA2* prompted studies exploring the roles of these genes. Male breast cancer was quickly identified as an important feature of the *BRCA2* phenotype.

Published estimates of the proportion of male breast cancer patients carrying germline *BRCA2* mutations vary greatly. As expected, given the presence of founder mutations within these populations, the highest reported frequencies are in Iceland (*BRCA2* mutations in 38 per cent of 34 male cases),[61] and in Israeli Ashkenazi Jews (mutations in 15 per cent of 89 cases).[95] Pooling the results of five studies from other populations gives a more modest *BRCA2* prevalence estimate of 11 per cent in cases unselected for family history.[96–100] The risk of male breast cancer associated with *BRCA2* mutations is estimated to be 2.8 per cent by age 70, and 6.9 per cent by age 80 (i.e. around 80 times higher than in the general population). This suggests that *BRCA2* mutations account for approximately 10 per cent of all male breast cancers, consistent with previous observations.[82]

The association between *BRCA1* mutations and male breast cancer appears to be considerably weaker. Although male breast cancer cases have been found in *BRCA1* linked families, the size of the male breast cancer risk is unclear.[80,95,97,101,102]

ESTIMATING CARRIER PROBABILITIES

Several attempts have been made to derive models that estimate the probability that an individual carries a mutation, given their personal and family history of cancer.

Couch *et al.* used logistic regression to model the probability of carrying a *BRCA1* mutation, based on a set of 263 women with breast cancer.[103] They found breast cancer diagnosed before 55 years of age, or ovarian cancer diagnosed at any age, or breast and ovarian cancer in the same woman each to be significant predictors of having a *BRCA1* mutation. Using information from around 600 women, each with a family history suggestive of a *BRCA1* mutation, Shattuck-Eidens *et al.* derived a logistic regression model for the probability of an affected woman carrying a *BRCA1* mutation, with covariates relating to her personal and family history of breast and ovarian cancer.[44] They estimated that the odds of carrying a mutation decrease by 8 per cent for every year added to the age at diagnosis of the proband, beyond age 30. The odds of a woman carrying a mutation are higher if ovarian cancer or bilateral breast cancer is present, or there are relatives

with breast or ovarian cancer. However, this model is only applicable to women who already have a cancer and does not make use of the woman's complete family history. When applied to a series of Ashkenazi Jewish families, the above two models considerably overestimated the number of mutations,[48] suggesting that the cases upon which they were based, drawn largely from breast cancer genetics clinics, are not representative of the wider population. This model has more recently been updated to provide *BRCA2* estimates (the 'Myriad II model').[104]

A Bayesian approach to *BRCA1* carrier-probability estimation has been proposed and implemented by Berry *et al.*[105] Using the BCLC penetrance estimates of Easton *et al.*,[76] they model the probability that a woman carries a *BRCA1* mutation, given her own incidence of breast and/or ovarian cancer and that of her first- and second-degree relatives. Estimates are available for affected and unaffected women, and the model takes into account the presence of unaffected relatives and the ages at which they were last known to be cancer-free. Subsequently, the model has been upgraded to include *BRCA2* (implemented in the program 'BRCAPRO'[106]). However, the penetrance estimates used are from a study of large, cancer-prone families chosen for use in linkage studies, and the model makes no allowance for the effect of other cancer predisposition genes.

The most recent model for estimating carrier probabilites is the result of a segregation analysis performed by Antoniou *et al.*,[93] based on data from a population series of women diagnosed with breast cancer before age 55, and a series of families with two or more cases of breast cancer, at least one of which was diagnosed before age 50. The model allows for the effects of other low-penetrance, multiplicatively acting genes, acting both in carriers and non-carriers of *BRCA1* or *BRCA2* mutations. Estimated carrier probabilities from this model for women with breast cancer unselected for family history are roughly consistent with the results of published population studies. For example, women diagnosed with breast cancer at ages 35, 45 or 55 years have estimated probabilities of 4.5 per cent, 2.2 per cent and 1.5 per cent, respectively, of carrying a mutation in *BRCA1* or *BRCA2*.

Estimated carrier probabilities for women from a range of family types are given in Figure 19.3. As expected, the carrier probabilities increase progressively with the numbers of women affected with breast and ovarian cancer under all models. However, it is notable that there are large discrepancies between the models. For families with few cases (e.g. Figure 19.3a), the Antoniou *et al.* model gives markedly lower probabilities than the other models, although the differences are less pronounced for families with larger numbers of cases (e.g. Figure 19.3g). The Antoniou *et al.* model generally gives lower *BRCA1* probabilities than the Myriad II model, but can give higher *BRCA2* probabilities for families with large numbers of

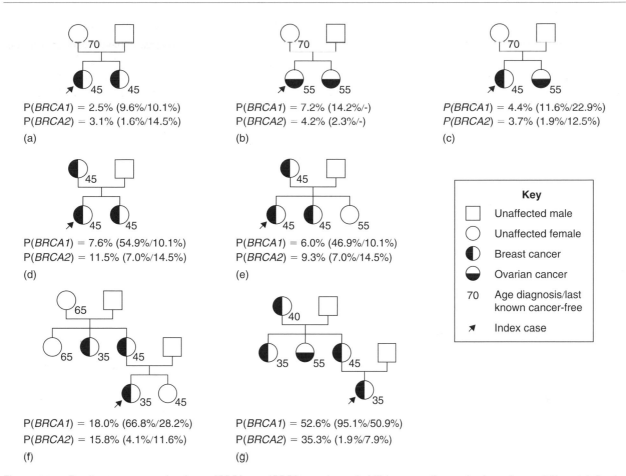

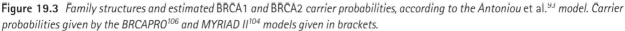

Figure 19.3 *Family structures and estimated* BRCA1 *and* BRCA2 *carrier probabilities, according to the Antoniou* et al.[93] *model. Carrier probabilities given by the BRCAPRO[106] and MYRIAD II[104] models given in brackets.*

cases. Clearly, further validation of these models is required before their routine use can be recommended.

PATHOLOGY AND CLINICAL OUTCOME

Breast cancer

The morphology of breast tumours arising in *BRCA1* carriers is markedly different from those occurring in non-carriers. In the largest study conducted to date, based on 114 breast tumours in *BRCA1* carriers and 528 tumours unselected for carrier status, *BRCA1* associated tumours were shown to be associated with higher average grade (i.e. usually grade 3) and, more specifically, with higher mitotic count.[107,108] While the large majority of *BRCA1*-associated tumours were infiltrating ductal, the frequency of tumours classified as medullary or atypical medullary type was significantly higher than in non-carriers (21 per cent vs. 2 per cent in this study). Conversely, *BRCA1* tumours were less likely to be lobular or to be associated with ductal or lobular carcinoma *in situ*. These

observations on the distribution of grade and the association with medullary type have been replicated by several studies.[109–114] Consistent with their higher grade, *BRCA1* tumours have been shown to be more often aneuploid with a higher average S-phase fraction.[111,112] Other studies have suggested that *BRCA1* tumours are larger[113,115,116] and more often associated with axillary lymph node involvement,[114] although the evidence for these associations is less convincing than for grade. Some studies have indicated that somatic p53 mutations are more common in these tumours,[117] although the evidence from immunohistochemical staining with TP53 antibodies is less clear.[118]

The above observations raised the possibility that some rather specific histological subtype diagnostic of *BRCA1* carrier status could be identified. However, the specific association with medullary breast cancer is problematic in that many of the *BRCA1* tumours appear to have some, but not all, of the features of medullary cancer. In an to attempt to clarify these associations, the BCLC conducted a further review in which more features, in particular those related to medullary breast cancer, were quantified. In this study, three factors were shown to be independently predictive of *BRCA1* status: mitotic count, the presence of continuous pushing margins, and lymphocytic infiltration.[107]

The other major difference between breast cancers in *BRCA1* carriers and non-carriers relates to oestrogen receptor (ER) status. Several studies have shown that *BRCA1* tumours are more likely to be ER negative (and progesterone receptor (PR) negative); in the largest study, over 90 per cent of *BRCA1* tumours exhibited no staining for ER.[118] ER-negative tumours tend to be of higher grade and some (but probably not all) of the difference in grade distribution may reflect this ER effect. This finding suggests that breast tumours arising in *BRCA1* carriers are less likely to be responsive to hormonal therapies, such as tamoxifen, and moreover that tamoxifen might be unable to prevent breast cancer in *BRCA1* carriers. Tumours in *BRCA1* carriers are also less likely to be c-erb-b2 positive.[111,118]

The observation that tumours in *BRCA1* carriers are high grade suggests that they are likely to develop rapidly, with the result that mammographic screening may be less effective in this group, although this has not been evaluated directly (see Chapter 20). Moreover, the distribution of clinical and pathological characteristics in *BRCA1* carriers (high grade, ER negative, node positive) would suggest that the prognosis in these patients is likely to be poor. Direct evidence of the prognosis in *BRCA1* carriers is, however, conflicting. Some studies have suggested that prognosis in *BRCA1* carriers is similar to or even better than prognosis in non-carriers.[112,119] However, these studies were based on following carriers identified in high-risk families; in most cases, the carriers were prevalent cases who had already survived some time after diagnosis before mutation testing, leading to an artefactually improved survival. One study that avoided these biases was based on testing for the Ashkenazi Jewish founder mutations in tumours from a consecutive series of breast cancer patients in Montreal.[120] This study observed a significantly poorer survival in the *BRCA1* carriers, an effect also observed in population-based studies in the UK and France[115,121] and, not significantly, in two other studies.[114,122]

The strong relationship between ER status, grade and *BRCA1* mutation status could provide an additional tool for targeting mutation testing. For example, Lakhani *et al.* estimate that the probability that a woman diagnosed below age 35 with a grade 3, ER-negative breast cancer carries a germline *BRCA1* mutation is 27 per cent compared to less than 1 per cent for a grade 1, ER-positive tumour.[118]

The pathological characteristics of tumours in *BRCA2* carriers are less clear than for *BRCA1*. The BCLC study found some evidence of a higher average grade in *BRCA2* tumours than those occurring in non-carriers, but the effect was weaker than for *BRCA1* and appeared to be related to lack of tubule formation rather than mitotic count.[108] However, this result has yet to be replicated elsewhere. Unlike in the case of *BRCA1*, there is no evidence for an excess of medullary-like features and the distribution of ER and PR is similar to that in non-carriers (i.e. the majority are ER positive).[118] As for *BRCA1*, there is some evidence that these tumours are less likely to be c-erb-b2 positive. Overall, however, the pattern of the pathology in *BRCA2* tumours is similar to that in non-carriers.

Reflecting these pathological differences, recent studies based on expression arrays have shown differences in the pattern of gene expression between *BRCA1* tumours and tumours arising in *BRCA2* carriers or non-carriers.[123–125]

Ovarian cancer

The pathology of ovarian tumours in carriers also shows some distinctive features. Cancers in carriers are invariably epithelial – there is no evidence of any risk of germ cell tumours. Moreover, the large majority are invasive; several studies have demonstrated that the proportion of borderline tumours is much lower than in non-carriers (consistent with the low rate of mutations in cases diagnosed below age 30, when borderline tumours are more common).[126–128] Tumours in *BRCA1* carriers are much less likely to be of mucinous type but more likely to be serous.[54,126–128] One study has suggested a better survival for ovarian cancers in *BRCA1* carriers[129] but others have found essentially no difference.[130]

RISKS OF OTHER CANCERS IN *BRCA1* AND *BRCA2* MUTATION CARRIERS

In addition to the marked excess of breast and ovarian cancer in *BRCA1* and *BRCA2* carriers, there is also evidence of more moderate risks of other cancer types. The largest study of cancer risks in *BRCA1* carriers was based on 699 families collected through the BCLC.[131] The overall cancer risk in male carriers was found to be very close to that in the general population, but the risk of cancers other than breast or ovarian in female carriers was increased by approximately twofold. Specifically, significant excesses were seen for cancers of the corpus uteri (relative risk; RR = 2.0), the cervix (RR = 3.8), the fallopian tubes (RR = 50) and the peritoneum (RR = 45). There was also some evidence of an excess risk of pancreatic cancer in carriers of both sexes (RR = 2.0) and prostate cancer below age 65 (RR = 1.8).

BRCA2 mutations are associated with increased risks of several other cancer types. In a parallel study, based on 173 *BRCA2* families, the risk of other cancers was approximately twofold greater than in the general population in both male and female carriers.[78] The largest excess risk was for prostate cancer, with an estimated 4.7-fold RR, increasing to sevenfold in men below age 65. A 3.5-fold RR of pancreatic cancer was also found, and significant excesses were also seen for cancers of the stomach, buccal cavity and pharynx, gallbladder, bileduct and fallopian tube, and for melanoma.

Other studies have also demonstrated an association between prostate cancer and *BRCA2* mutations. In particular, two Icelandic studies found prostate cancer relative risks of 4.6 and 3.5, respectively, among the first-degree relatives of *BRCA2* mutation carriers.[60,132] A study of 263 prostate cancer cases diagnosed below age 56 years, unselected for family history, identified 6 *BRCA2* mutations; this equates to a frequency of 2.9 per cent, allowing for the sensitivity of the mutation detection technique.[133] Several other studies have failed to detect any elevation in the frequency of *BRCA1* or *BRCA2* mutations in prostate cancer patients overall.[134-141] However, this is not inconsistent given the low population frequency of mutations. It is also notable that the relative risk of prostate cancer in the BCLC was significantly higher in European populations than in North America. Prostate specific antigen (PSA) screening is far more prevalent in North America, and it may be that *BRCA2* mutations predispose to tumours not readily detectable by screening. The excess of pancreatic cancer in *BRCA2* carriers (and, to a lesser extent, *BRCA1*) is also supported by other anecdotal reports.[14,142-147]

RISK-MODIFYING FACTORS

The age-specific penetrance estimates for carriers define the average risks to carriers in defined populations, but these risks may be adjusted by knowledge of other risk factors. Epidemiological studies have identified a number of important risk factors for breast and ovarian cancer, and a key issue is to determine whether any of these are also risk factors in carriers. Some of these, such as oral contraceptive use and early oophorectomy, may be important in the context of disease prevention in carriers. Evaluating such lifestyle factors in carriers presents a number of difficulties as a result of the limited sample size and potential biases inherent in studying risk factors in high-risk women. As a result, the effects of most lifestyle risk factors are still a matter of debate.

In addition, the differences in penetrance estimates between studies based on high risk families and those based on population studies suggest that the risks to carriers are also modified by other familial, most likely genetic, factors. Although risks vary by *BRCA1/BRCA2* mutation position and type, these variations in risk are probably too small to explain the apparent familial effects and a more plausible explanation is modification of risk by polymorphisms in other genes.

Hormonal and reproductive factors

In the general population, increasing parity is protective for both breast cancer and ovarian cancer.[148,149] The effect of parity in carriers is less clear, in part because of limited sample sizes and the fact that the decision to undergo testing may be influenced by parity. A study of 33 inferred *BRCA1* mutation carriers found increasing parity to reduce breast cancer risk but to increase the risk of ovarian cancer,[150] although the opposite effect on ovarian cancer risk was seen in a more recent study of Ashkenazi Jewish *BRCA1/2* mutation carriers (a 12 per cent reduction in risk with every birth).[151] Based on nearly 450 women with *BRCA1/2* mutations, Rebbeck et al. found a threefold increase in breast cancer risk in carriers who were nulliparous or were 30 years or older at their first live birth, but found no association with age at menarche.[152] In contrast, a large case-control study of early-onset breast cancer in *BRCA1* and *BRCA2* mutation carriers found women with a previous pregnancy to be at significantly increased breast cancer risk up to age 40 years.[153] While parity is generally protective against breast cancer, there is a transient increase in risk immediately following a pregnancy. It is possible that the increased breast cancer risk in mutation carriers is a result of this risk-increase being greater and more prolonged than usual, perhaps because the protective differentiation of breast epithelial cells occurring in the later stages of pregnancy has less effect on predisposed cells. An elevated risk of pregnancy-associated breast cancer has been reported in *BRCA1* mutation carriers, although this was based on small numbers.[154]

Oral contraceptive use has been shown to be associated with a small increase in breast cancer risk, although this ceases to be detectable 10 years after last use.[1] Conversely, the use of oral contraceptives is protective against ovarian cancer and the risk decreases with increasing years of use.[149] A collaborative study based on 207 affected *BRCA1* carriers and 166 controls found that ever use of oral contraceptives was associated with a 50 per cent reduction in ovarian cancer risk (i.e. similar to that in the general population).[155] However, a more recent population-based study in Ashkenazi Jewish women found no evidence of a risk reduction in carriers.[151] In the largest study to date on the risk of breast cancer associated with oral contraceptive use, based on 1311 cases and matched controls, use of oral contraceptives was associated with a slight increased risk in *BRCA1* carriers (odds ratio 1.2, rising to

1.33 for 5 or more years use). No increased risk was observed in *BRCA2* carriers, but the numbers involved were smaller and the relative risks in both groups would appear compatible with those observed in non-carriers.[156]

Other environmental risk factors

While cigarette smoking is strongly associated with cancer at many sites, it has little if any association with breast cancer risk.[157] One report has suggested that smoking reduces the risk of breast cancer in carriers of *BRCA1* and *BRCA2* mutations, with the degree of protection increasing with the number of pack-years smoked;[158] however, this has not been replicated.

No clear evidence has yet emerged with regard to a number of other factors known to affect the overall risk of breast cancer. These include alcohol consumption, body mass index, age at menarche, breast feeding and hormone replacement therapy.

Genetic risk-modifiers

Polymorphisms in a number of other genes have been suggested to be associated with breast or ovarian cancer risk in carriers, although none has been convincingly replicated to date. Perhaps the clearest result in this area relates to the 1100delC allele in *CHEK2*, which is associated with an approximately twofold risk of breast cancer overall, but does not appear to be associated with any increased risk in *BRCA1* or *BRCA2* carriers, presumably as a result of functional redundancy[159] (see Chapter 18).

The androgen receptor (AR) is known to mediate the growth and progression of breast tumours, and is thought to be co-activated by *BRCA1*.[160] Long versions of a CAG repeat within *AR* are associated with reduced androgen transactivation activity, and have been reported to reduce the risk of prostate cancer.[161] A case-control study of over 300 women carrying *BRCA1* mutations revealed an increased risk of breast cancer in women with at least one *AR* allele longer than 28 repeats,[162] although this result was not replicated in one subsequent study.[163] Longer alleles at a polyglutamine repeat sequence within the *AIB1* gene (a gene overexpressed in human breast tumours[164]) have been shown to be associated with an increased risk of breast cancer in carriers of *BRCA1*, and possibly *BRCA2*, mutations.[152]

Germline mutations in the gene *APC* are responsible for the familial adenomatous polyposis syndrome.[165,166] The I1307K polymorphism in *APC*, found in the Ashkenazi Jewish population and known to be associated with a moderate risk of colorectal cancer, has been found in one study to be associated with breast cancer, but only in the presence of a germline *BRCA1* or *BRCA2* mutation,

suggesting a role as a risk-modifier.[167] The C allele of the *RAD51* 135G > C single nucleotide polymorphism has been found to be associated with increased breast cancer risk, although only in *BRCA2* mutation carriers.[168,169] Recent linkage evidence has suggested that the risk of breast cancer in *BRCA1* carriers may be linked to a locus on chromosome 5q33–34.[170]

Finally, rare alleles at a minisatellite (VNTR) locus close to the *HRAS1* oncogene have been reported to be associated with an increased risk of several types of cancer. In a series of over 300 female *BRCA1* mutation carriers, women with ovarian cancer were significantly more likely to carry a 'rare' allele at the VNTR locus than unaffected women.[171]

Prophylactic surgery and chemoprevention

Prophylactic surgery is widely used in the management of women at high risk of breast or ovarian cancer. Two studies have indicated that prophylactic bilateral mastectomy is likely to be extremely effective in reducing *BRCA1/2*-associated breast cancer risk. Neither study observed any breast cancers in mutation carriers following this procedure, although the average lengths of follow-up were just 3 years and 13 years, respectively[172,173] (see Chapter 21). Prophylactic oophorectomy has also been shown to be effective at reducing the risk of ovarian and fallopian tube cancer. Although some cases of extraovarian peritoneal cancer following oophorectomy have been observed, the overall reduction in the risk of coelomic epithelial cancer has been estimated to be greater than 90 per cent.[174–176] Furthermore, prophylactic oophorectomy has been estimated to reduce the risk of breast cancer by approximately 50 per cent.[177] Tubal ligation has also been shown to reduce the risk of ovarian cancer.[178]

The value of tamoxifen as a chemopreventive agent in mutation carriers remains unclear. One retrospective study found that tamoxifen was associated with a reduced rate of contralateral breast cancer in *BRCA1* carriers. However, a recent analysis of mutations in breast cancer cases arising in the large US tamoxifen prevention study found no evidence of a preventative effect in *BRCA1* carriers, with some weak evidence of an effect in *BRCA2* carriers.[179] This result, albeit based on a very small number of cases, would be consistent with the pathological differences between *BRCA1*- and *BRCA2*-associated tumours described above.

BRCA1 AND *BRCA2* CHARACTERIZATION AND FUNCTION

Both *BRCA1* and *BRCA2* encode large proteins (molecular weights 220 kDa[12] and 384 kDa[17,18]) that exhibit little homology to other proteins. In comparison to other tumour suppressor genes, *BRCA1* and *BRCA2* are both poorly conserved between species; human *BRCA1* and murine *brca1* cDNA have an overall amino-acid sequence identity of just 58 per cent.[180] Both genes are ubiquitously expressed, with the highest levels in the testes, and also in the thyroid and the ovaries.

Studies of breast and ovarian tumours in *BRCA1* carriers have shown that a high proportion show loss of heterozygosity at the *BRCA1* locus.[181] This loss has been shown to invariably involve the wild-type chromosome, consistent with a classic loss of function tumour suppressor gene model. Essentially identical observations have been made for *BRCA2* tumours.[182]

RING domain missense mutations suggests that it is of some functional significance.[180] Two novel proteins have been identified on the basis of their association with BRCA1 via the RING domain, namely, BARD1 ('BRCA1-associated RING domain') and BAP1 ('BRCA1-associated protein').[183,184] The carboxyl-terminal end of BRCA1 contains a BRCT motif characteristic of proteins that bind to p53, and a transcriptional activation domain. A RAD51 binding region is located within the central portion of BRCA1.[185–187] Exon 11 contains nuclear localization signals, implying that the protein is nuclearized rather than secreted, as had been previously proposed.[188,189]

Features of *BRCA1*

Some of the more well-characterized domains of *BRCA1* and *BRCA2* are illustrated in Figure 19.4 (a more detailed analysis of the hypothesized functional domains of *BRCA1* and *BRCA2* is given by Welcsh and King[35]). An important feature of *BRCA1* is the presence of a cysteine-rich RING zinc-finger domain at the amino-terminus, a feature thought to be associated with DNA binding or protein–protein interactions.[11] The perfect homology between human *BRCA1* and murine *brca1* in this region, and the clear disease-causing potential of

Features of *BRCA2*

A major feature of the BRCA2 protein is a group of eight 30–80 amino-acid repeat motifs, named BRC1 to BRC8, located within the central third of BRCA2 encoded by exon 11.[190] The BRC repeats are conserved to a far higher extent than the rest of exon 11, and have been shown to bind to RAD51, suggesting an important role in the functionality of BRCA2.[191–194] Evidence that BRCA2 is also a nuclear protein is supported by the discovery of nuclear localization signals towards the 3′ terminus of the gene.[194,195]

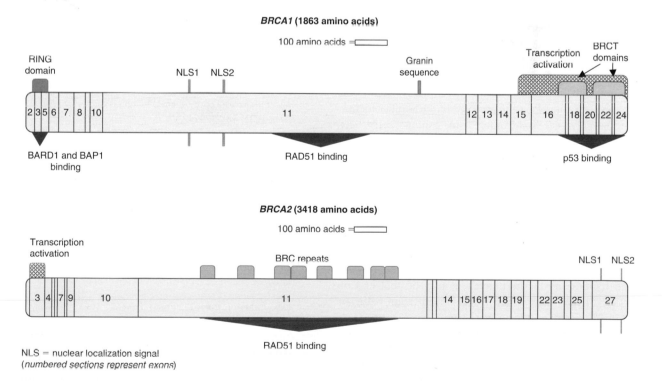

Figure 19.4 *Structural and functional features of BRCA1 and BRCA2.*

Possible functions

Many different functions have been proposed for BRCA1 and BRCA2 (reviewed by Venkitaraman[196]). BRCA1 is phosphorylated by ATM after exposure to γ-radiation, and possibly by other mechanisms in different contexts.[197] It is induced chiefly in the G1/S phase of the cell-cycle, suggesting a role in cell-cycle checkpoint control, loss of which is implicated in cancer development.[198] BRCA1 and BRCA2 are coordinately upregulated in rapidly proliferating cells and in tissue experiencing differentiation, for example, in the breast epithelium during puberty, pregnancy and lactation.[199] Recent evidence suggests that BRCA1 activates CHEK1 (and is activated by CHEK2) and hence is also implicated in G2/M checkpoint control.[200]

There is strong evidence that both BRCA1 and BRCA2 interact with RAD51, a protein involved in recombination and in the repair of double-strand DNA damage.[185,201] It appears that BRCA1, BRCA2 and RAD51 form a complex, which acts as a 'caretaker', repairing DNA damage by homologous recombination.[202] Mutations in *BRCA1* or *BRCA2* inactivate this complex, leaving DNA damage unrepaired, which in certain circumstances may lead to unrestricted proliferation and thus to tumorigenesis.[203] Although BRCA1 and BRCA2 are generally believed to function via the same pathway, the differences in the risks and in the typical tumour pathologies associated with the two genes imply that each must play a distinct role, possibly in addition to their common participation in this pathway. As an example of this, BRCA2 has been implicated in repair of DNA crosslinks, as evidenced by its involvement in Fanconi anaemia.[70]

Many tumour-suppressor genes involved in hereditary cancer syndromes are also frequently mutated in sporadic tumours, e.g. the *APC* gene involved in the familial adenomatous polyposis syndrome.[204] In contrast, very few sporadic breast or ovarian tumours have been found to contain somatic point mutations in *BRCA1* or *BRCA2*.[205,206] It has recently been proposed that the high density of Alu repeats in and around *BRCA1* increases the chance of a non-homologous recombination, deleting some or all of the gene.[35] These large mutations would not be detected in tumour DNA by conventional techniques, but may explain some proportion of sporadic cancers. Other mechanisms by which alleles could be somatically inactivated have also been hypothesized. Alternatively, it may be that loss of BRCA1 or BRCA2 function is not an important pathway in non-*BRCA1/2* mutation carriers.

Finally, although many hypotheses have been proposed, it is still not known why *BRCA1* and *BRCA2*, despite being expressed in almost every tissue type, predispose to cancers at such a restricted group of sites. This may suggest other functions for *BRCA1/2*, in addition to their roles in DNA repair.

KEY POINTS

- Mutations in *BRCA1* and *BRCA2* account for about 3 per cent of all breast-cancer families, and for about 80 per cent of large breast- and ovarian-cancer families. These figures are higher in some founder populations (e.g. the Ashkenazim).
- *BRCA1* and *BRCA2* are on 17q and 13q respectively.
- *BRCA1* mutations confer a higher risk of ovarian cancer than those in *BRCA2*.
- Mutations in *BRCA2* are associated with male breast cancer.
- Breast cancer in *BRCA1* mutation carriers is more often of grade 3, ER negative histology and stains positive for basal keratins. It is less often associated with DCIS.

REFERENCES

1. Collaborative Group on Hormonal Factors in Breast Cancer. Familial breast cancer: collaborative reanalysis of individual data from 52 epidemiological studies including 58 209 women with breast cancer and 101 986 women without the disease. *Lancet* 2001; **358**:1389–1399.
2. Lichtenstein P, Holm NV, Verkasalo PK, *et al.* Environmental and heritable factors in the causation of cancer – analyses of cohorts of twins from Sweden, Denmark, and Finland. *N Engl J Med* 2000; **343**:78–85.
3. Peto J, Mack TM. High constant incidence in twins and other relatives of women with breast cancer. *Nature Genet* 2000; **26**:411–414.
4. Claus EB, Risch N, Thompson WD. Genetic analysis of breast cancer in the cancer and steroid hormone study. *Am J Hum Genet* 1991; **48**:232–242.
5. Schildkraut JM, Risch N, Thompson WD. Evaluating genetic association among ovarian, breast, and endometrial cancer: evidence for a breast/ovarian cancer relationship. *Am J Hum Genet* 1989; **45**:521–529.
6. Easton DF, Matthews FE, Ford D, *et al.* Cancer mortality in relatives of women with ovarian cancer: the OPCS Study. Office of Population Censuses and Surveys. *Int J Cancer* 1996; **65**:284–294.
7. Fraumeni JF Jr, Grundy GW, Creagan ET, Everson RB. Six families prone to ovarian cancer. *Cancer* 1975; **36**:364–369.
8. Narod SA, Feunteun J, Lynch HT, Watson P, *et al.* Familial breast–ovarian cancer locus on chromosome 17q12–q23. *Lancet* 1991; **338**:82–83.
9. Hall JM, Lee MK, Newman B, *et al.* Linkage of early-onset familial breast cancer to chromosome 17q21. *Science* 1990; **250**:1684–1689.
10. Easton DF, Bishop DT, Ford D, Crockford GP, The Breast Cancer Linkage Consortium. Genetic linkage analysis in familial breast and ovarian cancer: results from 214 families. *Am J Hum Genet* 1993; **52**:678–701.

11. Online Mendelian Inheritance in Man (OMIM). http://www.ncbi.nlm.nih.gov, for inherited breast cancer type 1.

12. Miki Y, Swensen J, Shattuck-Eidens D, et al. A strong candidate for the breast and ovarian cancer susceptibility gene BRCA1. Science 1994; **266**:66–71.

13. Friedman LS, Ostermeyer EA, Szabo CI, et al. Confirmation of BRCA1 by analysis of germline mutations linked to breast and ovarian cancer in ten families. Nature Genet 1994; **8**:399–404.

14. Simard J, Tonin P, Durocher F, et al. Common origins of BRCA1 mutations in Canadian breast and ovarian cancer families. Nature Genet 1994; **8**:392–398.

15. Online Mendelian Inheritance in Man (OMIM). http://www.ncbi.nlm.nih.gov, for inherited breast cancer type 2.

16. Wooster R, Neuhausen SL, Mangion J, et al. Localization of a breast cancer susceptibility gene, BRCA2, to chromosome 13q12–13. Science 1994; **265**:2088–2090.

17. Wooster R, Bignell G, Lancaster J, et al. Identification of the breast cancer susceptibility gene BRCA2. Nature 1995; **378**:789–792.

18. Tavtigian SV, Simard J, Rommens J, et al. The complete BRCA2 gene and mutations in chromosome 13q-linked kindreds. Nature Genet 1996; **12**:333–337.

19. http://www.nchgri.nih.gov/Intramural_research/Lab_transfer/Bic/

20. Mazoyer S, Dunning AM, Serova O, et al. A polymorphic stop codon in BRCA2. Nature Genet 1996; **14**:253–254.

21. Eng C, Brody LC, Wagner TM, et al. Interpreting epidemiological research: blinded comparison of methods used to estimate the prevalence of inherited mutations in BRCA1. J Med Genet 2001; **38**:824–833.

22. Ford D, Easton DF, Stratton M, et al. Genetic heterogeneity and penetrance analysis of the BRCA1 and BRCA2 genes in breast cancer families. Am J Hum Genet 1998; **62**:676–689.

23. Montagna M, Santacatterina M, Torri A, et al. Identification of a 3 kb Alu-mediated BRCA1 gene rearrangement in two breast/ovarian cancer families. Oncogene 1999, **18**:4160–4165.

24. Payne SR, Newman B, King MC. Complex germline rearrangement of BRCA1 associated with breast and ovarian cancer. Genes Chromosomes Cancer 2000; **29**:58–62.

25. Petrij-Bosch A, Peelen T, van Vliet M, et al. BRCA1 genomic deletions are major founder mutations in Dutch breast cancer patients. Nature Genet 1997; **17**:341–345.

26. Puget N, Torchard D, Serova-Sinilnikova OM, et al. A 1-kb Alu-mediated germline deletion removing BRCA1 exon 17. Cancer Res 1997; **57**:828–831.

27. Rohlfs EM, Puget N, Graham ML, et al. An Alu-mediated 7.1 kb deletion of BRCA1 exons 8 and 9 in breast and ovarian cancer families that results in alternative splicing of exon 10. Genes Chromosomes Cancer 2000; **28**:300–307.

28. Rohlfs EM, Chung CH, Yang Q, et al. In-frame deletions of BRCA1 may define critical functional domains. Hum Genet 2000; **107**:385–390.

29. Swensen J, Hoffman M, Skolnick MH, Neuhausen SL. Identification of a 14 kb deletion involving the promoter region of BRCA1 in a breast cancer family. Hum Mol Genet 1997; **6**:1513–1517.

30. Unger MA, Nathanson KL, Calzone K, et al. Screening for genomic rearrangements in families with breast and ovarian cancer identifies BRCA1 mutations previously missed by

31. conformation-sensitive gel electrophoresis or sequencing. Am J Hum Genet 2000; **67**:841–850.

31. BRCA1 Exon 13 Duplication Screening Group. The exon 13 duplication in the BRCA1 gene is a founder mutation present in geographically diverse populations. Am J Hum Genet 2000; **67**:207–212.

32. Smith TM, Lee MK, Szabo CI, et al. Complete genomic sequence and analysis of 117 kb of human DNA containing the gene BRCA1. Genome Res 1996; **6**:1029–1049.

33. Nordling M, Karlsson P, Wahlstrom J, et al. A large deletion disrupts the exon 3 transcription activation domain of the BRCA2 gene in a breast/ovarian cancer family. Cancer Res 1998; **58**:1372–1375.

34. Wang T, Lerer I, Gueta Z, et al. A deletion/insertion mutation in the BRCA2 gene in a breast cancer family: a possible role of the Alu-polyA tail in the evolution of the deletion. Genes Chromosomes Cancer 2001; **31**:91–95.

35. Welcsh PL, King MC. BRCA1 and BRCA2 and the genetics of breast and ovarian cancer. Hum Mol Genet 2001; **10**:705–713.

36. Dunning AM, Chiano M, Smith NR, et al. Common BRCA1 variants and susceptibility to breast and ovarian cancer in the general population. Hum Mol Genet 1997; **6**:285–289.

37. Wagner TM, Hirtenlehner K, Shen P, et al. Global sequence diversity of BRCA2: analysis of 71 breast cancer families and 95 control individuals of worldwide populations. Hum Mol Genet 1999; **8**:413–423.

38. Durocher F, Shattuck-Eidens D, McClure M, et al. Comparison of BRCA1 polymorphisms, rare sequence variants and/or missense mutations in unaffected and breast/ovarian cancer populations. Hum Mol Genet 1996; **5**:835–842.

39. Healey CS, Dunning AM, Teare MD, et al. A common variant in BRCA2 is associated with both breast cancer risk and prenatal viability. Nature Genet 2000; **26**:362–364.

40. Spurdle AB, Hopper JL, Chen X, et al. The BRCA2 372 HH genotype is associated with risk of breast cancer in Australian women under age 60 years. Cancer Epidemiol Biomarkers Prev 2002; **11**:413–416.

41. Friedman LS, Szabo CI, Ostermeyer EA, et al. Novel inherited mutations and variable expressivity of BRCA1 alleles, including the founder mutation 185delAG in Ashkenazi Jewish families. Am J Hum Genet 1995; **57**:1284–1297.

42. Struewing JP, Brody LC, Erdos MR, et al. Detection of eight BRCA1 mutations in 10 breast/ovarian cancer families, including 1 family with male breast cancer. Am J Hum Genet 1995; **57**:1–7.

43. Tonin P, Serova O, Lenoir G, et al. BRCA1 mutations in Ashkenazi Jewish women. Am J Hum Genet 1995; **57**:189.

44. Shattuck-Eidens D, Oliphant A, McClure M, et al. BRCA1 sequence analysis in women at high risk for susceptibility mutations. Risk factor analysis and implications for genetic testing. JAMA 1997; **278**:1242–1250.

45. Bar-Sade RB, Kruglikova A, Modan B, et al. The 185delAG BRCA1 mutation originated before the dispersion of Jews in the diaspora and is not limited to Ashkenazim. Hum Mol Genet 1998; **7**:801–805.

46. Berman DB, Costalas J, Schultz DC, et al. A common mutation in BRCA2 that predisposes to a variety of cancers is found in both Jewish Ashkenazi and non-Jewish individuals. Cancer Res 1996; **56**:3409–3414.

47. Fodor FH, Weston A, Bleiweiss IJ, et al. Frequency and carrier risk associated with common BRCA1 and BRCA2 mutations in

Ashkenazi Jewish breast cancer patients. *Am J Hum Genet* 1998; **63**:45–51.

48. Hartge P, Struewing JP, Wacholder S, *et al*. The prevalence of common *BRCA1* and *BRCA2* mutations among Ashkenazi Jews. *Am J Hum Genet* 1999; **64**:963–970.

49. FitzGerald MG, MacDonald DJ, Krainer M, *et al*. Germ-line *BRCA1* mutations in Jewish and non-Jewish women with early- onset breast cancer. *N Engl J Med* 1996; **334**:143–149.

50. Warner E, Foulkes W, Goodwin P, *et al*. Prevalence and penetrance of *BRCA1* and *BRCA2* gene mutations in unselected Ashkenazi Jewish women with breast cancer. *J Natl Cancer Inst* 1999; **91**:1241–1247.

51. Satagopan JM, Offit K, Foulkes W, *et al*. The lifetime risks of breast cancer in Ashkenazi Jewish carriers of *BRCA1* and *BRCA2* mutations. *Cancer Epidemiol Biomarkers Prev* 2001; **10**:467–473.

52. Neuhausen S, Gilewski T, Norton L, *et al*. Recurrent *BRCA2* 6174delT mutations in Ashkenazi Jewish women affected by breast cancer. *Nature Genet* 1996; **13**:126–128.

53. Offit K, Gilewski T, McGuire P, *et al*. Germline *BRCA1* 185delAG mutations in Jewish women with breast cancer. *Lancet* 1996; **347**:1643–1645.

54. Moslehi R, Chu W, Karlan B, *et al*. *BRCA1* and *BRCA2* mutation analysis of 208 Ashkenazi Jewish women with ovarian cancer. *Am J Hum Genet* 2000; **66**:1259–1272.

55. Abeliovich D, Kaduri L, Lerer I, *et al*. The founder mutations 185delAG and 5382insC in *BRCA1* and 6174delT in *BRCA2* appear in 60 per cent of ovarian cancer and 30 per cent of early-onset breast cancer patients among Ashkenazi women. *Am J Hum Genet* 1997; **60**:505–514.

56. Gudmundsson J, Johannesdottir G, Arason A, *et al*. Frequent occurrence of *BRCA2* linkage in Icelandic breast cancer families and segregation of a common *BRCA2* haplotype. *Am J Hum Genet* 1996; **58**:749–756.

57. Thorlacius S, Olafsdottir G, Tryggvadottir L, *et al*. A single *BRCA2* mutation in male and female breast cancer families from Iceland with varied cancer phenotypes. *Nature Genet* 1996; **13**:117–119.

58. Johannesdottir G, Gudmundsson J, Bergthorsson JT, *et al*. High prevalence of the 999del5 mutation in Icelandic breast and ovarian cancer patients. *Cancer Res* 1996; **56**:3663–3665.

59. Ford D, Easton DF, Peto J. Estimates of the gene frequency of *BRCA1* and its contribution to breast and ovarian cancer incidence. *Am J Hum Genet* 1995; **57**:1457–1462.

60. Thorlacius S, Sigurdsson S, Bjarnadottir H, *et al*. Study of a single *BRCA2* mutation with high carrier frequency in a small population. *Am J Hum Genet* 1997; **60**:1079–1084.

61. Thorlacius S, Struewing JP, Hartge P, *et al*. Population-based study of risk of breast cancer in carriers of *BRCA2* mutation. *Lancet* 1998; **352**:1337–1339.

62. Vehmanen P, Friedman LS, Eerola H, *et al*. A low proportion of *BRCA2* mutations in Finnish breast cancer families. *Am J Hum Genet* 1997; **60**:1050–1058.

63. Boyd M, Harris F, McFarlane R, *et al*. A human *BRCA1* gene knockout. *Nature* 1995; **375**:541–542.

64. Kuschel B, Gayther SA, Easton DF, *et al*. Apparent human *BRCA1* knockout caused by mispriming during polymerase chain reaction: implications for genetic testing. *Genes Chromosomes Cancer* 2001; **31**:96–98.

65. Friedman E, Bar-Sade BR, Kruglikova A, *et al*. Double heterozygotes for the Ashkenazi founder mutations in *BRCA1* and *BRCA2* genes. *Am J Hum Genet* 1998; 63:1224–1227.

66. Connor F, Bertwistle D, Mee PJ, *et al*. Tumorigenesis and a DNA repair defect in mice with a truncating *Brca2* mutation. *Nature Genet* 1997; **17**:423–430.

67. Gowen LC, Johnson BL, Latour AM, *et al*. *Brca1* deficiency results in early embryonic lethality characterized by neuroepithelial abnormalities. *Nature Genet* 1996; **12**:191–194.

68. Ludwig T, Chapman DL, Papaioannou VE, Efstratiadis A. Targeted mutations of breast cancer susceptibility gene homologs in mice: lethal phenotypes of *Brca1*, *Brca2*, *Brca1/Brca2*, *Brca1/p53*, and *Brca2/p53* nullizygous embryos. *Genes Dev* 1997; **11**:1226–1241.

69. Suzuki A, de la Pompa JL, Hakem R, *et al*. *Brca2* is required for embryonic cellular proliferation in the mouse. *Genes Dev* 1997; **11**:1242–1252.

70. Howlett NG, Taniguchi T, Olson S, *et al*. Biallelic inactivation of *BRCA2* in Fanconi anemia. *Science* 2002; **297**:606–609.

71. Liede A, Rehal P, Vesprini D, *et al*. A breast cancer patient of Scottish descent with germline mutations in *BRCA1* and *BRCA2*. *Am J Hum Genet* 1998; **62**:1543–1544.

72. Ramus SJ, Friedman LS, Gayther SA, *et al*. A breast/ovarian cancer patient with germline mutations in both *BRCA1* and *BRCA2*. *Nature Genet* 1997; **15**:14–15.

73. Elston RC. Man bites dog? The validity of maximizing lod scores to determine mode of inheritance. *Am J Med Genet* 1989; **34**:487–488.

74. Greenberg DA. Inferring mode of inheritance by comparison of lod scores. *Am J Med Genet* 1989; **34**:480–486.

75. Antoniou AC, Pharoah PD, Narod SA, *et al*. Average risks of breast and ovarian cancer associated with *BRCA1* or *BRCA2* mutations detected in case series unselected for family history: a combined analysis of 22 studies. *Am J Hum Genet* 2003; **72**:1117–1130.

76. Easton DF, Ford D, Bishop DT. Breast Cancer Linkage Consortium. Breast and ovarian cancer incidence in *BRCA1*-mutation carriers. *Am J Hum Genet* 1995; **56**:265–271.

77. Ford D, Easton DF, Bishop DT, Narod SA, Goldgar DE, Breast Cancer Linkage Consortium. Risks of cancer in *BRCA1*-mutation carriers. *Lancet* 1994; **343**:692–695.

78. Breast Cancer Linkage Consortium. Cancer risks in *BRCA2* mutation carriers. *J Natl Cancer Inst* 1999; **91**:1310–1316.

79. Gayther SA, Warren W, Mazoyer S, *et al*. Germline mutations of the *BRCA1* gene in breast and ovarian cancer families provide evidence for a genotype-phenotype correlation. *Nature Genet* 1995; **11**:428–433.

80. Thompson D, Easton D, Breast Cancer Linkage Consortium. Variation in *BRCA1* cancer risks by mutation position. *Cancer Epidemiol Biomarkers Prev* 2002; **11**:329–336.

81. Gayther SA, Mangion J, Russell P, *et al*. Variation of risks of breast and ovarian cancer associated with different germline mutations of the *BRCA2* gene. *Nature Genet* 1997; **15**:103–105.

82. Thompson D, Easton D. Variation in cancer risks, by mutation position, in *BRCA2* mutation carriers. *Am J Hum Genet* 2001; **68**:410–419.

83. Serova OM, Mazoyer S, Puget N, *et al*. Mutations in *BRCA1* and *BRCA2* in breast cancer families: are there more breast

cancer-susceptibility genes? *Am J Hum Genet* 1997; **60**:486–495.

84. Shih HA, Couch FJ, Nathanson KL, *et al.* BRCA1 and BRCA2 mutation frequency in women evaluated in a breast cancer risk evaluation clinic. *J Clin Oncol* 2002; **20**:994–999.

85. Peto J, Collins N, Barfoot R, *et al.* Prevalence of BRCA1 and BRCA2 gene mutations in patients with early-onset breast cancer. *J Natl Cancer Inst* 1999; **91**:943–949.

86. Anglian Breast Cancer Study Group. Prevalence and penetrance of BRCA1 and BRCA2 mutations in a population-based series of breast cancer cases. *Br J Cancer* 2000; **83**:1301–1308.

87. Gayther SA, Russell P, Harrington P, *et al.* The contribution of germline BRCA1 and BRCA2 mutations to familial ovarian cancer: no evidence for other ovarian cancer-susceptibility genes. *Am J Hum Genet* 1999; **65**:1021–1029.

88. Antoniou AC, Gayther SA, Stratton JF, *et al.* Risk models for familial ovarian and breast cancer. *Genet Epidemiol* 2000; **18**:173–190.

89. Risch HA, McLaughlin JR, Cole DE, *et al.* Prevalence and penetrance of germline BRCA1 and BRCA2 mutations in a population series of 649 women with ovarian cancer. *Am J Hum Genet* 2001; **68**:700–710.

90. Takahashi H, Behbakht K, McGovern PE, *et al.* Mutation analysis of the BRCA1 gene in ovarian cancers. *Cancer Res* 1995; **55**:2998–3002.

91. Stratton JF, Gayther SA, Russell P, *et al.* Contribution of BRCA1 mutations to ovarian cancer. *N Engl J Med* 1997; **336**:1125–1130.

92. Takahashi H, Chiu HC, Bandera CA, *et al.* Mutations of the BRCA2 gene in ovarian carcinomas. *Cancer Res* 1996; **56**:2738–2741.

93. Antoniou AC, Pharoah PD, McMullan G, *et al.* A comprehensive model for familial breast cancer incorporating BRCA1, BRCA2 and other genes. *Br J Cancer* 2002; **86**: 76–83.

94. Parkin DM, Whelan SL, Ferlay J, *et al.* Cancer incidence in five continents. Lyon: IARC, 1997.

95. Struewing JP, Coriaty ZM, Ron E, *et al.* Founder BRCA1/2 mutations among male patients with breast cancer in Israel. *Am J Hum Genet* 1999; **65**:1800–1802.

96. Couch FJ, Farid LM, Deshano ML, *et al.* BRCA2 germline mutations in male breast cancer cases and breast cancer families. *Nature Genet* 1996; **13**:123–125.

97. Friedman LS, Gayther SA, Kurosaki T, *et al.* Mutation analysis of BRCA1 and BRCA2 in a male breast cancer population. *Am J Hum Genet* 1997; **60**:313–319.

98. Haraldsson K, Loman N, Zhang QX, *et al.* BRCA2 germline mutations are frequent in male breast cancer patients without a family history of the disease. *Cancer Res* 1998; **58**:1367–1371.

99. Kwiatkowska E, Teresiak M, Lamperska KM, *et al.* BRCA2 germline mutations in male breast cancer patients in the Polish population. *Hum Mutat* 2001; **17**:73.

100. Mavraki E, Gray IC, Bishop DT, Spurr NK. Germline BRCA2 mutations in men with breast cancer. *Br J Cancer* 1997; **76**:1428–1431.

101. Stratton MR, Ford D, Neuhausen S, *et al.* Familial male breast cancer is not linked to the BRCA1 locus on chromosome 17q. *Nature Genet* 1994; **7**:103–107.

102. Csokay B, Udvarhelyi N, Sulyok Z, *et al.* High frequency of germ-line BRCA2 mutations among Hungarian male breast cancer patients without family history. *Cancer Res* 1999; **59**:995–998.

103. Couch FJ, Deshano ML, Blackwood MA, *et al.* BRCA1 mutations in women attending clinics that evaluate the risk of breast cancer. *N Engl J Med* 1997; **336**:1409–1415.

104. Frank TS, Manley SA, Olopade OI, *et al.* Sequence analysis of BRCA1 and BRCA2: correlation of mutations with family history and ovarian cancer risk. *J Clin Oncol* 1998; **16**:2417–2425.

105. Berry DA, Parmigiani G, Sanchez J, *et al.* Probability of carrying a mutation of breast-ovarian cancer gene BRCA1 based on family history. *J Natl Cancer Inst* 1997; **89**:227–238.

106. Parmigiani G, Berry D, Aguilar O. Determining carrier probabilities for breast cancer-susceptibility genes BRCA1 and BRCA2. *Am J Hum Genet* 1998; **62**:145–158.

107. Lakhani SR, Jacquemier J, Sloane JP, *et al.* Multifactorial analysis of differences between sporadic breast cancers and cancers involving BRCA1 and BRCA2 mutations. *J Natl Cancer Inst* 1998; **90**:1138–1145.

108. Breast Cancer Linkage Consortium. Pathology of familial breast cancer: differences between breast cancers in carriers of BRCA1 or BRCA2 mutations and sporadic cases. *Lancet* 1997; **349**:1505–1510.

109. Armes JE, Egan AJ, Southey MC, *et al.* The histologic phenotypes of breast carcinoma occurring before age 40 years in women with and without BRCA1 or BRCA2 germline mutations: a population-based study. *Cancer* 1998; **83**:2335–2345.

110. Karp SE, Tonin PN, Begin LR, *et al.* Influence of BRCA1 mutations on nuclear grade and estrogen receptor status of breast carcinoma in Ashkenazi Jewish women. *Cancer* 1997; **80**:435–441.

111. Johannsson OT, Idvall I, Anderson C, *et al.* Tumour biological features of BRCA1-induced breast and ovarian cancer. *Eur J Cancer* 1997; **33**:362–371.

112. Marcus JN, Watson P, Page DL, *et al.* Hereditary breast cancer: pathobiology, prognosis, and BRCA1 and BRCA2 gene linkage. *Cancer* 1996; **77**:697–709.

113. Turchetti D, Cortesi L, Federico M, *et al.* BRCA1 mutations and clinicopathological features in a sample of Italian women with early-onset breast cancer. *Eur J Cancer* 2000; **36**:2083–2089.

114. Robson M, Gilewski T, Haas B, *et al.* BRCA-associated breast cancer in young women. *J Clin Oncol* 1998; **16**:1642–1649.

115. Stoppa-Lyonnet D, Ansquer Y, Dreyfus H, *et al.* Familial invasive breast cancers: worse outcome related to BRCA1 mutations. *J Clin Oncol* 2000; **18**:4053–4059.

116. Hamann U, Sinn HP. Survival and tumor characteristics of German hereditary breast cancer patients. *Breast Cancer Res Treat* 2000; **59**:185–192.

117. Phillips KA, Nichol K, Ozcelik H, *et al.* Frequency of p53 mutations in breast carcinomas from Ashkenazi Jewish carriers of BRCA1 mutations. *J Natl Cancer Inst* 1999; **91**:469–473.

118. Lakhani SR, van de Vijver MJ, Jacquemier J, *et al.* The pathology of familial breast cancer: predictive value of immunohistochemical markers estrogen receptor, progesterone receptor, HER-2, and p53 in patients with

118. mutations in *BRCA1* and *BRCA2*. *J Clin Oncol* 2002; **20**:2310–2318.

119. Verhoog LC, Brekelmans CT, Seynaeve C, *et al*. Survival and tumour characteristics of breast-cancer patients with germline mutations of *BRCA1*. *Lancet* 1998; **351**:316–321.

120. Foulkes WD, Chappuis PO, Wong N, *et al*. Primary node negative breast cancer in *BRCA1* mutation carriers has a poor outcome. *Ann Oncol* 2000; **11**:307–313.

121. Goode EL, Dunning AM, Kuschel B, *et al*. Effect of germ-line genetic variation on breast cancer survival in a population-based study. *Cancer Res* 2002; **62**:3052–3057.

122. Eerola H, Vahteristo P, Sarantaus L, *et al*. Survival of breast cancer patients in *BRCA1*, *BRCA2*, and non-*BRCA1/2* breast cancer families: a relative survival analysis from Finland. *Int J Cancer* 2001; **93**:368–372.

123. Jazaeri AA, Yee CJ, Sotiriou C, *et al*. Gene expression profiles of *BRCA1*-linked, *BRCA2*-linked, and sporadic ovarian cancers. *J Natl Cancer Inst* 2002; **94**:990–1000.

124. Berns EM, van Staveren IL, Verhoog L, *et al*. Molecular profiles of *BRCA1*-mutated and matched sporadic breast tumours: relation with clinico-pathological features. *Br J Cancer* 2001; **85**:538–545.

125. Hedenfalk I, Duggan D, Chen Y, *et al*. Gene-expression profiles in hereditary breast cancer. *N Engl J Med* 2001; **344**:539–548.

126. Werness BA, Ramus SJ, Whittemore AS, *et al*. Histopathology of familial ovarian tumors in women from families with and without germline *BRCA1* mutations. *Hum Pathol* 2000; **31**:1420–1424.

127. Narod S, Tonin P, Lynch H, *et al*. Histology of *BRCA1*-associated ovarian tumours. *Lancet* 1994; **343**:236.

128. Ramus SJ, Fishman A, Pharoah PD, *et al*. Ovarian cancer survival in Ashkenazi Jewish patients with *BRCA1* and *BRCA2* mutations. *Eur J Surg Oncol* 2001; **27**:278–281.

129. Rubin SC, Benjamin I, Behbakht K, *et al*. Clinical and pathological features of ovarian cancer in women with germ-line mutations of *BRCA1*. *N Engl J Med* 1996; **335**:1413–1416.

130. Pharoah PD, Easton DF, Stockton DL, *et al*. Survival in familial, *BRCA1*-associated, and *BRCA2*-associated epithelial ovarian cancer. United Kingdom Coordinating Committee for Cancer Research (UKCCCR) Familial Ovarian Cancer Study Group. *Cancer Res* 1999; **59**:868–871.

131. Thompson D, Easton DF. Cancer Incidence in *BRCA1* mutation carriers. *J Natl Cancer Inst* 2002; **94**:1358–1365.

132. Sigurdsson S, Thorlacius S, Tomasson J, *et al*. *BRCA2* mutation in Icelandic prostate cancer patients. *J Mol Med* 1997; **75**:758–761.

133. Edwards SM, Kote-Jarai Z, Meitz J, *et al*. Two per cent of men with early-onset prostate cancer harbor germline mutations in the *BRCA2* gene. *Am J Hum Genet* 2003; **72**:1–12.

134. Gayther SA, de Foy KA, Harrington P, *et al*. The frequency of germ-line mutations in the breast cancer predisposition genes *BRCA1* and *BRCA2* in familial prostate cancer. *Cancer Res* 2000; **60**:4513–4518.

135. Langston AA, Stanford JL, Wicklund KG, *et al*. Germline *BRCA1* mutations in selected men with prostate cancer. *Am J Hum Genet* 1996; **58**:881–884.

136. Lehrer S, Fodor F, Stock RG, *et al*. Absence of 185delAG mutation of the *BRCA1* gene and 6174delT mutation of the *BRCA2* gene in Ashkenazi Jewish men with prostate cancer. 1998; **78**:771–773.

137. Nastiuk KL, Mansukhani M, Terry MB, *et al*. Common mutations in *BRCA1* and *BRCA2* do not contribute to early prostate cancer in Jewish men. *Prostate* 1999; **40**:172–177.

138. Sinclair CS, Berry R, Schaid D, *et al*. *BRCA1* and *BRCA2* have a limited role in familial prostate cancer. *Cancer Res* 2000; **60**:1371–1375.

139. Vazina A, Baniel J, Yaacobi Y, *et al*. The rate of the founder Jewish mutations in *BRCA1* and *BRCA2* in prostate cancer patients in Israel. *Br J Cancer* 2000; **83**:463–466.

140. Wilkens EP, Freije D, Xu J, *et al*. No evidence for a role of *BRCA1* or *BRCA2* mutations in Ashkenazi Jewish families with hereditary prostate cancer. *Prostate* 1999; **39**:280–284.

141. Hubert A, Peretz T, Manor O, *et al*. The Jewish Ashkenazi founder mutations in the *BRCA1/BRCA2* genes are not found at an increased frequency in Ashkenazi patients with prostate cancer. *Am J Hum Genet* 1999; **65**:921–924.

142. Struewing JP, Hartge P, Wacholder S, *et al*. The risk of cancer associated with specific mutations of *BRCA1* and *BRCA2* among Ashkenazi Jews. *N Engl J Med* 1997; **336**:1401–1408.

143. Lal G, Liu G, Schmocker B, *et al*. Inherited predisposition to pancreatic adenocarcinoma: role of family history and germline *p16*, *BRCA1*, and *BRCA2* mutations. *Cancer Res* 2000; **60**:409–416.

144. Goggins M, Schutte M, Lu J, *et al*. Germline *BRCA2* gene mutations in patients with apparently sporadic pancreatic carcinomas. *Cancer Res* 1996; **56**:5360–5364.

145. Ozcelik H, Schmocker B, Di Nicola N, *et al*. Germline *BRCA2* 6174delT mutations in Ashkenazi Jewish pancreatic cancer patients. *Nature Genet* 1997; **16**:17–18.

146. Katagiri T, Nakamura Y, Miki Y. Mutations in the *BRCA2* gene in hepatocellular carcinomas. *Cancer Res* 1996; **56**:4575–4577.

147. White K, Held KR, Weber BH. A *BRCA2* germ-line mutation in familial pancreatic carcinoma. *Int J Cancer* 2001; **91**:742–744.

148. Clavel-Chapelon F, E3N-EPIC Group. Differential effects of reproductive factors on the risk of pre- and postmenopausal breast cancer. Results from a large cohort of French women. *Br J Cancer* 2002; **86**:723–727.

149. Whittemore AS, Harris R, Itnyre J. Characteristics relating to ovarian cancer risk: collaborative analysis of 12 US case-control studies. II. Invasive epithelial ovarian cancers in white women. Collaborative Ovarian Cancer Group. *Am J Epidemiol* 1992; **136**:1184–1203.

150. Narod SA, Goldgar D, Cannon-Albright L, *et al*. Risk modifiers in carriers of *BRCA1* mutations. *Int J Cancer* 1995; **64**:394–398.

151. Modan B, Hartge P, Hirsh-Yechezkel G, *et al*. Parity, oral contraceptives, and the risk of ovarian cancer among carriers and noncarriers of a *BRCA1* or *BRCA2* mutation. *N Engl J Med* 2001; **345**:235–240.

152. Rebbeck TR, Wang Y, Kantoff PW, *et al*. Modification of *BRCA1*- and *BRCA2*-associated breast cancer risk by AIB1 genotype and reproductive history. *Cancer Res* 2001; **61**:5420–5424.

153. Jernstrom H, Lerman C, Ghadirian P, *et al*. Pregnancy and risk of early breast cancer in carriers of *BRCA1* and *BRCA2*. *Lancet* 1999; **354**:1846–1850.

154. Johannsson O, Loman N, Borg A, Olsson H. Pregnancy-associated breast cancer in *BRCA1* and *BRCA2* germline mutation carriers. *Lancet* 1998; **352**:1359–1360.

155. Narod SA, Risch H, Moslehi R, *et al*. Oral contraceptives and the risk of hereditary ovarian cancer. *N Engl J Med* 1998; **339**:424–428.

156. Narod SA, Dube MP, Klijn J, *et al*. Oral contraceptives and the risk of breast cancer in *BRCA1* and *BRCA2* mutation carriers. *J Natl Cancer Inst* 2002; **94**:1773–1779.

157. Baron JA, Newcomb PA, Longnecker MP, *et al*. Cigarette smoking and breast cancer. *Cancer Epidemiol Biomarkers Prev* 1996; **5**:399–403.

158. Brunet JS, Ghadirian P, Rebbeck TR, *et al*. Effect of smoking on breast cancer in carriers of mutant *BRCA1* or *BRCA2* genes. *J Natl Cancer Inst* 1998; **90**:761–766.

159. Meijers-Heijboer H, van den OA, Klijn J, *et al*. Low-penetrance susceptibility to breast cancer due to *CHEK2*(*)1100delC in noncarriers of *BRCA1* or *BRCA2* mutations. *Nature Genet* 2002; **31**:55–59.

160. Park JJ, Irvine RA, Buchanan G, *et al*. Breast cancer susceptibility gene 1 (*BRCA1*) is a coactivator of the androgen receptor. *Cancer Res* 2000; **60**:5946–5949.

161. Giovannucci E, Stampfer MJ, Krithivas K, *et al*. The CAG repeat within the androgen receptor gene and its relationship to prostate cancer. *Proc Natl Acad Sci USA* 1997; **94**(7):3320–3323.

162. Rebbeck TR, Kantoff PW, Krithivas K, *et al*. Modification of *BRCA1*-associated breast cancer risk by the polymorphic androgen-receptor CAG repeat. *Am J Hum Genet* 1999; **64**:1371–1377.

163. Kadouri L, Easton DF, Edwards S, *et al*. CAG and GGC repeat polymorphisms in the androgen receptor gene and breast cancer susceptibility in *BRCA1/2* carriers and non-carriers. *Br J Cancer* 2001; **85**:36–40.

164. Anzick SL, Kononen J, Walker RL, *et al*. AIB1, a steroid receptor coactivator amplified in breast and ovarian cancer. *Science* 1997; **277**:965–968.

165. Groden J, Thliveris A, Samowitz W, *et al*. Identification and characterization of the familial adenomatous polyposis coli gene. *Cell* 1991; **66**:589–600.

166. Kinzler KW, Nilbert MC, Vogelstein B, *et al*. Identification of a gene located at chromosome 5q21 that is mutated in colorectal cancers. *Science* 1991; **251**:1366–1370.

167. Redston M, Nathanson KL, Yuan ZQ, *et al*. The *APC*I1307K allele and breast cancer risk. *Nature Genet* 1998; **20**:13–14.

168. Levy-Lahad E, Lahad A, Eisenberg S, *et al*. A single nucleotide polymorphism in the *RAD51* gene modifies cancer risk in *BRCA2* but not *BRCA1* carriers. *Proc Natl Acad Sci USA* 2001; **98**:3232–3236.

169. Wang WW, Spurdle AB, Kolachana P, *et al*. A single nucleotide polymorphism in the 5′ untranslated region of *RAD51* and risk of cancer among *BRCA1/2* mutation carriers. *Cancer Epidemiol Biomarkers Prev* 2001; **10**:955–960.

170. Nathanson KL, Shugart YY, Omaruddin R, *et al*. CGH-targeted linkage analysis reveals a possible *BRCA1* modifier locus on chromosome 5q. *Hum Mol Genet* 2002; **11**:1327–1332.

171. Phelan CM, Rebbeck TR, Weber BL, *et al*. Ovarian cancer risk in *BRCA1* carriers is modified by the *HRAS1* variable number of tandem repeat (VNTR) locus. *Nature Genet* 1996; **12**:309–311.

172. Hartmann LC, Sellers TA, Schaid DJ, *et al*. Efficacy of bilateral prophylactic mastectomy in *BRCA1* and *BRCA2* gene mutation carriers. *J Natl Cancer Inst* 2001; **93**:1633–1637.

173. Meijers-Heijboer H, van Geel B, van Putten WL, *et al*. Breast cancer after prophylactic bilateral mastectomy in women with a *BRCA1* or *BRCA2* mutation. *N Engl J Med* 2001; **345**:159–164.

174. Tobacman JK, Greene MH, Tucker MA, *et al*. Intra-abdominal carcinomatosis after prophylactic oophorectomy in ovarian-cancer-prone families. *Lancet* 1982; **2**:795–797.

175. Kauff ND, Satagopan JM, Robson ME, *et al*. Risk-reducing salpingo-oophorectomy in women with a *BRCA1* or *BRCA2* mutation. *N Engl J Med* 2002; **346**:1609–1615.

176. Rebbeck TR, Lynch HT, Neuhausen SL, *et al*. Prophylactic oophorectomy in carriers of *BRCA1* or *BRCA2* mutations. *N Engl J Med* 2002; **346**:1616–1622.

177. Rebbeck TR, Levin AM, Eisen A, *et al*. Breast cancer risk after bilateral prophylactic oophorectomy in *BRCA1* mutation carriers. *J Natl Cancer Inst* 1999; **91**:1475–1479.

178. Narod SA, Sun P, Ghadirian P, *et al*. Tubal ligation and risk of ovarian cancer in carriers of *BRCA1* or *BRCA2* mutations: a case-control study. *Lancet* 2001; **357**:1467–1470.

179. King MC, Wieand S, Hale K, *et al*. Tamoxifen and breast cancer incidence among women with inherited mutations in *BRCA1* and *BRCA2*: National Surgical Adjuvant Breast and Bowel Project (NSABP-P1) Breast Cancer Prevention Trial. *JAMA* 2001; **286**:2251–2256.

180. Abel KJ, Xu J, Yin GY, *et al*. Mouse *Brca1*: localization sequence analysis and identification of evolutionarily conserved domains. *Hum Mol Genet* 1995; **4**:2265–2273.

181. Smith SA, Easton DF, Evans DG, Ponder BA. Allele losses in the region 17q12–21 in familial breast and ovarian cancer involve the wild-type chromosome. *Nature Genet* 1992; **2**:128–131.

182. Collins N, McManus R, Wooster R, *et al*. Consistent loss of the wild type allele in breast cancers from a family linked to the *BRCA2* gene on chromosome 13q12–13. *Oncogene* 1995; **10**:1673–1675.

183. Jensen DE, Proctor M, Marquis ST, *et al*. BAP1: a novel ubiquitin hydrolase which binds to the *BRCA1* RING finger and enhances *BRCA1*-mediated cell growth suppression. *Oncogene* 1998; **16**:1097–1112.

184. Wu LC, Wang ZW, Tsan JT, *et al*. Identification of a RING protein that can interact in vivo with the *BRCA1* gene product. *Nature Genet* 1996; **14**:430–440.

185. Chapman MS, Verma IM. Transcriptional activation by *BRCA1*. *Nature* 1996; **382**:678–679.

186. Scully R, Chen J, Plug A, *et al*. Association of *BRCA1* with Rad51 in mitotic and meiotic cells. *Cell* 1997; **88**:265–275.

187. Koonin FV, Altschul SF, Bork P. *BRCA1* protein products … Functional motifs…*Nature Genet* 1996; **13**:266–268.

188. Jensen RA, Thompson ME, Jetton TL, *et al*. *BRCA1* is secreted and exhibits properties of a granin. *Nature Genet* 1996; **12**:303–308.

189. Thakur S, Zhang HB, Peng Y, *et al*. Localization of *BRCA1* and a splice variant identifies the nuclear localization signal. *Mol Cell Biol* 1997; **17**:444–452.

190. Bork P, Blomberg N, Nilges M. Internal repeats in the *BRCA2* protein sequence. *Nature Genet* 1996; **13**:22–23.

191. Bignell G, Micklem G, Stratton MR, *et al*. The BRC repeats are conserved in mammalian *BRCA2* proteins. *Hum Mol Genet* 1997; **6**:53–58.

192. Wong AK, Pero R, Ormonde PA, *et al.* RAD51 interacts with the evolutionarily conserved BRC motifs in the human breast cancer susceptibility gene *brca2*. *J Biol Chem* 1997; **272:**31941–31944.

193. Chen PL, Chen CF, Chen Y, *et al.* The BRC repeats in *BRCA2* are critical for RAD51 binding and resistance to methyl methanesulfonate treatment. *Proc Natl Acad Sci USA* 1998; **95:**5287–5292.

194. Bertwistle D, Swift S, Marston NJ, *et al.* Nuclear location and cell cycle regulation of the *BRCA2* protein. *Cancer Res* 1997; **57:**5485–5488.

195. Spain BH, Larson CJ, Shihabuddin LS, *et al.* Truncated *BRCA2* is cytoplasmic: implications for cancer-linked mutations. *Proc Natl Acad Sci USA* 1999; **96:**13920–13925.

196. Venkitaraman AR. Multiplying functions for *BRCA1* and *BRCA2?*. Meeting report, The Breakthrough Breast Cancer Second International Workshop on the function of *BRCA1* and *BRCA2*, Cambridge, UK, 9–10 September 1999. *Biochim Biophys Acta* 2000; **1470:**R41–R47.

197. Cortez D, Wang Y, Qin J, Elledge SJ. Requirement of ATM-dependent phosphorylation of *brca1* in the DNA damage response to double-strand breaks. *Science* 1999; **286:**1162–1166.

198. Vaughn JP, Cirisano FD, Huper G, *et al.* Cell cycle control of *BRCA2*. *Cancer Res* 1996; **56:**4590–4594.

199. Rajan JV, Wang M, Marquis ST, Chodosh LA. *Brca2* is coordinately regulated with *Brca1* during proliferation and differentiation in mammary epithelial cells. *Proc Natl Acad Sci USA* 1996; **93:**13078–13083.

200. Yarden RI, Pardo-Reoyo S, Sgagias M, *et al.* BRCA1 regulates the G2/M checkpoint by activating Chk1 kinase upon DNA damage. *Nature Genet* 2002; **30:**285–289.

201. Mizuta R, LaSalle JM, Cheng HL, *et al.* RAB22 and RAB163/mouse *BRCA2*: proteins that specifically interact with the RAD51 protein. *Proc Natl Acad Sci USA* 1997; **94:**6927–6932.

202. Chen JJ, Silver D, Cantor S, Livingston DM, Scully R. BRCA1, BRCA2, and Rad51 operate in a common DNA damage response pathway. *Cancer Res* 1999; **59**(7 Suppl): 1752s–1756s.

203. Brugarolas J, Jacks T. Double indemnity: *p53*, *BRCA* and cancer. *p53* mutation partially rescues developmental arrest in *Brca1* and *Brca2* null mice, suggesting a role for familial breast cancer genes in DNA damage repair. *Nature Med* 1997; **3:**721–722.

204. Miyoshi Y, Nagase H, Ando H, *et al.* Somatic mutations of the *APC* gene in colorectal tumors: mutation cluster region in the *APC* gene. *Hum Mol Genet* 1992; **1:**229–233.

205. Futreal PA, Liu Q, Shattuck-Eidens D, *et al.* BRCA1 mutations in primary breast and ovarian carcinomas. *Science* 1994; **266:**120–122.

206. Lancaster JM, Wooster R, Mangion J, *et al.* BRCA2 mutations in primary breast and ovarian cancers. *Nature Genet* 1996; **13:**238–240.

207. Krainer M, Silva-Arrieta S, FitzGerald MG, *et al.* Differential contributions of *BRCA1* and *BRCA2* to early-onset breast cancer. *N Engl J Med* 1997; **336:**1416–1421.

208. Eccles DM, Englefield P, Soulby MA, Campbell IG. BRCA1 mutations in southern England. *Br J Cancer* 1998; **77:**2199–2203.

209. Malone KE, Daling JR, Thompson JD, *et al.* BRCA1 mutations and breast cancer in the general population: analyses in women before age 35 years and in women before age 45 years with first-degree family history. *JAMA* 1998; **279:**922–929.

210. Newman B, Mu H, Butler LM, *et al.* Frequency of breast cancer attributable to *BRCA1* in a population-based series of American women. *JAMA* 1998; **279:**915–921.

211. Hopper JL, Southey MC, Dite GS, *et al.* Population-based estimate of the average age-specific cumulative risk of breast cancer for a defined set of protein-truncating mutations in *BRCA1* and *BRCA2*. *Cancer Epidemiol Biomarkers Prev* 1999; **8:**741–747.

212. Loman N, Johannsson O, Kristoffersson U, *et al.* Family history of breast and ovarian cancers and *BRCA1* and *BRCA2* mutations in a population-based series of early-onset breast cancer. *J Natl Cancer Inst* 2001; **93:**1215–1223.

213. Langston AA, Malone KE, Thompson JD, *et al.* BRCA1 mutations in a population-based sample of young women with breast cancer. *N Engl J Med* 1996; **334:**137–142.

20

Screening for breast cancer in high-risk populations

SUE MOSS

INTRODUCTION

This chapter addresses the subject of screening for breast cancer in women identified as being at high risk of the disease. The definition of screening is taken to be a test that identifies those subjects likely to have a disease from those who do not. This chapter does not, therefore, consider the issues surrounding the use of genetic testing to identify carriers of known breast cancer predisposition genes; these, together with the development of models to identify women at high risk, are considered elsewhere in this volume.

The evidence from randomized controlled trials that screening by mammography for breast cancer is effective in reducing mortality from the disease has led a number of countries to introduce nationwide population screening programmes, and many others to introduce pilot projects.[1] While it is recognized that screening will have costs and disadvantages as well as beneficial effects, the rationale for introducing population screening is that the benefits will outweigh the disadvantages in the population being targeted. Potential disadvantages of breast screening include: the increased time that a women with screen-detected disease will live with the knowledge that she has the disease and with the side effects of any treatment; the anxiety caused in those women with false-positive mammograms and possible more invasive procedures, such as cytology or biopsy;

the potential for radiation-induced cancers from mammography; and the possibility of overdiagnosis, particularly from the detection of carcinoma *in situ*. There are also considerable financial costs involved in a screening programme covering a general population. The attraction of targeting a high-risk group, rather than the whole population is that benefits are more likely to outweigh the costs.

However, while targeting a high-risk population might be financially more cost effective, excluding a group of women at lower risk might not be politically or ethically acceptable. To some extent, the value of targeted screening is already recognized by the fact that most population screening programmes only invite women in a certain age range. For example, in the UK women between the ages of 50 and 64 are currently invited for screening every 3 years. Women above age 64 have been able to self-refer; however, a decision has now been made in the UK to include women aged 65–70 in the invitation system, and there is increasing pressure not to exclude women who might potentially benefit.

In the USA, guidelines for screening vary between organizations. The American Cancer Society currently recommends that women begin monthly breast self-examination (BSE) at age 20, should have a clinical breast examination (CBE) every 3 years between ages 20 and 39, and an annual mammogram and CBE beginning at age 40.[2]

Most of the interest in screening high-risk women for breast cancer is centred on those at increased risk owing to a family history of the disease and, in particular, in those with identified cancer predisposition genes, such as *BRCA1* or *BRCA2*. However, other high-risk groups exist, for example, women treated by radiation for early-stage Hodgkin's disease.[3] It is estimated that between 5 and 10 per cent of breast cancers occur in women with a genetic predisposition.[4] Such women will be at increased risk from a young age, whereas, at present, the majority of the evidence on the effectiveness of the breast cancer screening is in women aged 50 and over. Much of the excess risk of familial breast cancer occurs before age 50[5] and it is generally recommended that screening start 5–10 years before the earliest age of diagnosis of affected family members.

This chapter, therefore, reviews the evidence from randomized controlled trials on the effectiveness of screening in the general population and then specifically on the effectiveness of screening below age 50. The evidence on screening by modalities other than mammography is also discussed. Results on the outcome of screening in high-risk women in terms of uptake and cancer detection rates are described. However, there is a lack of evidence on the effectiveness of screening in high-risk women. The extent to which results from the general population can be extrapolated to this group depends on whether the natural history of the disease and/or the sensitivity of different screening tests varies in such women. Finally, the various disadvantages of screening, and the extent to which these may vary in high-risk women, are discussed.

EVIDENCE FOR EFFECTIVENESS OF BREAST SCREENING

The effectiveness of population breast screening by mammography in reducing mortality in women at average risk of the disease has been demonstrated by a number of population-based randomized controlled trials. There has been no randomized controlled trial of breast screening in high-risk women. The original Health Insurance Plan (HIP) trial, carried out in New York in the 1960s, showed a reduction of 30 per cent in those women invited for four annual screens by mammography and clinical examination.[6] Five of the subsequent trials have been conducted in Sweden, with variations in protocol in terms of number of mammographic views and interval between screens. The randomized trials are summarized in Table 20.1, which gives the relative risk of breast cancer death in women invited to screening compared to the control group.

In 1993, an overview of the five Swedish trials was performed, using a standard endpoint and with the cause of death in all fatal breast cancer cases reviewed by an independent review committee.[7] The overview showed consistent relative risks of between 0.68 and 0.84 in the study groups of the five trials with an overall relative risk of 0.74 (95 per cent confidence interval (CI) 0.67–0.88). This analysis excluded breast cancer deaths in cases diagnosed after the date at which the control groups had been invited for screening. The largest benefit was shown in women aged 50–69 at entry to the trials, with a reduction of 29 per cent, with a non-significant reduction of 13 per cent in women age 40–49 (relative risk (RR) 0.87, CI

Table 20.1 *Randomized controlled trials of breast screening*

				Women aged			
				≥50		<50	
Study	Screening interval (months)	CBE included	Number of women	Length of follow-up (years)	RR (95% CI)	Length of follow-up (years)	RR (95% CI)
Health Insurance Plan[6]	12	Yes	62 000	10	0.68 (0.49–0.96)	18	0.77 (0.53–1.11)
Two County[58]	24–33	No	133 000	13	0.66 (0.46–0.93)	13	0.87 (0.54–1.41)
Gothenburg[61]	18	No	52 000			12	0.56 (0.32–0.98)
Stockholm[62]	30	No	60 300	11.4	0.62 (0.38–1.00)	11.4	1.08 (0.54–2.17)
Edinburgh[63,64]	24	Yes (annual)	50 000	10	0.85 (0.62–1.15)	14	0.78 (0.46–1.32)
Malmo[59,60]	18–24	No	42 300	8	0.79[a] (0.51–1.24)	12.7	0.64 (0.45–0.89)
NBSS 1[24]	12	Yes	50 000			11	1.14 (0.83–1.56)
NBSS 2[65 b]	12	Yes	40 000	13	1.02 (0.78–1.33)		

CBE, clinical breast examination; CI, confidence interval; NBSS, (Canadian) National Breast Screening Study; RR, relative risk.
[a] Age 55+.
[b] Mammography + CBE vs. CBE alone.

These include a possible lower sensitivity of mammography owing to the higher prevalence of mammographically dense tissue in premenopausal women, and the effect of age in the process of differentiation, with a transition to high-grade malignancy occurring earlier in women below age 50.[28]

Boyd *et al.* used data from the Canadian NBSS (National Breast Screening Study)[29] to show that mammographic density was strongly associated with a risk of breast cancer in women with a family history, suggesting potential approaches to prevention in this group.[30] Another possible reason for a lesser benefit is a tendency for breast cancers in younger women to be faster growing. This has implications for the frequency of screening.

Frequency of screening

Randomized trials of screening for breast cancer have generally used intervals of between 12 and 33 months. In the Swedish Two County study, a shorter interval of 26 months was used in women aged 40–49 at entry to that in women aged 50 plus where an interval of 33 months was used. Analysis of interval cancers in this study showed a lower sensitivity of mammography in the younger women than those aged 50 plus. The greatest benefit of screening in women below aged 50 has been shown in the trial carried out in Gothenburg, which used an annual screening interval. Most population-screening programmes have adopted a 2-year screening interval. In the UK, however, the programme has a 3-year interval. A randomized trial comparing an annual with a 3-yearly interval, based on surrogate outcome measures, found that shortening the screening interval was predicted to have only a small effect on mortality in the age group 50–64. Early results from two regions in England on interval cancers showed high rates in the third year.[31,32] Results from the Miscan simulation model have suggested that growth rates of breast cancer are higher in younger women, implying a need for a shorter screening interval, but again more information is needed on the natural history of breast cancer in high-risk women.

Even if the effectiveness of screening in younger women is established, the cost effectiveness in terms of cost per life years saved needs to be considered in comparison to that of screening in older women. A lesser reduction in the absolute reduction in number of deaths owing to the lower incidence at younger ages needs to be balanced against the increase in life years saved per death prevented. Clearly, however, in high-risk populations the cost effectiveness will be greater if the effectiveness is the same.

Screening by magnetic resonance imaging

Magnetic resonance imaging (MRI) of the breast is a technique that provides an *in vivo* image of the soft tissue.

The use of tissue-specific contrast agents has been shown to improve the sensitivity of the technique. While a number of studies have shown high sensitivity of contrast enhanced MRI, many have shown fairly low specificity of between 37 per cent and 89 per cent. The use of dynamic techniques in which data are collected, for example, every 60 seconds has been reported to increase specificity considerably. The sensitivity of the technique for detecting preinvasive lesions requires further assessment. In addition, the detection of mammographically occult lesions raises potential problems for subsequent biopsy. MRI does not involve the use of ionizing radiation and, therefore, may be particularly important in younger women where the potential increased risk of cancer from the radiation associated with conventional mammography may be greatest. A limiting factor at present in the use of MRI is the cost of the technique. However, in high-risk women, the cost–benefit ratio will be lower. A trial is currently in progress in the UK.[33] This is being carried out in high-risk women identified from genetic clinics who are being randomized to screening either by MRI imaging or by mammography. The trial is comparing the sensitivity of the two screening techniques in this population.

UPTAKE AND OUTCOME OF SCREENING IN HIGH-RISK WOMEN

A number of studies have now reported on the outcome of screening in women at high risk. Uptake of invitations or compliance with recommendations is likely to be high in women at increased risk. One study in Sydney, Australia, collected self-reported data from 461 women who approached a familial cancer clinic.[34] The women were allocated to moderate or high-risk groups according to their reported family history. They found that 89 and 90 per cent of women reported screening in line with age- and risk-specific recommendations, for mammography and CBE, respectively. A total of 51 per cent reported practising BSE monthly or more frequently. Among women aged less than 30, compliance with recommendations for screening was significantly lower (56 per cent) than in older women. Lalloo *et al.* studied 1259 women attending the family history clinic in Manchester, UK, all of whom had been referred by their general practitioner or surgeon.[35] Women with an estimated lifetime risk of one in six or greater were offered an appointment for annual mammography and CBE between the ages of 35 and 50, or from 5 years younger than the earliest age of diagnosis of breast cancer in the family. The mean age of women at entry to the programme was 39.1 years. Attendance rates at first and subsequent screens were 95.2 per cent and 98.9 per cent, respectively.

Chart and Franssen reported on a series of women evaluated for breast cancer risks at two clinics in Toronto

Canada between 1990 and 1996.[36] Women considered at high risk were recommended surveillance by annual mammography and 6-monthly CBE. Annual mammography and CBE were recommended for those at moderate risk; in both cases, mammography was started at 10 years before the earliest age of diagnosis of breast cancer in the family. For women at slightly increased risk, annual mammography and CBE were recommended from age 40; monthly BSE was recommended to all women. The average length of follow-up was 21.9 months and a total of 29 breast cancers were detected in 986 patients at increased risk with a mean age at diagnosis of 47.

MacMillan summarized results from 22 breast units in the UK (including the data from two of the above studies), including 8783 women screened and 9075 years of follow-up.[37] The median age at diagnosis was 43. Cancer detection rates were 4.8 per 1000 at prevalent screens and 4.5 at incident screens, comparable to those observed in women aged over 50 in the NHS Breast Screening Programme (NHSBSP). In the Manchester study, the ratio of total observed to expected invasive cancers was 1.42; the authors concluded that screening of high-risk younger women requires an annual screening policy and that lead time gained from screening in this group is likely to be short.[35]

PROGNOSIS OF BREAST CANCER

Women with a family history compared with those in the general population have been reviewed by Chappuis et al.[38] They found conflicting data as to whether the prognosis of familial breast cancer varied from that of sporadic cases, with 4 of 18 family history-based studies showing a significantly better survival and two significantly worse, in patients with a family history. No studies have shown a definitive survival analysis in BRCA1 carriers and some indicate worse survival (see Chapter 19).

A recent study in Rotterdam looked at 294 women at moderate risk of breast cancer with a mean age of 43.3, who were screened with yearly physical examination and mammography from 5 years before youngest age of onset in the family, and also 384 women with higher risk, mean age of 42.9, who were screened by physical examination every 6 months and yearly mammography.[39] From September 1995, MRI was also carried out for high-risk women with dense breasts. A comparison was made with patients with breast cancer referred because of symptoms, who appeared to have a positive family history, and also with patients detected during the national screening programme and referred to the clinic, who appeared to have a positive family history. Cancers in the surveillance group were detected significantly more often at early stage than in the other groups and were also more often node negative.

Moller et al. summarized data from seven centres participating in the EU Demonstration Project on Clinical Services for Familial Breast Cancer.[40] Of 162 cancers, 75 per cent were screen-detected, and mean age at diagnosis was 48.6 years. Overall 5-year survival was 89 per cent.

DISADVANTAGES OF SCREENING

One possible harmful effect of mammography is the potential to induce cancers through radiation. In the early years of mammographic screening, it was claimed that screening could induce as many breast cancers as were detected.[41] Uncertainties surrounding the exact level of risk arise from the fact that estimates of the dose–response effect of radiation at low doses are primarily obtained by extrapolating results from studies of very large dose effects, such as in atomic bomb survivors or in medical radiation treatment. The average radiation dose for mammography has reduced considerably over the past 15–20 years and concern is correspondingly less. However, the risk due to radiation is greater at younger ages of exposure, and the risk due to radiation has, therefore, been a particular issue in the debate on screening below aged 50. Most recent calculations have estimated that the benefit is still likely to outweigh the risk of screening even in younger women,[42,43] although the importance of a low dose exposure is emphasized.[44] In the UK NHSBSP, the current dose is 1–2 mGy per film, even with increased mean film density, which increases sensitivity but also dose levels. It has also been suggested that, for a small subgroup of women with large thick breasts, the ratio may be reversed.[45] While in women at increased risk of the disease the benefit due to mammography is likely to be greater, it is also possible that the risk side of the equation may also be increased in that it is possible that genetically predisposed women may have an increased sensitivity to radiation. Such women are also likely to be recommended to have screening at more frequent intervals and start at a younger age, thus increasing the total exposure to radiation.

As an example, ataxia telangiectasia (A-T) is an inherited autosomal recessive disease, one of the characteristics of which is increased sensitivity to ionizing radiation. Women who are AT–gene mutation carriers are also at an increased risk for breast cancer development. It has been suggested that exposure to ionizing radiation can increase the breast cancer risk in these women,[46] but these results have also been disputed.[47]

One mathematical model, which has been developed for cancer predisposition and radio sensitivity, has been used to predict the risk in BRCA1 carriers and has concluded that the benefits of mammography will outweigh the risks of radiation in this population.[48] However, it is generally considered that more data are required on increased susceptibility to radiation induced cancers in high-risk women.[49] The possibility of increased radio sensitivity in women at high risk owing to genetic mutations also has implications for the treatment of any breast cancer detected or diagnosed.

Anxiety

The process of inviting women in the general population to attend for breast screening does not appear to result in increased anxiety or psychological morbidity. However, the notification of a positive screening result and recall for further investigation is likely to result in increased anxiety. A study that compared anxiety and depression levels in a group of such women attending for further investigation with groups attending for routine screening and referred because of breast symptoms found higher anxiety levels in the symptomatic group, but also higher levels in the women attending because of positive screening findings than in those attending for routine screening.[50] However, after 3 months, anxiety levels in those women with false-positive screening mammograms were no different from those originally screened negative. A more recent study, which aimed to assess the psychological impact of screening by measuring psychometric scores in groups of women (1) invited to screening, (2) attending for routine screening, (3) attending for a further investigation after a positive mammogram and (4) at open biopsy, found no significant increase in anxiety in the latter two groups.[51]

Women with a family history of breast cancer may already have increased anxiety and the interaction with effect of screening may be difficult to determine. A number of studies have looked at anxiety in women identified at high risk from breast cancer and the implications for compliance with recommendations for screening. Lerman et al. found that most women at high risk followed National Cancer Institute guidelines for mammography, but this varied by age and was lower in those age 50 and over.[52] Compliance was also lower in women with a lower level of education and with increasing time since diagnosis of the women's first degree relative. However, only age and worry about breast cancer significantly reduced compliance. Kash et al. studied 270 women enrolled in their breast protection programme;[53] 94 per cent attended for regular mammograms but only 69 per cent for regular CBE. Overall, 40 per cent of women performed monthly BSE, but increased anxiety was related to poorer adherence with regular BSE.

Overdiagnosis

In screening for breast cancer, there is a possibility of overdiagnosis of cancers that would not otherwise have presented clinically. In particular, there is uncertainty over the natural history of ductal carcinoma in situ (DCIS), which is infrequently diagnosed in the absence of screening. In the original HIP screening trial, 2–3 years after the end of screening in the intervention group, the cumulative numbers of breast cancers in the intervention and control groups were similar, indicating that no overdiagnosis had occurred.[1] However, little in situ disease was detected in this trial and the sensitivity of modern-day mammography is much higher. In a population-screening study in Nijmegen, 11 per cent more cancers were initially found in a screen population compared with geographical controls. However, after 8–12 years, the cumulative breast cancer rates within the two groups were similar, suggesting that the additional cancers diagnosed by screening would eventually have presented symptomatically.[54] Results from the Swedish Two County Trial have been interpreted as suggesting that overdiagnosis was limited to cases diagnosed at the first screen, and that most overdiagnosis was occurring in women below aged 50.[55] However, in this study, the rate of detection of DCIS was comparatively low. In the current UK screening programme, approximately 17–20 per cent of cancers detected at each screen are DCIS and there is no reduction in this rate at repeat rounds of screening.[56] One study of screening of high-risk women in Nottingham has reported 21 per cent of detected cancers being in situ.

CONCLUSIONS

There is, at present, insufficient evidence on the efficacy of screening mammography in the general population below age 50 to draw conclusions about the benefit in high-risk women. If a beneficial effect on breast cancer mortality does become apparent, then it may be that the absolute reduction in high-risk women will be greater than that in the general population. However, more information is needed on the natural history of the disease in such women in order to determine the level of benefit, the recommended screening interval and the extent of any overdiagnosis. There is also uncertainty about the possible harmful effect of radiation from mammography in some women. Techniques such as MRI may be more sensitive but this remains to be proven. There is no evidence that routine breast self-examination has a beneficial effect in reducing mortality.

Meanwhile, advice is needed for high-risk women on whether or not to be screened.[57] They should be given as much information as possible in order for them to make an 'informed choice', which should include information on the disadvantages of screening as discussed above. The fact that screening will not detect all breast cancers, and the importance of continuing awareness of symptoms, should be emphasized.

REFERENCES

1. Shapiro S, Coleman EA, Broeders M, *et al*. For the International Breast Cancer Screening Network (IBSN) and the European Network of Pilot Projects for Breast Cancer Screening. Breast cancer screening programmes in 22 countries: current policies, administration and guidelines. *Int J Epidemiol* 1998; **27:**735–742.

2. Smith RA, Mettlin CJ, Davis KJ, Eyre H. American Cancer Society Guidelines for the Early Detection of Cancer. *Cancer J Clinicians* 2000; **50:**34–49.

3. Clemons M, Loijens L, Goss P. Breast cancer risk following irradiation for Hodgkin's disease. *Cancer Treat Rev* 2000; **26:**2910–2302.

4. Eeles RA. Screening for hereditary cancer and genetic testing, epitomised by breast cancer. *Eur J Cancer* 1999; **35:**1954–1962.

5. Houlston RS, McCarter E, Parbhoo S, *et al*. Family history and risk of breast cancer. *J Med Genet* 1992; **29:**154–157.

6. Shapiro S, Venet W, Strax P, *et al*. Ten-to fourteen-year effect of screening on breast cancer mortality. *J Natl Cancer Inst* 1982; **69:**349–355.

7. Nystrom L, Rutqvist LE, Wall S, *et al*. Breast cancer screening with mammography: overview of Swedish randomised trials. *Lancet* 1993; **341:**973–978.

8. Kerlikowske K, Grady D, Rubin SM, *et al*. Efficacy of screening mammography. A meta-analysis. *JAMA* 1995; **273:**149–154.

9. Gotzche PC, Olsen O. Is screening for breast cancer with mammography justified? *Lancet* 2000; **355:**129–134.

10. Quinn M, Allen E, on behalf of the United Kingdom Association of Cancer Registries. Changes in incidence of and mortality from breast cancer in England and Wales since introduction of screening. *Br Med J* 1995; **311:**1391–1395.

11. Blanks RG, Moss SM, McGahan CE, *et al*. Effect of NHS breast screening programme on mortality from breast cancer in England and Wales: comparison of observed with predicted mortality. *Br Med J* 2000; **321:**665–669.

12. Hakama M, Pukkala E, Heikkila, Kallio M. Effectiveness of the public health policy for breast cancer screening in Finland: population based cohort study. *Br Med J* 1997; **314:**864–867.

13. Sjonell G, Stahle L. Halsokontroller med mammografi minskar inte dodlighet i brostcancer. *Lakartidningen* 1999; **96:**904–913.

14. Rosen M, Rehnqvist N. No need to reconsider breast screening programme on basis of results from defective study. *Br Med J* 1999; **318:**809–810.

15. Tabar L, Vitak B, Chen HH, *et al*. Beyond randomized controlled trials. *Cancer* 2001; **91:**1724–1731.

16. Moss SM, Coleman DA, Ellman R, *et al*. Interval cancers and sensitivity in the screening centres of the UK Trial of Early Detection of Breast Cancer. *Eur J Cancer* 1993; **29A:**225–228.

17. Moss SM, Ellman R, Coleman D, Chamberlain J, for the United Kingdom Trial of Early Detection of Breast Cancer Group. Survival of patients with breast cancer diagnosed in the United Kingdom trial of early detection of breast cancer. *J Med Screening* 1994; **1:**193–198.

18. Baines CJ, Miller AB. Mammography versus clinical examination of the breasts. *J Natl Cancer Inst* 1997; **22:**125–129.

19. Mittra I, Baum M, Thornton H, Houghton J. Is clinical breast examination an acceptable alternative to mammographic screening? *Br Med J* 2000; **321:**1071–1073.

20. UK Trial of Early Detection of Breast Cancer Group. Breast cancer mortality after 10 years in the UK trial of early detection of breast cancer. *Breast* 1993; **2:**13–20.

21. Ellman R, Moss SM, Coleman D, Chamberlain J. Breast self-examination programmes in the trial of early detection of breast cancer: ten year findings. *Br J Cancer* 1993; **68:**208–212.

22. Gastrin G, Miller AB, To T, *et al*. Incidence and mortality from breast cancer in the Mama Program for breast screening in Finland, 1973–1986. *Cancer* 1994; **73:**2168–2174.

23. Thomas DB, Gao DL, Self SG, *et al*. Randomized trial of breast self-examination in Shanghai: methodology and preliminary results. *J Natl Cancer Inst* 1997; **89:**355–365.

24. Miller AB, To T, Baines CJ, Wall C. The Canadian National Breast Screening Study: Update on Breast Cancer Mortality. *J Natl Cancer Inst Monogr* 1997; **22:**37–41.

25. Hendrick RE, Smith RA, Rutledge JH, Smart CR. Benefit of screening mammography in women aged 40–49; a new meta-analysis of randomized controlled trials. *Monogr Natl Cancer Inst* 1997; **22:**87–92.

26. de Koning HJ, Boer R, Warmerdam PG, *et al*. Quantitative interpretation of age-specific mortality reductions from the Swedish breast cancer-screening trials. *J Natl Cancer Inst* 1995; **87:**1217–1223.

27. Moss S, for the Trial Steering Group. A trial to study the effect on breast cancer mortality of annual mammographic screening in women starting at age 40. *J Med Screening* 1999; **6:**144–148.

28. Day N, Warren R. Mammographic screening and mammographic patterns. *Breast Cancer Res* 2000; **2:**247–251.

29. The Breast Screening Frequency Trial Group. The future of breast cancer screening: results from the UKCCCR Randomised Trial. *Eur J Cancer* 2002; **38:**1458–1464.

30. Boyd NF, Lockwood GA, Martin LJ, *et al*. Mammographic densities and risk of breast cancer among subjects with a family history of this disease. *J Natl Cancer Inst* 1999; **91:**1404–1408.

31. Day N, McCann J, Camilleri-Ferrante C, *et al*. Monitoring interval cancers in breast screening programmes: the East Anglian experience. *J Med Screening* 1995; **2:**180–185.

32. Woodman CBJ, Threlfall A, Boggis CRM, Prior P. Is the three year breast screening interval too long? Occurrence of interval cancers in NHS breast screening programme's north western region. *Br Med J* 1995; **310**:224–226.

33. The UK MRI Breast Screening Study Advisory Group. (Brown J, Coulthard A, Dixon AK, *et al.*). Protocol for a national multi-centre study of magnetic resonance imaging screening in women at genetic risk of breast cancer. *Breast* 2000; **9**:78–82.

34. Meiser B, Butow P, Barratt A, *et al.* Breast cancer screening uptake in women at increased risk of developing hereditary breast cancer. *Breast Cancer Res Treat* 2000; **59**:101–111.

35. Lalloo F, Boggis CRM, Evans DGR, *et al.* Screening by mammography, women with a family history of breast cancer. *Eur J Cancer* 1998; **34**:937–940.

36. Chart PL, Franssen E. Management of women at increased risk for breast cancer: preliminary results from a new program. *Can Med Assoc J* 1997; **157**:1235–1242.

37. MacMillan RD. Screening women with a family history of breast cancer – results from the British Familial Breast Cancer Group. *Eur J Surg Oncol* 2000; **26**:149–152.

38. Chappuis PO, Rosenblatt J, Foulkes WD. The influence of familial and hereditary factors on the prognosis of breast cancer. *Ann Oncol* 1999; **10**:1163–1170.

39. Tilanus-Linthorst MM, Bartels CC, Obdeijn AI, Oudkerk M. Earlier detection of breast cancer by surveillance of women at familial risk. *Eur J Cancer* 2000; **36**:514–519.

40. Moller P, Reis MM, Evans G, *et al.* Efficacy of early diagnosis and treatment in women with a family history of breast cancer. *Disease Markers* 1000; **16**:179–186.

41. Bailar JC. Mammography: a contrary view. *Ann Intern Med* 1976; **84**:77–84.

42. Feig SA, Hendrick RE. Radiation risk from screening mammography of women aged 40–49 years. *J Natl Cancer Inst* 1997; **22**:119–124.

43. Beemsterboer PMM, Warmerdam PG, Boer R, de Koning HJ. Radiation risk of mammography related to benefit in screening programmes: a favourable balance? *J Med Screening* 1998; **5**:81–87.

44. Mattsson A, Leitz W, Rutqvist L-E. Radiation risk and mammographic screening of women from 40 to 49 years of age: effect on breast cancer rates and years of life. *Br J Cancer* 2000; **82**:220–226.

45. Law J. Risk and benefit associated with radiation dose in breast screening programmes – an update. *Br J Radiol* 1995; **68**:870–876.

46. Swift M, Morrell D, Massey RB, Chase CL. Incidence of cancer in 161 families affected by ataxia-telangiectasia. *N Engl J Med* 1991; **325**:1831–1836.

47. Wagner LK. To the editor. *N Engl J Med* 1992; **326**:1358.

48. Chakraborty R, Sankaranarayanan K. Mutations in the *BRCA1* gene: implications of inter-population differences for predicting the risk of radiation-induced breast cancers. *Genet Res Camb* 1998; **72**:191–198.

49. Law J. Cancers detected and induced in mammographic screening: new screening schedules and younger women with family history. *Br J Radiol* 1997; **70**:62–69.

50. Ellman R, Angeli N, Christians A, *et al.* Psychiatric morbidity associated with screening for breast cancer. *Br J Cancer* 1989; **60**:781–784.

51. Bull AR, Campbell MJ. Assessment of the psychological impact of a breast screening programme. *Br J Radiol* 1991; **64**:510–515.

52. Lerman C, Daly M, Sands C, *et al.* Mammography adherence and psychological distress among women at risk for breast cancer. *J Natl Cancer Inst* 1993; **85**:1074–1080.

53. Kash KM, Holland JC, Halper MS, Miller DG. Psychological distress and surveillance behaviors of women with a family history of breast cancer. *J Natl Cancer Inst* 1992; **84**:24–30.

54. Peeters PH. Evaluation of overdiagnosis of breast cancer in screening with mammography: results of the Nijmegen programme. *Int J Epidemiol* 1989; **18**:295–299.

55. Tabar L, Fagerberg G, Duffy SW, *et al.* Update of the Swedish Two-County Program of Mammographic Screening for Breast Cancer. *Radiol Clin North Am* 1992; **30**:187–210.

56. Blanks RG, Moss SM, Patnick J. Results From UK NHS breast screening programme 1992–1999. *J Med Screen* 2000; **7**:195–198.

57. Lucassen A, Watson E, Eccles D. Advice about mammography for a young woman with a family history of breast cancer. *Br Med J* 2001; **322**:1040–1042.

58. Tabar L, Fagerberg G, Chen HH, *et al.* Efficacy of breast cancer screening by age. *Cancer* 1995; **75**:2507–2517.

59. Andersson I, Aspegren K, Janzon L, *et al.* Mammographic screening and mortality from breast cancer: the Malmo mammographic screening trial. *Br Med J* 1988; **297**:943–948.

60. Andersson I, Janzon L. Reduced breast cancer mortality in women under age 50: updated results from the Malmo Mammographic Screening Program. *J Natl Cancer Inst Monogr* 1997; **22**:63–67.

61. Bjurstam N, Bjorneld L, Duffy SW, *et al.* The Gothenburg Breast Screening Trial. First results on mortality, incidence, and mode of detection for women ages 39–49 years at randomization. *Cancer* 1997; **80**:2091–2099.

62. Frisell J, Lidbrink E, Hellstrom L, Rutqvist L-E. Follow up after 11 years – update of mortality results in the Stockholm mammographic screening trial. *Breast Cancer Res Treat* 1997; **45**:263–270.

63. Alexander FE, Anderson TJ, Brown HK, *et al.* The Edinburgh randomised trial of breast cancer screening: results after 10 years of follow-up. *Br J Cancer* 1994; **70**:542–548.

64. Alexander FE, Anderson TJ, Brown HK, *et al.* 14 years of follow-up from the Edinburgh randomised trial of breast-cancer screening. *Lancet* 1999; **353**:1903–1908.

65. Miller AB, To T, Baines CJ, Wall C. Canadian National Breast Screening Study-2: 13-year results of a randomized trial in women aged 50–59 years. *J Natl Cancer Inst* 2000; **92**:1490–1499.

21

Risk-reducing mastectomy

TIMOTHY I. DAVIDSON AND NIGEL P.M. SACKS

INTRODUCTION

The controversy surrounding the operation of prophylactic mastectomy, usually with immediate reconstruction, has been of interest to surgeons and oncologists for a number of decades but, in recent years, has become highly topical.[1,2] In other areas of cancer management, prophylactic surgery has an established role. For example, in patients with the multiple endocrine neoplasia (MEN 2) syndrome and a mutation in *RET*, prophylactic total thyroidectomy is advocated to avoid the development of medullary thyroid carcinoma.[3] Prophylactic colectomy is routinely advised in patients with familial adenomatous polyposis (FAP) syndrome to avoid the inevitable progression of colonic adenomas to invasive carcinomas;[4] in patients with total ulcerative colitis with severe dysplasia on biopsy, the high risk of large bowel cancer is an additional reason for advising proctocolectomy in severely affected patients.

The role of prophylactic oophorectomy in women at risk of familial ovarian cancer is discussed in greater detail in Chapter 23, but has considerable relevance to breast cancer risk in, for example, woman carrying a *BRCA1* and *BRCA2* mutation. The risk of subsequent breast cancer development in *BRCA1* mutation carriers who undergo bilateral prophylactic oophorectomy has been found to be reduced by 50 per cent.[5] Women at risk of both breast and ovarian cancer will often be faced with the prospect of both prophylactic oophorectomy and mastectomy.

The debate over the role of prophylactic mastectomy in women at high risk of breast cancer spans several issues. The first is identifying which subgroup of women will have an acceptable cost–benefit ratio in relation to subsequent risk of breast cancer to justify offering them surgery. The second centres on the debate regarding which surgical technique should be used, subcutaneous or total mastectomy. The third issue, until recently largely unresolved, is to what extent prophylactic mastectomy can adequately remove all breast tissue and so reduce the risk of subsequent development of invasive breast cancer.

As increasingly robust evidence now emerges that a significant reduction in breast cancer risk can be achieved with surgery of this nature,[6] there is a move to use the term 'risk-reducing mastectomy'. This has the advantage of informing both the woman considering surgery, and the health professionals involved in her counselling both before and after such surgery, that her risk of breast cancer may successfully be reduced by this strategy, but cannot be abolished, whereas the term 'prophylactic mastectomy' may give the erroneous impression that prevention is guaranteed.

It is worthwhile remembering that the practice of subcutaneous mastectomy initially arose as an alternative to the Halsted radical mastectomy. Halsted mastectomy remained the standard operation for carcinoma of the breast until the acceptance of the modified radical mastectomy and, more recently, breast-conserving surgery. It is easy to imagine how a contour-saving operation, which also preserved the nipple–areolar complex, would be welcomed by women with a strong family history or borderline lesions who were in the past at high risk of being disfigured by radical mastectomy should an invasive cancer subsequently be diagnosed. Subcutaneous mastectomy with reconstruction fulfilled this need.

In the past two decades, however, both the cosmetic morbidity and the overall survival following breast cancer treatment has improved dramatically and, even if a mastectomy is necessary for breast cancer, immediate reconstruction with a good cosmetic result is now standard practice. Today, the majority of patients with invasive breast cancer can be treated with breast conservation surgery and will be alive 10 years after diagnosis. This has ironically allowed the procedure of risk-reducing surgery, or bilateral prophylactic mastectomy, to be viewed as a relatively radical surgical option.

INDICATIONS FOR RISK-REDUCING MASTECTOMY

There is, as yet, no consensus among surgeons, oncologists or epidemiologists on the absolute indications for prophylactic mastectomy, nor are firm guidelines likely to be formulated. The most common relative indications arise in women with a genetic predisposition to breast cancer,[6,7] those who have been found on biopsy to harbour specific premalignant proliferative lesions,[8] such as lobular carcinoma in situ or atypical lobular or ductal hyperplasia, and those who have been treated for a contralateral invasive breast carcinoma and who remain concerned about the risk in the untreated breast.

Familial breast cancer

With the awareness of family history as a risk factor in the development of breast cancer, the general practitioner and the breast specialist are both confronted by increased numbers of women who are anxious about their perceived increased risk. In the majority of women, the perceived risk greatly exceeds the actual increase in the odds ratio of developing breast cancer[9] and, after taking a careful family history and performing a clinical breast examination, the majority of women can be reassured in this respect. The relative risk to an individual woman is assessed from the number of members in her family affected by breast cancer, whether they are first- or second-degree relatives, the age at which the relatives were affected and whether the breast cancers were bilateral. Feuer et al., using surveillance, epidemiology and end result (SEER) data from the USA, have tabulated the eventual risk of developing and dying from breast cancer over given time intervals,[10] so that, when counselling women with a family history of breast cancer, some attempt can be made to quantify the degree of risk for an individual patient. It is estimated that 2–5 per cent of

cases of breast cancer are due to an inherited predisposing gene mutation.[11] It is now recognized that proven BRCA1 and BRCA2 mutation gene carriers have a high lifetime risk of developing breast cancer. Work is currently under way on identification of further breast cancer genes[12] (and see Chapter 18).

These data provide a useful basis for counselling those women at risk of familial breast cancer, and who, in considering risk-reducing surgery, wish to evaluate the risk–benefit ratio associated with bilateral prophylactic mastectomy and/or prophylactic oophorectomy.[5,7] In the UK, there is now evidence that women with a known BRCA1 or BRCA2 mutation within their family are increasingly opting for bilateral mastectomy and reconstruction as a risk-reducing strategy.[11] However, even though a large percentage of BRCA1 and BRCA2 mutation carriers will develop breast cancer by the age of 75, some will never do so, and it is inevitable that some women, even in this high-risk group, will be offered and will undergo unnecessary surgery. In addition, a number of breast cancer-predisposing genes remain to be identified, so the currently available genetic testing will not assist all the families with a strong family history of breast cancer.[12]

Management of the contralateral breast

It is important to remember that BRCA1/2 mutation carriers, who develop and are successfully treated for a breast cancer, subsequently face a considerably higher risk of developing contralateral disease than patients treated for sporadic breast cancer. The risk of developing a new primary tumour in the contralateral breast in a woman with primary breast cancer and a hereditary predisposition approaches 35 per cent at 10 years,[13] with a lifetime risk of contralateral disease as high as 64 per cent.[14]

For a woman undergoing breast cancer treatment, the management of the contralateral breast is complicated because the prognosis of the presenting disease has to be taken into consideration. Clearly, the poorer the prognosis as inferred from tumour grade, size, stage and receptor status, the less appropriate radical treatment of the contralateral breast. For a woman at genetic risk of contralateral disease, a recommendation of contralateral mastectomy might seem illogical, if the primary breast cancer management had been with breast conservation surgery to the affected breast. Genetic testing is now widely available to families at risk of an inherited predisposition, and a woman known to have a BRCA1 or BRCA2 mutation in her family, and who subsequently develops breast cancer, may well opt for bilateral mastectomy as the primary surgical procedure, the rationale being to provide treatment of the affected side and prevention on the contralateral side.

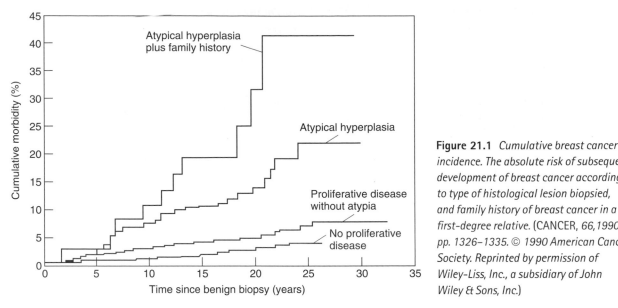

Figure 21.1 *Cumulative breast cancer incidence. The absolute risk of subsequent development of breast cancer according to type of histological lesion biopsied, and family history of breast cancer in a first-degree relative. (CANCER, 66,1990, pp. 1326–1335. © 1990 American Cancer Society. Reprinted by permission of Wiley-Liss, Inc., a subsidiary of John Wiley & Sons, Inc.)*

Borderline or premalignant lesions

The histological factors for subsequent development of breast cancer have in recent years been clarified[8] and borderline lesions can be stratified according to the degree of risk. When proliferative lesions with cellular atypia occur in the presence of a strong family history of breast cancer, this risk becomes disproportionately high (Figure 21.1). It would seem intuitive that, with an increasing postulated relative risk in an individual, the option of risk reducing surgery should be more strongly considered.

However, the problem remains of the threshold risk as *when* to advise surgery. For example, should a woman with a fivefold relative risk of developing breast cancer be counselled to consider prophylactic mastectomy while a woman with relative risk of twofold or threefold that of the age-matched population be counselled against this form of surgery? The ultimate decision to undergo surgery rests with the patient herself after appropriate counselling by the surgeon, geneticist and breast care nurse in the light of all the information available to her (Table 21.1).

SOCIAL ATTITUDES TO RISK-REDUCING MASTECTOMY

In severely affected families in the USA, a significant proportion of relatives at risk of breast cancer have chosen risk-reducing mastectomy. Until recent years, a smaller minority of women in the UK chose this option but, since the introduction of *BRCA1* and *BRCA2* gene mutation testing, there has been a recent rapid rise in interest in risk-reducing surgery on both sides of the Atlantic.[15] The willingness of many North American women to undergo mastectomy for benign breast conditions, such as mastalgia, as well as the large number of women in the US opting for cosmetic breast surgery, may possibly reflect the extent to which these treatment choices are surgeon-led in a society where health care is more radical, and prevention at all costs is more readily pursued and accepted.

One of the most potent arguments in favour of risk-reducing surgery is of course the lack of a proven alternative prevention strategy. In high-risk groups of women, there is scant evidence of substantial long-term overall health benefit from either intensive screening at an earlier age or the use of chemopreventative agents, such as tamoxifen[16] or retinoids.[17]

The breast cancer prevention trial (NSABP-P1) reported a 45 per cent reduction in breast cancer incidence with prophylactic use of tamoxifen.[18] A meta-analysis of several trials has shown a smaller but similar protective effect, but the overall health care benefit is uncertain owing to potential side effects of tamoxifen and the fact that it preferentially prevents hormone-responsive tumours, which would, in any case, have a more favourable prognosis.[19] More worrying is the suggestion that, in young women at risk and in those proven gene carriers, there may be little or no benefit from tamoxifen, particularly for *BRCA1* carriers.[20] While not currently advocated as a chemopreventative agent in breast cancer, the possible use of raloxifene has stimulated considerable interest and may have a future useful role beyond its current indication for prevention of osteoporosis. The role of raloxifene versus tamoxifen is currently being tested in the STAR prospective NIH/NSABP study (see Chapter 22).

The shortcomings of radiological surveillance with mammography in premenopausal women, where mammography detects significantly fewer cancers within dense glandular breast parenchyma, has led to a search for other

Table 21.1 *Factors affecting the relative risk of breast cancer in later life*

Factor	Relative risk
Family history	
Two relatives affected by breast cancer with an average age at diagnosis <40	
One relative with both breast and ovarian cancer at any age	
One or more relatives <50 with breast cancer and Ashkenazi ancestry	
Male breast cancer	>4
Menstrual history	
Age at menarche <12	1.3
Age at menopause 55 with 40 menstrual years	1.5
Pregnancy	
First child after age 35	3
Nulliparous	2–3
Previous benign breast biopsy	2
Atypical lobular hyperplasia	4
Lobular carcinoma *in situ*	7
Contralateral breast cancer	>5

Table 21.2 *Essential components of counselling prior to risk-reducing mastectomy*

Accurate assessment of risk/genetic predisposition including option of genetic testing (many centres have a threshold residual absolute breast cancer risk of 25%)

Full knowledge of all available non-surgical options

Full understanding of the extent of surgery and operative complications

Appreciation of the limitations of breast reconstruction including:

   loss of sensitivity of breasts/nipples

   possible dissatisfaction with cosmesis

   expected durability of implants

Understanding of the likely extent of risk reduction after surgery

screening strategies.[21] A multicentre MRC trial of breast magnetic resonance imaging (MRI) screening in high-risk women in the UK has been initiated to evaluate whether improved detection of early breast cancers with breast MRI can justify the introduction of this expensive, time-consuming and often uncomfortable examination as an alternative (or an adjuvant) to mammography (see Chapter 20). These uncertain measures will be insufficient for some high-risk women who will, therefore, consider prophylactic mastectomy.

It is essential that the patient considering risk-reducing surgery is comprehensively counselled (Table 21.2), and a specialist multidisciplinary team should be available to provide information and evaluate the suitability of women prior to any undertaking of risk reducing surgery.[22] The specialist breast surgeon, breast care nurse, clinical psychologist and clinical geneticist should all be involved in this process, and a formal protocol is recommended.[23] Risk-reducing mastectomy is ideally carried out in units where expertise in these disciplines in concentrated, and there is now a consensus amongst breast specialists that this form of surgery should not be undertaken on an occasional basis by a breast or reconstructive surgeon without the support of this multidisciplinary team. Verification of family history with hospital records, cancer registry data and review of histopathology may be an advisable step to avoid the risk of operating on the rare case of Munchausen's syndrome.[23]

SURGICAL TECHNIQUE

Once the patient who has been considered for risk-reducing surgery has decided to proceed with the operation, the choice needs to be made as to the type of operation that is most appropriate. It must be remembered that the surgical aim is mastectomy with reconstruction and *not* an operation primarily to enhance the appearance of the breast. The goal of preventing subsequent breast cancer in high-risk woman has to be balanced against a good lasting cosmetic result in someone who is, at the time of surgery, usually a young woman with apparently normal breasts, albeit carrying a mutation in a breast cancer predisposition gene. The two surgical options are subcutaneous mastectomy and total mastectomy, with immediate or delayed reconstruction.

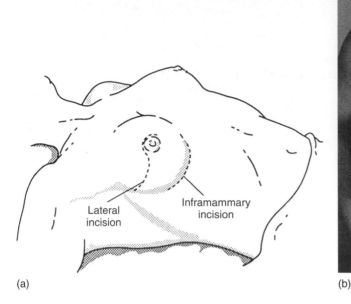

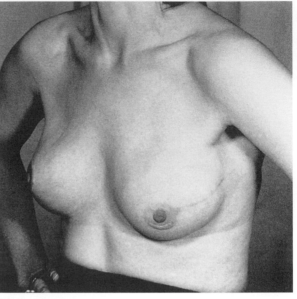

(a)   (b)

Figure 21.2 *(a) Skin incisions for subcutaneous mastectomy showing inframammary and lateral S-shaped incisions. (b) Postoperative appearances following bilateral subcutaneous mastectomy and subpectoral implants via lateral skin incisions.*

While the breast is a subcutaneous organ, the difference between the two operations is largely one of the underlying surgical aim. Subcutaneous mastectomy is an operation designed to remove the underlying breast parenchyma and minimize the subsequent risk of breast cancer development. The aim in total mastectomy on the other hand is to remove *all* the breast tissue, including the ducts within the nipple–areolar complex, with the intent of avoiding any subsequent breast cancer development.

A simple debulking procedure, incorporating thick skin flaps with inevitable retained large islands of breast tissue, has no place as a risk-reducing operation, and is to be condemned. In experimental animals, reduction in the volume of breast tissue does not lead to a reduced risk of breast cancer[24] and attention to surgical technique must be every bit as meticulous when the purpose of surgery is risk reduction, as it is in therapeutic surgery for breast cancer.

Technique for subcutaneous mastectomy

The surgical techniques for subcutaneous mastectomy have been widely reviewed.[25–27] Whether the operation is performed by a general surgeon with an interest in oncological and breast surgery, or by a plastic surgeon with an interest in reconstruction, is immaterial, so long as the operator is well trained in the technical requirements for this demanding operation.

The most appropriate skin incision is dependent to some extent on the size of the breasts. A 10–12 cm inframammary incision may occasionally be adequate in small-sized breasts, but we generally favour an 'S-shaped' incision that skirts around the edge of the areola and extends laterally to allow the operator to clear fully the upper breast quadrants and, in particular, the axillary tail (Figure 21.2). In pendulous breasts that necessitate skin reduction, a skin incision similar to that for reduction mammoplasty can be used (Figure 21.3), but underlying breast tissue must not be left deep to the nipple–areolar complex, which may either be sacrificed or resited as a free nipple graft. Up to one-third of patients may need reduction of the skin envelope to achieve optimal cosmetic results.

From these various incisions, thin skin flaps are dissected off the gland to allow removal of all visible breast tissue. The tissue under the nipple–areolar complex can at the time of surgery be examined histologically for atypical epithelial change to determine whether sacrifice of the nipple would be prudent. Any remaining islands of breast tissue are identified and removed by everting the skin envelope of the breast. Particular care must be taken to include the entire axillary tail of the breast, but axillary node dissection is not appropriate and confers an extra unnecessary morbidity.

Immediate reconstruction involves the fashioning of a submuscular pocket deep to the pectoralis major, serratus anterior and upper rectus abdominis muscles. This may be approached through an oblique incision in the pectoralis major muscle, or between the serratus anterior and pectoralis major muscle laterally. A large pocket is created with blunt dissection and a textured silicone-gel prosthesis is implanted. Anatomical-shaped implants, which provide greater projection in the lower pole of the

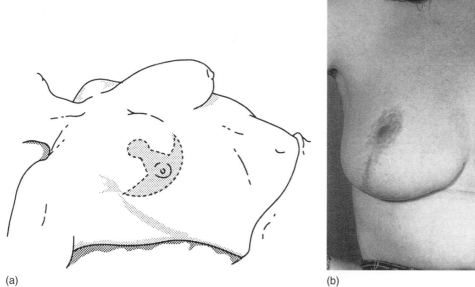

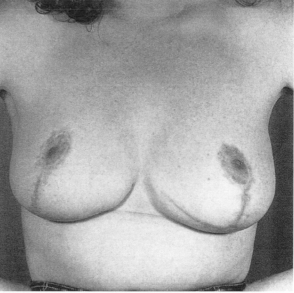

(a)   (b)

Figure 21.3 *(a) Skin incisions for subcutaneous mastectomy with marking pattern as for reduction mammoplasty. (b) Postoperative result following bilateral subcutaneous mastectomy with skin reduction and subpectoral implants.*

breast, may confer a slightly more natural profile to the reconstructed breast. For optimal cosmesis, it is important to position the implant medially and low enough.

In those patients where the volume of the submuscular pocket is not initially adequate, a temporary tissue expander or permanent expander-prosthesis (such as the Becker or McGhan 150 devices) can be used instead of a fixed-volume implant. The volume of this prosthesis can rapidly be increased over a period of weeks by injecting saline via a laterally placed subcutaneous filling port, which is subsequently removed.

To avoid the complications of capsule contracture and implant extravasation associated with subcutaneous placement, it is important that total muscular cover of the implant (or expander) be achieved with subpectoral placement. The use of a latissimus dorsi pedicled muscle flap may provide an alternative method of implant cover and has the advantage of achieving a greater degree of immediate ptosis, particularly when reconstructing the fuller breast. A myocutaneous flap technique with a small skin island can be used for reconstruction with replacement of the nipple–areolar complex following skin sparing mastectomy performed via a circumareolar incision.[28]

Early and long-term complications of subcutaneous mastectomy are not inconsiderable and those reported in a number of series have been reviewed.[29,30] Complications including flap and/or nipple loss, haematoma, implant exposure and infection, have been noted in up to 20 per cent of patients in some series. Some years ago the most frequent long-term complication was capsular contracture secondary to subcutaneous placement of the prosthesis. However, with submuscular placement of the

implant this complication is now very much less common, although displacement of the prosthesis, usually in an upward direction, may occur and need later correction. The use of textured implants has helped to reduce the problems of migration and encapsulation of the implant.

Technique for total mastectomy

With a total mastectomy the entire breast gland is removed, together with a small ellipse of skin bearing the nipple–areolar complex (Figure 21.4), or with a circular skin incision placed 2–3 mm outside the areolar margin to allow maximal skin sparing. The breast tissue, including the axillary tail, is dissected from the skin flaps under direct vision, and the likelihood of leaving residual islands of breast tissue is less than with subcutaneous or skin-sparing mastectomy. Reconstruction of the breast mound is performed in the same way as for subcutaneous mastectomy, with a prosthesis inserted into the submuscular pocket deep to the pectoralis major muscle, or alternatively using the transposed latissimus dorsi muscle to provide total muscular cover for the expander or implant.

Nipple–areola reconstruction can be performed immediately or as a second-stage procedure, and a variety of techniques have been described. Nipple projection is obtained by forming local flaps, such as the skate or tripod flaps in the central areolar area. The areola can be reconstructed using a full thickness skin graft from the inner medial thigh, or a good result can be achieved with careful skin tattooing.

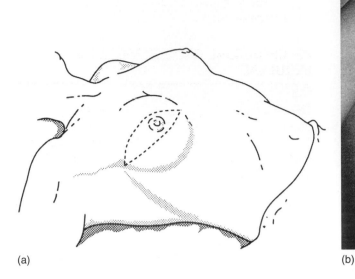

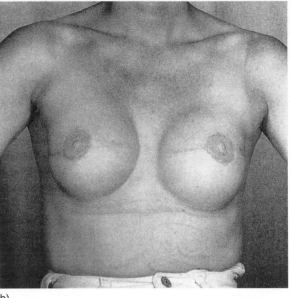

(a) (b)

Figure 21.4 *(a) Skin incision for total mastectomy. (b) Postoperative result following bilateral total mastectomy with subpectoral implants and nipple–areolar complex reconstruction.*

The disadvantages of total mastectomy as opposed to subcutaneous mastectomy include the inevitable shortcomings of the reconstructed nipple with loss of nipple sensation, less nipple projection, and the presence of a central linear mammary scar, which will remain obtrusive. The advantages are more complete clearance of breast tissue, particularly the axillary tail and avoidance of the theoretical risk associated with retention of the nipple–areolar complex.

In the recently updated Mayo Clinic study of 639 moderate and high-risk women,[6] 90 per cent of the patients underwent subcutaneous mastectomy with nipple preservation. Because the number of total mastectomy procedures was small, the study was, therefore, unable to demonstrate a statistical difference between the two techniques with regard to the risk of subsequent cancer development, but no patients developed breast cancer after total mastectomy. However, in the seven patients who went on to develop breast cancer following risk reducing surgery, the tumour occurred more often laterally in the breast than in relation to the retained nipple–areolar complex. We would advocate total mastectomy if the indication was *in situ* lobular or ductal carcinoma (LCIS or DCIS) or if the patient expressed anxiety about the risk of cancer development in the retained nipple–areolar complex.

Following some initial concerns arising from uncontrolled case studies, the whole question of long-term safety of silicone gel implants has now been extensively reviewed in Europe, the UK and North America.[31] This comprehensive review has shown no statistical link between silicone gel and connective tissue diseases, development of breast cancer or other distant complications. In view of this, the Chief Medical Officer has approved their continued use in the UK. The use of fixed-volume silicone gel implants remains restricted in the USA where reconstructive techniques require the use of either saline-filled implants (which have a higher leak rate) or reliance on autologous tissue transfer, such as a TRAM (transverse rectus abdominis muscle) flap.

In both subcutaneous and total mastectomy techniques, delayed reconstruction after a period of several months is an alternative approach to immediate reconstruction, and some patients, having reviewed all the available options, prefer not to undergo reconstruction at all. The cosmetic results of reconstruction are variable even in the hands of expert surgeons and, although excellent results can be achieved, it is important when counselling a woman to show good, average and poor results, so that her expectations from breast reconstruction are realistic. To this end, it is often very helpful for prospective patients to meet and see other women who have undergone risk-reducing mastectomy and reconstruction.

HOW EFFECTIVE IS RISK-REDUCING MASTECTOMY?

Until recently, there has been considerable uncertainty about the efficacy of both subcutaneous and total mastectomy procedures in reducing subsequent breast cancer in high-risk woman. Concerns have been raised about the amount of tissue left behind after subcutaneous mastectomy, assessed in the past as being as high as 10–15 per cent,[26] although other authors assess this figure to be much lower.[25]

Historically, retention of the nipple–areolar complex has been a source of anxiety with regard to possible subsequent breast cancer.[32] Incomplete follow-up data in many large series have meant that, while several reported cases of breast cancer have been documented following prophylactic subcutaneous mastectomy,[33] the incidence was unknown.

Hartmann's study from the Mayo Clinic has provided the most comprehensive data available to date,[6] with evidence of a reduction in both the incidence and mortality of breast cancer of at least 90 per cent following risk-reducing mastectomy (Table 21.3). The women in their study were divided into two groups – high risk and moderate risk – on the basis of family history. A control study of the sisters of the high-risk probands and the Gail model were used to predict the number of breast cancers expected in these two groups in the absence of prophylactic mastectomy. The authors concluded that, in a woman with a high risk of breast cancer on the basis of family history, prophylactic surgery could significantly reduce the incidence of breast cancer.

The surgeon, breast care nurse and genetic counsellor can discuss with the patient considering risk-reducing surgery what extent of risk reduction in her case is likely to be achieved. It should always be borne in mind, however, that many woman will need to undergo surgery to save relatively few lives. In the original Mayo Clinic study, 639 woman underwent surgery and, as a result, two breast cancer deaths were observed instead of the 20 expected. The 621 women who probably underwent unnecessary surgery paid a significant price to save those 18 lives.[2]

Several groups have now published on the efficacy of such surgery in known carriers of mutations in the BRCA1 and BRCA2 genes.[7,34–58] They have shown that both BRCA1 and BRCA2 mutation carriers have about a 90 per cent reduction in risk of breast cancer after prophylactic mastectomy.

PSYCHOSOCIAL AND PSYCHOSEXUAL SEQUELAE

The psychological importance of risk-reducing surgery cannot be overestimated.[34] A woman who is fearful of developing breast cancer, and who may have seen close relatives who have died from the disease, may indeed become mentally crippled by her anxiety and often, not surprisingly, grossly overestimates her own future breast cancer risk. Women at high risk of breast cancer need expert counselling and, likewise, those undergoing prophylactic surgery need psychological support, even after they have accepted the idea of surgery, and have undergone mastectomy and reconstruction. There is little doubt that the inherent psychosexual problems known to be associated with mastectomy can indeed be reproduced by prophylactic mastectomy and reconstruction.[39–41]

Postoperative difficulties in accepting the surgical result, sexual dysfunction, and high levels of depression and anxiety have all been observed following surgery, related in some cases to specific personality characteristics.[41] Among the variables suggested as being of importance in predicting adverse psychological reactions are: previous dissatisfaction after surgery, previous psychiatric treatment and insufficient social support. Previous marital problems, lack of information, vacillation of the woman in her view of risk-reducing surgery and physician initiated discussion of the subject may also be relevant factors.[9]

One year after surgery, the majority of patients rate their marital relations as similar to their preoperative situation, but almost half of patients undergoing subcutaneous mastectomy change their sexual habits regarding

Table 21.3 Bilateral prophylactive mastectomy in 639 moderate and high-risk women (modified from Hartmann et al.[6])

	Moderate risk (n = 425)	High risk (n = 214)
Median age at mastectomy	42	42
Type of mastectomy (%)		
Subcutaneous	90	89
Total	10	11
Subsequent breast cancer (total number)		
Expected	37.4	52.9
Observed	4	3
Risk reduction (%)	89.5	94.3
Breast cancer deaths		
Expected	10.4	19.4
Observed	0	2
Risk reduction (%)	100	89.7

their breasts after surgery. Frost *et al.* have reviewed the long-term satisfaction, and psychological and social function in over 600 patients following bilateral prophylactic mastectomy at the Mayo clinic.[39] Most woman (70 per cent) were satisfied with the procedure, 11 per cent were neutral and 19 per cent were dissatisfied. Two-thirds of respondents said that they would have the procedure again and three-quarters said that the operation had made them worry less about breast cancer. The majority of women reported no change in their levels of self-esteem, sexual relationships and feelings of femininity.

The psychological consequences for women of silicone implants have proved to be of major concern in the USA.[42] While the relationship between silicone-gel prostheses and systemic ill health (in particular, connective tissue disease) has been a major litigation issue in the USA, there is no scientific evidence to implicate implants in many of the disorders postulated. Current guidelines for the use of silicone breast implants in the UK reflect this viewpoint,[31] but individual patient concerns or anxieties about prosthetic implants should always be acknowledged and respected. Websites (e.g. www.facingourrisk.org) now carry a wide range of information, including personal accounts and photographs of women who have already made the difficult decision about risk-reducing mastectomy.

CONCLUSIONS

The concept of risk-reducing surgery is appealing, especially in proven *BRCA1/2* gene mutation carriers who have very few other options of comparable efficacy currently available to them. In practice, risk-reducing mastectomy remains somewhat flawed both in terms of its cosmetic and psychological morbidity, and its ability to guarantee absolute freedom from breast cancer in all patients. The Mayo Clinic study, while demonstrating a reduction in both breast cancer incidence and deaths in the order of 90 per cent, also illustrated the other side of the equation, namely that 639 woman underwent bilateral mastectomy and reconstruction to save an estimated 18 lives during the period of observation.[6] There is no doubt that this form of surgery should be undertaken only by surgeons with the relevant expertise and training in this field, and expert counselling for patients is required at every stage.[43]

The results of ongoing intensive screening and further chemoprevention studies are awaited with great interest and these should prove of major relevance to the role of risk-reducing surgery in high-risk groups of women. Our ability to screen for breast cancer mutations and to identify accurately a subgroup of women at very high risk of developing breast cancer[44] has led to increased acceptance of this procedure as an effective, though undoubtedly radical, strategy for significantly reducing the risk of breast cancer in carefully selected women.

KEY POINTS

- A protocol is recommended for women who request prophylactic mastectomy that involves genetic counselling, confirmation of family history, psychological assessment and careful pre-operative evaluation by both the breast care nurse as well as the surgeon.
- Such surgery should be carried out in units with experience of managing these women.
- Further prospective studies are needed to monitor efficacy and psychosocial effects of risk-reducing mastectomy.

REFERENCES

1. Fentiman IS. Prophylactic mastectomy: deliverance or delusion? *Br Med J* 1998; **317**:1402–1403.
2. Eisen A, Weber BL. Prophylactic mastectomy – the price of fear. *N Engl J Med* 1999; **340**:137–138.
3. Robbins J, Merino MJ, Boice JD Jr, *et al.* Thyroid cancer: a lethal endocrine neoplasm. *Ann Intern Med* 1991; **115**:133.
4. Herrea-Irbelas L. Familial polyposis coli. *Semin Oncol* 1987; **3**:66–139.
5. Rebbeck TR, Levin AM, Eisen A, *et al.* Breast cancer risk after bilateral prophylactic oophorectomy in *BRCA1* mutation carriers. *J Natl Cancer Inst* 1999; **91**:1475–1479.
6. Hartmann LC, Schaid DJ, Woods JE, *et al.* Efficacy of bilateral prophylactic mastectomy in women with a family history of breast cancer. *N Engl J Med* 1999; **340**:77–84.
7. Eisen A, Rebbeck TR, Wood WC, Weber BL. Prophylactic surgery in women with a hereditary predisposition to breast and ovarian cancer. *J Clin Oncol* 2000; **18**:1980–1995.
8. Page DL, Dupont WD. Anatomic markers of human pre-malignancy and breast cancer. *Cancer* 1990; **66**:1326–1335.
9. Fallowfield L, Hatcher MB, Fallowfield L, A'Hern R. The psychosocial impact of bilateral prophylactic mastectomy: prospective study using questionnaires and semistructured interviews. *Br Med J* 2001; **322**:76–79.
10. Fuer JE, Lap-Ming W, Boring C, *et al.* The lifetime risk of developing breast cancer. *J Natl Cancer Inst* 1993; **85**:892–897.
11. Sacks NPM, Gogas H. Familial breast cancer. *Cancer J* 1996, **9**:115–119.
12. Antoniou AC, Pharoah PD, McMullan G, *et al.* Evidence for further breast cancer susceptibility genes in addition to *BRCA1* and *BRCA2* in a population-based study. *Genet Epidemiol.* 2001; **21**:1–18
13. Chabner E, Nixon A, Gelman R, *et al.* Family history and treatment outcomes in young woman after breast conserving surgery and radiation therapy for early-stage breast cancer. *J Clin Oncol* 1998; **16**:2045–2051.

14. Easton D, Ford D, Bishop TD. Breast Cancer Linkage Consortium. Breast and ovarian cancer incidence in *BRCA1* carriers. *Am J Hum Genet* 1995; **56**:265–271.

15. Eisinger F, Geller G, Burke W, Holtzman NA. Cultural basis for differences between US and clinical recommendations for women at increased risk of breast and ovarian cancer. *Lancet* 1999; **353**:1993–2000.

16. Editorial. Is tamoxifen effective in prevention of breast cancer? *Lancet* 1998; **352**:80–81.

17. Veronesi U, De-Palo G, Costa A, *et al*. Chemoprevention of breast cancer with retinoids. *Monogr Natl Cancer Inst* 1992; **12**:93–97.

18. Fisher JB, Costantino JP, Wickerham DL, *et al*. Tamoxifen for prevention of breast cancer: report of the National Surgical Adjuvant Breast and Bowel Project P-I Study. *J Natl Cancer Inst* 1998; **90**:1371–1388.

19. Fisher B, Powles TJ, Pritchand KJ. Current controversies in cancer: tamoxifen for the prevention of breast cancer. *Europ J Cancer* 2000; **36**:142–150.

20. Osin P, Crook T, Powles T, *et al*. Hormone status of *in situ* cancer in *BRCA1/BRCA2* mutation carriers. *Lancet* 1998; **351**:1487.

21. Klijn JGM, Janin N, Cortes-Funes H, Colomer R. Should prophylactic surgery be used in women with a high risk of Breast Cancer. *Eur J Cancer* 1997; **33**:2149–2165.

22. Josephson U, Wickman M, Sandelin K. Initial experiences of women from hereditary breast cancer families after bilateral prophylactic mastectomy: a retrospective study. *Eur J Surg Oncol* 2000; **26**:351–356.

23. Eccles M, Evans DG. Management of the contralateral breast in patients with hereditary breast cancer. *Breast* 2000; **9**:301–305.

24. Wong JH, Jackson CF, Swanson JS, *et al*. Analysis of the risk reduction of prophylactic partial mastectomy in Sprague–Dawley rats with 7,12-dimethylbenzathracene-induced breast cancer. *Surgery* 1986; **99**:67–71.

25. Woods JE. Subcutaneous mastectomy: current state of the art. *Ann Plast Surg* 1983; **11**:541–550.

26. Hobby JA. Plastic surgery techniques for non-malignant breast disease. In: Smallwood JA, Taylor I (eds) *Benign breast disease*. London: Edward Arnold, 1990:155–179.

27. Malata CM, McIntosh SA, Purushotham AD. Immediate breast reconstruction after mastectomy for cancer. *Br J Surg* 2000; **87**:1455–1472.

28. Slavin SA, Schnitt SJ, Duda RB, *et al*. Skin-sparing mastectomy and immediate reconstruction: oncological risks and aesthetic results in patients with early-stage breast cancer. *Plast Reconstr Surg* 1998; **102**:49–62.

29. Slade LC. Subcutaneous mastectomy: acute complications and long-term follow-up. *Plast Reconstr Surg* 1984; **73**:84–88.

30. Fisher J, Maxwell GP, Woods J. Surgical alternatives in subcutaneous mastectomy reconstruction. *Clin Plast Surg* 1988; **15**:667–676.

31. Independent Review Group. *Silicone gel breast implants*. Crown copyright 1998. Cambridge: Jill Rogers Associates.

32. Parry RG, Cochran TC. When is there nipple involvement in carcinoma of the breast? *Plast Reconstr Surg* 1977; **59**:535–537.

33. Pennis VR, Capozzi A. Subcutaneous mastectomy data: a final statistical analysis of 1500 patterns. *Aesth Plast Surg* 1989; **13**:15–21.

34. Meijers-Heijboer EJ, Verhoog LC, Brekelmans CT, *et al*. Presymptomatic DNA testing and prophylactic surgery in families with a *BRCA1* or *BRCA2* mutation. *Lancet* 2000; **355**:2015–2020.

35. Offit K, Robson M, Schrag D. Prophylactic mastectomy in carriers of *BRCA* mutations. *N Engl J Med* 2001; **345**:1498–1499.

36. Hartmann LC, Sellars TA, Schaid DJ, *et al*. Efficacy of bilateral prophylactic mastectomy in *BRCA1* and *BRCA2* gene mutation carriers. *J Natl Cancer Inst* 2001; **93**:1633–1637.

37. Meijers-Heijboer H, Van Geel B, van Patten WLJ, *et al*. Breast cancer after prophylactic bilateral mastectomy in women with a *BRCA1* or *BRCA2* mutation. *N Engl J Med* 2001; **345**:159–164.

38. Rebbeck TR, Friebel T, Lynch HT, *et al*. Bilateral prophylactic mastectomy reduces breast cancer risk in *BRCA1* and *BRCA2* mutation carriers: the PROSE Study Group. *J Clin Oncol*. 2004; **22**:1055–1062.

39. Frost MH, Schaid DJ, Sellers TA, *et al*. Long-term satisfaction and psychological and social function following bilateral prophylactic mastectomy. *JAMA* 2000; **284**:319–324.

40. Stefanek M, Kelzlgauer K, Wilcox P, *et al*. Predictors of satisfaction with bilateral prophylactic mastectomy. *Prev Med* 1995; **24**:412–419.

41. Meyere L, Ringberg A. A prospective study of psychiatric and psychosocial sequelae of bilateral subcutaneous mastectomy. *Scand J Plast Reconstr Surg* 1986; **20**:101–107.

42. Hatcher M, Brooks L, Love C. Breast cancer and silicone implants: psychological consequences for women. *J Natl Cancer Inst* 1993; **85**:1361.

43. Borgen PI, Hill ADK, Tran KN, *et al*. Patient regrets after bilateral prophylactic mastectomy. *Ann Surg Oncol* 1998; **5**:603–606.

44. Phillips KA, Glendon G, Knight JA. Putting the risk of breast cancer in perspective. *N Engl J Med* 1999; **340**:141–144.

22

The role of chemoprevention in breast cancer

PAUL J. ROSS AND TREVOR J. POWLES

INTRODUCTION

Breast cancer affects about one in nine women in the Western world. Consequently, there has been considerable interest in developing strategies to prevent breast cancer. The model of endocrine promotion of breast cancer, in which oestrogen is able to activate the development of a single transformed cell into a clinical cancer, offers an opportunity for chemoprevention by use of antioestrogens, such as tamoxifen.

For women at high risk of breast cancer because of a positive family history, the issue of chemoprevention is particularly important. In healthy women at very high risk because of proven germline *BRCA1* or *BRCA2* gene mutations, randomized clinical trials may be unacceptable and they may need to be offered mastectomy and/or oophorectomy. Generally, it would be more acceptable to evaluate all preventative interventions in prospective randomized clinical trials and, for healthy women at a lesser risk, randomized trials of tamoxifen for chemoprevention have been underway for nearly 15 years.[1]

EXPERIMENTAL AND CLINICAL RATIONALE FOR TAMOXIFEN USE

Tamoxifen is an antioestrogen that inhibits the oestrogen-dependent proliferation of MCF7 cells *in vitro*.[2] Furthermore, in rats and mice, tamoxifen will inhibit the promotion by oestrogen of mammary tumours.[3,4] It also has *in vitro* agonist properties and is able to stimulate proliferation in suitably developed MCF7 cell lines in the absence of oestrogen.

In vivo, tamoxifen has been shown to prevent the development of experimental hormone dependent tumours, but has an agonist effect on bones and lipid metabolism.[3] Tamoxifen has been used for the treatment of advanced breast cancer since 1971[5] and as adjuvant therapy in women with primary breast cancers since 1974. Three randomized trials demonstrated a reduction in the risk of a cancer in the contralateral breast from adjuvant therapy with tamoxifen following primary surgery of breast cancer.[6–8] A meta-analysis of all adjuvant clinical trials has indicated a 47 per cent reduction in the risk of contralateral breast cancer when adjuvant tamoxifen was continued for 5 years ($p < 0.00001$).[9] This endorses the rationale for studying tamoxifen as a possible chemopreventive agent for breast cancer in healthy women at increased risk of the disease.

DURATION OF TREATMENT AND DOSAGE

Animal carcinogenesis experiments, together with epidemiological data of cancer incidence in Japan after the nuclear bomb explosions in 1945, indicate that breast cancer in humans may have a latent period of 10–30 years. The incidence of breast cancer in the Western world peaks at about 55 years and continues through to old age, indicating that much of the initiation and promotion of breast cancer occurs at or before the menopause when oestrogen levels are relatively high. This suggests that endocrine intervention should begin prior to the menopause.

In vivo data indicate that tamoxifen may only be cytostatic and halt tumour development for as long as the drug is used. However, clinical adjuvant data indicate that reduction in risk of relapse continues beyond 5 years, even when tamoxifen was used for only about 1 year.[9] A similar effect may occur in endocrine promotion of breast cancer and hence, at present, it would be best to administer tamoxifen for at least 5 years in order to maximize any possible preventive effect.

The issue of tamoxifen dosage may be critical in considering the overall health benefit, if this strategy is effective in reducing the incidence of breast cancer. It can be assumed that both acute side effects and long-term risks will be less at a dose of 10 mg/day than with 20 mg/day, and trials are planned to evaluate this dose in a chemoprevention setting. However, at the present time, the therapeutic dose of 20 mg/day has been used in chemoprevention trials.

TAMOXIFEN CHEMOPREVENTION TRIALS
(Table 22.1)

The Royal Marsden tamoxifen chemoprevention trial was a feasibility study to determine whether it was possible to use such an intervention in healthy women. Women at increased risk owing to a moderate/strong family history were eligible for this double-blind placebo-controlled study. The eligibility criteria included at least one first-degree relative aged less than 50 years with breast cancer, or one first-degree relative with bilateral breast cancer, or one affected first-degree relative of any age plus another affected first- or second-degree relative. Women with a history of a benign breast biopsy who had a first-degree relative with a breast cancer were also eligible. An initial analysis published in 1989 confirmed that tamoxifen had selective antioestrogenic activity with reduced serum cholesterol and prevention of bone mineral density loss in postmenopausal women. These findings encouraged the commencement of multicentre trials including the National Surgical Adjuvant Breast and Bowel Project (NSABP) P-1 trial in 1992; the Italian National Cancer Institute trial and the International Breast Cancer Intervention Study (IBIS), both in 1993.

In 1998, the NSABP P-1 trial, which included 13 000 women at risk of breast cancer, reported a 49 per cent reduction in the incidence of invasive breast cancer in the 6881 women randomized to tamoxifen compared to the 6707 women randomized to placebo ($p < 0.00001$).[10]

In addition, there was a 50 per cent reduction in the incidence of non-invasive ductal breast cancer with tamoxifen ($p < 0.002$). This effect was considered sufficient to stop the trial, unblind the randomization and offer tamoxifen to all participants on placebo. Publication of this finding initiated a debate on the significance of this reduction in breast cancer incidence in the context of long-term health benefit.

The eligibility criteria for the P-1 trial were based on the Gail model,[11] indicating at least a 1.66 per cent 5-year projected risk of breast cancer, or a previous history of lobular carcinoma *in situ* (LCIS). All categories of risk within the Gail model based on age, previous benign histology and family history of breast cancer appeared to benefit. The greatest benefit was observed in women who have a previous benign histology of atypical hyperplasia (relative risk 0.14) and LCIS (relative risk 0.44). The reduction in early breast cancer incidence for participants defined by the Gail model, excluding atypical hyperplasia or LCIS, was about 40 per cent.

Concerns about the application of the P-1 results to all risk groups of healthy women arose from the interim results of the smaller Royal Marsden and Italian breast cancer chemoprevention trials. The Royal Marsden trial reported 34 breast cancers in 1238 women on tamoxifen compared to 36 breast cancers in the 1233 women randomized to placebo.[12] The Italian trial observed 19 breast cancers in tamoxifen-treated women compared to 22 in women receiving placebo amongst the 5408 women randomized within this study.[13] Although considerably smaller than the P-1 trial, it is unlikely that lack of power, low compliance or use of hormone replacement therapy contributed significantly to these negative results. It has been suggested that difference in the results of the three trials may relate to differences in risk characteristics of participants in the US trial compared to the two European trials.[14] The inclusion criteria for the Royal Marsden trial make it more likely that participants have a genetic predisposition to breast cancer due to genes that could predispose, at least in part, to tamoxifen resistance. In the Italian trial, 74 per cent of women had undergone oophorectomy at the time of hysterectomy, which could have compromised any subsequent tamoxifen effect. The negative results at that time, therefore, indicated that there may be subgroups of healthy women in whom tamoxifen will not reduce the early incidence of breast cancer.

In the Royal Marsden trial, about 30 per cent of women were likely to have inherited a breast cancer predisposition gene according to the Claus model. In the NSABP P-1 trial, risk factors as defined by the Gail model were less likely to indicate genetic risk.[11] Furthermore, some non-genetic risk factors, such as LCIS and atypical hyperplasia, used as entry criteria in the NSABP P-1 trial, are likely to indicate endocrine sensitivity. In contrast, in genetically inherited breast cancers, loss or aberration of

Table 22.1 *Summary of the randomized tamoxifen chemoprevention of breast cancer trials*

Trial name (reference)	Number of women	Age limit (years)	Breast cancer risk criteria for entry	Previous LCIS or ADH	% post menopausal	Use of HRT	Median follow-up (months)	Total no. of breast cancers (relative risk and confidence intervals) Placebo Tam	Comments
NSABP-P1[10]	13 388	>34	Gail estimated risk of 1.66% over 5 years or previous LCIS	17%	61%	No	69	124 (RR 0.51, CI 0.39–0.66)	Most benefit for LCIS and ADH. Reduction in fractures
Italian National Trial[13,18]	5408	35–70	Hysterectomy (74% had also had an ovariectomy) with no special risk factors for breast cancer	0%	NA	Yes	94	34 (RR 0.76, CI 0.47–1.60)	Only women taking HRT had a significant benefit
Royal Marsden Trial[1,2]	2494	30–70	Estimated age adjusted fourfold risk based on family history	0%	34%	Yes	120	62 (RR 0.83, CI NA)	66% premenopausal higher proportion of women in families likely to harbour a breast cancer predisposition gene
International Breast Intervention Study[19]	7140	35–70	Estimated age adjusted 2–3-fold risk based on family history and other factors	5%	49.9%	Yes	50	68 (RR 0.67, CI 0.49–0.91)	Lesser effect than NSABPP-1, especially for invasive cancers

ADH, atypical ductal hyperplasia; CI, confidence interval; HRT, hormone replacement therapy; LCIS, lobular carcinoma *in situ*; NA, not applicable; RR, relative risk.

oestrogen receptor function may occur earlier in the carcinogenic process than in sporadic cancers,[15] resulting in tamoxifen resistance or even tamoxifen-stimulated proliferation.[14] However, this hypothesis could imply that tamoxifen could still prevent development of these breast cancers if given early enough in the carcinogenic process. This raised the possibility that a reduction in long-term breast cancer incidence could be observed with further follow-up in the Royal Marsden trial.

The beneficial effect of tamoxifen on early breast cancer incidence in the P-1 trial was similar in participants with one, two or more affected relatives. However, a full pedigree analysis was not undertaken. Consequently, it is not possible to predict the likelihood of these groups carrying a high-risk breast cancer gene. This means that continued accrual and follow-up of the European trials are needed in order to further define groups, who may or may not benefit from tamoxifen chemoprevention.

ADVERSE EFFECTS OF TAMOXIFEN AND THE OVERALL HEALTH BENEFIT

At the time of reporting the NSABP P-1 trial, there was a balance of risks and benefits. The risk of pulmonary embolus and deep vein thrombosis was significantly increased in the tamoxifen group, for the most part in women over 50 years of age. Cerebrovascular events were also increased in women receiving tamoxifen therapy. Women who received tamoxifen had a 2.5-fold increased relative risk of endometrial cancer compared with women who received placebo. Invasive cancers at sites other than breast and endometrium were equally distributed. In particular, no liver cancers occurred in either group and there was no increase in the incidence of colon, rectal, ovarian or other genitourinary tumours. Osteoporotic fragility fractures were reduced 19 per cent in women who received tamoxifen compared to placebo. In spite of previous reports of a favourable effect of tamoxifen on the lipid profile,[16] no reduction in events related to ischaemic heart disease was observed. There was an increase in the incidence of cataracts and cataract surgery and in the incidence of vasomotor symptoms. Overall, it is difficult to summate all of these potentially beneficial and adverse effects of tamoxifen in order to make a prediction of the overall health benefit. At this time, it is even more difficult to predict how the risk–benefit ratio of tamoxifen chemoprevention in healthy women will alter with longer follow-up. This is particularly important because the 86 fewer breast cancers were all oestrogen-receptor positive, mostly less than 2 cm in diameter, and axillary node negative, indicating an 80–90 per cent curability.

A further problem relates to the lack of evidence indicating a survival advantage by taking tamoxifen in the NSABP P-1 trial.[1] At the time of reporting, the number of deaths was small, and the unblinding and offered crossover of the NSABP P-1 study at this time has rendered it impossible to evaluate mortality data from this study in the future. Long-term mortality data will now only become available from the continued follow-up of other placebo-controlled tamoxifen chemoprevention studies. The Italian trial initially showed no risk reduction for breast cancer[13] but, with longer follow-up, it now shows a marginal benefit that occurs predominantly in women on hormone replacement therapy (HRT).[17] The Italian trial only recruited women who had a hysterectomy, and most of these women had also had their ovaries removed. The incidence of breast cancer in this trial was therefore low, so it was only those women who had an increased breast cancer risk due to HRT that received the preventative benefit of tamoxifen. The IBIS trial found a significant risk reduction for breast cancer, particularly for non-invasive cancers though the risk reduction was smaller than in the NSABP P-1 study.[19] The participants in the IBIS trial had a low likelihood of inheriting a breast cancer predisposition gene and had not, for the most part, had their ovaries removed. Toxicity in the IBIS trial was similar to that in the other reported trials, with a twofold increase in endometrial cancer and a 2.6-fold increase in the incidence of venous thrombosis and pulmonary embolus. There was no observed increase in cardiac events, but there was a significant increase in deaths for women on tamoxifen ($p = 0.01$), not obviously related to tamoxifen toxicity.

An overview meta-analysis of the four tamoxifen breast cancer prevention trials has recently been undertaken to review the main outcomes of breast and endometrial cancer incidence, vascular events and mortality.[19] The combined data indicate a decrease in the overall relative risk (RR) for breast cancer of about 40 per cent (RR 0.61, 95 per cent confidence interval (CI) 0.52–0.71). For the development of oestrogen receptor (ER)-positive cancers, the RR was 0.50 (CI 0.40–0.63), whereas for ER-negative cancers, the RR was 1.16 (CI 0.84–1.60), indicating that tamoxifen was only effective for preventing the development of ER-positive cancers after this short follow-up time. It is possible that some breast cancers start as ER-positive but become ER-negative during development, by which time tamoxifen would be ineffective at prevention. The meta-analysis confirms an increase in endometrial cancer events (RR 2.4, CI 1.5–4.0) and thromboembolic events (RR 1.8, CI 1.4–2.4), but not in cardiovascular events. Overall, there was no effect on mortality (RR 0.91, CI 0.70–1.18), although there have been very few breast cancer deaths so far. From these data and from the mortality data from the very large breast cancer treatment trials[9] it seems unlikely that non-cancer deaths are increased by tamoxifen.

In conclusion, many women, especially in North America, may consider the reduction in early incidence of breast cancer worth the risk of taking tamoxifen, even though there is no evidence of an overall health or survival benefit.[20] The drug has, therefore, been approved by the FDA for *reduction in the early incidence* of breast cancer for use in the USA. In Europe, the licensing authorities have not approved the use of tamoxifen in healthy women at this time and trial follow-up continues.

CHEMOPREVENTION USING SELECTIVE OESTROGEN-RECEPTOR MODULATORS

Consequent to the detrimental side effects of tamoxifen, particularly on the endometrium, other agents with a spectrum of oestrogenic and antioestrogenic activity on various tissues of the body have been sought. One such selective oestrogen-receptor modulator (SERM) is raloxifene. Experimentally raloxifene has been shown *in vivo* to be antioestrogenic on breast and uterus, but oestrogenic for bone and lipid profiles.[4,21,22] A double-blind placebo-controlled trial of raloxifene (at 60 mg or 120 mg/day) involving 12 512 healthy postmenopausal women at increased risk of osteoporosis owing to reduced bone mineral density (Multiple Outcomes of Raloxifene Evaluation or MORE trial) demonstrated a reduced risk of osteoporotic fragility fractures.[23] Participants in this trial had biannual mammography in order to evaluate a secondary endpoint of breast cancer incidence. An interim analysis with a median follow-up of 40 months showed a 76 per cent reduction in the early incidence of breast cancer in women on raloxifene compared to placebo ($p < 0.001$).[24] Further analysis revealed that raloxifene reduced the incidence of ER-positive, but not ER-negative breast cancer. In contrast to tamoxifen, raloxifene did not result in a significant increase in the incidence of endometrial cancer relative to placebo, but it was associated with an increased incidence of vasomotor symptoms and thromboembolic events. Although breast cancer incidence was not a primary endpoint in this trial and, therefore, cannot be used at this time for licensing raloxifene for use for chemoprevention of breast cancer, the result is very encouraging and was the basis for the NSABP starting the Study of Tamoxifen versus Raloxifene (STAR) trial. This trial aims to recruit 22 000 healthy women in a randomized comparison of raloxifene with tamoxifen. The primary endpoints for this study will be breast cancer incidence and toxicity. The clear evidence from these prevention trials is that tamoxifen and raloxifene have differential oestrogenic or antioestrogenic effects on different tissues, and that these effects can change with time and exposure to oestrogen. An ideal SERM should be able to reduce the risk of breast cancer, osteoporosis, cardiovascular disease, vasomotor symptoms, uterine prolapse, urinary incontinence,

loss of cognitive function and possibly Alzheimer's disease without increasing the risk of thromboembolism or carcinogenesis. An alternative approach would be to use drugs to block the production of oestrogen in the body.

In addition to raloxifene, the use of other SERMs for breast cancer chemoprevention is being studied. Toremifene, a synthetic tamoxifen analogue, has been used as adjuvant treatment for primary breast cancer and for the treatment of advanced breast cancer. Its efficacy is similar to tamoxifen, but it may have a better effect on bone mineral density and it may also reduce cholesterol with a possible added benefit over tamoxifen on the cardioprotective lipid profile.[25] Its effects on the endometrium have not been fully evaluated. The Royal Marsden has, therefore, commenced a small pilot studying the spectrum of activity of evaluating toremifene in healthy women.

AROMATASE INHIBITORS

Clinical trials have shown that the third-generation aromatase inhibitors, such as letrozole and anastrozole, are sufficiently powerful inhibitors of oestrogen synthesis to produce undetectable levels of circulating oestrogen.[26] They have also been shown to be more effective than tamoxifen for treatment of metastatic or locally advanced breast cancer.[27–30] Similarly, when used after surgery for treatment of operable breast cancer, anastrozole was shown to be more effective than tamoxifen or a combination of the two drugs at reducing both relapse and the risk of developing a new breast cancer.[31] These results strongly indicate that the therapeutic activity of tamoxifen is impeded by its oestrogenic activity, even when used in combination with an aromatase inhibitor. It is, therefore, likely that, for chemoprevention, an aromatase inhibitor will be more active than tamoxifen. However, although more efficacious, the side effects for an aromatase inhibitor may be substantially greater than for tamoxifen in healthy women who are treated for many years. The very low circulating and tissue levels of oestrogen that are achieved with aromatase inhibitors, such as anastrozole or letrozole, are unique in biology, and long-term medication might give rise to adverse effects on the brain, pelvic floor, cardiovascular system, the bones and other tissues. Only a few thousand women have received these drugs for a relatively short follow-up period compared with the millions of women who have received tamoxifen over the last 30 years. An increased fracture rate has already been reported with arimidex.[31]

A SERM such as raloxifene that has less oestrogenic activity than tamoxifen may also be more active than tamoxifen for preventing breast cancer, but may still retain some of the beneficial oestrogenic properties on bone and the heart. Newer SERMs, such as lasofoxifene or arzoxifene, are under evaluation in clinical trials and may have a better spectrum of activity than raloxifene. Whether an aromatase inhibitor or a SERM will prove to be better for chemoprevention of breast cancer will depend on the results of the next generation of prevention trials.

In order to develop the concept of prevention of multiple diseases in women further by the use of SERMS or aromatase inhibitors, it is necessary to explore the mechanisms of how the oestrogen receptor functions.

In the USA, the NSABP are now accruing to the 22 000 women P2 trial, directly comparing the efficacy and toxicity of tamoxifen with raloxifene but no placebo in healthy women at a similar risk to P1. In the UK, the proposed IBIS II trial will probably compare anastrozole with placebo in women at similar risk to IBIS I. A direct comparison of raloxifene with an aromatase inhibitor is needed. There are other proposals for evaluating newer SERMs, such as lasofoxifene, in a prevention setting. It is also essential that the phenotypic and genetic risk factors that predispose to oestrogen promoted breast cancer are identified in order to maximize the benefit versus toxicity ratio and obviate the need to treat everybody. The trials must address this issue by more clearly defining risk groups, including phenotypic features of risk, such as breast density, and by undertaking carefully planned genetic research. Unless these questions are answered, the exciting possibility that breast cancer could substantially be prevented will never be a reality.

KEY POINTS

- The results of the NSABP P-1 trial have shown a 49 per cent reduction in the early incidence of breast cancer in healthy women at risk, as defined by the Gail model, and who are given tamoxifen.
- At the present time, no overall health benefit or improvement in survival from tamoxifen chemoprevention has been shown.
- Other trials also now show a reduction in incidence of breast cancer with tamoxifen chemoprevention; however, at present, it is unclear which subgroups of women will have greater benefit than others.
- Early data suggest that tamoxifen chemoprevention may be more effective in *BRCA2* rather than *BRCA1* mutation carriers and also may only prevent oestrogen receptor-positive tumours.
- In the UK, the proposed IBIS II trial will compare anastrozole with placebo in women at similar risk to IBIS I and who are postmenopausal.
- A direct comparison of raloxifene with an aromatase inhibitor is needed. There are other proposals for evaluating newer SERMs in a prevention setting.
- It is essential that the phenotypic and genetic risk factors that predispose to oestrogen promoted

breast cancer are identified in order to maximize the benefit versus toxicity ratio and obviate the need to treat everyone. The trials must address this issue by more clearly defining risk groups, including phenotypic features of risk, such as breast density, and by undertaking carefully planned genetic analyses using family history and genotypic data.

- In the USA, tamoxifen is licensed for breast cancer chemoprevention in healthy women, with at least a 1.66 per cent risk over 5 years of developing breast cancer. In Europe, the consensus remains that healthy women should not be offered tamoxifen chemoprevention outside of a clinical trial, until a significant health benefit or survival advantage has been demonstrated.
- It is essential that follow-up of the Royal Marsden trial, and accrual and follow-up of the IBIS trial continue. It may be possible to have an overview meta-analysis of all trials in 2005, in order to identify the long-term effects of tamoxifen on incidence and mortality. Such an analysis may also help define which subgroups of healthy at risk benefit from tamoxifen chemoprevention.
- Continued follow up of the MORE trial will be important, as will accrual and follow-up of the STAR trial.
- New initiatives will continue to be needed, including evaluation of new SERMs as they become available.
- The role of endocrine agents without agonist effects on the breast including luteinizing hormone-releasing hormone agonists, aromatase inhibitors, and pure oestrogen antagonists will need evaluation.
- In future, it will be important that trials can clearly show an overall health benefit and/or survival benefit before recommending widespread use in healthy women in the general population.

REFERENCES

1. Powles T, Hardy J, Ashley S, et al. A pilot trial to evaluate the acute toxicity and feasibility of tamoxifen for prevention of breast cancer. *Br J Cancer* 1989; **60**:126–131.
2. Lippman M, Bolan G, Huff K. The effects of androgens and antiandrogens on the hormone-responsive human breast cancer in long-term tissue culture. *Cancer Res* 1976; **36**:4595–4601.
3. Jordan V. Effect of tamoxifen (ICI 46 474) on initiation and growth of DMBA-induced rat mammary carcinomata. *Eur J Cancer* 1976; **12**:419–425.
4. Gottardes M, Jordan V. Antitumour actions of keoxifene and tamoxifen in the N-nitrose-methylurea-induced rat mammary carcinoma model. *Cancer Res* 1987; **47**:4020–4024.
5. Ward H. Anti-oestrogen therapy for breast cancer. A trial of tamoxifen at low dose levels. *Br Med J* 1973; **i**:13.

6. Rutquist L, Cedermark B, Glas U, *et al*. Contralateral primary tumours in breast cancer patients in a randomized trial of adjuvant tamoxifen therapy. *J Natl Cancer Inst* 1991; **83**:1299–1306.

7. Fisher B, Redmond C. New perspective on cancer of the contralateral breast: a marker for assessing tamoxifen as a preventive agent. *J Natl Cancer Inst* 1991; **83**:1278–1280.

8. Party CABTW. Cyclophosphamide and tamoxifen therapy as adjuvant therapies in the management of breast cancer. *Br J Cancer* 1988; **57**:604–607.

9. Group EBCTC. Tamoxifen for early breast cancer: an overview of the randomised trials. *Lancet* 1998; **351**:1451–1467.

10. Fisher B, Costantino J, Wickerham D, *et al*. Tamoxifen for prevention of breast cancer: report of the National Surgical Adjuvant Breast and Bowel Project P-1 Study. *J Natl Cancer Inst* 1998; **90**:1371–1388.

11. Gail M, Brintom L, Byar D, *et al*. Projecting individualised probabilities of developing breast cancer for white females who are examined annually. *J Natl Cancer Inst* 1989; **81**:1879–1886.

12. Powles T, Eeles R, Ashley S, *et al*. Interim analysis of the incidence of breast cancer in the Royal Marsden Hospital tamoxifen randomised chemoprevention trial. *Lancet* 1998; **352**:98–101.

13. Veronesi U, Maisonneuve P, Costa A, *et al*. Prevention of breast cancer with tamoxifen: preliminary findings from the Italian randomised trial among hysterectomised women. Italian Tamoxifen Prevention Study. *Lancet* 1998; **352**:93–97.

14. Powles T. Re: Tamoxifen for prevention of Breast cancer: report of the National Surgical Adjuvant Breast and Bowel Project P-1 Study [letter]. *J Natl Cancer Inst* 1999; **91**:730.

15. Osin P, Crook T, Powles T, *et al*. Hormone status of an *in situ* cancer in *BRCA1/BRCA2* mutation carriers. *Lancet* 1998; **351**:1487.

16. Love R, Newcomb P, Wiebe D, *et al*. Effects of tamoxifen on lipid and lipoprotein levels in postmenopausal patients with node-negative breast cancer. *J Natl Cancer Inst* 1990; **82**:1327–1332.

17. Veronesi U, Maisonneuve P, Sacchini V, *et al*. Tamoxifen for breast cancer among hysterectomised women. *Lancet* 2002; **359**:1122–1124.

18. IBIS Working Party and Principal Investigators. First results from the IBIS Breast Cancer Prevention Trial. *Lancet* 2002; **360**:817–824.

19. Cusick J, Powles T, Veronesi U, *et al*. Overview of the main outcomes in breast-cancer prevention trials. *Lancet* 2003; **361**:296–300.

20. Chlebowski R, Collyar D, Somerfield M, *et al*. American Society of Clinical Oncology: Technology assessment on breast cancer risk reduction strategies: tamoxifen and raloxifene. *J Clin Oncol* 1999; **17**:1939–1995.

21. Black L, Jones C, Falcone J. Antagonism of estrogen action with new benzothiophene derived antiestrogen. *Life Sci* 1983; **11**:835–842.

22. Draper M, Flowers D, Huster W, *et al*. A controlled trial of raloxifene (LY 139481) HCl: impact on bone turnover and serum lipid profile in healthy postmenopausal women. *J Bone Miner Res* 1997; **11**:835–842.

23. Delmas P, Bjarnason N, Mitlak B, *et al*. Effects of raloxifene on bone mineral density, serum cholesterol concentrations, and uterine endometrium in postmenopausal women. *N Engl J Med* 1997; **337**:1641–1647.

24. Cummings S, Eckert S, Krueger K, *et al*. The effect of raloxifene on risk of breast cancer in postmenopausal women. Results from the MORE randomized trial. *JAMA* 1999; **281**:2189–2197.

25. Saarto T, Blomqvist C, Ehnholm C, *et al*. Antiatherogenic effects of adjuvant antiestrogens: A randomized trial comparing the effects of tamoxifen and toremifene on plasma lipid levels in postmenopausal women with node–positive breast cancer. *J Clin Oncol* 1996; **14**:429–433.

26. Bonneterre J, Thurlimann B, Robertson J. Anastrozole versus tamoxifen as first-line therapy for advanced breast cancer in 668 postmenopausal women: results of the tamoxifen or arimidex randomised group efficacy and tolerability study. *J Clin Oncol* 2000; **18**:3748–3757.

27. Goss P, Strasser K. Aromatase inhibitors in the treatment and prevention of breast cancer. *J Clin Oncol* 2001; **19**:881–894.

28. Nabholtz J, Budzar A, Pollack M. Anastrozole is superior to tamoxifen as first-line therapy for advanced breast cancer in post-menopausal women: results of a North American multicenter randomised trial. *J Clin Oncol* 2000; **18**:3758–3767.

29. Mourisden H, Gershanovich M, Sun Y. Superior efficacy of letrozole versus tamoxifen as first-line therapy for postmenopausal women with advanced breast cancer: results of a phase III study of the International Letrozole Breast Cancer Group. *J Clin Oncol* 2001; **19**:2596–2606.

30. McDonnell D, Clemm D, Hermann T. Analysis of oestrogen receptor function *in vitro* reveals at least three distinct classes of antioestrogens. *Mol Endocrinol* 1995; **9**:659–668.

31. ATAC Trialists' Group. Anastrozole alone or in combination with tamoxifen versus tamoxifen alone for adjuvant treatment of postmenopausal women with early breast cancer: first results of the ATAC randomised trial. *Lancet* 2002; **359**:2131–2139.

23

Familial ovarian cancer: genetics and management

PAUL D.P. PHAROAH AND BRUCE A.J. PONDER

INTRODUCTION

Ovarian cancer, like most common cancers, tends to cluster in families, a fact that has been recognized since Roman times. Mendelian transmission of ovarian cancer in families was first described in the 1950s and, during the 1960s and 1970s, a variety of hereditary cancer syndromes were defined, including the Lynch syndrome[1] and the Hereditary Breast Ovarian Cancer Syndrome,[2] which include ovarian cancer as part of the characteristic phenotype. Since then, the genetic basis for many of these families has been identified.

In this chapter, we review the literature quantifying the risks associated with a family history of ovarian cancer and assess the evidence that this familial clustering of ovarian cancer is genetically determined. We describe the known susceptibility genes and their contribution to ovarian cancer in families and in the general population. The evidence for the existence of other ovarian cancer genes is then considered, followed by a summary of the results of the published case-control studies of polymorphisms in candidate low-penetrance ovarian cancer susceptibility genes. In the final section, we consider the options for risk management in women at increased risk because of a family history and propose a framework for the management of these women.

FAMILIAL RISK OF OVARIAN CANCER

A large body of epidemiological data has shown that a family history of ovarian cancer in a first-degree relative is associated with an increased risk of ovarian cancer. A meta-analysis using data from 15 case-control and cohort studies has estimated that, compared to the general population, the relative risk of developing ovarian cancer for women with a single first-degree relative affected with ovarian cancer is 3.1 (95 per cent confidence interval (CI) 2.6–3.7).[3] Based on ovarian cancer incidence rates typical in northern Europe and north America, this risk equates to a cumulative risk of 4 per cent by age 70. The relative risk estimate represents an average across all ages, but there is some evidence that the familial risk declines with the age of the at-risk woman and with the age at which the relative was affected. Auranen et al. reported that the relative risk of ovarian cancer in sisters of a woman diagnosed with ovarian cancer before age 55 was 5.2 compared with 3.6 for sisters of women diagnosed after the age of 55, although this difference was not statistically significant.[4] Similarly, the relative risk for women aged under 50 was 5.1 compared to 3.4 for older women.

The evidence for the magnitude of the familial risks associated with a family history of more than one affected relative is less extensive. Three studies have estimated the ovarian cancer risk in women with two or more affected relatives, but these estimates have had wide confidence limits.[5–7] Easton et al. used data from a population-based cohort study of women with two first-degree relatives with confirmed ovarian cancer and found the relative risk of death from ovarian cancer to be 24 (CI 6.6–62).[5] Another population-based study estimated the relative risk of developing ovarian cancer to be 2.1 (0.20–13) for women with two affected relatives, using a case–control study design.[6] The third published study used data from the UKCCCR Familial Ovarian Cancer Register to obtain risk estimates for ovarian and breast cancer in women from 316 families with at least two first-degree relatives with ovarian cancer.[7] A cohort of unaffected women in these families was followed for up to 8 years, and the number of observed incident cancers compared with the number expected based on national-, age-, sex- and period-specific incidence rates for England and Wales. The average relative risk of ovarian cancer was found to be 7.2 (CI 3.8–12), declining from 16 (6.4–33) in women under 50 to 4.4 (1.6–9.5) in women 50 years of age and older. This corresponds to an absolute risk of ovarian cancer by age 70 of 11 per cent.

GENETIC MODELS OF OVARIAN CANCER SUSCEPTIBILITY

In principle, the familial aggregation of cancer may be the result of genetic or non-genetic factors that are shared within families. Twin studies compare the concordance of cancer between monozygotic and dizygotic twins, and provide some information on the relative importance of the two alternatives. The largest twin study of ovarian cancer included data on nearly 10 000 pairs of twins.[8] The ovarian cancer risk to a monozygotic twin of an affected woman was found to be increased by sixfold, which is twice the sibling risk. This is what would be expected if most of the excess familial risk were due to genetic factors, rather than shared environmental factors.

Genetic models to explain familial aggregation can be formally tested using segregation analysis. This involves a detailed mathematical modelling of the patterns of transmission of disease within families. However, the result of any segregation analysis is likely to reflect the effects of several susceptibility genes within a population, given that it is unlikely that all familial ovarian cancer is due to a single gene. Furthermore, susceptibility gene frequencies may differ between populations. These problems may explain the different results reported by the two published segregation analyses of ovarian cancer. Houlston et al. analysed 462 pedigrees ascertained through an unaffected relative. They found the observed pattern of ovarian cancer was compatible with an autosomal dominant gene. The gene frequency of the abnormal allele was predicted to be 0.0015–0.0026.[9] In contrast, an analysis of ovarian cancer families ascertained from a population-based series of ovarian cancer cases found evidence for a recessive gene.[10] The elucidation of the molecular basis for some ovarian cancer families has subsequently provided support for the dominant model but no recessive genes for ovarian cancer have yet been identified.

HIGH-PENETRANCE OVARIAN CANCER SUSCEPTIBILITY GENES

Ovarian cancer is a characteristic of the phenotype of two distinct familial cancer syndromes: hereditary breast/ovarian cancer syndrome and Lynch syndrome.

Site-specific familial ovarian cancer and the hereditary breast ovarian cancer syndrome

No gene that confers increased susceptibility to ovarian cancer alone has yet been isolated, and so site-specific familial ovarian cancer and the hereditary breast–ovarian cancer syndrome are considered to be part of the same spectrum.

BRCA1 on chromosome 17q12–21 was the first major breast–ovarian cancer susceptibility gene locus to be identified. Convincing evidence for the locus was first published in 1990, and came from a linkage study of 23 families with multiple cases of breast cancer among relatives.[11] BRCA1 was subsequently cloned in 1994.[12,13] Prior to its identification, other linkage studies had indicated that BRCA1 was responsible for a large proportion of families with cases of breast cancer only (45 per cent) and virtually all families with cases of breast cancer in association with epithelial ovarian cancer, and site-specific ovarian cancer families. A second major breast–ovarian cancer locus (BRCA2) was mapped to chromosome 13q12–13 in 1995[14] and the gene isolated one year later.[15] Initial studies indicated that the majority of breast–ovarian cancer families with evidence against linkage to the BRCA1 locus were linked to BRCA2.

PROPORTION OF OVARIAN CANCER FAMILIES DUE TO BRCA1 AND BRCA2

There have been many studies of the contribution of BRCA1 and BRCA2 to hereditary breast and ovarian cancer families.[16] Most of these studies have been based on families that have been ascertained because of the aggregation of breast cancer. An analysis of 237 families with at least four cases of breast cancer has been performed by the Breast Cancer Linkage Consortium to estimate the proportion of families that are due to BRCA1 and BRCA2.[17] Families were selected without regard to the occurrence of ovarian or other cancers. Using a combination of mutation data and linkage data, it was estimated that 52 per cent of families were due to *BRCA1*, 32 per cent of families were due to *BRCA2* and 16 per cent of families were not due to either gene. As predicted from previous studies using linkage data alone, almost all families with breast and ovarian cancer were due either to *BRCA1* (81 per cent of families) or *BRCA2* (14 per cent of families). However, these results may not apply to families ascertained because of clustering of ovarian cancer.

There have been two studies of families ascertained because of ovarian cancer clustering.[18] The largest study was based on 112 families registered with the UKCCCR Familial Ovarian Cancer Register, that have been tested for mutations in *BRCA1* and *BRCA2*.[18] The proportion of these families that were found to have a mutation varied according to the extent of the family history (Table 23.1).

Thus, the majority of families with an extensive family history (at least four members affected with ovarian or breast cancer) can be accounted for by *BRCA1* with a handful due to *BRCA2*. Nevertheless, even in these families, no mutation was found in nearly a third of families. In the two case only ovarian cancer families, *BRCA1* and *BRCA2* accounted for only one-fifth of families. It is likely that in some families mutations are missed because of the insensitivity of the mutation testing.

BRCA1 AND *BRCA2* IN UNSELECTED OVARIAN CANCER CASE SERIES

The prevalence of *BRCA1* mutations in ovarian cancer cases unselected for family history has been reported by five studies.[19–23] The first published study reported found

Table 23.1 *Proportion of families with mutations in* BRCA1 *and* BRCA2 *according to extent of family history*

Family history category[a]	No. of families	BRCA1 (%)	BRCA2 (%)
At least two cases of ovarian cancer and at least two cases of breast cancer	18	56	5
At least three cases of ovarian cancer and not more than one case of breast cancer	27	63	7
Two cases of ovarian cancer and one case of breast cancer	17	29	18
Two cases of ovarian cancer and no cases of breast cancer	50	16	4
Total	112	36	7

[a] Confirmed cases of ovarian cancer diagnosed at any age, breast cancer diagnosed at age ≤60.

12 truncating mutations in 374 cases (3 per cent) from Southern England.[20] A subsequent larger study reported a higher prevalence, with 39 mutations (8 per cent) in 515 patients from Canada.[23] However, a substantial proportion of these mutations were in cases from the Ashkenazi Jewish or French-Canadian ethnic groups, in whom common founder mutations are known to be prevalent. In the 316 cases of British origin, only eight (2.5 per cent) were *BRCA1* mutation carriers. The other studies, two from the USA and one from Japan, were smaller: one reported 10 mutations in 116 patients,[21] another reported 4 mutations in 120 cases[24] and the third found 4 mutations in 76 patients.[19] Fewer data are available for *BRCA2*, but the Canadian study reported 21 truncating mutations out of the total of 515 cases (4 per cent) of which seven occurred in the 316 cases of British origin (2.2 per cent prevalence). The study reported by Rubin *et al.* found only one *BRCA2* mutation carrier in 116 cases.[21]

Prevalence studies have also been carried out in unselected case series from populations with founder mutations. Seven studies have reported the prevalence of these mutations in Ashkenazi Jewish patients with ovarian cancer.[25–31] The *BRCA1* 185delAG mutation has been reported to be present in 25–30 per cent of cases, *BRCA1* 5382insC was found in 0–9 per cent of cases, and *BRCA2* 6174delT was present in 3–19 per cent of cases. Tonin *et al.* tested 99 French-Canadian women with ovarian cancer unselected for family history for the most common mutations that have been described in French-Canadian breast cancer and breast–ovarian cancer families.[32] Germline mutations were found in eight cases, five of whom carried the *BRCA1* C4446T mutation and two carried the *BRCA2* 8765delAG mutation. A similar study of 615 women with ovarian cancer from Norway found 13 (2 per cent) carried *BRCA1* 1675delA and 5 (1 per cent) carried *BRCA1* 1135insA.

CANCER RISKS ASSOCIATED WITH *BRCA1* AND *BRCA2* MUTATIONS

This is covered in Chapter 19.

GENE–GENE AND GENE–ENVIRONMENT INTERACTIONS

The published estimates of ovarian cancer risk for *BRCA1* and *BRCA2* mutation carriers have varied depending on the methods used to derive them (see Chapter 19). Those derived from family-based studies appear to be somewhat higher than those derived from population-based studies. The cause of this difference is not clear. Assuming that the difference is not simply due to chance, there must be some variation in penetrance between carriers. In principle, this could be due to allelic heterogeneity in risk, but the effects of allelic heterogeneity are unlikely to account for the magnitude of the difference observed. A more important potential explanation is that there may be other factors that modify risk. These could be modifier genes or non-genetic factors, some of which may be related to lifestyle. There is mounting evidence to support the assertion that the risks of cancer in *BRCA1* and *BRCA2* families are modified both by genetic background and environmental factors.

Low parity is a well-established risk factor for sporadic breast cancer and has also been shown to be associated with an increased breast cancer risk in women found by haplotype analysis to carry *BRCA1* mutations.[33] More recent studies have suggested an increased risk of *BRCA1*-associated breast cancer with pregnancy.[34,35] In one study, the risk of ovarian cancer in *BRCA1* carriers was found to increase significantly with increasing parity, which is also the opposite effect to that seen in the general population.[33] Cigarette smoking is thought to have minimal effect on sporadic breast cancer risk but, in one study, subjects with *BRCA1* or *BRCA2* gene mutations and breast cancer were significantly more likely to have been non-smokers than control (unaffected) subjects with mutations.[36] As with sporadic cancer, oral-contraceptive use may reduce the risk of ovarian cancer in women with pathogenic mutations in the *BRCA1* or *BRCA2* gene.[37] A case-control study from Israel failed to confirm these data,[38] but this may have been because the controls were poorly matched to the cases in terms of age. Ligation of the fallopian tubes has been found to be protective against ovarian cancer in the general population. A similar effect has been observed in *BRCA1* mutation carriers but not in *BRCA2* mutation carriers.[39]

Genes that have been shown to alter cancer risks in mutation carriers include *HRAS1* and the androgen receptor gene (*AR*). Rare alleles of a variable number tandem repeat (VNTR) polymorphism located about 1 kb downstream of the *HRAS1* proto-oncogene on chromosome 11p15.5 confer an increased risk of breast cancer.[40] These alleles do not seem to be associated with an increased risk of breast cancer in *BRCA1* carriers, but they may be associated with an increased risk of ovarian cancer.[41] Breast cancer risk may be altered by a polymorphism in the *AR* gene; one study showed that age at breast cancer diagnosis is earlier among *BRCA1* mutation carriers with very long AR-CAG repeats.[42] Another study has reported that short AR-CAG repeats are associated with early diagnosis of ovarian cancer.[43] A preliminary report from the same group has also suggested that the steroid hormone metabolism gene, *AIB1*, may alter breast cancer risk in *BRCA1* mutation carriers.[44]

CLINICAL FEATURES OF *BRCA1*- AND *BRCA2*-ASSOCIATED OVARIAN CANCERS

The clinicopathological characteristics of familial and inherited epithelial ovarian cancer are broadly similar to those of non-familial cancer, although some minor differences have been reported. In one small study of site-specific familial ovarian cancer, no difference in grade was found between familial and sporadic ovarian tumours.[45] Another study of familial ovarian cancer found a significantly higher proportion of serous cystadenocarcinoma in familial cases (83 per cent) compared to controls (49 per cent).[46] A high proportion of serous adenocarcinoma has also been reported for *BRCA1* associated ovarian tumours[47,48] and ovarian cancers occurring in *BRCA1*-positive families are more likely to be high grade and non-mucinous than cancers arising in women from *BRCA1*-negative families.[49,50]

The influence of mutations in *BRCA1* and *BRCA2* on outcome in ovarian cancer has been studied by several groups with conflicting results. An early report described improved survival of *BRCA1*-associated ovarian cancer patients compared to sporadic controls[48] but was subsequently criticised for possible selection bias. However, support for this finding has emerged from two larger studies. Boyd *et al.* found improved survival in *BRCA1/2*-associated ovarian cancer patients presenting with Stage III disease, although the result was no longer significant when early-stage cases were included in a multivariate analysis that also adjusted for age at diagnosis.[29] Ramus *et al.* found a slightly improved survival, which was not statistically significant, for 27 Ashkenazi ovarian cancer patients with one of the founder mutations in *BRCA1* or *BRCA2* compared to 71 patients with no mutation.[31] Other studies have found no difference in survival of *BRCA1*-associated ovarian cancer in breast cancer families compared with population controls,[51] and no survival difference in ovarian cancer patients from *BRCA1* and *BRCA2* ovarian cancer families compared to patients from families in which no mutation could be found.[49] Finally, a small study of Ashkenazi Jewish patients found no difference in the survival of ten individuals with ovarian cancer who were relatives of *BRCA1* or *BRCA2* carriers compared with the survival of 116 ovarian cancer cases who were relatives of individuals who were not carriers.[52] Larger studies in unselected case series that have been tested for mutation in *BRCA1* and *BRCA2* will be needed to settle the issue.

Hereditary non-polyposis colorectal cancer and the mismatch repair genes

The Lynch syndrome or hereditary non-polyposis colorectal cancer (HNPCC) was first described in 1966.[1] The syndrome is characterized by marked susceptibility to malignancies of the large bowel but cancers in other organs, including the ovary, also occur frequently.[53] Cancer susceptibility in HNPCC families has been shown to be due to defects in the mismatch repair (MMR) system, which is responsible for the repair of nucleotide mismatches during DNA replication, and prevents the propagation of potentially harmful mutations. The first MMR gene to be cloned in humans was MSH2[54,55] and MLH1 was cloned a year later.[56,57] Mutations in MSH2 and MLH1 account for 70 per cent of reported HNPCC cases with PMS1, PMS2 and MSH3 accounting for some of the rest.[58] The cumulative risk of colorectal cancer in MMR gene mutation carriers from HNPCC families is over 80 per cent and that of ovarian cancer is 12 per cent.[59] The role of the MMR genes in ovarian cancer other than that occurring in known HNPCC families has rarely been studied. One analysis of ovarian cancer cases diagnosed before the age of 30 found no mutations in MSH2 and only two MLH1 mutations in 101 patients.[60]

EVIDENCE FOR OTHER OVARIAN CANCER SUSCEPTIBILITY GENES

Assuming that most of the familial aggregation of ovarian cancer is due to inheritance and not shared environment, evidence for the existence of other ovarian cancer susceptibility genes comes from considering the extent to which the known susceptibility genes can explain all the observed excess familial risk. Any familial risk that is not explained by the known susceptibility genes provides evidence for other genes. The excess familial risk associated with a specific genetic variant depends on the frequency of the variant in the population and the size of the disease risks associated with that gene. If we assume mutant alleles of BRCA1 occur in the population with a frequency of 1:1000[61,62] and confer a 20-fold risk of ovarian cancer, they will account for 16 per cent of the excess familial risk. Similarly, BRCA2 accounts for 8 per cent of the excess familial risk assuming a 1:500 frequency of alleles conferring a tenfold increase in risk. Thus, less than 30 per cent of the known excess risk of familial ovarian cancer can be accounted for by the known susceptibility genes. This implies that there are other susceptibility genes yet to be identified.

Evidence for the existence of other ovarian cancer genes comes from the observation that BRCA1 and BRCA2 mutations were identified in less than half the families registered with the UKCCCR Familial Ovarian Cancer Registry.[18] This possibility is supported by the finding that the risk of ovarian cancer to women in the families that had tested negative for mutations in BRCA1 and BRCA2 was substantially elevated (relative risk of 12 (3.1–30)).[7] However, an alternative scenario to explain these findings was suggested by a segregation analysis of data from these families, which found that a combination of chance clustering of sporadic cases and insensitivity of the mutation detection methods may account for the BRCA1/2 negative families.[63] Nevertheless, the possibility that other susceptibility genes (as yet unidentified) are involved could not be excluded.

Drawing these strands of evidence together, it seems likely that other susceptibility genes do exist but the range of plausible genetic models is wide. Data from the large multiple case families suggest that any other very high-penetrance genes will be rare but the possibility remains for several genes conferring a tenfold increase in risk. For example, several moderate risk genes with a combined frequency of 5 per cent could account for the excess familial risk and the remaining multiple case families. An alternative model predicts multiple common low-risk (low-penetrance) genetic variants conferring relative risks of less than five.

LOW–PENETRANCE OVARIAN CANCER SUSCEPTIBILITY

Parametric and non-parametric linkage studies on multiple case pedigrees have proved very successful at identifying rare, high-risk cancer susceptibility genes. However, low-penetrance alleles may not be expressed in multiple members of a single family and are, therefore, not amenable to identification by linkage analysis.[64] An alternative to gene finding by linkage is the association study in which polymorphic genotype frequencies are compared between groups with different phenotypes (cases and controls) in order to estimate the risk associated with each genotype.[65] An association study can be used to identify polymorphisms, which are either causally related to disease risk or are in strong linkage disequilibrium with disease causing variants. There are several types of polymorphism in the human genome. Of these, single nucleotide polymorphisms (SNPs) in the coding sequence of a gene, leading to amino-acid substitution in the protein product, seem the most likely candidates for low-penetrance cancer susceptibility. Polymorphisms in regulatory sequences and inactivating polymorphisms in non-essential genes may also be important. There are at least 2 million SNPs distributed throughout the genome. Most of these are in the non-coding sequence but 60 000 SNPs are predicted in the coding sequences of approximately 30 000 genes.[66] Given the large number of polymorphisms present in the human genome, it would, in theory, be possible to carry out a genome wide search for common low-penetrance alleles. However, the number of neutral markers that would be needed is unknown because the extent of linkage disequilibrium across the human genome is not known. It is likely that a minimum of several markers per gene would be required and such an approach is not technically feasible at present. Thus, the association study is currently limited to the analysis of a few polymorphisms in candidate susceptibility genes. These are genes that are plausible candidates because they function in molecular pathways that are known to be important in the development of ovarian cancer. Examples include genes in the sex steroid-hormone metabolism pathway, carcinogen metabolism genes, cell-cycle control genes and DNA repair genes.

The number of published association studies has increased rapidly over the past 5 years. The results of these studies are summarized in Table 23.2. Two of the polymorphisms studied alter genes in the sex steroid-hormone signalling and metabolism pathways. The androgen receptor is involved in various pathways, including those of differentiation, development and regulation of cell growth. Exon 1 of AR encodes two expressed polymorphic repeats. One of these, the polyglutamine tract ($[CAG]_n$), is in the transactivation domain and *in vitro* studies have shown that smaller repeat lengths are associated with greater transactivation capabilities.[67] CYP17

encodes a cytochrome P450 enzyme, which functions at two points in the steroid biosynthesis pathway. A 5′ promoter T to C substitution creates an additional SP1-type promoter site but this has not been shown to bind the Sp1 transcription factor.[68] Neither of these polymorphisms have been shown to alter ovarian cancer risk.

The glutathione-S-transferase (GST) family are phase II enzymes that detoxify carcinogens and their reactive intermediates, by facilitating their conjugation to glutathione and subsequent excretion. For both *GSTM1* and *GSTT1* (reviewed in Rebbeck[69]), a high percentage of the Caucasian population are homozygous for null alleles (up to 60 per cent and 20 per cent, respectively) and have no detoxifying GST activity. Levels of DNA adducts, sister-chromatid-exchange and somatic genetic mutations may be increased in carriers of *GSTM1* and *GSTT1* null

Table 23.2 *Case-control studies of polymorphisms in candidate ovarian cancer susceptibility genes*

Gene/ polymorphism	Cases	Controls	Rare allele frequency	Heterozygote risk (95% CI)	Rare homozygote risk (95% CI)	Rare allele carrier risk	Reference
CYP2D6							
2367delA	258	231	0.20	1.2 (0.8–1.8)	1.6 (0.8–3.1)	1.3 (0.9–1.8)	86
TP53							
IVS3 16 bp dup	62	424	0.14	1.6 (0.9–3.0)	8.8 (2.9–26)	2.1 (1.2–3.60)	71
IVS3 16 bp dup	82	100	0.13	0.7 (0.3–1.5)	0.6 (0.1–6.4)	0.7 (0.3–1.4)	73
IVS3 16 bp dup	216	113	0.15	1.2 (0.7–2.0)	0.7 (0.2–3.3)	1.1 (0.7–1.9)	74
IVS3 16 bp dup	310	364	0.12	1.7 (1.2–2.3)	3.8 (1.0–14)	1.7 (1.2–2.4)	72
IVS6 G>A	225	254	0.10	2.0 (1.3–3.0)	2.0 (0.6–7.2)	2.0 (1.3–3.0)	75
IVS6 G>A	310	364	0.11	1.7 (1.2–2.5)	3.2 (0.8–13)	1.9 (1.3–2.9)	72
Arg72Pro	151	52	0.25	1.1 (0.6–2.2)	1.1 (0.3–3.6)	1.1 (0.6–2.1)	70
GSTM1							
GSTM1 deletion	103	115	0.38[a]		0.8 (0.4–1.3)		87
GSTM1 deletion	241	295	0.55		0.9 (0.6–1.3)		88
GSTT1							
GSTT1 deletion	103	115	0.14[a]		0.9 (0.4–1.9)		87
GSTT1 deletion	241	295	0.19[a]		1.0 (0.6–1.6)		88
GSTP1							
Ile105Val	238	292	0.38	1.0 (0.7–1.5)	0.9 (0.5–1.5)	1.0 (0.6–1.6)	88
AR							
Exon 1 Poly(CAG)	319	853	Not applicable	0.9 (0.6–1.2)[b]	1.1 (0.8–1.6)[c]	1.0 (0.7–1.3)[d]	89
CYP17							
Promoter T>C	319	298	0.38	1.1 (0.7–1.5)	1.1 (0.7–1.8)	1.1 (0.8–1.5)	90
PR							
Val660Leu	551	298		0.8 (0.6–1.1)	1.4 (0.5–4.1)		91
HRAS1							
Minisatellite	136	108	Not applicable	1.7 (0.9–3.0)[e]	2.9 (0.8–11)[f]		92

[a] null genotype frequency.
[b] carrier of one allele ≥ 22 repeats.
[c] carrier of two alleles ≥ 22 repeats.
[d] carrier of one or two alleles ≥ 22 repeats.
[e] carrier of one rare allele.
[f] carrier of two rare alleles.
CI, confidence interval.

genotypes.[69] CYP2D6 is a non-essential phase I enzyme responsible for the metabolism of environmental carcinogens and a polymorphic single base pair deletion in exon 5 produces a non-functioning protein. Again, none of these polymorphisms have been shown to be associated with ovarian cancer.

TP53 is critical for DNA repair through its influence on the G1/s cell-cycle checkpoint and for upstream regulation of apoptotic pathways of programmed cell death that are essential for a response to ionizing radiation and chemotherapeutic agents. Several polymorphisms in the TP53 gene have been described including a 16 base pair duplication in intron 3, a substitution of proline for arginine at codon 72 in exon 4 and a G to A substitution in intron 6. None of these variants have been convincingly shown to alter TP53 function but several association studies have investigated their role in ovarian cancer. The only study to investigate Arg72Pro failed to detect an association of the Pro allele with ovarian cancer.[70] The results of four studies of the intron 3 duplication have been inconsistent, with two studies reporting a significant increase in ovarian cancer risk associated with carriers of the Pro allele[71,72] and two studies reporting no effect.[73,74] Both studies that have investigated the intron 6 polymorphisms reported a significant increase in risk associated with carriers of the A allele.[72,75]

There are several problems that need to be considered in the interpretation of the results of these studies. Few of the published studies report results that are statistically significant. However, few studies have sufficient statistical power to detect moderate risks even for common genetic variants. For example, 400 cases and 400 controls would be needed to have 80 per cent power to identify a susceptibility gene at the 0.05 level of significance, if the risk allele had a population frequency of 0.3, acted in a dominant manner and conferred a 1.5-fold increase in ovarian cancer risk. If the allele were recessive, 1000 cases and 1000 controls would be needed. The sample sizes required for rarer alleles or lesser risks are even greater. It is evident that most published studies are seriously underpowered and false-negative results may occur. Gene–gene and gene–environment interactions may also be important, but the power to detect these is even more limited.

Allied to this, there is a potential problem with false positives because the number of true positives is likely to be very small compared with the total number of SNPs tested. The problem of false positives is then likely to be aggravated by publication bias – the preferential publication of results that are 'statistically significant'. Of the genes studied so far, TP53 would appear to be the best candidate for ovarian cancer susceptibility, although the case for this is by no means proven. Of the remaining, only GSTM1 can be excluded as being unlikely to confer a risk of 1.5 or more.

REDUCING RISK OF OVARIAN CANCER IN WOMEN AT HIGH RISK

In principle, two approaches are available to reduce the risk of morbidity and mortality from ovarian cancer. These are the prevention of incident disease (primary prevention) and the early detection of prevalent disease (secondary prevention). Primary prevention includes interventions, such as hormonal manipulation/chemoprophylaxis and prophylactic surgery. Several methods, such as serum markers and/or ultrasound examination of the ovaries, can be used for surveillance with a view to early detection of ovarian cancer. The following section provides a brief discussion of effectiveness of these interventions with specific reference to women at high risk of ovarian cancer.

Prophylactic surgery

Prophylactic bilateral salpingo-oophorectomy (BPO) is perhaps the most common prophylactic procedure used in women at high risk of ovarian cancer. Indeed, the NIH Consensus Statement on Ovarian Cancer recommended that women at risk of inherited ovarian cancer undergo prophylactic oophorectomy after completion of childbearing or at age 35 years.[76] However, a rather different view was taken by the Cancer Genetic Studies Consortium, which concluded that 'there was insufficient evidence to recommend for or against prophylactic oophorectomy as a measure for reducing ovarian cancer risk'.[77]

Removal of both the ovaries would seem a rational way to reduce the risk of ovarian cancer in women at high risk. Unfortunately this operation does not eliminate the risk of developing primary peritoneal ovarian cancer. In addition, ovarian ablation is associated with important side effects, including hot flushes, impaired sleep habits, vaginal dryness, and increased risk of osteoporosis and heart disease. Hormone replacement therapy is often necessary to counteract these adverse effects.

Two studies have estimated the effect of BPO on reducing ovarian cancer risk in women who may be at elevated ovarian cancer risk because of family history. Struewing et al. studied 346 non-oophorectomized and 44 oophorectomized women in 'high risk' families.[78] Two post-BPO cases of intra-abdominal carcinomatosis and eight ovarian cancers in the non-BPO group were observed. After adjusting for age and duration of follow-up, these results suggested a 50 per cent risk reduction but the study was too small to achieve statistical significance. Piver et al. studied 324 women from the Gilda Radner Familial Ovarian Cancer Registry who underwent BPO and reported six cases of intra-abdominal carcinomatosis 1–27 years following surgery.[79] These data suggest that BPO may reduce risk in women with *BRCA1* or *BRCA2* mutations, although no studies of BPO in women who are known to carry a mutation in *BRCA1* or *BRCA2* have been reported.

An additional consideration is that ovarian ablation also seems to reduce the risk of breast cancer.[80] A universal recommendation for or against BPO cannot be made and, when a woman is making a decision about the value of ovarian ablation, all the possible benefits and risks should be considered on an individual patient basis.

Chemoprophylaxis

It is well established that the combined oestrogen–progestin oral contraceptive pill is associated with a decreased risk of ovarian cancer in the general population. Several studies have now shown that hormonal manipulation with the oral contraceptive pill also reduces ovarian cancer risk in women with a family history of ovarian cancer[81] and women with a mutation in *BRCA1* or *BRCA2*.[37] However, the benefit in mutation carriers, who are at substantial risk of breast cancer, may be outweighed by the enhancement of the breast cancer risk by exogenous estrogens.[82] Until further data are available to evaluate the overall risks and benefits, the oral contraceptive pill should not be recommended as an option for reducing ovarian cancer risk.

Early detection

Currently available screening strategies for ovarian cancer consist of transvaginal ultrasound (TVS) and measurement of serum levels of CA125. The efficacy of these in the general population has been widely discussed, but the data available on screening high-risk women are scanty. In a study of both transabdominal and transvaginal ultrasonography in self-referred women with a first- or second-degree relative with ovarian cancer, abnormalities requiring surgical exploration were found in 3.8 per cent of screened women, of whom only 10 per cent were found to have ovarian cancer (five of six had stage I disease).[83] Five additional cases of cancer not detected by screening (three ovarian and two peritoneal) were reported 2–44 months after the last ultrasound.

In another study of 386 women with a first-degree relative or multiple second-degree relatives with ovarian cancer using ultrasound and CA125, 15 women underwent exploratory laparotomies, ten as a result of abnormal ultrasound findings alone, three as a result of abnormal CA125 levels and ultrasound findings and two women because of rising CA125 levels. No cancer was identified in any of these women, one of whom sustained unrecognized small bowel damage requiring further surgery.[84] In a more recent study, 1261 women with a significant family history were followed up with transvaginal ultrasound with colour Doppler imaging and tumour-marker estimation including CA125, initially every 2 years and then annually from 1995, giving a total of 6082 screening visits.[85] Three stage I ovarian cancers and seven cases of peritoneal serous papillary carcinoma were identified. All three cases of ovarian cancer were identified because of an abnormal ultrasound and four of the seven peritoneal carcinoma cases were identified because of abnormal ultrasound (two cases) or elevated CA125 levels (two cases). The other three cases of peritoneal cancer were identified because of the development of abdominal or pelvic pain at 5, 6 and 15 months after their last normal screening visit. The authors do not clarify details of the family history inclusion criteria needed before volunteers were offered a place on this screening program and it is unclear how many truly high-risk women were involved.

The results of these studies suggest that, even if screening strategies involving serial CA125 measurement and regular ultrasound imaging are not cost effective in the postmenopausal normal-risk population, this may not be the case in the high- and moderate-risk population. Large, robust prospective clinical trials examining different screening strategies in the high- and moderate-risk groups are urgently required.

Suggested management framework

This framework is based on the strategy of stratifying women presenting with a family history of ovarian cancer into two risk categories based on the strength of that history: high risk and low risk.

CRITERIA FOR DEFINING HIGH RISK WOMEN

Families fulfilling the following criteria are classified as high risk.

- One woman with ovarian cancer at any age and one individual with breast cancer diagnosed under 50 years who are first-degree relatives. Families in which affected individuals are connected by a second-degree relationship through an unaffected male are also eligible.
- Two women with ovarian cancer at any age connected by a second-degree relationship.

When appropriate, offer to refer them to a cancer genetics clinic for a *BRCA1* or *BRCA2* mutation search (see later). If a mutation search is not possible, the suggested management of unaffected women who are first-degree relatives of an affected woman from these families includes the discussion of the advantages and disadvantages of BPO, emphasizing particularly the important age-related issues, that is, that the risk of developing ovarian cancer below the age of 40 is low, and the incidence of short- and long-term side effects is higher in women undergoing oophorectomy at a younger age. The implications of the results outlined in the paper of Karlan et al.[85] discussed under the section on screening, for the practice of prophylactic oophorectomy remain unclear, but should be mentioned.

In the UK, women from these families who are over 35 and who have an affected first-degree relative may be offered entry into the UKCCCR familial ovarian screening study, a single arm prospective study of annual CA125 estimation and annual ultrasonography after a full discussion of the potential false-negative and false-positive results.

CRITERIA FOR DETERMINING WHO IS ELIGIBLE FOR GENETIC TESTING

The availability of *BRCA1* and *BRCA2* testing varies from country to country, and even from clinic to clinic within a country. Typical criteria for identifying eligible families that are used in family cancer clinics in the UK are as follows:

- four or more relatives affected at any age by ovarian or breast cancer;
- two or more individuals with ovarian cancer who are first-degree relatives;
- one individual with ovarian cancer at any age and two individuals with breast cancer diagnosed under 60 years who are connected by first-degree relationships;
- one relative with both breast and ovarian cancer at any age.

Eligible families should be referred to a specialist in cancer genetics for genetic counselling. A search for *BRCA1/2* mutations may then be undertaken if there is a living affected family member available for testing. If a mutation is then identified in the family, direct genetic testing is offered to unaffected family members. As described above, unaffected individuals who have been identified as carriers have a variety of options to manage their breast and ovarian cancer risk from which to choose. The pros and cons of these have to be considered on an individual basis. Women who are non-carriers from these families have the same ovarian cancer risks as the general population.

Rarely, ovarian cancer occurs as part of the hereditary non-polyposis colorectal cancer syndrome. This should be suspected in families with three individuals with colorectal cancer with at least one case diagnosed before 50 years as well as one case of ovarian cancer, and all of these individuals are connected by first-degree relationships. These families should also be referred for specialist genetic counselling and management.

LOW RISK

This category includes individuals with a family history of ovarian cancer that does not fit the high-risk criteria. These women should be informed that their risk of developing ovarian cancer is higher than that of an individual of the same age without a family history but that, at present, this increased risk is not considered sufficient to warrant screening, given that there is no formal evidence that it is effective.

Giving consistent information through primary care, secondary care in breast and gynaecology units, and tertiary care in cancer genetics centres is particularly important in gaining and retaining public confidence. Different strategies for achieving this remain high on the research agenda.

KEY POINTS

- There is evidence for familial clustering of ovarian cancer either alone or in combination with other cancers (the breast/ovarian syndrome and the Lynch syndromes).
- Ovarian cancer which has a genetic predisposition may not necessarily occur at younger ages, unlike many other cancer predisposition situations.
- *BRCA1* and *BRCA2* account for the majority of families with breast and ovarian cancer.
- Germline mutations in *BRCA1/2* are uncommon in single cases of ovarian cancer.
- The oral contraceptive pill is protective against the development of ovarian cancer.
- The role of transvaginal ultrasound for screening in high-risk women is unproven and the subject of study.

REFERENCES

1. Lynch HT, Shaw MW, Magnuson CW, et al. Hereditary factors in cancer. Study of two large midwestern kindreds. *Arch Intern Med* 1966; **117**:206–212.

2. Lynch HT, Guirgis HA, Albert S. Familial association of carcinoma of the breast and ovary. *Surg Gynecol Obstet* 1974; **138**:717.

3. Stratton JF, Pharoah PDP, Smith SK, et al. A systematic review and meta-analysis of family history and risk of ovarian cancer. *Br J Obstet Gynaecol* 1998; **105**:493–499.

4. Auranen A, Pukkala E, Makinen J, et al. Cancer incidence in the first-degree relatives of ovarian cancer patients. *Br J Cancer* 1996; **74**:280–284.

5. Easton DF, Matthews FE, Ford D, et al. Cancer mortality in relatives of women with ovarian cancer: the OPCS study. *Int J Cancer* 1996; **65**:284–294.

6. Schildkraut JM, Thompson WD. Familial ovarian cancer: a population-based case-control study. *Am J Epidemiol* 1988; **128**:456–466.

7. Sutcliffe S, Pharoah PD, Easton DF, Ponder BA. Ovarian and breast cancer risks to women in families with two or more cases of ovarian cancer. *Int J Cancer* 2000; **87**:110–117.

8. Lichtenstein P, Holm NV, Verkasalo PK, *et al*. Environmental and heritable factors in the causation of cancer – analyses of cohorts of twins from Sweden, Denmark, and Finland. *N Engl J Med* 2000; **343**:78–85.

9. Houlston RS, Collins A, Slack J, *et al*. Genetic epidemiology of ovarian cancer: segregation analysis. *Ann Hum Genet* 1991; **55**:291–299.

10. Auranen A, Iselius L. Segregation analysis of epithelial ovarian cancer in Finland. *Br J Cancer* 1998; **77**:1537–1541.

11. Hall JM, Lee MK, Newman B, *et al*. Linkage of early onset familial breast cancer to chromosome 17q21. *Science* 1990; **266**:120–122.

12. Miki Y, Swensen J, Shattuck-Eidens D, *et al*. A strong candidate for the 17 linked breast and ovarian cancer susceptibility gene *BRCA1*. *Science* 1994; **266**:66–71.

13. Futreal PA, Liu Q, Shattuck-Eidens D, *et al*. *BRCA1* mutations in primary breast and ovarian carcinomas. *Science* 1994; **266**:120–122.

14. Wooster R, Neuhausen SL, Mangion J, *et al*. Localization of a breast cancer susceptibility gene, *BRCA2*, to chromosome 13q12–13. *Science* 1994; **265**:2088–2090.

15. Wooster R, Bignell G, Lancaster J, *et al*. Identification of the breast cancer susceptibility gene *BRCA2*. *Nature* 1995; **378**:789–792.

16. Gayther SA, Pharoah PDP, Ponder BAJ. The genetics of inherited breast cancer. *J Mamm Gland Biol Neoplasia* 1998; **3**:365–376.

17. Ford D, Easton DF, Stratton M, *et al*. Genetic heterogeneity and penetrance analysis of the *BRCA1* and *BRCA2* genes in breast cancer families. *Am J Hum Genet* 1998; **62**:676–689.

18. Gayther SA, Russell P, Harrington P, *et al*. The contribution of germline *BRCA1* and *BRCA2* mutations to familial ovarian cancer: no evidence for other ovarian cancer-susceptibility genes. *Am J Hum Genet* 1999; **65**:1021–1029.

19. Matsushima M, Kobayashi K, Emi M, *et al*. Mutation analysis of the *BRCA1* gene in 76 Japanese ovarian cancer patients: four germline mutations, but no evidence of somatic mutation. *Hum Mol Genet* 1995; **4**:1953–1956.

20. Stratton JF, Gayther SA, Russell P, *et al*. Contribution of *BRCA1* mutations to ovarian cancer. *N Engl J Med* 1997; **336**:1125–1130.

21. Rubin SC, Blackwood MA, Bandera C, *et al*. *BRCA1*, *BRCA2*, and hereditary nonpolyposis colorectal cancer gene mutations in an unselected ovarian cancer population: relationship to family history and implications for genetic testing. *Am J Obstet Gynecol* 1998; **178**:670–677.

22. Janezic SA, Ziogas A, Krumroy LM, *et al*. Germline *BRCA1* alterations in a population-based series of ovarian cancer cases. *Hum Mol Genet* 1999; **8**:889–897.

23. Risch HA, McLaughlin JR, Cole DE, *et al*. Prevalence and penetrance of germline *BRCA1* and *BRCA2* mutations in a population series of 649 women with ovarian cancer. *Am J Hum Genet* 2001; **68**:700–710.

24. Anton Culver H, Cohen PF, Gildea ME, Ziogas A. Characteristics of *BRCA1* mutations in a population-based case series of breast and ovarian cancer. *Eur J Cancer* 2000; **36**:1200–1208.

25. Abeliovich D, Kaduri L, Lerer I, *et al*. The founder mutations 185delAG and 5382insC in *BRCA1* and 6174delT in *BRCA2* appear in 60 per cent of ovarian cancer and 30 per cent of early-onset breast cancer patients among Ashkenazi women. *Am J Hum Genet* 1997; **60**:505–514.

26. Beller U, Halle D, Catane R, *et al*. High frequency of *BRCA1* and *BRCA2* germline mutations in Ashkenazi Jewish ovarian cancer patients, regardless of family history. *Gynecol Oncol* 1997; **67**:123–126.

27. Gotlieb WH, Friedman E, Bar Sade RB, *et al*. Rates of Jewish ancestral mutations in *BRCA1* and *BRCA2* in borderline ovarian tumors. *J Natl Cancer Inst* 1998; **90**:995–1000.

28. Lu KH, Cramer DW, Muto MG, *et al*. A population-based study of *BRCA1* and *BRCA2* mutations in Jewish women with epithelial ovarian cancer. *Obstet Gynecol* 1999; **93**:34–37.

29. Boyd J, Sonoda Y, Federici MG, *et al*. Clinicopathologic features of *BRCA*-linked and sporadic ovarian cancer. *JAMA* 2000; **283**:2260–2265.

30. Moslehi R, Chu W, Karlan B, *et al*. *BRCA1* and *BRCA2* mutation analysis of 208 Ashkenazi Jewish women with ovarian cancer. *Am J Hum Genet* 2000; **66**:1259–1272.

31. Ramus SJ, Fishman A, Pharoah PDP, *et al*. Ovarian cancer survival in Ashkenazi Jewish patients with *BRCA1* and *BRCA2* mutations. *Eur J Surg Oncol* 2001; **27**:278–281.

32. Tonin PM, Mes Masson AM, Narod SA, *et al*. Founder *BRCA1* and *BRCA2* mutations in French Canadian ovarian cancer cases unselected for family history. *Clin Genet* 1999; **55**:318–324.

33. Narod SA, Goldgar D, Cannon Albright L, *et al*. Risk modifiers in carriers of *BRCA1* mutations. *Int J Cancer* 1995; **64**:394–398.

34. Johannsson O, Loman N, Borg A, Olsson H. Pregnancy-associated breast cancer in *BRCA1* and *BRCA2* germline mutation carriers. *Lancet* 1998; **352**:1359–1360.

35. Jernstrom H, Lerman C, Ghadirian P, *et al*. Pregnancy and risk of early breast cancer in carriers of *BRCA1* and *BRCA2*. *Lancet* 1999; **354**:1846–1850.

36. Brunet JS, Ghadirian P, Rebbeck TR, *et al*. Effect of smoking on breast cancer in carriers of mutant *BRCA1* or *BRCA2* genes. *J Natl Cancer Inst* 1998; **90**:761–766.

37. Narod SA, Risch H, Moslehi R, *et al*. Oral contraceptives and the risk of hereditary ovarian cancer. *N Engl J Med* 1998; **339**:424–428.

38. Modan B, Hartge P, Hirsh-Yechezkel G, *et al*. Parity, oral contraceptives, and the risk of ovarian cancer among carriers and noncarriers of a *BRCA1* or *BRCA2* mutation. *N Engl J Med* 2001; **345**:235–240.

39. Narod SA, Sun P, Ghadirian P, *et al*. Tubal ligation and risk of ovarian cancer in carriers of *BRCA1* or *BRCA2* mutations: a case-control study. *Lancet* 2001; **357**:1467–1470.

40. Krontiris TG, Devlin B, Karp DD, *et al*. An association between the risk of cancer and mutations in the *HRAS1* minisatellite locus. *N Engl J Med* 1993; **329**:517–523.

41. Phelan CM, Rebbeck TR, Weber BL, *et al*. Ovarian cancer risk in *BRCA1* carriers is modified by the *HRAS1* variable number of tandem repeat (VNTR) locus. *Nature Genet* 1996; **12**:309–311.

42. Rebbeck TR, Kantoff PW, Krithivas K, *et al*. Modification of *BRCA1*-associated breast cancer risk by the polymorphic

androgen-receptor CAG repeat. *Am J Hum Genet* 1999; **64**:1371–1377.

43. Levine DA, Boyd J. The androgen receptor and genetic susceptibility to ovarian cancer: results from a case series. *Cancer Res* 2001; **61**:908–911.

44. Modification of breast cancer risk in *BRCA1* mutation carriers by the *AIB1* gene. *American Association for Cancer Research Annual Meeting*, March 1999; Philadelphia.

45. Buller RE, Anderson B, Connor JP, Robinson R. Familial ovarian cancer. *Gynecol Oncol* 1993; **51**:160–166.

46. Chang J, Fryatt I, Ponder B, *et al.* A matched control study of familial epithelial ovarian cancer: patient characteristics, response to chemotherapy and outcome. *Ann Oncol* 1995; **6**:80–82.

47. Johannsson OT, Idvall I, Anderson C, *et al.* Tumour biological features of *BRCA1*-induced breast and ovarian cancer. *Eur J Cancer* 1997; **33**:362–371.

48. Rubin SC, Benjamin I, Behbakht K, *et al.* Clinical and pathological features of ovarian cancer in women with germline mutations of *BRCA1*. *N Engl J Med* 1996; **335**:1413–1416.

49. Pharoah PDP, Easton DF, Stockton DL, *et al.* Survival in familial, *BRCA1* and *BRCA2* associated epithelial ovarian cancer. *Cancer Res* 1999; **59**:868–871.

50. Werness BA, Ramus SJ, Whittemore AS, *et al.* Histopathology of familial ovarian tumors in women from families with and without germline *BRCA1* mutations. *Hum Pathol* 2000; **31**:1420–1424.

51. Johannsson OT, Ranstam J, Borg A, Olsson H. Survival of *BRCA1* breast and ovarian cancer patients: a population-based study from southern Sweden. *J Clin Oncol* 1998; **16**:398–404.

52. Lee JS, Wacholder S, Struewing JP, *et al.* Survival after breast cancer in Ashkenazi Jewish *BRCA1* and *BRCA2* mutation carriers. *J Natl Cancer Inst* 1999; **91**:259–263.

53. Aarnio M, Mecklin JP, Aaltonen IA, *et al.* Life time risk of different cancers in hereditary non-polyposis colorectal cancer (HNPCC) syndrome. *Int J Cancer* 1995; **64**:430–433.

54. Fishel R, Lescoe MK, Rao MR, *et al.* The human mutator gene homolog *MSH2* and its association with hereditary nonpolyposis colon cancer. *Cell* 1993; **75**:1027–1038.

55. Leach FS, Nicolaides NC, Papadopoulos N, *et al.* Mutations of a mutS homolog in hereditary nonpolyposis colorectal cancer. *Cell* 1993; **75**:1215–1225.

56. Bronner CE, Baker SM, Morrison PT, *et al.* Mutation in the DNA mismatch repair gene homologue *hMLH1* is associated with hereditary non-polyposis colon cancer. *Nature* 1994; **368**:258–261.

57. Papadopoulos N, Nicolaides NC, Wei YF, *et al.* Mutation of a mutL homolog in hereditary colon cancer. *Science* 1994; **263**:1625–1629.

58. Wheeler JM, Bodmer WF, Mortensen NJ. DNA mismatch repair genes and colorectal cancer. *Gut* 2000; **47**:148–153.

59. Aarnio M, Sankila R, Pukkala E, *et al.* Cancer risk in mutation carriers of DNA-mismatch-repair genes. *Int J Cancer* 1999; **81**:214–218.

60. Stratton JF, Thompson D, Bobrow L, *et al.* The genetic epidemiology of early-onset epithelial ovarian cancer: a population-based study. *Am J Hum Genet* 1999; **65**:1725–1732.

61. Anglian Breast Cancer Study Group. Prevalence and penetrance of *BRCA1* and *BRCA2* in a population based series of breast cancer cases. *Br J Cancer* 2000; **83**:1301–1308.

62. Peto J, Collins N, Barfoot R, *et al.* Prevalence of *BRCA1* and *BRCA2* gene mutations in patients with early-onset breast cancer. *J Natl Cancer Inst* 1999; **91**:943–949.

63. Antoniou AC, Gayther SA, Stratton JF, *et al.* Risk models for familial breast and ovarian cancer. *Genet Epidemiol* 2000; **18**:173–190.

64. Risch N, Merikangas K. The future of genetic studies of complex diseases. *Science* 1996; **273**:1516–1517.

65. Khoury MJ. Genetic epidemiology. In: Rothman K, Greenland S (eds) *Modern epidemiology*, 2nd edn. Philadelphia: Lippincott-Raven, 1997.

66. International SNP Map Working Group. A map of human genome sequence variation containing 1.42 million single nucleotide polymorphisms. *Nature* 2001; **409**:928–933.

67. Chamberlain NL, Driver ED, Miesfeld RL. The length and location of CAG trinucleotide repeats in the androgen receptor N-terminal domain affect transactivation function. *Nucl Acids Res* 1994; **22**:3181–3186.

68. Kristensen VN, Haraldsen EK, Anderson KB, *et al.* CYP17 and breast cancer risk: the polymorphism in the 5' flanking area of the gene does not influence binding to Sp-1. *Cancer Res* 1999; **59**:2825–2828.

69. Rebbeck TR. Molecular epidemiology of the human glutathione S-transferase genotypes *GSTM1* and *GSTT1* in cancer susceptibility. *Cancer Epidemiol Biomarkers Prev* 1997; **6**:733–743.

70. Buller RE, Sood A, Fullenkamp C, *et al.* The influence of the p53 codon 72 polymorphism on ovarian carcinogenesis and prognosis. *Cancer Gene Ther* 1997; **4**:239–245.

71. Runnebaum IB, Tong XW, Konig R, *et al.* p53-based blood test for p53PIN3 and risk for sporadic ovarian cancer. *Lancet* 1995; **345**:994.

72. Wang Gohrke S, Weikel W, Risch H, *et al.* Intron variants of the p53 gene are associated with increased risk for ovarian cancer but not in carriers of *BRCA1* or *BRCA2* germline mutations. *Br J Cancer* 1999; **81**:179–183.

73. Lancaster IM, Brownlee HA, Wiseman RW, Taylor J. p53 polymorphism in ovarian and bladder cancer. *Lancet* 1995; **346**:182.

74. Campbell IG, Eccles DM, Dunn B, *et al.* p53 polymorphism in ovarian and breast cancer. *Lancet* 1996; **347**:393–394.

75. Mavridou D, Gornall R, Campbell IG, Eccles DM. TP53 intron 6 polymorphism and the risk of ovarian and breast cancer. *Br J Cancer* 1998; **77**:676–677.

76. NIH Consensus Development Panel on Ovarian Cancer. NIH consensus conference. Ovarian cancer. Screening, treatment, and follow-up. *JAMA* 1995; **273**:491–497.

77. Burke W, Daly M, Garber J, *et al.* Recommendations for follow-up care of individuals with an inherited predisposition to cancer. II. *BRCA1* and *BRCA2*. *JAMA* 1997; **277**:997–1003.

78. Struewing JP, Watson P, Easton DF, *et al.* Prophylactic oophorectomy in inherited breast/ovarian cancer families. *J Natl Cancer Inst Monogr* 1995; **17**:33–35.

79. Piver MS, Jishi MF, Tsukada Y, Nava G. Primary peritoneal carcinoma after prophylactic oophorectomy in women with a family history of ovarian cancer. A report of the Gilda Radner Familial Ovarian Cancer Registry. *Cancer* 1993; **71**:2751–2755.

80. Rebbeck TR, Levin AM, Eisen A, *et al.* Breast cancer risk after bilateral prophylactic oophorectomy in *BRCA1* mutation carriers. *J Natl Cancer Inst* 1999; **91**:1475–1479.

81. Piver MS, Baker TR, Jishi MF, *et al*. Familial ovarian cancer. A report of 658 families from the Gilda Radner Familial Ovarian Cancer Registry 1981–1991. *Cancer* 1993; **71**(2 Suppl):582–588.

82. Collaborative group on hormonal factors in breast cancer. Breast cancer and hormonal contraceptives: collaborative reanalysis of individual data on 53297 women with breast cancer and 100239 women without breast cancer from 54 epidemiological studies. *Lancet* 1996; **347**:1713–1727.

83. Bourne IH, Campbell S, Reynolds KM, *et al*. Screening for early familial ovarian cancer with transvaginal ultrasonography and colour blood flow imaging. *Br Med J* 1993; **306**:1025–1029.

84. Einhorn N, Sjovall K, Knapp RC. Prospective evaluation of serum CA 125 levels for early detection of ovarian cancer. *Obstet Gynecol* 1992; **80**:14–18.

85. Karlan BY, Baldwin RL, Lopez-Luevanos E, *et al*. Peritoneal serous papillary carcinoma, a phenotypic variant of familial ovarian cancer: implications for ovarian cancer screening. *Am J Obstet Gynecol* 1999; **180**:917–928.

86. Bryan EJ, Thomas NA, Palmer K, *et al*. Refinement of an ovarian cancer tumour suppressor gene locus on chromosome arm 22q and mutation analysis of *CYP2D6*, *SREBP2* and *NAGA*. *Int J Cancer* 2000; **87**:798–802.

87. Hengstler JG, Kett A, Arand M, *et al*. Glutathione S-transferase T1 and M1 gene defects in ovarian carcinoma. *Cancer Lett* 1998; **130**:43–48.

88. Spurdle AB, Webb PM, Purdie DM, *et al*. Polymorphisms at the glutathione S-transferase *GSTM1*, *GSTT1* and *GSTP1* loci: risk of ovarian cancer by histological subtype. *Carcinogenesis* 2001; **22**:67–72.

89. Spurdle AB, Webb PM, Chen X, *et al*. Androgen receptor exon 1 CAG repeat length and risk of ovarian cancer. *Int J Cancer* 2000; **87**:637–643.

90. Spurdle AB, Chen X, Abbazadegan M, *et al*. *CYP17* promotor polymorphism and ovarian cancer risk. *Int J Cancer* 2000; **86**:436–439.

91. Spurdle AB, Webb PM, Purdie DM, *et al*. No significant association between progesterone receptor exon 4 Val660Leu G/T polymorphism and risk of ovarian cancer. *Carcinogenesis* 2001; **22**:717–721.

92. Weitzel JN, Ding S, Larson GP, *et al*. The *HRAS1* minisatellite locus and risk of ovarian cancer. *Cancer Res* 2000; **60**:259–261.

24

Familial colon cancer syndromes and their genetics

SUSAN M. FARRINGTON AND MALCOLM G. DUNLOP

INTRODUCTION

Colorectal cancer is a major public health problem in the Western world, being the most common cause of early cancer death in the non-smoking population. In the UK, there are 34 000 new cases of colorectal cancer and more than 20 000 deaths annually. Recent developments in the field of genetics have led to the isolation of a number of cancer predisposition genes with moderate to high-risk penetrance. Identifying people who carry such high-risk alleles offers real opportunities for application of preventative measures. Intensive surveillance to detect early cancer or to effect prevention by polyp removal can be targeted by information from the genotype. Prophylactic surgery and chemoprevention guided by genetic information are also likely to be part of the future armamentarium in combating the disease. Understanding key molecular events involved in susceptibility to colorectal cancer is already providing new insight into the fundamental molecular basis of colorectal carcinogenesis. The last 10 years has seen a number of exciting developments in understanding the molecular basis of colorectal cancer, which are beginning to have a clinical impact on the disease. In this chapter, we will describe the major advances, and discuss how they are making an impact on the diagnosis and clinical management of colorectal cancer.

The multifactorial aetiology of colorectal cancer involves environmental factors as well as genetic susceptibility, as indicated by marked differences in the prevalence of the disease worldwide. For the majority of individuals, an ill-defined increased risk of the disease is indicated by having an affected relative with around 20–25 per cent of all colorectal cancer cases being associated with a family history of the disease.[1] Screening studies suggest that cancer susceptibility is due to predisposition to the development of colorectal adenomas.[2] Fortunately, not all adenomas progress to cancer because the population frequency of the 'adenoma-prone' allele was calculated as 19 per cent. The effects of diet clearly must influence the expression of such an allele in terms of both adenoma and cancer, but the trait could probably be thought of as a 'normal' variation of the human constitution. Perhaps the most radical suggestion is that colorectal neoplasms only occur in the presence of a genetic predisposition.[2]

It is clear that colorectal cancer susceptibility is complex. Dominant predisposition genes have been identified, but there may also be autosomal recessive alleles and a polygenic inheritance. Such alleles are likely to be associated with a marginally increased risk. This review is restricted to genes of major effect in the interests of clarity and brevity. However, it is likely that new risk alleles will be identified, especially in light of the human genome project and the development of new dense genetic marker maps.

A number of well-defined clinical syndromes are characterized by a strong family history and evidence of germline transmission as an autosomal dominant genetic trait. Of these hereditary syndromes, familial adenomatous polyposis (FAP) and hereditary non-polyposis colorectal cancer (HNPCC) have been extensively studied and their genetic bases are beginning to be understood. There are also other variants or rarer predisposition syndromes where the genes involved have more recently been described. The prevalence of colorectal cancer due to FAP depends greatly on the assiduousness of screening programs of those at risk but is around 0.2 per cent in most developed countries. HNPCC makes up a more substantial proportion of all cases, accounting for 2–5 per cent[3,4] but, owing to the lack of definitive biomarkers for HNPCC, diagnostic criteria have been pragmatic and are not inclusive of all cases. Clinical criteria such as the Amsterdam criteria[5] will only identify families where the gene defect is highly penetrant and the families are of sufficient size to allow the appropriate number of cases to arise. Thus, there is a bias, which tends to exclude small families inappropriately.

As HNPCC and FAP are high-penetrance genetic traits, genotype information can be translated to a reduction in the death rate from malignancy. Through the improved awareness of patients and clinicians, and the development of local FAP registries and colonic screening, FAP gene carriers should less frequently present with invasive cancer. HNPCC kindreds are usually identified because several family members have already died from colorectal cancer before the familial nature of the problem is understood. With the identification of a number of genes responsible for HNPCC and also the genes involved in rarer predisposition syndromes, it will be of great interest to elucidate the true prevalence of familial colorectal cancer.

FAMILIAL ADENOMATOUS POLYPOSIS

Familial adenomatous polyposis is an autosomal dominant disorder characterized by the development of more than 100, but frequently thousands of adenomatous polyps of the colon and rectum. The population frequency depends on the accuracy and completeness of the registration of cases, but the annual incidence is around 1/7000 live births.[6] Malignancy is virtually inevitable if prophylactic colectomy is not undertaken. The syndrome is also associated with extracolonic features, such as multiple craniofacial and long bone osteomata, epidermoid cysts, retinal pigmentation, gastroduodenal polyposis and malignancy, desmoid tumours and an increased risk of peri-ampullary, papillary thyroid, brain tumours, hepatoblastoma and sarcomas.

Localization of the gene responsible for FAP to the long arm of chromosome 5 was aided by cytogenetic analysis of a FAP patient who carried a constitutional deletion of the region. Genetic linkage studies demonstrated that the gene lay in the region 5q21–22.[7,8] Positional cloning

strategies, including genetic linkage, deletion mapping in sporadic colorectal cancers and mapping of constitutional microdeletions in FAP patients, isolated a number of candidate genes. The adenomatous polyposis coli (APC) gene was cloned and a number of FAP patients were shown to carry germline mutations.[9–12] It was the first gene to be identified that confers germline susceptibility to colorectal neoplasia. The majority of germline mutations reported in FAP families result in premature truncation of the APC product by either base substitution or deletion/insertion with frameshift, causing a downstream premature stop codon.[13–15]

APC comprises an 8.5 kb transcript encoding a 2843-amino-acid polypeptide in 15 exons. The function of the APC gene product is a focus of intense research and the complexities of APC function have yet to be fully understood. Antibodies to the APC protein have identified a 312 kDa protein expressed in colonic epithelial cells in the upper portions of the colonic crypts, suggesting involvement in colonocyte maturation.[16,17] Several functional domains are revealed in the protein sequence.[18] Short repeat sequences at the amino terminus of APC are predicted to form coiled-coil structures, suggesting that normal APC product functions as a homodimer. Other domains indicate that APC is involved in numerous cellular processes, including cellular adhesion, cell-cycle regulation, apoptosis, differentiation and intracellular signal transduction. The central part of the APC protein contains β-catenin binding and regulation domains and also binding domains for the axin family of proteins. APC may, therefore, affect the interaction between catenins and E-cadherin, thus influencing cellular adhesion and promoting the shedding and migration of epithelial cells. In conjunction with other proteins, such as axin, glycogen synthase kinase 3β (GSK) and a recently identified GSK-binding protein (GBP), APC plays a critical role in intracellular communication by modulating the levels of β-catenin dependent transcription (see reviews[19,20]). The downstream targets of β-catenin include oncogenic proteins, such as cyclin D1 and c-myc.[21] Extensive studies are under way in model organisms to fully define the APC/β-catenin signalling pathway (Figure 24.1) but the pivotal role of this pathway in colorectal tumorigenesis is exemplified by the identification of somatic mutations in many of the components, such as APC, β-catenin and axin.[22,23] Hence, although each of these genes are candidate germline susceptibility alleles predisposing to colorectal cancer, to date, only germline mutations of the APC gene have been identified.

Other functions of wild-type APC involve the microtubule cytoskeleton. In vitro studies indicate that wild-type APC not only binds to microtubules, but promotes their formation and bundling.[17,24] The organization and structure of microtubules are vital to cell division and migration, and an APC protein missing its carboxy terminus,

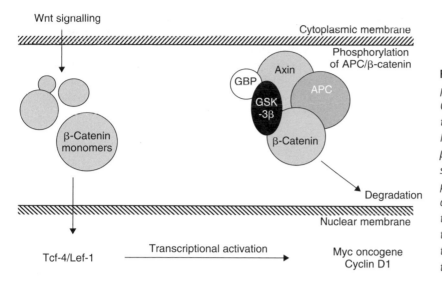

Wnt signalling

Cytoplasmic membrane

Phosphorylation
of APC/β-catenin

Axin

GBP

APC

GSK
-3β

β-Catenin
monomers

β-Catenin

Degradation

Nuclear membrane

Tcf-4/Lef-1

Transcriptional activation

Myc oncogene
Cyclin D1

Figure 24.1 *The APC/β-catenin signalling pathway. A protein complex of APC, axin, GSK-3β, GBP and β-catenin are present in the cytoplasm. Phosphorylation events lead to the subsequent degradation of β-catenin via the proteosome. Extracellular signals, e.g. Wnt, or mutations of the protein members, increase the cytoplasmic accumulation of β-catenin, which is then transported to the nucleus where it aids transcriptional activation of downstream targets including c-Myc and cyclin D1 via the transcription factors Tcf-4/Lef-1.*

owing to premature truncation, appears to be unable to bind microtubules.[25] The carboxy terminus of the protein not only binds microtubules, but also the proteins EB1 and the tumour suppressor protein Dlg,[26,27] which are both implicated in tumorigenesis. Once the underlying function of APC has been clearly determined, it may be possible to restore or augment the effects of deleterious mutations by pharmacological means.

Modifiers of *APC*

The wide spectrum of clinical presentation of FAP, even within a single family where affected individuals all carry the same *APC* mutation, indicates that there are factors that affect the phenotypic expression of the disease.[28] It is postulated that these may include modifier genes. Mouse models are beginning to aid the understanding of colorectal carcinogenesis. The Min (for multiple intestinal neoplasia) mouse was generated by germline mutagenesis that fortuitously mutated the murine *apc* gene.[29,30] The resulting phenotype includes the development of multiple neoplastic lesions mainly affecting the foregut. Phenotypic expression was shown to be modulated by an unlinked locus[31] and a modifier locus was identified called *mom1*.[32] *mom1* encodes for a secretory phospholipase A2,[33] a gene involved in lipid metabolism and prostaglandin production. The homologous human gene was found to be located on chromosome 1p35–36.[34] Evidence suggests a modifier locus in this region,[35,36] but no correlation for phospholipase A2 gene mutation with observed phenotype has been established and, therefore, it is unlikely to be the modifier involved in FAP.[37,38] Other candidate mouse modifier loci have also been identified in *apc* mutant mice, which may encode for genes imparting X-ray responsiveness.[39] A number of *Apc* mouse models now exist and these will allow specific investigation of

gene–environment interactions and also novel treatments for preventing the development of colorectal neoplasia in FAP. The effects of the environment, especially diet, are already being addressed. *Apc* mutant mice that were fed a Western-style diet (high fat, low calcium and vitamin D), were found to have an increased tumour incidence. Interestingly, there was also a shift in tumour site to the large intestine, consistent with the clinical presentation of FAP.[40,41]

Mutation spectrum of *APC* in FAP patients

Around 80 per cent of the *APC* mutations identified to date are in exon 15. Two specific exon 15 mutations occurring at codons 1061 and 1309 account for 15–20 per cent of all *APC* mutations, but the remainder are spread throughout the gene with no particular 'hot spots'.[12,42–45] The mutations detected are mainly deletions or insertions of short sequences,[46] suggesting they are due to replication errors rather than to the action of environmental mutagens. Indeed, there is evidence that colorectal tumours from patients with HNPCC and/or germline DNA mismatch repair (*MMR*) gene mutations, which are defective in replication error repair (i.e. MMR defective), show a propensity for deletions and insertions of repeat sequences of the *APC* gene.[47] There are conflicting data on this finding,[48] which may be due to germline versus somatic *MMR* gene inactivation. Most *APC* mutations generate a STOP codon, either directly or by frameshift, and hence result in premature termination of transcription and resultant truncation of the protein. Truncated APC protein may then interact with the normal APC product, resulting in a heterodimer, which may abrogate the function of the normal protein in a dominant-negative manner.[49]

Correlation of the type of mutation, or its location within the *APC* gene, may help inform the clinical decision on optimum timing for prophylactic surgery and also in predicting whether extracolonic manifestations, such as desmoid disease, are likely. Indeed, the common 1309 mutation is associated with a dense polyp phenotype and a high cancer risk in the retained rectum. Hence, the best surgical option may be proctocolectomy and ileoanal pouch rather than colectomy and ileorectal anastomoses, where the rectum is retained and so remains at risk for the rest of the patient's life. However, it is important to note that genotype–phenotype correlations are not well defined. One study of 22 unrelated Japanese FAP patients predicted that the site of mutation might determine the number of colorectal polyps,[46] while other groups have identified families with identical *APC* mutations, but diverse phenotype in terms of both colorectal polyposis and extracolonic disease.[50] A number of clinically described variant syndromes are known to be caused by germline *APC* mutations. Gardner's variant encompasses florid polyposis with epidermoid cysts of the skin, osteomas of the mandible and congenital hypertrophy of the retinal pigment epithelium. Attenuated FAP (AAPC or AFAP) describes patients who develop colorectal disease at a later age, where the polyp numbers are greatly reduced and of a slightly flatter type. The *APC* mutations responsible for this phenotype tend to be found upstream of codon 200 and downstream of codon 1600. Turcot syndrome manifests as multiple colonic adenomas with a young onset of colorectal cancer and also tumours of the central nervous system, particularly brain tumours. If the brain tumour is cerebellar medulloblastoma, the genetic defect is likely to be in the *APC* gene, whereas if the family display glioblastoma multiforme, the fault is likely to be defective DNA mismatch repair.[51] Although general phenotype–genotype correlations are being drawn, there are still many variables to be considered, especially in view of the potential modifier loci.

Identification of the mutation responsible for the FAP syndrome in a family has obvious advantages for presymptomatic diagnosis. Once the *APC* mutation has been identified in an affected individual, all at-risk offspring can be screened and prediction of carrier status based on mutation analysis can be made with extreme accuracy. However, the lack of a specific mutation or a small number of mutational 'hot spots' as the underlying genetic aetiology of FAP means that the entire gene must be laboriously screened for each different FAP family. Once the mutation has been identified, mutation-specific polymerase chain reaction (PCR) primers can be generated and used for each generation at risk. Owing to the rapid introduction of mutation detection into the clinical sphere, it seems likely that only FAP family members who are known to carry a mutant *APC* gene will undergo regular surveillance to determine the optimum timing for prophylactic surgery.

Future research into the molecular genetics of FAP will lead to better and more user friendly methods of carrier status assessment. Greater understanding of the structure, function and interactions of the APC protein, combined with the use of mouse models, will undoubtedly lead to new treatments of not only FAP but also sporadic colorectal cancer.

HEREDITARY NON–POLYPOSIS COLORECTAL CANCER

HNPCC is an autosomal dominant disorder with high penetrance in which colorectal cancer develops in gene carriers but without the myriads of adenomas seen in FAP.[52] Adenomatous polyps are found in HNPCC patients but these are in numbers comparable to that of the general population (usually less than ten). In classically defined HNPCC, there is a propensity for both adenomas and carcinomas to develop in the proximal part of the colon. Expression of the HNPCC phenotype is diverse in terms of the age of onset and also the organs that develop malignancy. It can be inherited as a site-specific colorectal cancer susceptibility trait or can also be associated with uterine, gastric, ovarian, upper urinary tract, small intestinal and other malignancies.

Large HNPCC families are fairly uncommon and so minimum criteria were drawn up to define HNPCC for research purposes. The stringency of inclusion criteria is intimately related to the prevalence of HNPCC. Thus, when diagnostic criteria are loosened, more cases of colorectal cancer will be attributed to HNPCC and vice versa. Conversely, simply because a family fulfils the minimum criteria for HNPCC does not unfailingly mean that the apparent familial aggregation is due to genetic predisposition. Colorectal cancer is a very common disease and so aggregation of cases in a family could occur by chance. The issue of diagnostic criteria has a major effect on the apparent prevalence of HNPCC and also considerably influences the apparent penetrance of the gene defect(s). HNPCC is said to be a disorder with high penetrance,[52] but it is the diagnostic criteria that demand a highly penetrant disease! Thus, diagnostic criteria create considerable circularity in the assignment of penetrance and indeed the prevalence of HNPCC. The criteria proposed by the International Collaborative Group on HNPCC require: (1) three or more relatives with histologically proven colorectal cancer, one being a first degree relative of the other two; (2) two or more generations affected; and (3) at least one family member affected before age 50 years (The 'Amsterdam Criteria').[53] Evidence from analysis of the genes responsible for the majority of HNPCC has led to the expansion of these criteria to include extracolonic cancers, such as endometrial, upper gastrointestinal tract and urinary tract cancers.[5] In addition to the predetermination of gene penetrance, such criteria will only identify families of sufficient size to allow the appropriate number of cases to arise. Therefore, as already stated, many small families will be inappropriately excluded. However, the recent identification of several causative genes will allow systematic assessment of the prevalence and penetrance of HNPCC on a whole population basis.

There are no robust biomarkers for HNPCC. Abnormalities of colonic epithelial cell proliferation and the crypt cell production rate have been reported in HNPCC.[54] These abnormalities appear to be more pronounced as the strength of family history increases.[55,56] This effect may be due to shared family environment but this cannot fully explain these observations because, although relatives of colorectal cancer patients are at increased risk, their spouses have the same risk as the general population.[57] There is a predominance of certain tumour histological features in HNPCC, such as a lymphoid response, mucinous histology and poor differentiation,[58,59] but these features are not specific and do not accurately identify all cases of familial colorectal cancer. One useful biomarker for HNPCC has been identified in recent years in light of elucidation of the molecular basis of cancer susceptibility in this syndrome, namely, tumour genetic instability or MSI. This is due to defective DNA mismatch repair (MMR). While not all MSI+ tumours are due to germline defects in *MMR* genes, patients with tumours exhibiting this phenotype are highly enriched for HNPCC. Systematic analysis of *MMR* genes and the further study of the prevalence of MSI+ tumours is now shedding light on the overall contribution of these genes to cancer susceptibility.

The DNA mismatch repair genes

Identification of colorectal tumours displaying widespread genomic instability at short repetitive DNA tracts suggested that defective DNA mismatch repair might be involved, in view of previous work in bacteria and yeast.[60–63] The best defined mismatch repair system is in *E. coli* (reviewed in Grilley *et al*[64]), where a number of gene products are required, namely MutL, MutH, MutS and MutU. Yeast also have a similar mismatch repair pathway, which requires a homologue of MutS and two MutL homologues, MLH1 and PMS1.[65,66] Around the same time that these observations of a mutator phenotype in HNPCC patients tumours were being made, a systematic linkage mapping strategy was in progress investigating a number of large HNPCC kindreds. In two families, linkage analysis identified a locus linked to the anonymous marker, D2S123, which maps to the short arm of chromosome 2.[67] Fourteen smaller families were also analysed and one-third

showed no evidence of linkage to D2S123. In addition, a second locus was identified by a report of linkage to a marker on chromosome 3p shortly afterwards,[68] clearly establishing locus heterogeneity in HNPCC.

A combination of positional cloning and candidate gene approaches to gene isolation was then employed by two groups to identify the human homologues of the yeast and bacterial DNA mismatch repair genes. The first to be isolated was *MSH2* on chromosome 2p. Using degenerate PCR primers for the yeast *MSH* genes, Fishel *et al*. identified the human homologue *MSH2* and localized it to the same region on chromosome 2p as the markers linked in HNPCC families.[69] Vogelstein's group generated multiple markers within a 25 cM region defined by the linkage studies.[70] When analysed in HNPCC families linked to the 2p gene, recombination events were identified that designated a minimum region containing the gene of interest. After extensive screening of candidate genes mapping to this region, germline mutations were identified in HNPCC kindreds in a gene homologous to the bacterial MutS gene. This was named *hMSH2* (human MutS homologue). A 2802 bp cDNA from *MSH2* was found to contain a highly conserved region between codons 615 and 788 with considerable cross-species homology between human, yeast and bacteria. Several mutations were identified within the highly conserved region, including stop codons, resulting in premature truncation of the protein product and a splice site alteration. Mutations were also shown to co-segregate with the disease in HNPCC families.

With the discovery that there was a dramatic increase in repetitive tract instability in yeast, when mutations were induced in the yeast MutL homologues MLH or PMS,[67] the human homologues of other genes involved in the MMR pathway were obvious candidates. Indeed, following their identification, mutations of other MMR genes were demonstrated to be responsible for the HNPCC syndrome.[71,72] *MLH1* was shown to be the gene segregating with chromosome 3p markers[68] and *PMS1* and *PMS2* lie on chromosomes 2q and 7q, respectively.[73] The other human *MSH* genes, *MSH6* (also known as *GTBP/p160*[74,75]) and *MSH3*[76] were initially only thought to be involved somatically in tumour formation. However, recent evidence has identified mutations in *MSH6* as a strong candidate for the germline defect in atypical HNPCC families, especially those families where endometrial cancer is a predominant feature.[77–79] A further *MMR* gene has been identified recently, *MLH3*,[80] which has higher homology to the bacterial and yeast proteins than to mammalian MMR proteins. As it is the 3rd MutL homologue to be identified, its role in HNPCC is questionable, due to the functional redundancy likely between *PMS2/PMS1* and the newly cloned *MLH3*, although it has been found to induce microsatellite instability (MSI) on mutation.[80] It is possible that, like *MSH6*, it may play a role in the less typical HNPCC cancer families.

MMR mutation spectrum and genotype–phenotype correlations

The mutational spectrum in *MSH*, *MLH* and *PMS* genes in HNPCC is influenced by case selection. However, reported mutations include base substitutions, and insertions/deletions, both short and of a few hundred basepairs. The proportion of HNPCC families due to mutations in each of the genes remains to be elucidated, but it would appear that around 58 per cent of mutations identified are in *MLH1* and 38 per cent in *MSH2* [ICG-HNPCC at www.nfdht.nl]. Very few germline mutations have been identified in the MutL homologues *PMS2* and *PMS1*. This may be due to redundancy between the participants in the DNA mismatch repair pathway, including *MLH3*, which has only recently been cloned.

Some evidence for genotype–phenotype correlations is coming to light for a number of the *MMR* genes. There are reports that *MSH2* mutations are associated with an excess risk of extracolonic cancers, such as transitional cell carcinoma of the renal-pelvis and ureter, as well as carcinoma of the stomach and ovaries.[81] *MSH2* and *MLH1* mutations impart a substantially elevated risk of endometrial and small bowel cancers.[81–83] Other reports suggest that gastric cancer is more prevalent in *MLH1* than in *MSH2* gene carriers (11.0 per cent vs. 4.5 per cent) and that these cancers are of intestinal type, a specific histological type associated with enviromental aetiology.[84] As already stated, the *MSH6* gene is associated with atypical HNPCC families that have an excess of endometrial cases, a delayed age of onset of the disease and incomplete penetrance.[77–79] Our own data indicate that gender also influences cancer risk – the lifetime risk of colorectal cancer in *MSH2/MLH1* gene carriers was significantly greater for males than females (74 per cent vs. 30 per cent). The endometrial risk in females was 42 per cent, and the lifetime risk for all cancers was 91 per cent for males and 69 per cent for females.[82,83]

Two other related syndromes are caused by germline mutations of the *MMR* genes. The rare autosomal dominant cancer susceptibility syndrome Muir–Torre is diagnosed by the presence of at least one sebaceous gland neoplasm (adenoma, epithelioma or carcinoma) and/or a keratoacanthoma and at least one internal malignancy. It is now thought that this syndrome is an allelic variant of HNPCC: germline mutations in either *MSH2* or *MLH1* (predominantly *MSH2*) have been identified but other genetic and enviromental factors may play a role in the differences in phenotypic expression.[85–87] Turcot syndrome, already described above, can be separated into two variants. Germline mutations of *PMS2* or *MLH1* are associated with the phenotypic expression of glioblastoma multiforme in HNPCC families, rather than the cerebellar medulloblastomas associated with defects in *APC*.[51]

Although there is considerable allelic heterogeneity, data so far have not indicated any clear link between phenotype and specific germline mutations at any given gene. However, work on a Danish founder mutation (*MLH1* intron 14 splice donor) in a family with a low frequency of extracolonic cancers, revealed that the allele was not transcribed and so the low rate of extracolonic cancer may be due to inability of the mutant protein to exert a dominant negative effect.[88] Another group has suggested that missense mutations in the *MMR* genes may result in a less severe phenotype or lower penetrance, as functionally relevant structural changes may be less severe.[89] Further studies of the relationship of mutation to clinical outcome using model animals and *in vitro* systems may help in this regard.[90,91]

Since inactivation of either *MSH*, *MLH* or *PMS* in humans and in yeast results in a mutator phenotype[60,65,66,72,73,92] and the true penetrance of HNPCC gene mutations may well be relatively low, this suggests that the population mutation frequency may be substantially higher than previously suspected. This has important implications for human population genetics. Lynch has calculated that the population gene frequency of an HNPCC allele may be around 0.005,[93] and recently we have indicated that the population prevalence could be as high as 1 in 2793.[94] Hence, it is perfectly reasonable to expect progeny from (say) an *MLH1*− and *MSH2*− pairing. This has intriguing implications for the DNA repair pathway in such progeny. It is possible that the *MLH1*−/*MSH2*− genotype may be lethal, but most of the evidence suggests that there is no effect of heterozygous inactivation of either gene and that homozygous inactivation is required for tumour formation.[95] In addition, *MLH1/PMS1* double mutants in yeast have very similar phenotypes to either *MLH1* or *PMS1* single mutants.[60,65,66] Clearly, individuals carrying such a genotype would be at an increased risk of HNPCC-related cancers. Indeed, there are now reports of homozygosity for mismatch repair deficiency. All three reports involve the *MLH1* gene alone. The first involved two different heterozygous missense mutations and the patient developed breast cancer at the age of 35;[96] the other two reports are of the progeny of consanguineous parents. In these families, the phenotype of the homozygous children was much more severe, with the development of early-onset haematological maligancies (also prevalent in mouse models deficient for *MMR*) and neurofibromatosis type 1.[97,98] MSI analysis of somatic tissues from the children demonstrated that there was indeed a constitutional mismatch repair deficiency in the normal tissues. It is also exciting to speculate that such a genotype may have a dramatic effect on repeat sequences in the germline of such double mutant gene carriers. Expansion of repeated sequences is known to cause disorders such as Huntington's chorea and Fragile X. It is intriguing to speculate that passage through the germline of such gene carriers, or even of the germline of a single mutant, might contribute to the expansion of triplet repeats characteristic of such genetic disorders. There is some evidence to suggest this may be the case, as a defined *MLH1* mutation has been reported in association with instability at the *FRAXA* locus.[99] However, work in model systems on the repair of triplet repeats has provided conflicting results. Work in bacteria has demonstrated that MMR acts to promote large deletions from triplet repeat sequences that are tract length dependent, but prevents smaller length changes.[100,101] Conversely, defective MMR increases the frequency of small changes in bacteria and yeast.[102–104] MMR has also been postulated to have a causal role in the instability of triplet repeats in human fetal tissues.[105] However, investigation of simple repeats in families suffering from Huntington's chorea demonstrated that only the triplet repeat associated with the disease showed any instability.[106] More work is required to provide further understanding of the influence of DNA MMR on genomic instability observed in many disorders.

Mismatch repair defects in humans and DNA instability in tumours

Tumours from HNPCC gene carriers exhibit a characteristic alteration in the stability of repetitive tract DNA in microsatellite markers[62,107,108] (an example of an MSI+ tumour is shown in Figure 24.2) and in tumour-promoting genes, such as *TGFβRII*, *BAX* and *APC*.[47,109,110] Such changes are also detectable in around one in six of apparently sporadic colorectal cancers.[61–63,111] These 'sporadic' tumours with MSI tend to be right sided, diploid, with an inverse relationship with *TP53* mutation and to be associated with good prognosis. A common mechanism of somatic inactivation of DNA mismatch repair in the sporadic cases is epigenetic silencing of *MLH1* by hypermethylation of CpG islands in the promoter.[112–115] Thus, deficiency of the DNA mismatch repair process can occur via different mechanisms – germline mutation and subsequent inactivation of the wild-type allele[70,72] or, in the true sporadic cases, by two somatic alterations, of which the majority are due to hypermethylation of *hMLH1* (now termed CpG Island methylator phenotype).[112,114]

Our own investigations of very early-onset colorectal cancer demonstrate that more than half display the MSI phenotype[116] and that the majority of these contain identifiable germline MMR gene mutations.[117] Therefore, identification of microsatellite instability in tumours on a prospective basis from the general population may have utility in understanding the influence of these different mechanisms on clinicopathological factors. Retrospective data from our own laboratory[118] suggests that inference of data from older cohorts to early-onset cases is not entirely valid. The tumour histopathology was significantly

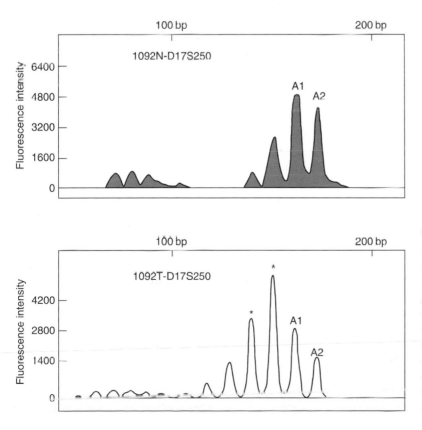

Figure 24.2 *A tumour showing microsatellite instability. The top panel shows colonic normal mucosal DNA from a patient amplified with the CA repeat marker D17S250. The presence of the two alleles is denoted by A1 and A2, the size of A1 is indicated as ~152 basepairs. The lower panel represents a colorectal tumour from the same patient, alleles A1 and A2 are shown and the extra alleles are denoted by *, the first extra allele being of ~150 base pairs. These traces are from an ABI Prism310.*

different between the two cohorts and MSI was only associated with better prognosis in the older cohort, and not with patients developing the disease under the age of 30. This indicates that the different molecular mechanisms of the MSI phenotype may play a significant role in survival. However, a recent study investigating MSI in colorectal cancer patients diagnosed when aged under 50[119] suggests that MSI is an independent predictor of a favourable outcome in this age group. This study only investigated tumour MSI and no germline analysis of MMR genes was performed; these results could, therefore, still demonstrate fundamental age-dependent differences in tumour MSI origin. Further studies are required to clarify the impact of germline mutation on prognosis.

The detection of microsatellite instability in endometrial cancer[120] and in a number of cancers of different tissue origin in HNPCC gene carriers[108] is of great interest. The underlying HNPCC gene mutation does appear to be responsible for the mutator phenotype, although the pathways may be different.[79] In addition, it has been shown that microsatellite instability occurs in tumours from patients with multiple different primary cancers,[121] suggesting that such individuals may well carry DNA repair gene mutations even without a family history of cancer.

MOLECULAR MECHANISMS OF COLORECTAL CARCINOGENESIS AND DEFECTIVE MMR

The human MMR system appears to be similar to that in yeast with MSH, MLH and PMS homologues. A homologue of the *E. coli* MutH gene has not been detected in yeast but has been recently reported for the human system. Bellacosa *et al.* demonstrated that the human DNA repair protein MED1/MBD4 (a methyl CpG binding protein with homology to bacterial DNA repair glycosylases/lyases[122]) forms a complex with MLH1[123] and displays endonuclease activity. It has been suggested that MED1 is the human equivalent of the bacterial endonuclease, MutH. Mismatch repair involves recognition and binding of mismatches by two separate MSH heterodimers. MutSα is a complex of MSH2/MSH6 and binds to G:T mismatches and small deletions/insertions, whereas MutSβ is a complex of MSH2/MSH3 and binds looped DNA, denoting larger deletions and insertions.[124,125] The correct strand for excision is recognized and the MLH and PMS complexes work in concert to direct excision of a segment of DNA some 1–2 kb in length, which is subsequently repaired by DNA polymerase. There may well be further mismatch repair systems, including a nucleotide-specific mismatch repair system that recognizes deaminated bases such as 5MeC, which produce G:T mismatches.[126] Such a system is of great interest because G:T mismatches will result in a C–T transition if allowed to progress through mitosis. Such transitions are frequently

seen in the *APC* gene in colorectal tumours in addition to short deletions or insertions at repetitive sequences. Hence this opens the intriguing possibility that many of the somatic changes that are involved in the genesis of colorectal cancer may be caused by defects in DNA MMR. Indeed, in tumours displaying MSI, we have observed a marked propensity for somatic mutations of the *APC* gene to occur at repeat tracts.[47] However, other studies have not observed any particular predominance of such mutations and this may be due to differences in the proportion of tumours arising in germline MMR gene mutation carriers.[48] Nonetheless, it is clear that MMR deficiency results in an elevated mutation rate in several key genes involved in colorectal carcinogenesis (reviewed in Kinzler and Vogelstein[127]). This is also supported by the finding that microsatellite instability is detectable in early adenomas of patients carrying HNPCC gene mutations.[108]

Mouse models have been created for all the MMR genes, but the inactivation of most is quite surprising, with lymphomas being the most prevalent tumour and then gastrointestinal tumours (reviewed in Heyer *et al*[128]). Interestingly, the Pms1 mouse model does not display any tumour burden and a number of the other MMR knockouts have meiotic phenotypes, resulting in reduced fertility or infertility, suggesting that these genes have unique roles in gametogenesis. Thus, these models are helping to reveal the other functions of the MMR genes, which include methylation tolerance and hyper-recombination between divergent sequences,[129] a role in the cell-cycle checkpoint mechanisms[130] and also in apoptosis.[131] Many of these functions have major implications for conventional chemotherapeutic regimes. MMR-deficient cells showing resistance to alkylating agents (methylation tolerance) are often resistant to other cytotoxic drugs, such as 5-fluorouracil,[132] although this toxicity has also been shown to be *p53*-dependent.[133] These drugs are commonly used in the treatment of colorectal cancer patients and may have genotoxic effects on normal tissues of patients with a MMR defect. Thus, in the future, treatment regimes may be tailored according to the genetic profile of a given tumour with respect to MMR status.

Much work remains to be done in understanding the effects of these HNPCC gene mutations in carcinogenesis, their effect on mutation rate in the homozygous and heterozygous state, on population gene frequency, penetrance and the question of other DNA repair systems that may be involved in heritable predisposition to colorectal cancer.

OTHER CANDIDATE SUSCEPTIBILITY GENES INVOLVED IN HNPCC

Not all HNPCC families are due to mutations of known MMR genes, suggesting that defects in other, as yet unidentified, MMR genes may be implicated in some

HNPCC families. There is intense research interest in fully defining the deranged cellular pathways involved in colorectal cancer at the somatic level and many of the components of these pathways are potential candidate susceptibility alleles.

The transforming growth factor β (TGFβ)/SMAD pathway is an interesting example of a deranged signalling transduction pathway, observed in sporadic and familial colorectal cancer, but with relevance to germline susceptibility. A total of 80–90 per cent MSI$^+$ colorectal tumours display mutations in a coding polyA tract in the TGFβRII gene,[109] resulting in inactivation of the TGFβ receptor and so downregulating the antiproliferative effects of soluble TGFβ. A proportion of MSI$^-$ cancers also harbour somatic mutations of the gene, although these arise in the kinase domain[134] and not the poly-A repeat. However, the consequence of each of these mutations is inactivation of receptor function, thereby emphasizing that dysregulation of TGFβ signalling plays a contributory role in colorectal tumorigenesis. A link with cancer susceptibility was established following identification of germline TGFβRII mutations in atypical colorectal cancer families. The mutations not only segregated with the disease but also resulted in disruption of TGFβ signalling.[135]

Only a small fraction of all familial colorectal cancer is due to mutations of TGFβRII, but this example serves to emphasize the importance of fully understanding each of the components of a signalling pathway, so that a comprehensive assessment of all the relevant potential candidates can be investigated. Thus, unravelling the complexities of TGFβ signalling resulted in characterization of the molecular basis of another colorectal cancer predisposition syndrome, namely juvenile polyposis (see later). That chromosome 18q harboured a tumour suppressor gene relevant to the development of colorectal cancer was first suggested by frequent cytogenetic deletions[136] and loss of heterozygosity in that region.[137] Subsequently, a number of genes have been identified from the region, including DCC (deleted in colorectal cancer[138]), JV18 and DPC4 (deleted in pancreatic cancer[139]). DPC4 is a homolog of a family of Drosophila genes, known as SMADs, which code for cytoplasmic proteins involved in TGFβ signalling. Heterozygous mutations of Smad4 gene in mice induce a cancer phenotype, although it is a fairly late age of onset.[140] Recently, germline mutations of SMAD4/DPC4 have been identified in a number of hereditary juvenile polyposis syndrome (JPS) familes.[141] JPS will be discussed in the next section but there is an elevated risk of colorectal cancer in JPS families, thereby authenticating the idea that disruption of the TGFβ signalling pathway has important implications for colorectal carcinogenesis and also emphasizing the complex inter-relationship of genes involved in colorectal neoplasia at the somatic and the germline level.

The involvement of the p53 gene in colorectal carcinogenesis has been investigated extensively and, while p53 mutations have been shown to be responsible for a proportion of Li–Fraumeni families,[142] colorectal cancer is rare in Li–Fraumeni gene carriers. Furthermore, constitutional p53 mutations have not been identified in patients who developed colorectal cancer at a very young age.[143] Hence, it seems highly unlikely that p53 mutations confer susceptibility to colorectal cancer despite frequent abnormalities of p53 in somatic colorectal cancer tissue.

HEREDITARY COLORECTAL CANCER AND ANEUPLOIDY

Although MMR gene defects play an important role in an appreciable fraction of all cases of colorectal cancer, the majority of tumours are proficient for DNA mismatch repair. However, these tumours often exhibit aneuploidy (Plate 3 shows an example of an aneuploid cell), perhaps due to defects in cell cycle control or chromosome segregation.[144–146] A number of mechanisms might explain aneuploidy in colon cancer cells including defective cell cycle checkpoint control, aberrant chromosome segregation, defects in any, or all, of cytokinesis, kinetochores and the centrosome cycle. Again colorectal cancer has provided a model system for investigation of the role of aneuploidy in tumour formation. Aneuploidy has recently been shown to be an ongoing process, termed the chromosomal instability (CIN) phenotype.[146] In some instances, CIN phenotype has been shown to be due to defects in the G2/M checkpoint genes BUB1 and BUBR1.[146] Somatic mutations have been demonstrated in these genes in CIN tumour cell lines, but a germline change has also been identified.[146] Thus, BUB genes are candidate susceptibility loci, although much work remains to be done and no other germline changes have been identified in any of the other checkpoint genes.[147] It seems likely that checkpoint control genes may play a role in somatic alterations of aneuploid tumours, but their involvement in cancer susceptibility remains to be defined.

THE GENETICS OF OTHER POLYPOSIS COLON CANCER SUSCEPTIBILITY SYNDROMES

There are a number of rarer syndromes that are associated with an elevated risk of colorectal cancer, usually markedly lower than the cancer risk in FAP and HNPCC. Each of the syndromes is characterized by benign polyposis of the intestine and the polyps are of unusual histology. The clinical phenotypes of these syndromes are heterogeneous and there is some clinical overlap between them. Genes involved in these hereditary syndromes have recently been described and are providing new insights into the molecular mechanisms involved in susceptibility to colorectal cancer.

Juvenile polyposis

Juvenile polyposis is an autosomal dominant syndrome with incomplete penetrance and manifests as diffuse harmatomatous polyps of the colon, small bowel and stomach, with onset at a very early age (less than 10 years) and another at ~55 years. Using genetic linkage studies, the JPS locus was mapped to chromosome 18q and analysis of candidate genes in the area demonstrated germline mutations of *SMAD4/DPC4* in a number of familes.[141] A small number of JPS families have also been associated with the *PTEN* gene and mutations in *BMPRIA*.[148,149,150] The complexities of the relationship of cancer susceptibility and the TGFβ/SMAD signalling pathway have been outlined earlier in the text.

Peutz–Jeghers syndrome

Peutz–Jeghers Syndrome (PJS) is a rare autosomal dominant condition with low penetrance, whose susceptibility defect has been recently identified. It is characterized by the development of hamartomatous polyposis of the gastrointestinal tract and, in 95 per cent of the patients, the hallmark feature is melanin spots on the lips and buccal mucosa. There is an increased risk of gastrointestinal, pancreatic, testis, ovarian, breast and uterine cancers.[151] The PJS gene was mapped to chromosome 19p13.3, cloned and mutations identified in a number of families.[152–154] The gene encodes a novel nuclear serine/threonine kinase and was named *LKB1* or *STK11*. This gene appears to be involved in signalling and regulation of cellular differentiation and it appears that a cAMP-dependent kinase is involved in the regulation of its function by phosphorylation.[153] Given the paradigms of the APC/β-catenin and the TGFβ/SMAD pathways, it seems likely that other components of this pathway may be involved in colorectal tumorigenesis and also perhaps in germline susceptibility.

Cowden disease (see Chapter 12)

Cowden disease is a rarely recognized autosomal dominant disorder characterized by the development of oral and facial papules in concert with harmatomatous lesions of the thyroid, breast, skin and digestive tract. Occasionally, there are also neurological features. The gene was mapped to chromosome 10q22–24[155] and then cloned, and mutations identified in affected family members.[156–158] *PTEN* encodes a dual specificity phosphatase, which is downregulated by TGFβ. PTEN also shares

homology to the focal adhesion protein tensin and is, therefore, implicated in many different regulatory roles, such as cell motility, migration, communication, etc., which on disruption lead to an increase in invasion and metastasis.[158] For both JPS and CD, the genes identified do not account for all the families and, thus, more genes may be identified as susceptibility genes for these syndromes.

CLINICAL RELEVANCE OF COLORECTAL CANCER SUSCEPTIBILITY GENES AND RISK ALLELES

Available data suggest that colorectal cancer is preventable by removal of premalignant polyps, while survival is related to stage at presentation. Hence, there is real potential to reduce colorectal cancer mortality by early detection through identifying individuals who carry susceptibility alleles, in order to instigate preventative measures, such as colonoscopic surveillance. In some circumstances, such as in FAP, the cancer risk is so high that prophylactic colectomy is indicated and so molecular screening is already under way in FAP kindreds. This has allowed targeting clinical screening to gene carriers and avoids unnecessary investigation of non-carriers.[159,160] Similarly, the effect of characterizing the mutations and identifying the gene carriers in HNPCC has great potential for substantial reduction in colon cancer mortality in such families. There is even the prospect for large-scale mutation detection in asymptomatic populations, targeting the screening to relatives of cancer cases.

Molecular analysis of colorectal cancer susceptibility syndromes is shedding new light on the complexities of pathways that control cellular proliferation and normal cellular function. The APC/β-catenin signalling pathway is of central importance to the development of both familial and sporadic colorectal cancer. Defining the genetic defects resulting in defective DNA mismatch repair as well as understanding the complex inter-relationships of TGFβ signalling pathways has already identified a number of susceptibility loci, and will doubtless continue to advance knowledge of the genetic basis of colorectal cancer. It seems likely that classification of hereditary syndromes will change from the current empirical, descriptive clinical definitions to incorporate a molecular description related to clinical phenotype. Animal models of key susceptibility genes will allow study of gene function, of regulatory elements and of the influence of modifier genes on colorectal cancer susceptibility. It may be possible to develop novel preventative treatment regimes by exploiting model systems, such as transgenic animals. Already such studies are underway in animal models of FAP in order to investigate non-steroidal anti-inflammatory agents, in view of the known effect of such agents on reducing colorectal cancer risk[161] and in causing polyp regression in FAP patients.[162] Given the scale of the problem of colorectal cancer throughout the industrialized world, there is already considerable commercial interest in developing chemopreventative agents, informed by understanding of the fundamental basis of colorectal carcinogenesis.

The current rapid progress in understanding colorectal carcinogenesis seems set to continue. Molecular genetics seem set to influence clinical management by targeting screening to those at risk of the disease and by affording the development of agents that will prevent the disease, which has, to date, resisted progress in conventional therapeutic approaches and the best efforts of medical research.

RECENT ADVANCES

Recently, a number of exciting major advances have been made in the understanding of the field of heritable susceptibility to colorectal cancer, and we briefly describe these here.

Intriguing data come from two publications regarding a new role for the APC protein in chromosome segregation.[163,164] Not only does APC bind to microtubules, but it presents them to the kinetochores – these are protein complexes that mediate the attachment of chromosomes to the spindle apparatus in order to accurately separate the sister chromatids during mitosis. Mouse cells which were homozygous for the truncating APC[min] mutation displayed abnormal chromosome patterns when compared with their wild-type counterparts. Thus, there is now evidence indicating that the APC protein plays an important role in maintaining fidelity of chromosome segregation and thereby contributes to the prevention of aneuploidy. This underscores the importance of observations that aneuploidy occurs in the majority of colorectal cancers and indicates further complexity in the role that APC mutations play in tumorigenesis and tumour progression.

As we previously hypothesized in the introduction, there is now concrete evidence for a recessive syndrome predisposing to colorectal neoplasia. The *MUTYH* gene has been identified as a recessive susceptibility gene for multiple adenoma formation.[165] A number of multiple adenoma families were screened and found to contain homozygous or compound heterozygous variants of the *MUTYH* gene.[166] The protein product, MYH, is an integral part of cellular DNA repair systems with a major role in base excision repair, expecially the repair of 8oxoG:A mispairs. Lack of MYH results in an increased frequency of G:C toT:A transversion mutations in coding and non-coding DNA sequences. Interestingly, a major source of these mispairs is through oxidative damage, which is prevalent in the gut. Future goals will be to determine the relevance of *MUTYH* as a colorectal cancer risk allele and assess the protein's function in carcinogenesis.

Another hot area of research is the identification of cancer risk alleles of moderate to low penetrance and also alleles that interact with major susceptibility alleles to modify the cancer susceptibility phenotype. Although many association studies are hampered by lack of statistical power, due to low effect and small cohort numbers, one robust candidate seems to be a variant in STK15.[167] This was found to be a low penetrant allele in an outbred murine model with some supporting human data. Interestingly, the gene resides in a chromosomal area showing allelic imbalance in Finnish familial colorectal cancer cases.[168] Other important candidate risk alleles include a variant in the transforming growth factor-beta receptor type I gene,[169] a gene involved in the TGF/SMAD signalling pathway. Interestingly TGF/SMAD signalling has already been implicated in colorectal carcinogenesis. Finally cyclin D1 is emerging as an important modifier of HNPCC[170] as well as a possible risk allele in itself. Future analysis of these risk and modifying alleles will require very large case-control cohorts to robustly assess their effect on colorectal cancer risk.

KEY POINTS

- FAP is an autosomal dominant disease with >100 colonic polyps. It is due to mutations in the *APC* gene. There is some genotype/phenotype correlation. Attenuated FAP with fewer polyps tends to have mutations in a different part of the gene from classical FAP.

- HNPCC is an autosomal dominant disease with <100 polyps and other features, often other cancers. A large proportion of classical families that have a certain phenotype, the 'Amsterdam' criteria, have mutations in mismatch repair genes. There are now antibodies for the products of these genes and loss of staining is associated with mutation. Increasingly, immunohistochemistry of tumour tissue is being used as a first step in the testing process.

- There are other rarer conditions, for example PJS, JP, which are due to mutations in other genes (*LKB1 or STK11; SMAD4*).

- It is now recognized that there are recessive multiple adenoma families with an increased risk of colon cancer in mutation carrier homozygotes (*MutYH*).

REFERENCES

1. Bonelli L, Martines H, Conio M, *et al.* Family history of colorectal cancer as a risk factor for benign and malignant tumours of the large bowel. A case control study. *Int J Cancer* 1988; **41**:513–517.

2. Cannon-Albright LA, Solnick MH, Bishop DT, *et al.* Common inheritance of susceptibility to colonic adenomatous polyps and associated colorectal cancers. *N Engl J Med* 1988; **319**:533–537.

3. Kee F, Collins BJ. How prevalent is cancer family syndrome? *Gut* 1991; **32**:509–512.

4. Lynch HT, de la Chapelle A. Genetic susceptibility to non-polyposis colorectal cancer. *J Med Genet* 1999; **36**:801–818.

5. Vasen HFA, Watson P, Mecklin J-P, *et al.* New clinical criteria for hereditary nonpolyposis colorectal cancer (HNPCC, Lynch syndrome) proposed by the International Collaborative Group on HNPCC. *Gastroenterology* 1999; **116**:1453–1456.

6. Bisgaard ML, Fenger K, Bulow S, *et al.* Familial adenomatous polyposis (FAP): frequency, penetrance, and mutation rate. *Hum Mutat* 1994; **3**:121–125.

7. Bodmer WF, Bailey CJ, Bodmer J, *et al.* Localisation of the gene for familial adenomatous polyposis on chromosome 5. *Nature* 1987; **328**:614–616.

8. Leppert M, Dobbs M, Scambler P, *et al.* The gene for familial polyposis maps to the long arm of chromosome 5. *Science* 1987; **238**:1411–1413.

9. Kinzler KW, Nilbert MC, Su L-K, *et al.* Identification of FAP locus genes from chromosome 5q21. *Science* 1991; **253**:661–664.

10. Joslyn L, Carlson M, Thliveris A, *et al.* Identification of deletion mutations and three new genes at the familial polyposis locus. *Cell* 1991; **66**:601–613.

11. Groden J, Thliveris A, Samowitz W, *et al.* Identification and characterization of the familial adenomatous polyposis coli gene. *Cell* 1991; **66**:589–600.

12. Miyoshi Y, Ando H, Nagase H, *et al.* Germ-line mutations of the *APC* gene in 53 familial adenomatous polyposis patients. *Proc Natl Acad Sci USA* 1992; **89**:4452–4456.

13. Nagase H, Miyoshi Y, Horii A, *et al.* Screening for germ-line mutations in familial adenomatous polyposis patients: 61 new patients and a summary of 150 unrelated patients. *Hum Mutat* 1992; **1**:467–473.

14. Nagase H, Nakamura Y. Mutations of the *APC* (adenomatous polyposis coli) gene. *Hum Mutat* 1993; **2**:425–434.

15. Mandl M, Paffenholz R, Friedl W, *et al.* Frequency of common and novel inactivating *APC* mutations in 202 families with familial adenomatous polyposis. *Hum Molec Genet* 1994; **3**:181–184.

16. Smith KJ, Johnson KA, Bryan TM, *et al.* The *APC* gene product in normal and tumour cells. *Proc Natl Acad Sci USA* 1993; **90**:2846–2850.

17. Nathke IS, Adams CL, Polakis P, *et al.* The adenomatous polyposis coli (APC) tumour suppressor protein localizes to plasma membrane sites involved in active cell migration. *J Cell Biol* 1996; **134**:165–180.

18. Rubinfeld B, Souza B, Albert I, *et al.* Association of the *APC* gene product with β-catenin. *Science* 1993; **262**:1731–1734.

19. Barth AIM, Nathke IS, Nelson WJ. Cadherins, catenins and APC protein: interplay between cytoskeletal complexes and signaling pathways. *Curr Opin Cell Biol* 1997; **9**:683–690.

20. Ben-Ze'ev A, Geiger B. Differential molecular interactions of β-catenin and plakoglobin in adhesion, signaling and cancer. *Curr Opin Cell Biol* 1998; **10**:629–639.

21. He T-C, Sparks AB, Rago C, *et al.* Identification of c-MYC as a target of the APC pathway. *Science* 1998; **281**:1509–1512.

22. Satoh S, Daigo Y, Furukawa Y, *et al.* AXIN1 mutations in hepatocellular carcinomas, and growth suppression in cancer cells by virus-mediated transfer of AXIN1. *Nature Genet* 2000; **24**:245–250.

23. Polakis P. The oncogenic activation of beta-catenin. *Curr Opin Genet Dev* 1999; **9**:15–21.

24. Munemitsu S, Souza B, Muller O, *et al.* The *APC* gene product associates with microtubules in vivo and promotes their assembly *in vitro*. *Cancer Res* 1994; **54**:3676–3681.

25. Smith KJ, Levy DB, Maupin P, *et al.* Wild-type but not mutant APC associates with microtubule cytoskeleton. *Cancer Res* 1994; **54**:3672–3675.

26. Su L-K, Burrell M, Hill DE, *et al.* APC binds to the novel protein EB1. *Cancer Res* 1995; **55**:2972–2977.

27. Matsumine A, Ogai A, Senda T, *et al.* Binding of APC to the human homolog of the Drosophila discs large tumour suppressor protein. *Science* 1996; **272**:1020–1023.

28. Burt RW. Familial risk and colorectal cancer. *Gastroenterol Clinics North Am* 1996; **25**:793–803.

29. Moser AR, Pitot HC, Dove WF. A dominant mutation that predisposes to multiple intestinal neoplasia in the mouse. *Science* 1990; **247**:322–324.

30. Su L-K, Kinzler KW, Vogelstein B, *et al.* Multiple intestinal neoplasia caused by a mutation in the murine homolog of the *APC* gene. *Science* 1992; **256**:668–670.

31. Moser AR, Dove WF, Roth KA, *et al.* The Min (Multiple Intestinal Neoplasia) Mutation: Its effect on gut epithelial cell differentiation and interaction with a modifier system. *J Cell Biol* 1992; **116**:1517–1526.

32. Dietrich WF, Lander ES, Smith JS, *et al.* Genetic identification of Mom-1, a major modifier locus affecting Min-induced intestinal neoplasia in the mouse. *Cell* 1993; **75**:631–639.

33. MacPhee M, Chepenik KP, Liddell RA, *et al.* The secretory phospholipase A2 gene is a candidate for the Mom1 locus, a major modifier of Apc(Min)-induced intestinal neoplasia. *Cell* 1995; **81**:957–966.

34. Praml C, Savelyeva L, Le Paslier D, *et al.* Human homologue of a candidate for the Mom1 locus, the secretory type II phospholipase A2 (PLA2S-II), maps to 1p35-36/D1S199. *Cancer Res* 1995; **55**:5504–5506.

35. Tomlinson IPM, Neale K, Talbot IC, *et al.* A modifying locus for familial adenomatous polyposis may be present on chromosome 1p35-p36. *J Med Genet* 1996; **33**:268–273.

36. Dobbie Z, Heinimann K, Bishop DT, *et al.* Identification of a modifier gene locus on chromosome 1p35-36 in familial adenomatous polyposis. *Hum Genet* 1997; **99**:653–657.

37. Spirio LN, Kutchera W, Winstead MV, *et al.* Three secretory phospholipase A2 genes that map to human chromosome 1P35-36 are not mutated in individuals with attenuated adenomatous polyposis coli. *Cancer Res* 1996; **56**:955–958.

38. Dobbie Z, Muller H, Scott RJ. Secretory phospholipase A2 does not appear to be associated with phenotypic variation in familial adenomatous polyposis. *Hum Genet* 1996; **98**:386–390.

39. Van der Houven van Oordt CW, Smits R, Schouten TG, *et al.* The genetic background modifies the spontaneous and X-ray-induced tumor spectrum in the Apc1638N mouse model. *Genes Chromosomes Cancer* 1999; **24**:191–198.

40. Wasan HS, Novelli M, Bee J, *et al.* Dietary fat influences on polyp phenotype in multiple intestinal neoplasia mice. *Proc Natl Acad Sci USA* 1997; **94**:3308–3313.

41. Yang K, Edelmann W, Fan K, *et al.* Dietary modulation of carcinoma development in a mouse model for human familial adenomatous polyposis. *Cancer Res* 1998; **58**:5713–5717.

42. Cottrell S, Bicknell D, Kaklamanis L, *et al.* Molecular analysis of *APC* mutations in familial adenomatous polyposis and sporadic colon carcinomas. *Lancet* 1992; **340**:626–630.

43. Olschwang S, Laurent-Puig P, Groden J, *et al.* Germ-line mutations in the first 14 exons of the adenomatous polyposis coli (*APC*) gene. *Am J Hum Genet* 1993; **52**:273–279.

44. Nagase H, Miyoshi Y, Horii A, *et al.* Screening for germ-line mutations in familial adenomatous polyposis patients: 61 new patients and a summary of 150 unrelated patients. *Hum Mutat* 1993; **1**:467–473.

45. Groden J, Gelbert L, Thliveris A, *et al.* Mutational analysis of patients with adenomatous polyposis: identical inactivating mutations in unrelated individuals. *Am J Hum Genet* 1993; **52**:263–272.

46. Nagase H, Miyoshi Y, Horii A, *et al.* Correlation between the location of germ-line mutations in the *APC* gene and the number of colorectal polyps in familial adenomatous polyposis patients. *Cancer Res* 1992; **52**:4055–4057.

47. Huang J, Papadopoulos N, McKinley AJ, *et al. APC* mutations in colorectal tumors with mismatch repair deficiency. *Proc Natl Acad Sci USA* 1996; **93**:9049–9054.

48. Homfray TFR, Cottrell SE, Ilyas M, *et al.* Defects in mismatch repair occur after *APC* mutations in the pathogenesis of sporadic colorectal tumours. *Hum Mutat* 1998; **11**:114–120.

49. Su L-K, Johnson KA, Smith KJ, *et al.* Association between wild-type and mutant *APC* gene products. *Cancer Res* 1993; **53**:2728–2731.

50. Paul P, Letteboer T, Gelbert L, *et al.* Identical *APC* exon 15 mutations result in a variable phenotype in familial adenomatous polyposis. *Hum Molec Genet* 1993; **2**:925–931.

51. Hamilton SR, Parsons RE, Papadopoulos N, *et al.* The molecular basis of Turcot's syndrome. *N Engl J Med* 1995, **332**:839–847.

52. Lynch HT, Kimberling WJ, Albano WA, *et al.* Hereditary nonpolyposis colorectal cancer (Lynch Syndromes 1 and 2). 1. Clinical description of resource. *Cancer* 1985; **56**:934–938.

53. Vasen HFA, Mecklin J-P, Meera-Khan P, *et al.* The International Collaborative Group on Hereditary Non-Polyposis Colorectal Cancer (ICG-HNPCC). *Dis Colon Rectum* 1991; **34**:424–425.

54. Lipkin N, Blattner WE, Fraumeni JF, *et al.* Tritiated thymidine labelling distribution as a marker for hereditary predisposition to colon cancer. *Cancer Res* 1983; **43**:1899–1904.

55. Gerdes H, Gillin JS, Zimbalist E, *et al.* Expansion of the epithlial cell proliferative compartment and frequency of adenomatous polyps in the colon correlate with the strength of family history of colorectal cancer. *Cancer Res* 1993; **53**:279–282.

56. Rooney PS, Robinson MHE, Clarke PA, *et al.* Individuals with a strong family history of colorectal cancer demonstrate abnormal rectal mucosal proliferation. *Br J Surg* 1993; **80**:249–251.

57. Jenson OM, Bolander AM, Sigtryggsson P, *et al.* Large-bowel cancer in married couples in Sweden. A follow-up study. *Lancet* 1980; **1**:1161–1163.

58. Smyrk TC, Lynch HT, Watson PA, Appelman HD. Histological features of hereditary non-polyposis colorectal cancer. In: Utsunomiya J, Lynch HT (eds) *Hereditary colorectal cancer.* Tokyo: Springer-Verlag, 1990:357–362.

59. Jass JR, Smyrk TC, Stewart SM, *et al.* Pathology of hereditary non-polyposis colorectal cancer. *Anticancer Res* 1994; **14**:1631–1634

60. Strand M, Prolla TA, Liskay RM, *et al.* Destabilization of tracts of simple repetitive DNA in yeasts by mutations affecting DNA mismatch repair. *Nature* 1993; **365**:274–276.

61. Ionov Y, Peinado MA, Malkhosyan S, *et al.* Ubiquitous somatic mutations in simple repeated sequences reveal a new mechanism for colonic carcinogenesis. *Nature* 1993; **363**:558–561.

62. Aaltonen LA, Peltomaki P, Leach FS, *et al.* Clues to the pathogenesis of familial colorectal cancer. *Science* 1993; **260**:812–816.

63. Thibodeau SN, Bren G, Schaid D. Microsatellite instability in cancer of the proximal colon. *Science* 1993; **260**:816–819.

64. Grilley M, Holmes J, Yashar B, Modrich P. Mechanisms of DNA-mismatch correction. *Mutation Res* 1990; **26**:253–267.

65. Prolla TA, Christie D-M, Liskay RM. Dual requirement in yeast DNA mismatch repair for *MLH1* and *PMS1*, two homologs of bacterial MutL Gene. *Molec Cell Biol* 1994; **14**:407–415.

66. Prolla TA, Pang Q, Alani E, *et al. MLH1, PMS1* and *MSH2* interactions during the initiation of DNA mismatch repair in yeast. *Nature* 1994; **365**:1091–1093.

67. Peltomaki L, Aaltonen LA, Sistonen P, *et al.* Genetic mapping of a locus predisposing to human colorectal cancer. *Science* 1993; **260**:810–812.

68. Lindblom A, Tannergard P, Werelius B, Nordenskjold M. Genetic mapping of a second locus predisposing to hereditary non-polyposis colon cancer. *Nature Genet* 1993, **5**:279–282.

69. Fishel R, Lescoe MK, Rao MRS, *et al.* The human mutator gene homolog *MSH2* and its association with hereditary nonpolyposis colon cancer. *Cell* 1993; **75**:1027–1038.

70. Leach FS, Nicolaides NC, Papadopolous N, *et al.* Mutations of a MutS homolog in hereditary non-polyposis colorectal cancer. *Cell* 1993; **75**:1215–1225.

71. Bronner CE, Baker SM, Morrison PT, *et al.* Mutation in the DNA mismatch repair gene homologue *MLH1* is associated with hereditary non-polyposis colon cancer. *Nature* 1994; **360**:258–261.

72. Papadopolous N, Nicolaides NC, Wei Y-F, *et al.* Mutation of a mutL homolog in hereditary colon cancer. *Science* 1994; **263**:1625–1629.

73. Nicolaides NC, Papadopoulos N, Wei Y-F, *et al.* Mutations of two PMS homologues in hereditary nonpolyposis colon cancer. *Nature* 1994; **371**:75–80.

74. Jiricny J, Hughes M, Corman N, *et al.* A human 200-kDa protein binds selectively to DNA fragments containing GT mismatches. *Proc Natl Acad Sci USA* 1988; **85**:8860–8864.

75. Palombo F, Gallinari P, Iccarino I, *et al.* GTBP, a 160-kilodalton protein essential for mismatch-binding activity in human cells. *Science* 1995; **268**:1913–1914.

76. Watanabe A, Ikejima M, Suzuki N, *et al.* Genomic organization and expression of the human *MSH3* gene. *Genomics* 1996; **31**:311–318.

77. Miyaki M, Konishi M, Tanaka K, *et al.* Germline mutation of *MSH6* as the cause of hereditary nonpolyposis colorectal cancer. *Nature Genet* 1997; **17**:271–272.

78. Akiyama Y, Sato H, Yamada T, *et al.* Germ-line mutations of the *hMSH6/GTBP* gene in an atypical hereditary nonpolyposis colorectal cancer kindred. *Cancer Res* 1997; **57**:3920–3923.

79. Wijnen JT, de Leeuw W, Vasen H, *et al.* Familial endometrial cancer in female carriers of *MSH6* germ line mutations. *Nature Genet* 1999; **23**:142–144.

80. Lipkin SM, Wang V, Jacoby R, *et al. MLH3*: A DNA mismatch repair gene associated with mammalian microsatellite instability. *Nature Genet* 2000; **24**:27–35.

81. Vasen HFA, Wijnen JT, Menko FH, *et al.* Cancer risk in families with hereditary nonpolyposis colorectal cancer diagnosed by mutation analysis. *Gastroenterology* 1996; **110**:1020–1027.

82. Dunlop MG, Farrington SM, Carothers AD, *et al.* Cancer risk associated with germline DNA mismatch repair gene mutations. *Hum Molec Genet* 1997; **6**:105–110.

83. Froggatt NJ, Green J, Brassett C, *et al.* A common *MSH2* mutation in English and North American HNPCC families: origin, phenotypic expression, and sex specific differences in colorectal cancer. *J Med Genet* 1999; **36**:97–102.

84. Aarnio M, Mecklin J-P, Aaltonen LA, *et al.* Life-time risk of different cancers in hereditary nonpolyposis colorectal cancer (HNPCC) syndrome. *Int J Cancer* 1995; **64**:430–433.

85. Kolodner R, Hall N, Lipford J, *et al.* Structure of the human *MSH2* locus and analysis of two Muir–Torre kindreds for *MSH2* mutations. *Genomics* 1994; **24**:516–526.

86. Bapat M, Xia L, Madlensky L, *et al.* The genetic basis of Muir–Torre syndrome includes the *MLH1* locus. *Am J Hum Genet* 1996; **59**:736–739.

87. Kruse R, Lamberti C, Wang Y, *et al.* Is the mismatch repair deficient type of Muir–Torre syndrome confined to mutations in the *MSH2* gene? *Hum Genet* 1996; **98**:747–750.

88. Jäger AC, Bisgaard M-L, Myrhøj T, *et al.* Reduced frequency of extracolonic cancers in hereditary nonpolyposis colorectal cancer families with monoallelic *MLH1* expression. *Am J Hum Genet* 1997; **61**:129–138.

89. Beck NE, Tomlinson IPM, Homfray T, *et al.* Genetic testing is important in families with a history suggestive of hereditary non-polyposis colorectal even if the Amsterdam criteria are not fulfilled. *Br J Surg* 1997; **84**:233–237.

90. Shimodaira H, Filosi N, Shibata H, *et al.* Functional analysis of human *MLH1* mutations in *Saccharomyces cerevisiae. Nature Genet* 1998; **19**:384–389.

91. Guerrette S, Acharya S, Fishel R. The interaction of the human mutL homologues in hereditary nonpolyposis colon cancer. *J Biol Chem* 1999; **274**:6336–6341.

92. Liu B, Parsons RE, Hamilton SR, *et al. MSH2* Mutations in hereditary nonpolyposis colorectal cancer kindreds. *Cancer Res* 1994; **54**:4590–4594.

93. Lynch HT, Smryk TC, Watson P, *et al.* Genetics, natural history, tumor spectrum, and pathology of hereditary nonpolyposis colorectal cancer: an updated review. *Gastroenterology* 1993; **104**:1535–1549.

94. Dunlop MG, Farrington SM, Nicholl ID, *et al.* Population carrier frequency of *MSH2* and *MLH1* mutations. *Br J Cancer* 2000; **83**:1643–1645.

95. Parsons RE, Li G-M, Longley MJ, *et al.* Hypermutability and mismatch repair deficiency in RER$^+$ tumour cells. *Cell* 1993; **75**:1227–1236.

96. Hackman P, Tannergard P, Osei-Mensa S, *et al.* A compound heterozygote for two *MLH1* missense mutations. *Nature Genet* 1997; **17**:135–136.

97. Ricciardone MD, Oezcelik T, Cevher B, *et al.* Human *MLH1* deficiency predisposes to hematological malignancy and neurofibromatosis type 1. *Cancer Res* 1999; **59**:290–293.

98. Wang Q, Lasset C, Desseigne F, *et al.* Neurofibromatosis and early onset of cancers in *MLH1*-deficient children. *Cancer Res* 1999; **59**:294–297.

99. Sharrock A, Bunyan DJ, Pond MC, *et al.* FRAXA instability in a family with HNPCC. *J Med Genet* 1997; **34**:S55.

100. Jaworski A, Rosche WA, Gellibolian R, *et al.* Mismatch repair in *Escherichia coli* enhances instability of (CTG)$_n$ triplet-repeats from human hereditary diseases. *Proc Natl Acad Sci USA* 1995; **92**:11019–11023.

101. Pareniewski P, Jaworski A, Wells RD, Bowater RP. Length of CTG. CAG repeats determines the influence of mismatch repair on genetic instability. *J Molec Biol* 2000; **299**:865–874.

102. Schumacher S, Fuchs RPP, Bichara M. Expansion of CTG repeats from human disease genes is dependent upon replication mechanisms in *Escherichia coli*: the effect of long patch repair revisited. *J Molec Biol* 1997; **279**:1101–1110.

103. Wells RD, Pareniewski P, Pluciennik A, *et al.* Small slipped register genetic instabilities in *Escherichia coli* in triplet-repeat sequences associated with hereditary neurological diseases. *J Biol Chem* 1998; **273**:19532–19541.

104. Schweitzer JK, Livingstone DM. Destabilization of CAG trinucleotide repeaty tracts by mismatch repair mutations in yeast. *Hum Molec Genet* 1997; **6**:349–355.

105. Wöhrle D, Kennerknecht I, Wolf M, *et al.* Heterogeneity of DM kinase repeat expansion in different foetal tissues and further expansion during cell proliferation *in vitro*: evidence for a causal involvement of methyl-directed DNA mismatch repair in triplet-repeat stability. *Hum Molec Genet* 1995; **4**:1147–1153.

106. Goellner GM, Tester D, Thibodeau S, *et al.* Different mechanisms underlie DNA instability in Huntington disease and colorectal cancer. *Am J Hum Genet* 1997; **60**:879–890.

107. Peltomaki P, Lothe RA, Aaltonen LA, *et al.* Microsatellite instability is associated with tumours that characterize the hereditary non-polyposis colorectal carcinoma syndrome. *Cancer Res* 1993; **53**:5853–5855.

108. Aaltonen LA, Peltomaki P, Mecklin J-P. Replication errors in benign and malignant tumours from hereditary non-polyposis colorectal cancer patients. *Cancer Res* 1994; **54**:1645–1648.

109. Markowitz S, Wang J, Myeroff L, *et al.* Inactivation of the type II TGF-beta receptor in colon cancer cells with microsatellite instability. *Science* 1995; **268**:1336–1338.

110. Ouyang H, Furukawa T, Abe T, *et al.* The *BAX* gene, the promoter of apoptosis, is mutated in genetically unstable cancers of the colorectum, stomach, and endometrium. *Clin Cancer Res* 1998; **4**:1071–1074.

111. Lothe RA, Peltomaki P, Meling GI, *et al.* Genomic instability in colorectal cancer: relationship to clinicopathological variables and family history. *Cancer Res* 1993; **53**:5849–5852.

112. Herman JG, Umar A, Polyak K, *et al.* Incidence and functional consequences of *MLH1* promoter hypermethylation in colorectal carcinoma. *Proc Natl Acad Sci USA* 1998; **95**:6870–6875.

113. Cunningham JM, Christensen ER, Tester DJ, *et al.* Hypermethylation of the *MLH1* promoter in colon cancer with microsatellite instability. *Cancer Res* 1998; **58**:3455–3460.

114. Toyota M, Ahuja N, Ohe-Toyota M, *et al.* CpG island methylator phenotype in colorectal cancer. *Proc Natl Acad Sci USA* 1999; **96**:8681–8686.

115. Kuismanen SA, Holmberg MT, Salovaara R, *et al.* Epigenetic phenotypes distinguish microsatellite-stable and -unstable colorectal cancers. *Proc Natl Acad Sci USA* 1999; **96**:12661–12666.

116. Liu B, Farrington SM, Petersen GM, *et al.* Genetic instability occurs in the majority of young patients with colorectal cancer. *Nature Med* 1995; **2**:348–352.

117. Farrington SM, Lin-Goerke J, Ling J, *et al.* Systematic analysis of *MSH2* and *MLH1* in young colon cancer patients and controls. *Am J Hum Genet* 1998; **63**:749–759.

118. Farrington SM, McKinley AJ, Carothers AD, *et al.* Evidence for an age-related influence of microsatellite instability on colorectal cancer survival. *Int J Cancer* 2002; **98**:844–850.

119. Gryfe R, Kim H, Hsieh ETK, *et al.* Tumor microsatellite instability and clinical outcome in young patients with colorectal cancer. *N Engl J Med* 2000; **342**:69–77.

120. Risinger JI, Berchuck A, Kohler MF, *et al.* Genetic instability of microsatellites in endometrial carcinoma. *Cancer Res* 1993; **53**:5100–5103.

121. Horii A, Han H-J, Shimada M, *et al.* Frequent replication errors at microsatellite loci in tumors of patients with multiple primary cancers. *Cancer Res* 1994; **54**:3373–3382.

122. Hendrich B, Bird A. Identification and characterization of a family of mammalian methyl-CpG binding proteins. *Molec Cell Biol* 1998; **18**:6538–6547.

123. Bellacosa A, Cicchillitti L, Schepis F, *et al.* MED1, a novel human methyl-CpG-binding endonuclease, interacts with DNA mismatch repair protein MLH1. *Proc Natl Acad Sci USA* 1999; **96**:3969–3974.

124. Acharya S, Wilson T, Gradia S, *et al.* MSH2 forms specific mispair-binding complexes with MSH3 and MSH6. *Proc Natl Acad Sci USA* 1996; **93**:13629–13634.

125. Marsischky GT, Filosi N, Kane MF, Kolodner R. Redundancy of Saccharomyces cerevisiae MSH3 and MSH6 in MSH2-dependent mismatch repair. *Genes Dev* 1996; **10**:407–420.

126. Wiebauer KM, Jiricny J. Mismatch-specific thymine DNA glysosylase and DNA polymerase B mediate the correction of G.T mispairs in nuclear extracts from human cells. *Proc Natl Acad Sci USA* 1990; **87**:5842–5845.

127. Kinzler KW, Vogelstein B. Gatekeepers and caretakers. *Nature* 1994; **386**:761–763.

128. Heyer J, Yang K, Lipkin M, *et al.* Mouse models for colorectal cancer. *Oncogene* 1999; **18**:5325–5333.

129. de Wind N, Dekker M, Berns A, *et al.* Inactivation of the mouse *Msh2* gene results in mismatch repair deficiency, methylation tolerance, hyperrecombination, and predisposition to cancer. *Cell* 1995; **82**:321–330.

130. Koi M, Umar A, Chauhan DP, *et al.* Human chromosome 3 corrects mismatch repair deficiency and microsatellite instability and reduces N-methyl-N'-nitro-N-nitrosoguanidine tolerance in colon tumor cells with homozygous *MLH1* mutation. *Cancer Res* 1994; **54**:4308–4314.

131. Zhang H, Richards B, Wilson T, *et al.* Apoptosis induced by overexpression of MSH2 or MLH1. *Cancer Res* 1999; **59**:3021–3027.

132. Carethers JM, Chauhan DP, Fink D, *et al.* Mismatch repair proficiency and *in vitro* response to 5-fluorouracil. *Gastroenterology* 1999; **117**:123–131.

133. Bunz F, Hwang PM, Torrance C, *et al.* Disruption of p53 in human cancer cells alters the responses to therapeutic agents. *J Clin Invest* 1999; **104**:263–269.

134. Grady WM, Myeroff LL, Swinler SE, *et al.* Mutational inactivation of transforming growth factor beta receptor type II in microsatellite stable colon cancers. *Cancer Res* 1999; **59**:320–324.

135. Lu S-L, Kawabata M, Imamura T, *et al.* HNPCC associated with germline mutation in the TGF-beta type II receptor gene. *Nature Genet* 1998; **19**:17–18.

136. Muleris M, Nordlinger B, Dutrillaux B, *et al.* Cytogenetic characterization of a colon adenocarcinoma from a familial polyposis coli patient. *Cancer Genet Cytogenet* 1989; **38**:249–253.

137. Vogelstein B, Fearon ER, Hamilton SR, *et al.* Genetic alterations during colorectal tumour development. *N Engl J Med* 1988; **319**:525–532.

138. Fearon ER, Cho KR, Nigro JM, *et al.* Identification of a chromosome 18q gene that is altered in colorectal cancers. *Science* 1990; **247**:49–56.

139. Hahn SA, Schutte M, Hoque ATMS, *et al.* DPC4, a candidate tumor-suppressor gene at human-chromosome 18q21.1. *Science* 1996; **271**:350–353.

140. Sirard C, de la Pompa JL, Elia A, *et al.* The tumor suppressor gene *SMAD4/DPC4* is required for gastrulation and later for anterior development of the mouse embryo. *Genes Dev* 1998; **12**:107–119.

141. Howe JR, Roth S, Ringold JC, *et al.* Mutations in the *SMAD4/DPC4* gene in juvenile polyposis. *Science* 1998; **280**:1086–1088.

142. Malkin D, Li FP, Strong LC, *et al.* Germ line *p53* mutations in a familial syndrome of breast cancer, sarcomas, and other neoplasms. *Science* 1990; **250**:1233–1238.

143. Bhagirath TH, Condie A, Dunlop MG, *et al.* Exclusion of constitutional *p53* mutations as a cause of genetic susceptibility to colorectal cancer. *Br J Cancer* 1993; **68**:712–714.

144. Carder P, Wyllie AH, Purdie CA, *et al.* Stabilised *p53* facilitates aneuploid clonal divergence in colorectal cancer. *Oncogene* 1993; **8**:1397–1401.

145. Lengauer C, Kinzler KW, Vogelstein B. Genetic instability in colorectal cancers. *Nature* 1997; **386**:623–627.

146. Cahill DP, Lengauer C, Yu J, *et al.* Mutations of mitotic checkpoint genes in human cancers. *Nature* 1998; **392**:300–303.

147. Cahill DP, da Costa LT, Carson-Walter EB, *et al.* Characterization of *MAD2B* and other mitotic spindle checkpoint genes. *Genomics* 1999; **58**:181–187.

148. Lynch ED, Ostermeyer EA, Lee MK, *et al.* Inherited mutations in *PTEN* that are associated with breast cancer, Cowden disease, and juvenile polyposis. *Am J Hum Genet* 1997; **61**:1254–1260.

149. Olschwang S, Serova-Sinilnikova OM, Lenoir GM, Thomas G. *PTEN* germ-line mutations in juvenile polyposis coli. *Nature Genet* 1998; **18**:12–14.

150. Zhou XP, Woodford-Richens K, Lehtonen R, *et al*. Germline mutations in *BMPRIA/ALK3* cause a subset of cases of juvenile polyposis syndrome and of Cowden and Bannayan–Riley–Ruvalcaba syndromes. *Am J Hum Genet* 2001; **69**: 704–711.

151. Giardello FM, Welsh SB, Hamilton SR, *et al*. Increased risk of cancer in the Peutz–Jeghers syndrome. *N Engl J Med* 1987; **316**:1511–1514.

152. Hemminki A, Tomlinson I, Markie D, *et al*. Localization of a susceptibility locus for Peutz–Jeghers syndrome to 19p using comparative genomic hybridization and targeted linkage analysis. *Nature Genet* 1997; **15**:87–90.

153. Hemminki A, Markie D, Tomlinson I, *et al*. A serine/threonine kinase gene defective in Peutz–Jeghers syndrome. *Nature* 1998; **391**:184–187.

154. Jenne DE, Reimann H, Nezu J, *et al*. Peutz–Jeghers syndrome is caused by mutations in a novel serine threonine kinase. *Nature Genet* 1998; **18**:38–44.

155. Nelen MR, Padberg GW, Peeters EA, *et al*. Localization of the gene for Cowden disease to chromosome 10q22–23. *Nature Genet* 1996; **13**:114–116.

156. Nelen MR, van Staveren WC, Peeters EA, *et al*. Germline mutations in the *PTEN/MMAC1* gene in patients with Cowden disease. *Hum Molec Genet* 1997; **6**:1383–1387.

157. Liaw D, Marsh DJ, Li J, *et al*. Germline mutations of the *PTEN* gene in Cowden disease, an inherited breast and thyroid cancer syndrome. *Nature Genet* 1997; **16**:64–67.

158. Li DM, Sun H. TEP1, encoded by a candidate tumor suppressor locus, is a novel protein tyrosine phosphatase regulated by transforming growth factor beta. *Cancer Res* 1997; **57**:2124–2129.

159. Petersen GM, Francomano C, Kinzler K, *et al*. Presymptomatic direct detection of adenomatous polyposis coli (*APC*) gene mutations in familial adenomatous polyposis. *Hum Genet* 1993; **91**:307–311.

160. Maher ER, Barton DE, Slatter R, *et al*. Evaluation of molecular genetic diagnosis in the management of familial adenomatous polyposis coli: a population based study. *J Med Genet* 1993; **30**:675–678.

161. Thun MJ, Namboodiri MM, Heath CW. Aspirin use and reduced risk of fatal colon cancer. *N Engl J Med* 1991; **325**:1593–1596.

162. Giardiello FM, Hamilton SR, Krush AJ, *et al*. Treatment of colonic and rectal adenomas with sulindac in familial adenomatous polyposis. *N Engl J Med* 1993; **328**: 1313–1316.

163. Kaplan KB, Burds AA, Swedlow JR, *et al*. A role for the Adenomatous Polyposis Coli protein in chromosome segregation. *Nat Cell Biol* 2001; **3**(4):429–432.

164. Fodde R, Kuipers J, Rosenberg C, *et al*. Mutations in the *APC* tumour suppressor gene cause chromosomal instability. *Nat Cell Biol* 2001; **3**(4):433–438.

165. Al-Tassan N, Chmiel NH, Maynard J, *et al*. Inherited variants of *MYH* associated with somatic G:C→T:A mutations in colorectal tumors. *Nature Genet* 2002; **30**(2):227–232.

166. Sieber OM, Lipton L, Crabtree M, *et al*. Multiple colorectal adenomas, classic adenomatous polyposis, and germ-line mutations in *MYH*. *N Engl J Med* 2003; **348**(9):791–799.

167. Ewart-Toland A, Briassouli P, de Koning JP, *et al*. Identification of *STK6/STK15* as a candidate low-penetrance tumor-susceptibility gene in mouse and human. *Nature Genet* 2003; **34**(4):403–412.

168. Laiho P, Hienonen T, Karhu A, *et al*. Genome-wide allelotyping of 104 Finnish colorectal cancers reveals an excess of allelic imbalance in chromosome 20q in familial cases. *Oncogene*, 2003; **22**(14):2206–2214.

169. Bian Y, Kaklamani V, Reich J, Pasche B. TGF-beta signaling alterations in cancer. *Cancer Treat Res* 2003; **115**:73–94.

170. Kong S, Wei Q, Amos CI, *et al*. Cyclin D1 polymorphism and increased risk of colorectal cancer at young age. *J Natl Cancer Inst* 2001; **93**(14):1106–1108.

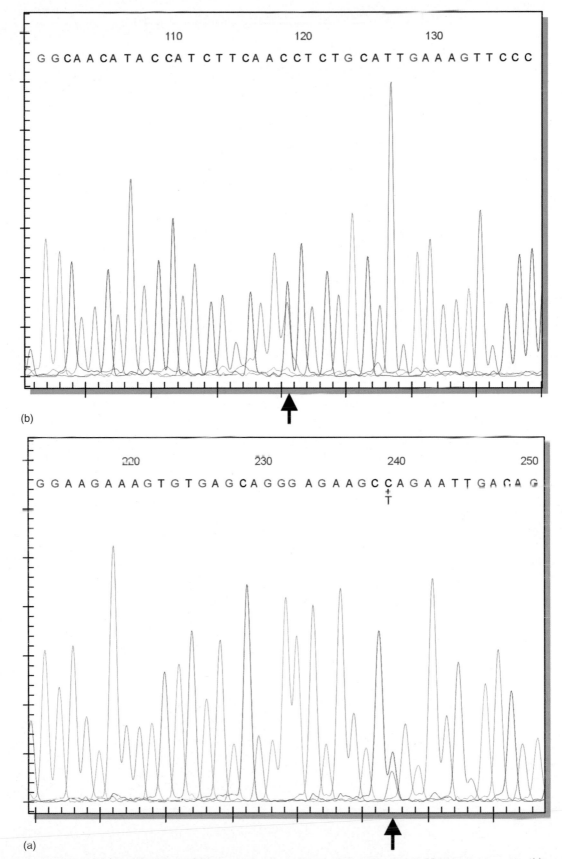

Plate 1 *Detection of a real (a) and artefactual (b) heterozygous mutation or polymorphism in the BRCA1 gene by nucleotide sequencing. (Courtesy Dr Nathalie van Orsouw.)*

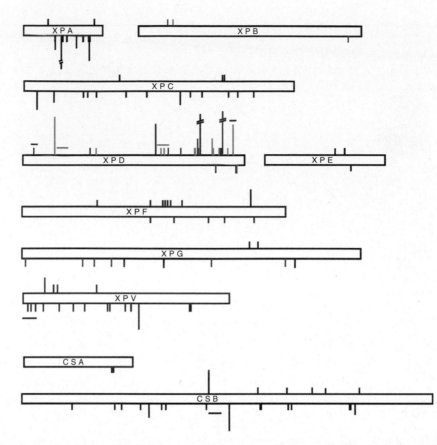

Plate 2 *Distribution of mutations in patients with Xeroderma pigmentosum, Cockayne syndrome and trichothiodystrophy. The XP and CS proteins are indicated as boxes, with lines depicting the positions of identified mutations. Bars above the proteins represent missense mutations, whereas those below result in protein truncations. Horizontal bars represent in-frame deletions. Lengths of the vertical bars are approximately proportional to number of individuals mutated at that site. Purple bars represent XP/CS mutations yellow denotes TTD mutations. In XPD, blue bars are XP mutations and black bars are mutations thought to be lethal.*

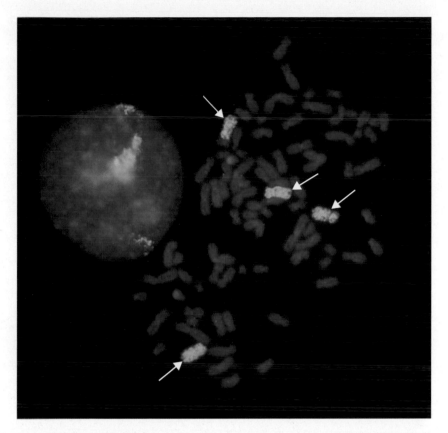

Plate 3 *An example of an aneuploid cell. This is a metaphase spread showing the presence of 87 chromosomes instead of the normal complement of 46. The arrows indicate four copies of chromosome 12 using fluorescent* in situ *hybridization.*

25

Screening and management of familial colon cancer

SHIRLEY V. HODGSON AND VICTORIA MURDAY

INTRODUCTION

About 5 per cent of colorectal cancers are thought to arise in individuals with a strong hereditary susceptibility to the condition. Inherited cancer susceptibility syndromes predisposing to colorectal cancer include familial adenomatous polyposis (FAP) and hereditary non-polyposis colorectal cancer (HNPCC). These conditions are inherited as autosomal dominant conditions characterized by early-onset bowel cancer. A larger proportion of familial clustering of colorectal cancer is characterized by a later age at onset of cancer and a less obvious mode of inheritance. Some of these familial cases may be due to less significant mutations in the genes causing FAP or HNPCC (APC and the mismatch repair genes), or other less penetrant susceptibility genes, interacting with environmental factors. Many genes involved in this type of susceptibility may as yet be unidentified.

Non-syndromic familial colorectal cancer

In the absence of a clear-cut predisposing syndrome, such as FAP, HNPCC or juvenile polyposis, it is still possible to observe familial clustering of colorectal cancer. A family history of colorectal cancer increases the empirical risk for an individual of developing colorectal cancer; this risk increases with increasing numbers of affected close relatives and with decreasing age at diagnosis in those

relatives. The risk of colorectal cancer does not increase at a much younger age than in the general population and there is no strong tendency to develop adenomatous polyps. Cancers that do occur have a distribution more similar to that seen in sporadic cancers than the proximal distribution characteristic of HNPCC, but there is still more right-sided neoplasia than in sporadic cancers.[1] One explanation for this proximal preponderance is that a small proportion of familial cases are due to HNPCC but are not obvious from the family history.[2,3,4]

First-degree relatives of cases of colorectal cancer have a 2–3-fold increased risk of developing the condition themselves. The risk increases with earlier age at diagnosis in a first-degree relative, such that, if the case was diagnosed at 45 years or below, the risk is 4–5 times the population risk (see Table 25.1 and Chapter 17), a similar risk to having two first-degree relatives affected at any age. In individuals with a family history of colorectal cancer, management depends in the first instance on ascertainment of an accurate personal and family history. Care should be taken to exclude evidence of diagnosable conditions in the consultand, such as ulcerative colitis or FAP. Cancer diagnoses should be verified in affected relatives and FAP excluded. If the cancer risk is 4–5 times the population risk, the consultand is appropriate for consideration of surveillance for colorectal neoplasia. Other individuals who could be offered surveillance because of a similarly increased colorectal cancer risk (CRC)[5–9] are women who themselves have had ovarian or

Table 25.1 *Relative risk of colon cancer in first degree relatives of a case*

Relative risk	Reference
3.3	Woolf (1958)[12]
2.9	Macklin (1960)[13]
3.5	Lovett (1976)[14]
6.3	Maire et al. (1984)[15]
3.1	Rozen et al. (1987)[16]
2.36	Bonelli et al. (1988)[17]
2.13	Kune et al. (1989)[18]
7.5	Ponz de Leon et al. (1989)[19]
4.6	Stephenson et al. (1991)[20]
1.9	Boutron et al. (1994)[21]

Table 25.2 *Families to be considered for screening*

	Relative risk	Reference
1 Individuals with a single first-degree relative diagnosed with CRC below 40 years of age	5	Lovett (1976)[14]
2 Individuals with two affected relatives at any age	5.7	St John et al. (1993)[22]
3 Individuals who have developed ovarian or endometrial cancer themselves and have a first-degree relative with CRC	4.5	Rozen et al. (1986)[23]

CRC, colorectal cancer.

endometrial cancer, and have a first-degree relative with colorectal cancer (4.5-fold increased risk of CRC) and, debatably, men or women who are carriers of a pathogenic mutation in the *BRCA1* and *BRCA2* genes (possibly increased risk; Table 25.2).[10,11]

RATIONALE FOR SCREENING STRATEGY

The aim of colorectal screening is firstly to reduce the incidence of CRC in susceptible individuals and, in addition, to detect early neoplasia at a stage when treatment is likely to be effective. Colorectal cancer often presents at a late stage in individuals not on surveillance, with a resulting poorer prognosis. Faecal occult blood testing (FOB) is used specifically to detect early cancer and is poor at detecting adenomas. It is thus unlikely to reduce the incidence of cancer, although it may reduce mortality. Endoscopic screening will detect adenomas and lead to a reduction in the incidence of the disease in susceptible individuals. A comparison of flexible sigmoidoscopy

and FOB in asymptomatic volunteers who went on to have colonoscopy demonstrated a sensitivity for neoplasia of 93.8 per cent for sigmoidoscopy compared with 20.8 per cent for FOB, and this poor predictive value of FOB relative to sigmoidoscopy has been confirmed by other studies. In addition, approximately 2 per cent of individuals will test positive on FOB testing and require follow-up colonoscopy.[16,24,25]

However, sigmoidoscopy alone is not considered to be appropriate in high-risk individuals because of the increased proportion of proximal neoplasia compared with controls, such that 50 per cent of colonic neoplasia occurs proximal to the sigmoid flexure. Synchronous distal neoplasia will occur in fewer than 30 per cent of cases of proximal cancer.[26–28] Colonoscopy is thus the method of choice for surveillance in this group.[29–31]

The age at which screening should be initiated is a matter of debate. Since the age at onset of CRC in familial non-HNPCC is only a little earlier than in sporadic cases, occurring predominantly in individuals over the age of 50 years,[24] surveillance should probably be initiated at 5–10 years before the earliest case in the family, or from 45 years of age. The adenoma–carcinoma transition is thought to take 5–10 years in the general population,[32] although the speed at which cancer develops from an adenoma in an individual with HNPCC is very much accelerated, documented to take 1–2 years (see later section on HNPCC). Endoscopy will have an effect in reducing mortality from CRC in individuals with a family history up to 10 years later, with a strong effect for 5 years.[33] It thus seems appropriate to offer colonoscopies at an interval of 5 years, unless adenomas are detected, in which case screening should be 3-yearly unless the pathology detected suggests the need for more frequent endoscopies (e.g. if multiple polyps suggestive of attenuated FAP are detected).[2,3,34]

Colonoscopy is only effective at reducing morbidity and mortality from cancer if it detects adenomas and early-stage cancers, and thus should be initiated 5–10 years before the age at which the risk of CRC becomes significant. In the case of sporadic CRC, the risk per 100 000 per year for men is 5 at 35–39 years of age, but rises to 51 at 50–54 years of age and 140 at 60–64 years of age. The incidence in females increases at a slightly later age (about 5 years later than in men). In individuals with a family history of CRC, these risks appear to apply 10 years earlier.[16,33,35,36] It could, therefore, be argued that colonoscopy should be initiated at 10–15 years before the risk exceeds 5 per cent, that is, approximately 45 years of age in men and 48 years of age in women with a relative risk (RR) of 5.

Most prospective studies of screening first-degree relatives of affected individuals have detected very low levels of neoplasia in individuals under 40 years of age. Screening should, therefore, probably be initiated at 40–45 years in this group.[22,35] The American Gastroenterological

Association performed a decision analysis in 1997, which suggested a reduction of colorectal cancer incidence by 72 per cent and deaths by 74 per cent would be achieved by colonoscopic surveillance,[36] but this must be balanced against the risk of bowel perforation and other complications from colonoscopy, estimated at 1 in 300 procedures (particularly when polypectomy is performed) and a risk of death at 1–3 per 10 000 procedures.[5–9]

In view of the fact that a screening programme of colonoscopic surveillance along the lines outlined above might apply to 1 per cent of the population, the costs of colonoscopic surveillance (both financial and the potential harmful side effects) must be weighed up against the potential gain in lives saved. The cost of a colonoscopy is approximately £150, but theatre and nursing/doctor time should also be costed.

HNPCC

This autosomal dominant condition is characterized by a high risk of developing colorectal cancer (80–85 per cent lifetime risk in men; 42–65 per cent in women) and an increased risk of certain extracolonic cancers, particularly endometrial (approximately 45 per cent risk), ovarian (10 per cent) and gastric cancers, but also urothelial, pancreatic and biliary tract cancers. Affected individuals develop few polyps[37–41] but the adenoma–carcinoma sequence is accelerated, such that interval cancers have been reported to occur in affected individuals on 2-yearly colonoscopic surveillance.[42–44] Since there are rarely any diagnostic phenotype features other than the skin lesions of the Muir–Torre syndrome that may occur in HNPCC (notably kerato-acanthomas) to facilitate diagnosis, the diagnostic Amsterdam criteria were drawn up to provide uniformity for collaborative studies (Table 25.3). More recently, modified Amsterdam II diagnostic criteria have been developed to take into account the likelihood that a family member with an extracolonic cancer of the HNPCC spectrum is affected[45] (Table 25.4).

A further set of criteria incorporating data about site and histopathology of CRC and adenomas diagnosed before the age of 40 years have been developed, known as the Bethesda guidelines, which are more sensitive but less specific than the Amsterdam criteria for diagnosing HNPCC.[46]

The condition is caused by inherited mutations in genes involved in DNA mismatch repair, the majority of cases being due to germline mutations in *MSH2* (45 per cent) and *MLH1* (51 per cent). Germline mutations in *PMS1*, *PMS2* and *MSH6/GTBP* together account for only approximately 3 per cent of cases.[38,47–51] Mutations in *MSH6* underly a small proportion of families, particularly where endometrial cancer has occurred and, in such families, the age at diagnosis may be later (mean age at

Table 25.3 *Amsterdam criteria I*

1 Three close relatives affected with colorectal cancer
2 One should be the first-degree relative of the other two
3 At least two generations affected
4 At least one diagnosis before 45 years of age
5 Familial adenomatous polyposis excluded

Table 25.4 *Amsterdam criteria II*

There should be at least three relatives with an HNPCC-associated cancer (colorectal cancer, endometrial, small bowel, ureter or renal pelvis) and:

1 One should be the first-degree relative of the other two
2 At least two successive generations should be affected
3 At least one diagnosed before age 50 years
4 Familial adenomatous polyposis excluded
5 Tumours pathologically verified

HNPCC, hereditary non-polyposis colorectal cancer.

diagnosis 61 years) and some associated cancers show low levels of microsatellite instability (MSI) (see later).[52,53] Mismatch repair deficiency results in the accumulation of mutations in genes that promote cancer development. Colorectal cancer characteristically develops at a young age (mean age at diagnosis 45 years) in HNPCC and is more often proximally sited in the colon, and synchronous and metachronous neoplasia is common. The risk of metachronous CRC is reported to be 30 per cent at 10 years after limited resection, and 50 per cent at 15 years.[26–28]

Colorectal cancers occurring in individuals with HNPCC tend to be replication-error (RER) positive, owing to MSI, particularly of mononucleotide repeats, which are poorly differentiated, diploid, mucinous with lymphocytic infiltration and *TP53* mutation negative.[54] These histopathological appearances, immunohistochemical staining for MSH2 and MLH1, and MSI can be used to identify cancers likely to be due to HNPCC.[55,56] Their prognosis may be better than in sporadic carcinoma, with a 5-year cumulative survival rate in HNPCC of 65 per cent (95 per cent confidence interval (CI) 57–72) compared with 44 per cent (CI 43–45) for patients with sporadic CRC.

Fulfilment of the Amsterdam criteria and the presence of endometrial cancer in the family are strong predictors of the presence of HNPCC.[57] The likelihood of HNPCC being present is increased if an endometrial cancer is present in the family, or an individual in the family has multiple CRCs.[55] First-degree relatives of individuals with HNPCC have a 50:50 risk of inheriting the condition. There is now convincing evidence for a reduction in morbidity and mortality from colorectal cancer in individuals with HNPCC on colonoscopic surveillance and removal of colonic adenomatous polyps during endoscopy.[34,42,43,58] Full colonoscopy to the caecum is clearly the screening method of choice in view of the preponderance of proximal neoplasia in this condition. Where significant neoplasia is detected, it is appropriate to consider subtotal colectomy. This form of surgery should also be considered if an individual with HNPCC is undergoing surgery for colonic neoplasia.

Some adenomas in HNPCC may be flat, and many develop very rapidly to cancer.[59] In addition, colonoscopists may miss about 15 per cent of neoplastic colorectal polyps. Prophylactic hysterectomy, possibly with oophorectomy, can also be considered if an affected woman is undergoing surgery.

Since the age of diagnosis of colorectal cancer is young in HNPCC, the international collaborative group for HNPCC has suggested that colonoscopic surveillance in individuals at risk of HNPCC be initiated at 25 years of age. Colonoscopy should be performed 2-yearly (1–3 years).[26,60] Surveillance for extracolonic cancers in HNPCC should be addressed. It is suggested that yearly vaginal ultrasound with endometrial sampling should be offered for female gene carriers from 25 years of age,[61–63] although this optimal method for screening has not yet been defined, but this method is thought to be 82–98 per cent sensitive in postmenopausal women.[26,64] There is no recommendation for screening for ovarian cancer although transvaginal ultrasound and serum CA-125 are usually performed annually.

Screening for gastric or urinary tract cancers is only recommended in families in which these cancers have occurred. In such families, the suggested regime is gastroscopy every 1–2 years, beginning at age 35 years, and early morning urine cytology every 1–2 years from 35 years of age, with supporting radiological examinations.[65]

In families where the mutation causing the condition has been identified in an affected individual, predictive testing may be offered to at-risk individuals in that family. This should only be done when the pathogenic nature of the mutation has been demonstrated, for example, by finding that it segregates with the disease in the family, has been reported to cause the condition in other families, and is likely to cause disruption of gene function. Genetic counselling protocols for predictive testing are being developed, and should include detailed discussions of the likely emotional, insurance and employment implications of the result. More than one pretest counselling session should be offered.

FAMILIAL ADENOMATOUS POLYPOSIS

Classical familial adenomatous polyposis is an autosomal dominant condition characterized by the development of hundreds of adenomas in the large bowel from the early teens. The risk of colorectal cancer is almost inevitable once the polyps are established, and the age at diagnosis of CRC is very early. Once the diagnosis has been made and polyps have begun to develop, the treatment of choice is to remove the large bowel, either by ileorectal anastamosis or total colectomy and pouch construction. Surveillance of the rectum is maintained if an ileorectal anastamosis has been performed. The offspring of an affected person have a 50:50 risk of inheriting the condition, and surveillance by annual sigmoidoscopy initially should, therefore, commence in the early teens. Sigmoidoscopy is sufficient for the early years of surveillance, since polyps almost always occur first in the sigmoid and rectum in classical FAP. However, colonoscopy should be performed at a later age with dye spray, if polyps have not been seen.

The occurrence of congenital hypertrophy of the retinal pigment epithelium (CHRPE) in affected individuals may be seen in some families, and be an adjunct to diagnosis in at-risk individuals, as may the other extracolonic features of the disorder, such as sebaceous cysts, desmoids and osteomas (Gardiner syndrome). However, affected individuals with certain *APC* mutations do not manifest the CHRPE. In many families it is now possible to identify the *APC* mutation in an affected individual, enabling a predictive test to be offered to their relatives. The most appropriate age at which to test children is uncertain, although many would advocate doing this in the early teens, at the time when screening would be initiated. Since no alteration in management would be advocated in a child testing positive at a younger age, it is probably not necessary to test earlier.

Initial studies of testing for FAP in children have shown no adverse psychological effects.[66]

Management of an affected adult postcolectomy should include annual upper gastrointestinal (GI) endoscopies from 25 years of age because of the risk of duodenal cancer. (Absolute risk of small bowel cancer is 3 per cent lifetime; RR > 300.[67]) Rectal surveillance is also imperative and consideration of conversion to a total colectomy with ileostomy could be made to avoid the risk of rectal carcinoma, which occurs mainly after the age of 40 years.[68] The risk of hepatoblastoma in childhood, although raised, is not sufficient to warrant screening. There is an increased risk of papillary thyroid cancer in young women with FAP, but this usually has a good prognosis and screening is not advocated for this. Women with FAP should be aware of early signs of the condition.[69]

Occasional families have been described with attenuated polyposis.[70] This is due to certain mutations in the *APC* gene – normally those sited in the extreme or 3′ regions of the gene. Affected individuals appear to have fewer and more variable numbers of polyps than in the classical form of FAP (usually fewer than 50) but still have an elevated risk of CRC. The onset of CRC may be later than in classical FAP. Surveillance in such individuals should include regular colonoscopies with consideration of colectomy and ileorectal anastamosis once the condition has been diagnosed. The offspring of affected individuals should undergo colonoscopic surveillance annually from their mid-teens. In many cases, however, a predictive test may be available.

A polymorphism in the *APC* gene has been described in 6 per cent of the Ashkenazi Jewish population, where an apparent neutral base-change, which converts an AAATAAAA sequence to $(A)^8$, renders the *APC* gene likely to undergo somatic mutations.[71] This is apparently associated with an increased relative risk of CRC, although the exact degree of risk has yet to be established.

Screening protocols for individuals from families with this common mutation are contentious because of the small increased relative risks of CRC in gene carriers. Predictive testing is possible because the mutation is known but, since there is no consensus for management and surveillance of such individuals, whose risk of CRC may only be 2–3-fold increased above the population risk, it is uncertain how such families should be managed.

MYH POLYPOSIS

This condition was recently described, and differs from most of the other single gene disorders causing colorectal cancer in that it is inherited as an autosomal recessive condition with a risk to sibs but low risk to offspring.[72,73] It is important to identify these families so that the appropriate people in the family are offered screening, and the offspring of affected individuals can be reassured that they are not at high risk. The condition is associated with multiple adenomas in affected individuals but the numbers of polyps vary from frank polyposis to as few as five, similar to the pattern seen in attenuated FAP. Families who resemble APC or AAPC but where there is no mutation or evidence of autosomal dominant transmission should undergo MYH mutation analysis: mutations are detected in about 20 per cent of these families and there are common founder mutations. Since MYH testing is relatively simple and cheap, laboratories have begun changing their strategy to test for MYH mutations before APC in selected families.

Since its elucidation many groups have looked at sporadic colorectal cancers and identify biallellic mutations in about 0.5 per cent. In general these cases are found with additional adenomas in the bowel. The carrier frequency for MYH mutations may be as high as 1 per cent.

Table 25.5 *Extracolonic cancer risks in hereditary non-polyposis colorectal cancer (adapted from Flanders and Foulkes[75])*

	Relative risk	Cumulative % risk to age 80 years
Endometrium	10.0	43
Hepatobiliary	5.0	18
Ovary	3.5	9
Pancreas	1.5	
Urothelial	3.5 (kidney), 22.0 (ureter)	<5

TURCOT SYNDROME

This is a rare condition characterized by colorectal adenomatous polyps (of variable numbers) and central nervous system malignancies (glioblastomas and medulloblastomas). This name has been applied to several different conditions. Medulloblastomas occur in FAP and glioblastomas in HNPCC (confirmed by mutation analysis). In addition, there is a severe childhood onset disorder with brain tumours associated with severe polyposis and café au lait patches, almost always fatal in childhood, for which the molecular basis is uncertain. However, consanguinity is common in the parents of these children, and it has been suggested that they are homozygous for mismatch repair gene mutations (Coles T, personal communication 2000).[74] Surveillance of relatives is as for HNPCC or FAP, depending on the underlying cause (Table 25.5).

OTHER RARE CONDITIONS PREDISPOSING TO COLORECTAL CANCER

Juvenile polyposis

This is an uncommon condition in which hamartomatous polyps develop throughout the GI tract. Severe cases tend to be sporadic, but some pedigrees have been described with autosomal dominant inheritance and there is a significantly increased risk of colorectal cancer in such cases (18–20 per cent).[76] Some families have been identified as having mutations in *SMAD4* and others have mutations in *BMPRIA*.[78–80]

Extracolonic abnormalities may also be found in affected individuals, suggesting that some cases of juvenile polyposis may actually have Ruvalcaba–Myhre–Smith or Cowden syndrome with germline mutations in *PTEN*.[81]

Colonoscopic surveillance should be offered to affected individuals and their first-degree relatives but, owing to the rarity of this condition, there is no consensus about the frequency with which this should be offered, although 2-yearly colonoscopy from 15 years of age has been suggested (Houlston R, personal communication).

Peutz–Jeghers syndrome

This is a rare autosomal dominant condition in which multiple hamartomatous polyps develop throughout the GI tract. Other features of the condition include striking melanin flecks on the lips and mucocutaneous borders. These tend to develop during childhood and fade in adult life. The risk of death from GI cancer is increased (RR 13, CI 2.7–38.1).[82] Colorectal cancer is the most frequent cancer diagnosed, but because of the increasing risk of duodenal, jejunal and gastric cancer in affected individuals,[83] affected individuals should have regular upper GI endoscopy with small bowel meal in addition to colonoscopy. There is no clear consensus about how to investigate first-degree relatives of affected individuals, but since the melanin freckling does not invariably occur, offspring of affected individuals should probably undergo one or more colonoscopies in their late teens to detect any signs of affection status. Affected individuals should have colonoscopy 2-yearly from adolescence and upper GI endoscopy with small bowel double-contrast radiology. Women with this syndrome should be offered regular breast examinations from age 20 years and mammography from 35 years of age, and gynaecological surveillance for ovarian cysts. Benign ovarian cysts may occur, so the detection of these requires careful evaluation.[68]

The gene responsible for the condition (STKII) has recently been identified, allowing predictive tests to be offered in families in which the mutation is known.[84]

Other rare inherited conditions in which variable numbers of hyperplastic or hamartomatous polyps may be found in the colon include the hereditary mixed polyposis syndrome, and hyperplastic polyposis associated with a family history of CRC.[85] Again, occasional colonoscopic surveillance in such individuals and their first-degree relatives would appear prudent, but no consensus for such management has been reached because of the rarity of these conditions, the variability of the extent of the polyposis and the uncertainty about the risk of progression to cancer.

CHEMOPREVENTION

There is now beginning to be evidence that aspirin and resistant starch/non-steroidal anti-inflammatories and cox-2 inhibitors may have an effect on reducing the incidence and development of colorectal cancer and may alter or retard tumour growth in patients with FAP and HNPCC.[86–88]

KEY POINTS

- About 5 per cent of colorectal cancers may arise in individuals with a strong hereditary predisposition.
- The main syndromes that have an autosomal dominant (AD) inheritance are FAP and HNPCC. There are also rarer AD syndromes, JP and PJS.
- There is also a recessive syndrome of multiple adenomas due to mutations in the *MYH* gene.
- Colonoscopy is the current screening tool of choice for the large bowel as it visualizes the right colon, except for FAP where sigmoidoscopy is performed until polyps appear and then total colectomy is recommended.
- Screening of other cancers is indicated in many of the syndromes.

REFERENCES

1. Cannon-Albright L, Thomas T, Bishop D, *et al.* Characteristics of familial colon cancer in a large population base. *Cancer* 1989; **64**:1971–1975.
2. Guillem JG, Forde KA, Treat MR, *et al.* Colonoscopic screening for neoplasms in asymptomatic first-degree relatives of colon cancer patients. A controlled, prospective study. *Dis Colon Rectum* 1992; **35**:523–529.
3. Rozen P, Fireman Z, Figer A, *et al.* Family history of colorectal cancer as a marker of potential malignancy within a screening programme. *Cancer* 1987; **60**:248–254.
4. Anderson D, Strong L. Genetics of gastrointestinal tumours. Proceedings of the XIth International Cancer Conference. *Excerpta Med* 1974; **351**:267–271.
5. Fuchs CS, Giovannucci EL, Colditz GA, *et al.* A prospective study of family history and the risk of colorectal cancer. *N Engl J Med* 1994; **331**:1669–1674.
6. Luchtefeld M, Syverson D, Solfelt M, *et al.* Is colonoscopic screening appropriate in asymptomatic patients with family history of colon cancer? *Dis Colon Rectum* 1991; **34**:763–768.
7. Houlston RS, Murday V, Haracopos C, *et al.* Screening and genetic counselling for relatives of patients with colorectal cancer in a family cancer clinic. [Published erratum appears in *Br Med J* 1990; **301**:446]. *Br Med J* 1990; **301**:366–368.
8. Odes HS, Rozen P, Ron E, *et al.* Screening for colorectal neoplasia: a multi-centre study in Israel (see comments). *Israel J Med Sci* 1992; **28**:21–38.
9. Stephenson B, Murday V, Finan P, *et al.* Feasibility of family-based screening for colorectal neoplasia experience in one general surgical practice. *Gut* 1993; **34**:96–100.
10. Ford D, Easton E, Bishop DT, *et al.* Breast Cancer Consortium. Risks of cancer in BRCA-1 mutation carriers. *Lancet* 1994; **343**:692–695.
11. Struewing JP, Hartge P, Wacholder S, *et al.* The risk of cancer associated with specific mutations of *BRCA1* and

BRCA2 among Ashkenazi Jews. *N Engl J Med* 1997; **336:** 1401–1408.

12. Woolf CM. A genetic study of carcinoma of the large intestine. *Am J Hum Genet* 1958; **10:**42–47.

13. Macklin MT. Inheritance of cancer of the stomach and large intestine in man. *J Natl Cancer Inst* 1960; **24:**551–557.

14. Lovett E. Family studies in cancer of the colon and rectum. *Br J Surg* 1976; **63:**13–18.

15. Maire P, Morichau-Beauchant M, Drucker J, *et al.* Familial occurrence of cancer of the colon and the rectum: results of a 3-year case-control survey. *Gastroenterologie clin biol* 1984; **8:**22–27.

16. Rozen P, Ron E, Fireman Z, *et al.* The relative value of faecal occult blood tests and flexible sigmoidoscopy in screening for large bowel neoplasia. *Cancer* 1987; **60:**2553–2558.

17. Bonelli L, Martines H, Conio M, *et al.* Family history of colorectal cancer as a risk factor for benign and malignant tumours of the large bowel. A case control study. *Int J Cancer* 1988; **41:**513–517.

18. Kune GA, Kune S, Watson LF. The role of heredity in the aetiology of large bowel cancer: data from the Melbourne Colorectal Cancer Study. *World J Surg* 1989; **13:**124–129; discussion 129–131.

19. Ponz de Leon M, Sassatelli R, Sacchetti C, *et al.* Familial aggregation of tumours in the 3-year experience of a population-based colorectal cancer registry. *Cancer Res* 1989; **49:**4344–4348.

20. Stephenson BM, Finan PJ, Gascoyne J, *et al.* Frequency of familial colorectal cancer. *Br J Surg* 1991; **78:**1162–1166.

21. Boutron MC, Faivre J, Quipourt V, *et al.* Family history of colorectal tumours and implications for the adenoma-carcinoma sequence: a case control study. *Gut* 1995; **37:**830–834.

22. St John D, McDermott F, Hopper J, *et al.* Cancer risk in the relatives of patients with common colorectal cancer. *Ann Intern Med* 1993; **118:**785–790.

23. Rozen P, Fireman Z. Figer A, Ron E. Colorectal tumour screening in women with a past history of breast, uterine, or ovarian malignancies. *Cancer* 1986; **57:**1235–1239

24. Hardcastle J, Robinson M, Mulrow CD, *et al.* Randomised controlled trial of faecal occult blood screening for colorectal cancer. *Lancet* 1996; **348:**1472–1477.

25. Kronberg O, Olsen J, Jorgensen O, Sondergaard O. Randomised study of screening for colon cancer with faecal-occult blood test. *Lancet* 1996; **348:**1467–1471.

26. Burke W, Petersen G, Lynch P, *et al.* Recommendations for following care of individuals with an inherited predisposition to cancer in HNPCC. *JAMA* 1997; **277:**915–919.

27. Mecklin JP, Jarvinen J. Treatment and follow-up strategies in HNPCC. *Dis Colon Rectum* 1993, **36.**927–929.

28. Lynch HT, Harris RE, Lynch PM, *et al.* Role of heredity in multiple primary cancer. *Cancer* 1977; **40:**1849–1854.

29. Levin TR, Palitz A, Grossman S, *et al.* Predicting advanced proximal colonic neoplasia with screening sigmoidoscopy. *JAMA* 1999; **281:**1611–1617.

30. Dinning L, Hixson L, Clark L. Prevalence of distal colonic neoplasia associated with proximal colon cancers. *Arch Intern Med* 1994; **154:**853–856.

31. Selby JV, Friedman GD, Queensbury CP, Weiss NS. A case-control study of screening sigmoidoscopy and mortality from colorectal cancer. *N Engl J Med* 1992; **326:**653–657.

32. Muto T, Bussey H, Morson BC. The evolution of cancer of the colon and rectum. *Cancer* 1975; **36:**2251–2270.

33. Muller A, Sonnerberg A. Protection by endoscopy against death from colorectal cancer. *Arch Intern Med* 1995; **155:**1741–1748.

34. Winawer SJ, Zauber AG, Ho MN, *et al.* Prevention of colorectal cancer by colonoscopic polypectomy: The National Polyp Study Workgroup. *New Engl J Med* 1993; **329:**1977–1981.

35. Brewer D, Fung C, Chapuis P, Bokey E. Should relatives of patients with colorectal cancer be screened. *Dis Colon Rectum* 1994; **37:**1328–1338.

36. Winawer SJ, Zauber AG, O'Brien MJ, *et al.* Randomised comparison of surveillance intervals after colonoscopic polypectomy. *N Engl J Med* 1993; **329:**901–906.

37. Vasen HFA, Mecklin JP, Meera Khan P, Lynch HT. HNPCC. *Lancet* 1991; **338:**877.

38. Aarnio M, Mecklin JP, Aaltonen LA, *et al.* Life-time risk of different cancers in HNPCC syndrome. *Int J Cancer* 1995; **64:**430–433.

39. Lynch HT, Smyrk TC. HNPCC (Lynch Syndrome): an updated review. *Cancer* 1996; **78:**1149–1167.

40. Mecklin JP, Jarvinen JJ. Clinical features of colorectal carcinoma in cancer family syndrome. *Dis Colon Rectum* 1986; **78:**160–164.

41. Marra G, Boland CR. HNPCC. *J Natl Cancer Inst* 1995; **87:**1114–1125.

42. Jarvinen JG, Mecklin JP, Sistonen P. Screening reduced colorectal cancer rate in families with HNPCC. *Gastroenterology* 1995; **108:**1405–1411.

43. Ahlquist DA. Aggressive polyps in HNPCC: targets for screening. *Gastroenterology* 1995; **108:**1590–1592.

44. Vasen HFA, Nagengast FM, Meera Khan P. Interval cancers in HNPCC (Lynch Syndrome). *Lancet* 1995; **345:**1183–1184.

45. Vasen HFA, Watson P, Mecklin J-P, Lynch HT. ICG-HNPCC. New clinical criteria for hereditary non-polyposis colorectal cancer (HNPCC, Lynch Syndrome) proposed by the international collaborative group on HNPCC. *Gastroenterology* 1999; **116:**1453–1456.

46. Rodriguez-Bigas MA, Bolan CR, Hamilton SR, *et al.* A national Cancer Institute workshop on hereditary non-polyposis colorectal cancer syndrome: meeting highlights and Bethesda guidelines. *J Natl Cancer Inst* 1997; **89:**1758–1761.

47. Viel A, Novella E, Gennard M, *et al.* Lack of *PMS2*-truncating mutations in patients with hereditary colorectal cancer. *Int J Onc* 1998; **13:**565–569.

48. Lin HH, Chen CD, Chen CK, *et al.* Is total abdominal hysterectomy with bilateral salpingo-oophorectomy adequate for new FIGO stage 1 endometrial carcinoma? *Br J Obstet Gynaecol* 1995; **102:**148–152.

49. Liu B, Parsons RE, Hamilton SR, *et al. MSH2* mutations in HNPCC kindreds. *Cancer Res* 1994; **54:**4590–4594.

50. Liu B, Parsons RE, Papadopoulos N, *et al.* Analysis of mismatch repair genes in HNPCC patients. *Nature Med* 1994; **2:**169–174.

51. Farrington S, Lin-Goeike J, Long J, *et al.* Systematic analysis of *MSH2* and *MLH1* in young colon cancer patients and controls. *Am J Hum Genet* 1998; **63:**749–759.

52. Boland CR, Thibodeau SN, Hamilton SR, *et al.* A National Cancer Institute Workshop on microsatellite instability for cancer detection and familial predisposition: development of interational criteria for the determination of microsatellite

instability in colorectal cancer. *Cancer Res* 1998; **58**:5248–5257.

53. de Leeuw WJ, Dierssan J, Vasen HF, *et al.* Prediction of a mismatch repair gene defect by microsatellite instability and immunohistochemical analysis in endometrial tumours from HNPCC patients. *J Pathol* 2000; **192**:328–335.

54. Lynch HT, Smyrk TC, Watson P, *et al.* Genetics, natural history, tumour spectrum, and pathology of HNPCC: an updated review. *Gastroenterology* 1993; **104**:1535–1549.

55. Wijnen JT, Vasen HFA, Meera-Khan P, *et al.* Clinical findings with implications for genetic testing in families with clustering of colorectal cancer. *N Engl J Med* 1998; **339**:511–518.

56. Jass JR. Pathology of hereditary nonpolyposis colorectal cancer. *Ann N Y Acad Sci* 2000; **910**:62–74.

57. Wijnen J, Khan P, Vasen H, *et al.* Hereditary non-polyposis colorectal cancer families not complying with the Amsterdam criteria show low frequency of mismatch-repair gene mutations. *Am J Hum Genet* 1997; **61**:329–335.

58. Fitzgibbons RJ, Lynch HT, Lanspa SJ, *et al.* Surgical strategies for management of the Lynch syndromes. *Hered Colorectal Cancer* 1990; 211–217.

59. Lynch HT, Lynch JF. Genetics of colonic cancer. *Digestion* 1998; **59**:481–492.

60. Jass JR, Stewart SM, Schroeder D, Lane MR. *Eur J Gastroenterol Hepatol* 1992; **4**:523–527.

61. Warner EA, Parson AK. Screening and early diagnosis of gynaecologic cancers. *Med Clin North Am* 1996; **80**:45–61.

62. Vasen HF, Watson P, Mecklin JP, *et al.* The epidemiology of endometrial cancer in hereditary non-polyposis colorectal cancer. *Anticancer Res* 1994; **14**:1675–1678.

63. Osmers RGW, Kuhn W. Vaginosonography for early detection of endometrial carcinoma? *Curr Opin Obstet Gynaecol* 1990; **6**:75–79.

64. Van den Bosch T, Van den Dael A. Combining vaginal ultrasonography and office endometrial sampling in the diagnosis of endometrial disease in postmenopausal women. *Obstet Gynaecol* 1995; **85**:349–352.

65. Weber T. Clinical surveillance recommendations adopted for HNPCC. *Lancet* 1996; **348**:465.

66. Michie S, Marteau T, on behalf of the FAP collaborative research group. Predictive genetic testing in children and adults: a study of emotional impact. *British Human Genetics Conference*, York, September 2000.

67. Giardello FM, Offerhaus JG. Phenotype and cancer risk of various polyposis syndromes. *Eur J Cancer* 1995; **31A**:1085–1087.

68. Tytgat GNJ. Surveillance of familial adenomatous polyposis after ileorectal anastomosis or ileoanal pouch anastamosis. *Gastrointest Endosc Clin North Am* 1997; **7**:111–127.

69. Fenton PA, Clarke SEM, Owen W, *et al.* Cribriform variant papillary thyroid cancer, a characteristic of familial adenomatous polyposis. *Thyroid* 2001; **11**:193–197.

70. Spirio L, Olschwang S, Groden J, *et al.* Alleles of the *APC* gene: an attenuated form of familial polyposis. *Cell* 1993; **75**:951–957.

71. Laken SJ, Peterson GM, Gruber SB, *et al.* Familial colorectal cancer in Ashkenazim due to a hypermutable tract in *APC*. *Nature Genet* 1997; **17**:79–83.

72. Sieber OM, Lipton L, Crabtree M, *et al.* Multiple colorectal adenomas, classical adenomatous polyposis and germline mutations in MYH. *NEJM* 2003; **348**:791–799.

73. Al-Tassan N, Chinnel NH, Maynard J, *et al.* Inherited variants of MYH associated with somatic G:C>T:A mutations in colorectal tumours. *Nat Genet* 2002; **30**:227–232.

74. Hamilton SR, Liu B, Parsons RE, *et al.* The molecular basis of Turcot syndrome. *N Engl J Med* 1995; **332**:839–847.

75. Flanders T, Foulkes W. Cancers of the digestive system. In: Foulkes WD, Hodgson SV (eds.) *Inherited susceptibility to cancer: clinical, predictive and ethical perspectives.* Cambridge: Cambridge University Press, 1998:Chapter 9.

76. Desai DC, Neale KF, Talbot IC, *et al.* Juvenile polyposis. *Br J Surg* 1995; **82**:14–17.

77. Jass JR, Williams CB, Bussey HJ, Morson BC. Juvenile polyposis – a precarious condition. *Histopathology* 1988; **13**:619–630.

78. Houlston R, Bevon R, Williams A, *et al.* Mutations in *DPC4/SMAD4* cause juvenile polyposis syndrome but only in a minority of cases. *Hum Molec Genet* 1998; **7**:1907–1912.

79. Howe JR, Roth S, Ringold JC, *et al.* Mutations in the *SMAD4/DPC4* gene in juvenile polyposis. *Science* 1998; **280**:1086–1088.

80. Zhou XP, Woodford-Richens K, Lehtonen R, *et al.* Germline mutations in *BMPR1A/ALK3* cause a subset of cases of juvenile polyposis syndrome and of Cowden and Bannayan-Riley-Ruvalcaba syndromes. *Am J Hum Genet* 2001; **69**:704–711.

81. Eng C, Peackocke M. *PTEN* and inherited hamartoma–cancer syndromes. *Nature Genet* 1998; **19**:223.

82. Spigelman AD, Murday V, Phillips RK. Cancer and the Peutz-Jeghers Syndrome. *Gut* 1989; **11**:1588–1590.

83. Konishi F, Wyse NE, Muto T, *et al.* Peutz-Jeghers polyposis associated with carcinoma of the digestive organs. Report of three cases and review of the literature. *Dis-Colon Rectum* 1987; **10**:790–799.

84. Rashid A, Houlihan PS, Booker S, *et al.* Phenotype and molecular characteristics of hyperplastic polyposis. *Gastroenterology* 2000; **119**:323–332.

85. Hemminki A, Markie D, Tomlinson I, *et al.* A serine/threanine kinase gene defective in Peutz-Jeghers syndrome. *Nature* 1998; **391**:184–187.

86. Gupta RA, DuBois RN, Wallace MC. New avenues for the prevention of colorectal cancer: targeting cyclo-oxygenase-2 activity. *Best Pract Clin Gastroenterol* 2002; **16**:945–956.

87. Huls G, Koornstra JJ, Kleibeuker JH. Non-steroidal anti-inflammatory drugs and molecular carcinogenesis of colorectal carcinomas. *Lancet* 2003; **362**:230–232.

88. Viner JL, Umar A, Hawk EZ. Chemoprevention of colorectal cancer: problems, progress and pospects. *Gastroenterol Clinics of North America* 2002; **31**:971–979.

26

Familial prostate cancer and its management

RASHMI SINGH, ROSALIND A. EELES, LISA CANNON-ALBRIGHT AND WILLIAM ISAACS

INTRODUCTION

Prostate cancer (PrCa) is an important public health problem, particularly in Western countries, where it is the most common malignancy among men, who have a lifetime risk of one in ten or more.[1] The highest incidence is in the USA and Jamaica. Both incidence and mortality have increased worldwide in the last few decades, even when the expected increase from PrCa screening is taken into account.[2] The prevalence of PrCa varies markedly between different ethnic groups, with the highest frequency found in African-Americans and the lowest frequency in the Asian populations.[1,3,4] The extent to which this ethnic disparity is attributable to environmental or genetic factors is unknown. One of the strongest risk factors for PrCa identified to date is a family history of disease, suggesting that genetic factors are important.

EPIDEMIOLOGICAL STUDIES

Although not widely recognized as a familial cancer until recently, evidence for familial aggregation of prostate cancer dates as far back as 1956.[5] Clustering of cases is classically observed in the large high-risk Utah kindreds, some with now over 60 cases[6,9] (L. Cannon-Albright, unpublished). Many epidemiological studies have been undertaken to investigate the role of family history as a

PrCa risk factor. There have been two types of case-control study: one compared the number of prostate cancer cases in relatives of cases vs. controls; the other compared the percentage of cases vs. controls with a positive family history of prostate cancer. These studies are summarized in Table 26.1.[5–18] The relative risk of prostate cancer in first-degree relatives of cases ranges from 1.76 to 11.00 in the first study type, and from 0.64 to 7.50 in the second. Only one study has a reduced relative risk in relatives but it has only 39 cases.[13] Woolf reported an increased incidence of prostate cancer of 3.00 in the first-degree relatives of 228 individuals with PrCa in the Utah population,[6] using data from death certificates. This is similar to the relative risks seen with other cancers (see Chapter 17), where there is a well-recognized genetic component. The largest study in this population by Cannon et al. used the Utah Population Data Base (UPDB) in conjunction with the Utah Cancer Registry to study the 'familiality' of a number of cancer sites, including 2821 cases of prostate cancer occurring in Utah from 1958 to 1981.[9] Their unique analytical method involved calculating the mean kinship coefficient (a measure of relatedness) between all possible pairs of cases and appropriate groups of age and race-matched controls. PrCa had the fourth highest mean kinship after lip cancer, melanoma and ovarian cancer. This was a stronger familial association than colon or breast cancer, both of which have a known genetic component (see Chapters 18 and 24). There have been two cohort studies, the first American[19] and the second Swedish;[20] these showed

Table 26.1 *A comparison of case-control studies*

| Reference | Number of cases | No. of cases in first-degree relatives of | | |
		Cases	Controls	Relative risk
Morganti *et al.* (1959)[5] [a]	183	11	1	11.0
Woolf (1960)[6] [b]	228	15	5	3.0
Krain (1974)[7] [a]	221	12	2	6.0
Fincham *et al.* (1990)[8] [a]	382	58	31	3.2
Cannon *et al.* (1982)[9] [b]	2824	[c]	[c]	2.4
Meikle *et al.* (1985)[10] [b]	150	11	1	4.0 (at age 80)
Brothers only				16.6 (at age < 49)
Isaacs *et al.* (1995)[11] [a]	690	119	55	1.76
Keetch *et al.* (1995)[12] [b]	1084	273[d]	85	3.40
% with positive family history		%	%	
Steele *et al.* (1971)[13] [a]	39	12.8	20.0	0.64
Schuman *et al.* (1977)[14] [a]	40	16.7	7.3	2.30
Steinberg *et al.* (1990)[15] [a]	691	15.0	8.0	1.90
Spitz *et al.* (1991)[16] [a]	378	13.0	5.7	2.30
Ghadirian *et al.* (1991)[17] [a]	140	15.0	2.0	7.50
Ghadirian *et al.* (1997)[18] [b]	640	15.0	5.0	3.32

[a] Information from patient/control questionnaire only.
[b] Diagnosis verified by hospital records, cancer registration or death certificate.
[c] Measured genealogical index; see article by Neuhausen *et al.*[146]
[d] First- and second-degree relatives.

relative risks of prostate cancer of 2.20 (95 per cent confidence interval (CI) 2.00–2.40) and 1.70 (CI 1.51–1.90), respectively.

While screening for PrCa in 6390 men aged 50–80 years, Narod *et al.* found a significantly higher prevalence (6.7 per cent) of the disease among men with any first-degree relative affected (relative risk; RR 1.72) in comparison with those with no first-degree relative affected (prevalence 3.89 per cent, RR 1.00), with the highest risk for brothers of affected men (prevalence 10.2 per cent; RR 2.62, *p* 0.0002).[21]

The increase in the size of the relative risk from the case-control studies as clustering becomes more dramatic suggests a genetic effect. The relative risks of prostate cancer due to other factors, such as age at first marriage, are all about 1.5, which is the level of risk in breast cancer aetiology from hormonal factors. All but one of the relative risk figures in the familial studies are higher than this, and all but three are higher than 2.0. The best evidence that there is a genetic effect is that the relative risk markedly increases as the age of the proband decreases (Table 26.2), as the closeness and number of affected members in the family increases (Tables 26.3 and 26.4), or when both factors are taken together (Table 26.5). Tables such as these are useful in risk assessment for genetic counselling. A change in relative risk of this magnitude as clustering increases cannot be explained solely by a common environmental effect in each cluster, although there may still be an environmental component

Table 26.2 *Relative odds for prostate cancer in brothers of prostate cancer cases by age. (Reproduced from Cannon et al.[9])*

| Age of affected case | Age of brother (years) | | |
	<65	65–79	80+
<65	5.97[b]	2.77[a]	2.29
65–79	2.77[a]	2.04[b]	2.52[a]
80+	2.29	2.52[a]	1.14

[a] *p* < 0.01; [b] *p* < 0.001.

Table 26.3 *Relative risks for prostate cancer in relatives of prostate cancer cases by degree of relationship. (Reproduced with permission from Blackwell Publishing from Steinberg et al.[15])*

Affected relatives	Relative risk (95% confidence interval)
First-degree	2.0 (1.2–3.3)
Second-degree	1.7 (1.0–2.9)
Both first and second	8.8 (2.8–28.1)

present. Twin studies also support the existence of an underlying genetic predisposition to PrCa. Monozygotic twins have a fourfold increased concordance rate for the development of PrCa compared with dizygotic twins, confirming the importance of genetic factors.[23]

Table 26.4 *Age-adjusted relative risk estimates for prostate cancer by number of additional affected family members. (Reproduced with permission from Blackwell Publishing from Steinberg et al.[15])*

Affected relatives (besides proband)	Odds ratio (95% confidence interval)
1	2.2 (1.4–3.5)
2	4.9 (2.0–12.3)
3	10.9 (2.7–43.1)

Table 26.5 *Estimated risk ratios for prostate cancer in first-degree relatives of probands, by age at onset in proband and additional family members. (Reproduced from Carter et al.[22])*

Age at onset of proband	Number of additional relatives affected	One or more additional first-degree relatives affected
50	1.9 (1.2–2.8)	7.1 (3.7–13.6)
60	1.4 (1.1–1.7)	5.2 (3.1–8.7)
70	1.0[a]	3.8 (2.4–6.0)

[a] Reference group.

SEGREGATION ANALYSES

Although the case-control studies above support the importance of genetic factors in PrCa development, the genetic mode of transmission has been much debated. Segregation analyses have been performed to model the mode of inheritance and the penetrance of the putative predisposing gene(s). A study of 691 families of PrCa patients performed by Carter et al. suggested that family clustering was best explained by an autosomal dominant inheritance of a highly penetrant gene, displaying a population frequency of 0.003 and predisposing to an early onset of the disease. The cumulative risk of PrCa by age 85 was estimated to be 88 per cent in carriers compared to only 5 per cent in non-carriers. The gene accounted for 43 per cent of cases by age 55 and for 9 per cent of cases by age 80.[22] However, this study was in nuclear families and there may have been a bias towards ascertainment of particularly strong close clustering.

Two further segregation analyses by Schaid et al.[24] and Grönberg et al.[25] also proposed similar transmission models; however, the Grönberg model proposed a more common gene with lower penetrance, although the penetrance is still high at 67 per cent by age 80. This latter study was subject to the least bias, since it was a systematic analysis of a population-based dataset from a cancer registry, although much of the risk is still accounted for by only a few large families. Whereas these three studies were consistent in supporting the presence of at least one highly penetrant autosomal dominant PrCa susceptibility

gene, Cui et al. recently proposed a model including a dominantly inherited increased risk that was greater, in multiplicative terms, at younger ages, as well as a recessively or X-linked risk that was greater at older ages. The model was the result of single- and two-locus segregation analyses of data from 1476 population-based Australian men diagnosed with PrCa < 70 years and from their male relatives. Penetrance to age 80 was about 70 per cent for the dominant effect and virtually 100 per cent for the recessive and X-linked effects.[26]

LINKAGE ANALYSES

There are several potential problems in the mapping of genes causing familial prostate cancer. The disease is common and so has a high phenocopy rate (i.e. several cases in each family may be sporadic). PrCa typically occurs at an older age and so it is often difficult to obtain DNA from living affected men for more than one generation. There is currently a debate as to whether the pathology of familial and 'sporadic' disease is different and, therefore, the pathology may not prove to be useful in linkage stratification. Despite these problems, several groups have been collecting information on PrCa families and performing linkage analysis to identify candidate genes. They have formed an International Consortium (the ICPCG; International Consortium for Prostate Cancer Genetics) and joint analyses of their linkage results are planned. Linkage has been a very successful approach for finding key genes that predispose to other common cancers, such as melanoma,[27] breast cancer[28,29] and colon cancer.[30,31] In contrast, it has become apparent that there are difficulties in finding one or a few high-risk genes that could account for the majority of hereditary PrCa families. In fact, numerous regions of the genome have now been identified as containing putative susceptibility loci for PrCa but confirmatory studies often produce inconsistent results.

HPC1 – 1q24–25

In 1996, Smith et al. performed a genomewide search of linkage analysis in 91 high-risk PrCa families from the USA and Sweden.[32] They found evidence for linkage on chromosome 1q24–25 with a maximum multipoint LOD score under heterogeneity of 5.43 (see Chapter 3). Interestingly, two of the linked families were African-American and contributed to over 1.00 of the total LOD score. Several other studies were performed in order to confirm these findings. Among these, four studies have shown only weak linkage to the locus using non-parametric methods.[33–36] In the study by Cooney et al., 6 out of 59 families were African-American and again contributed disproportionately to the observation of linkage, although this did not reach statistical significance.[33] Other studies, however, have failed to find evidence of linkage.[37–40]. An analysis by the UK/Canadian/Texan Linkage Consortium[37] failed to find evidence for linkage in the 1q24–25 region in 136 PrCa families; the estimated proportion of families linked was 4 per cent and there was no evidence in families with three or fewer cases, but among families with four or more cases up to 20 per cent could have been linked on the heterogeneity analysis. This led to the hypothesis that *HPC1* may be more likely to be involved in larger PrCa clusters, which was supported by other results, which reported that linkage to 1q was more likely if families displayed male-to-male disease transmission and a mean age at diagnosis of younger than 65 years.[41,42] Furthermore, the study by Grönberg *et al.* provided some clues for correlations between *HPC1* genotype and clinicopathological phenotype;[41] 1q-linked families had earlier-onset, grade 3 and later stage disease compared with those cases in non-linked families. The hypothesis of an aggressive phenotype for *HPC1*-linked tumours is also supported by Goode *et al.*, who assessed linkage at four loci (*HPC1, PCAP, HPCX, CABP*) in PrCa families stratified by age of diagnosis, grade and stage of disease, and found the strongest evidence of *HPC1* linkage was in families with higher grade or more advanced-stage PrCa and which were not likely to be linked to loci other than 1q. However, in this study, the strongest evidence for *HPC1* linkage was displayed by older-onset families.[43]

The inconsistency of the studies so far performed hampers the assessment of the actual contribution of *HPC1* to hereditary PrCa. Although the initial report of linkage to *HPC1* proposed that up to 34 per cent of PrCa families could be linked to this locus, the pooled analysis of 772 families by Xu found much weaker evidence of linkage, with the estimated proportion of linked families being 6 per cent.[42] *HPC1* involvement in the predisposition to cancer sites other than prostate appears to be limited, although a slight excess of breast and colon cancer has been observed in potentially-linked families.[41] Loss of heterozygosity (LOH) studies at this locus in prostate tumours initially suggested that *HPC1* is not a tumour suppressor gene;[44] however, recently Carpten *et al.* have reported mutations in a candidate gene in the region (*RNASEL*).[44] This gene is involved in interferon-induced apoptosis and LOH was seen at this locus in linked families. This publication prompted a lot of interest; however, subsequent studies have failed to confirm that it is a high-risk susceptibility gene, but there may be variants within it that confer a more moderate, if any, PrCa risk. Many studies failed to confirm segregation of variants within *RNASEL* in PrCa cases and this was evidence that the gene was unlikely to be *HPC1*, at least in the highly penetrant form predicted by the segregation analyses and the linkage data.[45–50] This illustrates the dilemma of causality when a mutation is found that disrupts protein

function, since this was clearly demonstrated in the first report. However, a disruption of protein function could theoretically be a normal variant of the function that has hitherto been undetected and may not be causal. A further publication from the Utah group[51] has supported a locus at 1q and so further studies of RNASEL are being conducted.

PCAP – 1q42.2–43

A second putative PrCa susceptibility locus (*PCAP*) was reported by Berthon *et al.* in 1998 at 1q42.2–43, a locus 60 cM downstream from *HPC1*.[52] This group obtained a two-point LOD score of 2.7 and estimated that as many as 40–50 per cent of their French and German families could be linked to this locus. Again the evidence for linkage came predominantly from families with early-onset cases (<60 years). Although four subsequent studies of the *PCAP* region failed to find any significant evidence of linkage,[36,53–55] a recent study by Cancel-Tassin *et al.* has reported evidence of linkage to *PCAP* in 64 PrCa families from southern and western Europe, whereas no evidence of linkage existed for *HPC1, CAPB* and *HPCX*. It is, therefore, possible that *PCAP* could play a role in PrCa susceptibility in specific geographical areas, but its contribution to the total burden of hereditary PrCa is likely to be considerably less than the 40–50 per cent originally reported.[56]

CAPB – 1p36

In 1999, evidence for a third locus on chromosome 1 linked to familial PrCa was reported by Gibbs *et al.*[57] The locus, 1p36, was identified through linkage studies in 12 high-risk PrCa families and was restricted to kindreds with at least one case of primary brain cancer. The overall LOD score in these families was 3.22, and after exclusion of 3 of the 12 families that had better evidence of linkage to other putative PrCa susceptibility loci, a two-point LOD score of 4.74 was achieved. This group, therefore, concluded that a significant proportion of the families with both a high risk for PrCa and a family member with primary brain cancer showed linkage to the 1p36 region. A subsequent study by Badzioch *et al.* failed to find evidence of linkage at 1p36 in 207 PrCa families, including nine prostate–brain cancer families, but the LOD scores were higher in families with younger average age at PrCa onset (<66 years), with or without a family history of brain cancer.[58] In addition, no correlation was found with tumours of any other primary site. These results led to the hypothesis that an early onset of PrCa, instead of the association with cancer of the brain or other sites, was responsible for the positive linkage to 1p36.[58] Subsequent studies failed to find evidence of linkage to *CABP*,[36] whereas another found positive linkage results in four out of six brain–prostate cancer families.[59] Based on such controversial results, no conclusions are possible regarding the role of this gene from the linkage evidence.

HPCX – Xq27–q28

In several case-control studies, the relative risk of PrCa has been higher for brothers than fathers of cases. In the study by Schaid *et al.*, PrCa was 1.5 times more common among brothers than fathers of men with PrCa.[24] These findings could be explained by an X-linked or recessive inheritance of PrCa susceptibility in some families; this is also supported by the segregation analysis by Cui *et al.*[26] Indeed, in 1998, Xu *et al.* proposed a PrCa susceptibility locus on the long arm of chromosome X at Xq27–28.[60] Evidence for linkage was found in a combined study population of 360 North American, Swedish and Finnish families, with a maximum two-point LOD score of 4.6. The proportion of families linked to *HPCX* was estimated to be 16 per cent. These findings have been confirmed by three subsequent independent studies.[61–63] Lange *et al.* reported that the greatest evidence for linkage on Xq was in the subset of families with no male-to-male transmission and an age at disease onset of <65 years.[61] An analysis of Finnish families found significant linkage at *HPCX* in association with the subgroup again of male to male transmission but, in contrast to the previous study, with a later age at PrCa diagnosis (>65 years).[63] The candidate for the Xq locus remains to be identified.

HPC2/ELAC2 – 17p11

In 2001, Tatvigian *et al.* demonstrated evidence of linkage of large PrCa pedigrees from Utah to 17p11 (LOD 4.60 assuming a recessive model). Positional cloning within the refined interval identified a gene known as *ELAC2*, which is homologous to *PSO2* (*SNM1*), that codes for a DNA interstrand cross-link repair protein, and *CPSF73*, a subunit of mRNA 3' end-cleavage and polyadenylation factor. Mutation screening of the gene detected two changes co-segregating with the disease; a frameshift mutation (1641insG) and a non-conservative amino acid change (Arg781His); and two common missense variants (Ser217Leu and Ala541Thr). All of the Thr541 variants were observed in Leu217 chromosomes.[64] Since then, several groups have investigated the association of these polymorphisms with PrCa. Rebbeck *et al.* studied 359 PrCa cases and 266 male controls from a large health-system population and found an increased risk for PrCa in men who carried the two variants Leu217 and Thr541 (odds ratio (OR) 2.37, CI 1.06–5.29), regardless of their family history.[65] Suarez *et al.* found an increased frequency

of the Thr541 allele in PrCa cases drawn from multiplex sibships, compared to healthy controls, but no excess clustering of the allele and little or no evidence of linkage to the *HPC2/ELAC2* region was evident in these families.[66] Overall, other studies have failed to uniformly confirm the association between the variants Leu217 and Thr541 and PrCa.[67–70] Two papers have reported meta analyses of the published data.[71,72] The latter shows that an increased relative risk of developing PrCa is only significantly seen when cases from family clusters are compared with controls. This suggests that lower penetrance genetic alterations should be investigated by comparing frequencies in familial clusters versus controls first, subsequently followed by large case-control analyses. However, the results for *HPC2* in such a familial analysis versus controls still only demonstrate an OR of 2.21 with carriage of both Leu217 and Thr541 versus carriage of neither.[72] This argues against a major role of *HPC2/ELAC2* polymorphisms in PrCa susceptibility. This is also supported by the observation that several genomewide linkage analyses have not found any evidence of linkage to chromosome 17p.[32,73–75]

Other candidate loci

Localization of further PrCa susceptibility loci has emerged from genomic searches of large sets of PrCa families; a genomewide search on 162 North American families with three or more members affected with PrCa has recently found evidence of linkage to a novel locus at chromosome 20q13 (*HPC20*), with a maximum two-point LOD score of 2.69, which is below statistical significance.[76] Interestingly, the strongest evidence of linkage was found in smaller families with less than five affected relatives, a later average age of diagnosis and no male to male transmission. Subsequent studies by Bock *et al.* and Cancel-Tassin *et al.* found no evidence of linkage,[77,78] whereas Zheng *et al.* found elevated non-parametric linkage scores in a study of 159 hereditary PrCa families,[79] with higher scores in subgroups of families with a later age at diagnosis (>64 years), fewer than five affected family members or without male-to-male transmission, consistent with the initial observation by Berry. A genomic screen of 504 brothers with PrCa performed by Suarez *et al.* identified five new regions of interest based on nominal evidence for linkage (i.e. a Z_{lr} score > 1.645) at 2q, 12p, 15q, 16p and 16q.[73] This latter region, which was found to have the highest signal (Z_{lr} = 3.15), has been reported as a candidate area for a tumour-suppressor gene in PrCa in several studies.[80–82] Stratification of the sample population in the Suarez study identified three further regions of interest; families with a history of breast cancer showed evidence of linkage to chromosome 1q35.1 (Z_{lr} = 3.78, corresponding to a LOD score > 3); those with no family history of breast cancer had linkage to a region proximal to *HPC1*

($Z_{lr} = 1.75–2.72$) and those with late-onset disease had linkage to chromosome 4q ($Z_{lr} = 1.92–2.85$).[73]

A third genomic scan of 94 PrCa families by Gibbs *et al.* has proposed multiple regions of interest, including loci on chromosomes 10, 12 and 14.[74] This study also provided some evidence for PrCa linkage on 8p, a region where there is frequently observed LOH in prostate tumour tissue. Xu *et al.* found evidence for linkage at 8p22–23, with a peak heterogeneity LOD (HLOD) of 1.84 ($p = 0.004$).[83] The estimated proportion of families linked (alpha; see Chapter 3) was 14 per cent; interestingly, Ashkenazi Jewish families appeared to be contributing disproportionately to the overall LOD score. They have subsequently reported that mutations in the gene encoding the macrophage scavenger receptor 1 (*MSR1*) are more frequently identified in men with PrCa than in controls.[84] The data presented in support of this are in several independent parts. First, variants were more common in cases than controls. In European populations, one nonsense mutation, R293X, was seen in 8 of 317 non-hereditary PrCa cases and in 1 of 256 unaffected men (OR 6.60, CI 0.87–294, $p = 0.047$). When all variants were combined, they were more common in non-*HPC* cases than in controls (14 of 317 among cases, compared with 2 of 256 in controls; OR 5.87, CI 1.33–53.6, $p = 0.009$). Second, among hereditary PrCa families, the HLOD was 1.40 in families carrying a mutation in *MSR1* compared with 0.05 in those without mutations. However, families carrying the mutation most likely to be disease-associated (R293X) did not show evidence of linkage in a parametric test ($p = 0.27$). Third, in a different population (African-Americans), similar results were obtained (for all variants: 8 of 48 in cases vs. 3 of 110 in controls; OR 7.13, CI 1.59–43.2, $p = 0.003$). Other groups have tried to confirm these high odds ratios without success;[85,86] however, other variants have been found in this gene and their role in PrCa will have to be assessed.

THE LINKAGE STORY SO FAR

A common theme is, therefore, emerging where a hint of linkage in PrCa cases from one or more collections are subsequently not confirmed by other groups.[87] The most likely explanation is that there is considerable genetic heterogeneity. In contrast to other common cancers, such as colon cancer and breast cancer, where a small number of very high-risk genes account for a proportion of the high-risk multiple case families, hereditary prostate cancer is likely to be caused by numerous different genes. There are several possible solutions to this problem: (i) meta analyses of all linkage searches worldwide; (ii) substratification by ethnic origin of the families and disease parameters. The former is being achieved by the creation of the ICPC G. Several of the component groups have published genome wide linkage searches recently in

a volume of *The Prostate*,[88] but no one locus is found consistently.

Several groups have used a stratification approach and a number of parameters have been hypothesized to be associated with specific genes. Among these, ethnicity definitely plays a major role. Ethnic differences in PrCa incidence may be explained by both genetic and environmental factors, but the higher risk of PrCa in Blacks compared with White men in the USA and the results of the 1q24 linkage studies that support the hypothesis that *HPC1* may be more frequently involved in African/American than in Caucasian PrCa families suggest a role for this gene in this ethnic group.[32,33] The number of affected family members is a critical factor for identifying predisposition genes to common cancers. Large clusters, such as those seen in familial breast cancer studies, are not common in PrCa families; the majority of families collected by different groups include three or four cases, few families with eight or more cases exist, and only in large Utah kindreds are up to 60 cases reported. A correlation with cluster size has been suggested for some of the loci to date identified, suggesting that the penetrance of the different PrCa loci may be different: *HPC1* has been reported to be more frequently involved in larger clusters,[37,41,42] whereas *HPC20* has been suggested to be more likely to be involved in small clusters.[76,79] In contrast with most hereditary cancer syndromes, hereditary PrCa in linked families appears to be mainly a site-specific condition, therefore, the association with other tumours in the family is not generally helpful in suggesting specific loci of susceptibility to PrCa. A possible exception could be the association with primary brain cancer, due to *CABP*, although this is debated.[57,58] A correlation between high-grade, advanced-stage PrCa and linkage at *HPC1* has been hypothesized,[41] and a study of families stratified by grade and stage has provided support to the hypothesis.[43] Stratification by grade and stage is particularly relevant because of the increasing number of PrCa cases detected by screening. Foci of PrCa are a common finding in specimens from autopsy and from surgery for benign disease, which has led to the conclusion that a proportion of PrCa, which may potentially include screen-detected cases, follows an indolent course; this could have a different genetic basis from clinically significant disease. This could be a confounding factor in the mapping of PrCa genes. One major concern of PrCa screening is that those cancers that would never have progressed are treated, leading to additional unnecessary treatment-related morbidity and mortality. Indeed, if hereditary PrCa, or at least the proportion linked at *HPC1*, was confirmed to be more aggressive than sporadic disease then, once genetic assessment became possible, we would have the opportunity of identifying a subset of individuals at high risk not only of developing PrCa but also of dying of it. Such individuals may gain more benefit from screening.

The other confounding factor in finding PrCa susceptibility genes is the ability to perform large-scale mutation screening. This is now a two-edged sword. On the one hand, large-scale mutation screening of genes in the regions of linkage can be performed more easily. However, conversely, these reveal variations in the code of candidate genes in the region whose effects are uncertain and which are not consistently associated with PrCa susceptibility. Certainly those that have been reported to date are not of the high relative risks that would be predicted by the linkage evidence.

KNOWN GENES POTENTIALLY INVOLVED IN GENETIC SUSCEPTIBILITY TO PROSTATE CANCER

Genes involved in steroid hormone metabolism

Androgens, steroid hormones that are essential for prostate development, growth and maintenance, are thought to play a role in prostate carcinogenesis. Therefore, several genes involved in androgen pathway have been investigated to assess their possible contribution to PrCa risk. Androgen receptor (AR) is a transcription factor that mediates the proliferative effects of androgens in the prostate by binding to androgen responsive elements (ARE) in target gene promoters. The AR gene, located at Xq11–12, is highly polymorphic in the human population and, in particular, the length of a CAG microsatellite in exon 1 displays ethnic variation mirroring the ethnic variation in PrCa rates. Several studies have shown an inverse association of CAG length with PrCa risk,[89–92] but the association has not been confirmed by other studies.[93–96] Edwards et al. reported an increased risk of relapse (RR 1.74, CI 1.08–2.79) and death (RR 1.98, CI 1.13–3.45) for PrCa cases with ≥ 16 GGC repeats, even after adjusting for stage and grade.[97] The function of the GGC is uncertain. The germline mutation R726L has been reported in the Finnish population, where it may contribute to cancer development in up to 2 per cent of PrCa cases.[98,99]

The GG genotype of PSA (prostate-specific antigen) has been reported recently to be associated with increased PrCa risk, especially when associated with short CAG allele of AR.[99]

HSD17β2 encodes 17β-hydroxysteroid dehydrogenase type II, which catalyses the conversion of active 17β-hydroxysteroids into their 17-keto forms and, therefore, inactivates both androgens and oestrogens.[100] The HSD17β2 gene maps to chromosome 16q24.1–q24.2,[101] a frequently deleted region in prostate tumours.[102] Moreover, the frequency of loss of heterozygosity at this region is significantly associated with metastatic and clinically aggressive behaviour of PrCa.[102]

SRD5A2 encodes 5α-reductase type II, which catalyses the conversion of testosterone into the more bioactive androgen dihydrotestosterone (DHT) and maps to 2p23–22.[103,104] DHT synthesis occurs in prostate tumours and modulation of its activity may be responsible for some of the variations in PrCa risk among ethnic groups.[105]

The frequency of the missense mutation V89L in different ethnic groups mirrors the incidence of PrCa in these populations, suggesting it may affect the risk for this disease.[106] A study has suggested that this variant reduces PrCa risk.[107] A second missense mutation, A49T, was found to be more common in PrCa cases, compared to asymptomatic controls, among African-American and Hispanic men[108,109] and in a sample of Italian men, although in this case the difference was not statistically significant.[107] In addition, the A49T variant, but not the V89L, appeared to be associated with more advanced disease in 275 Caucasian PrCa patients.[110]

The CYP17 gene, mapping to 10q24, encodes the enzyme cytochrome P45017α, which mediates both 17α-hydroxylase and 17,20-lyase activity, playing a key role for sex steroid and cortisol biosynthesis. A polymorphism (T > C) in the 5′-untranslated region of the gene has been hypothesized to result in increased expression of the gene, leading to elevated serum levels of sexual hormones,[111] which could increase the risk for hormone-related cancers, such as prostate and breast cancer. However, studies evaluating the correlations between CYP17 genotype and increased risk for these cancers yield contradictory results. For PrCa, some authors report a positive association between the variant (allele A2) and an increased risk,[112–115] whereas other studies found the risk to be higher in carriers of the wild-type (A1) allele.[116,117] Chang et al. recently reported evidence for linkage to the CYP17 gene region in 159 PrCa families, but failed to find differences in the frequency of either allele between PrCa cases (hereditary and sporadic) and healthy controls. Their results suggest that the CYP17 gene or other genes in the region may increase the susceptibility to PrCa, but the polymorphism in the 5′ promoter region is unlikely to be associated with an increased risk.[118]

Finally, some evidence exists that polymorphisms in other genes of the CYP family, such as CYP1A1 and CYP3A4 may affect PrCa risk and prognosis, presumed to be due to the role of these enzymes in the metabolism of a number of substrates, including chemical carcinogens and chemotherapeutic drugs.[119–121]

BRCA1 and BRCA2

Familial co-aggregation of prostate and breast cancer has been reported[122–125] and carriers of mutations in the breast cancer predisposition genes BRCA1 and BRCA2 in breast/ovarian cancer families have been shown to have a

3–7-fold increased risk of PrCa in some studies.[126–128] Moreover, the 185delAG Ashkenazi mutation in *BRCA1* has been reported in one family of that origin with four cases of PrCa,[129] although studies analysing the frequency of the founder Askenazi *BRCA1* and *BRCA2* mutations among Azhkenazi Jewish PrCa patients suggest that these *particular* mutations do not have a significant role in the disease in this ethnic group.[130–132] A truncating mutation in *BRCA2* has been identified in a Swedish family with five cases of early-onset, aggressive PrCa and three cases of breast cancer.[133] In the Icelandic population, the founder *BRCA2* mutation 999del5 has been reported to be associated with a more aggressive form of PrCa.[134] The UK/Canadian/Texan Consortium has analysed the contribution of *BRCA1* and *BRCA2* to small prostate cancer clusters in a study of 100 clusters. Up to 30 per cent may be linked to *BRCA1/2*; however, the confidence intervals were wide and included zero.[135] Direct mutation analysis of 38 prostate cancer clusters from the UK Familial Prostate Cancer Study has not revealed any *BRCA1* mutation; however, germline mutations were found in *BRCA2* in two men belonging to sibling pairs affected by early-onset PrCa.[136] A subsequent study by this group[137] screened the complete coding sequence of *BRCA2* for germline mutations in 263 men diagnosed with prostate cancer diagnosed at ⩽55 years. Protein-truncating mutations were found in six men (2.3 per cent, CI 0.8–5.0 per cent); all of these mutations were clustered outside the ovarian cancer cluster region. The relative risk of developing prostate cancer by the age of 60 from a deleterious germline *BRCA2* mutation was 23-fold. Three of the six patients with mutations did not have a family history of breast or ovarian cancer. These results confirm that *BRCA2* is a high-risk prostate cancer susceptibility gene and has potential implications for the management of early-onset prostate cancer cases and their relatives. This would warrant further screening of the *BRCA2* gene in other young-onset PrCa series.

Nevertheless, Sinclair *et al.* failed to find truncating mutations in *BRCA1* and *BRCA2* by screening 22 high-risk PrCa families, but at the low level of mutation (2.3 per cent of cases) this could have been undetectable in a sample set of this size or the result may only pertain to particularly young onset disease.[138]

MANAGEMENT

When advising individuals in prostate cancer families about their risk, Tables 26.1–26.5 can be useful to give general levels of relative risk according to the numbers of affected individuals in the family and their ages at diagnosis. For example, if there are two first-degree relatives affected with prostate cancer aged about 60 years, the relative risk in the unaffected, related individual is about

fivefold. The population risk in a Western Caucasian population is 0.5 per cent by age 64 and 2 per cent by age 74,[139] so the absolute risk is 2.5 per cent and 10 per cent by these ages, respectively.

Since relatives of prostate cancer patients are at increased risk of the disease, the question arises whether they should be offered targeted screening. It has been shown that earlier diagnosis results in a better survival,[140] but improvement in mortality as a result of prostate cancer screening remains to be proven, although some studies are suggestive of an effect.[141–143] There is debate as to whether measurement of the blood marker, prostate-specific antigen (PSA), alone is sufficient or whether rectal examination would also be needed. If a higher risk population would be identified, in theory, PSA screening should result in a higher yield of cancer cases detected per number screened. McWhorter *et al.* have studied first-degree relative of 17 sets of brother pairs, both with prostate cancer.[144] A total of 34 relatives were screened (sons and brothers, aged 55–80 years) with an intensive programme of PSA, rectal examination (DRE), transrectal ultrasound (TRUS) and systematic as well as clinically directed biopsies. Six (18 per cent) had a raised PSA but only three had cancer. Both PSA and DRE were abnormal in four individuals and TRUS showed a lesion in seven. Although eight cancers were found on histology in this study, in only seven was the TRUS abnormal. The other problem with such intensive screening is that it may detect cancer that would not become clinically relevant in the lifetime of the individual. However, one of the cancers was a stage C and, after radical prostatectomy, the other seven were four stage C and four stage B. The overall cancer detection rate was, therefore, 8 out of 34 (or 9 per cent) and all had clinically significant disease. Using a similar screening protocol in the general population, with the difference that biopsy was only undertaken if indicated, the cancer detection rate in a population of 1630 men was 2.2 per cent.[145] Catalona *et al.* have shown that targeted screening in ethnic groups with a higher risk and those men with a family history does reveal prostate cancer which is clinically important.[146] Neuhausen *et al.* also reported a similar result.[147]

In conclusion, the search for PrCa predisposing genes has been to date complicated by the discovery of multiple loci on linkage, but subsequent mutation detection does not bear out the presence of deleterious mutations that can be substantiated, as occurred in the discovery of *BRCA1* and *BRCA2* in breast cancer genetic predisposition. This is probably due to the heterogeneity of the disease. The discovery of a small proportion of individuals with early-onset disease who have germline deleterious *BRCA2* mutations needs to be followed up further and would imply that high-risk prostate cancer predisposition genes do exist, but are each only present in a small proportion of cases. A recent example of this is the finding that mutations in the Nijmegen breakage syndrome gene in the slavic population confer a 16-fold increased risk of prostate cancer *in this particular population*.[148] These findings will make the identification of genes difficult by linkage and they will be found by candidate approaches.

KEY POINTS

- Epidemiological and twin studies suggest prostate cancer predisposition genes do exist.
- Linkage analyses have suggested numerous loci but few candidate genes.
- The candidate genes thus identified have on further analyses proved to be moderate/lower penetrance genes.
- There is debate about the role of targeted prostate cancer screening and studies are in progress. Blacks have a higher risk and should be screened at an earlier age if a screening programme is offered.
- *BRCA2* mutations have been found by using a candidate genetic analysis approach in young onset prostate cancer cases. This result needs to be confirmed and, if so, it has implications for screening of relatives and genetic testing of this gene.

REFERENCES

1. Hsing AW, Tsao L, Devesa S: International trends and patterns of prostate cancer incidence and mortality. *Int J Cancer* 2000; **85**:60–67.
2. Greenlee RT, Hill-Harmon MB, Muttay T, Thun M. Cancer statistics, 2001. *CA Cancer J Clin* 2001; **51**:15–38.
3. Parkin DM, Pisani P, Ferlay J. Estimates of the worldwide incidence of 18 major cancers in 1985. *Int J Cancer* 1993; **54**:594–606.
4. Whittemore AS, Kolonel LN, Wu AH, *et al*. Family history and prostate cancer risk in black, white and Asian men in the United States and Canada. *Am J Epidemiol* 1995; **141**: 732–740.
5. Morganti G, *et al*. Recherches clinico-statistiques et éétiques sur les éopasies de la prostate. *Acta Genetica Statistica* 1959; **6**:304–305.
6. Woolf CM. An investigation of the familial aspects of carcinoma of the prostate. *Cancer* 1960; **13**:739–744.
7. Krain LS. Some epidemiologic variables in prostatic carcinoma in California. *Prev Med* 1974; **3**:154–159.
8. Fincham SM, Hill GB, Hanson J, Wijayasinghe C. Epidemiology of prostate cancer: a case control study. *Prostate* 1990; **17**:189–206.
9. Cannon LA, Bishop DT, Skolnick M, *et al*. Genetic epidemiology of prostate cancer in the Utah Mormon Genealogy. *Cancer Surv* 1982; **1**:47–69.
10. Meikle AW, Smith JA, West DW. Familial factors affecting prostatic cancer risk and plasma sex-steroid levels. *Prostate* 1985; **6**:121–128.
11. Isaacs SD, Kiemeney LA, Baffoe-Bonnie A, *et al*. Risk of cancer in relatives of prostate cancer probands. *J Natl Cancer Inst* 1995; **87**:991–996.
12. Keetch DW, Rice JP, Suarez BK, Catalona WJ. Familial aspects of prostate cancer: a case control study. *J Urol* 1995; **154**:2100–2102.
13. Steele R, Lees REM, Kraus AS, Rao C. Sexual factors in the epidemiology of cancer of the prostate. *J Chron Dis* 1971; **24**:29–37.
14. Schuman LM, Mandel J, Blackard C, *et al*. Epidemiologic study of prostatic cancer: preliminary report. *Cancer Treat Rep* 1977; **61**:181–186.
15. Steinberg GD, Carter BS, Beaty TH, *et al*. Family history and the risk of prostate cancer. *Prostate* 1990; **17**:337–347.
16. Spitz MR, Currier RD, Fueger JJ, *et al*. Familial patterns of prostate cancer: a case-control analysis. *J Urol* 1991; **146**:1305–1307.
17. Ghadirian P, Cadotte M, Lacroix A, Perret C. Family aggregation of cancer of the prostate in Quebec: the tip of the iceberg. *Prostate* 1991; **19**:43–52.
18. Ghadirian P, Howe GR, Hislop TG, Maisonneuve P. Family history of prostate cancer: a multi-centre case-control study in Canada. *Int J Cancer* 1997; **70**:679–681.
19. Goldgar DE, Easton DF, Cannon-Albright LA, Skolnick MH. Systematic population-based assessment of cancer risk in first-degree relatives of cancer probands *J Natl Cancer Inst* 1994; **86**:1600–1608.
20. Grönberg H, Damber L, Damber JE. Familial Prostate cancer in Sweden. *Cancer* 1996; **77**:138–143.
21. Narod SA, Dupont A, Cusan L, *et al*. The impact of family history on early detection of prostate cancer. *Nature Med* 1995; **1**:99–101.
22. Carter BS, Beaty TH, Steinberg GD, *et al*. Mendelian inheritance of familial prostate cancer. *Proc Natl Acad Sci USA* 1992; **89**:3367–3371.
23. Gronberg H, Damber L, Damber JE. Studies of genetic factors in prostate cancer in a twin population. *J Urol* 1994; **152**:1484–1487.
24. Schaid DJ, McDonnell SK, Blute ML, Thibodeau SN. Evidence for autosomal dominant inheritance of prostate cancer. *Am J Hum Genet* 1998; **62**:1425–1438.
25. Grönberg H, Damber L, Damber JE, Iselius L. Segregation analysis of prostate cancer in Sweden: support for dominant inheritance. *Am J Epidemiol* 1997; **146**:552–557.
26. Cui J, Staples MP, Hopper JL, *et al*. Segregation analyses of 1,476 population-based Australian families affected by prostate cancer. *Am J Hum Genet* 2001; **68**:1207–1218.
27. Cannon-Albright IA, Goldgar DE, Meyer LJ, *et al*. Assignment of a locus for familial melanoma, MLM, to chromosome 9p13–p22. *Science* 1992; **258**:1148–1152.
28. Hall JM, Lee MK, Newman B, *et al*. Linkage of early-onset familial breast cancer to chromosome 17q21. *Science* 1990; **250**:1684–1689.
29. Wooster R, Neuhausen S, Mangion J, *et al*. Localization of a breast cancer susceptibility gene, *BRCA2*, to chromosome 13q12–13. *Science*. 1994; **265**:2088–2090.

30. Nakamura Y, Lathrop M, Leppert M, et al. Localization of the genetic defect in familial adenomatous polyposis within a small region of chromosome 5. Am J Hum Genet 1988; 43:638–644.

31. Peltomaki P, Aaltonen LA, Sistonen P, et al. Genetic mapping of a locus predisposing to human colorectal cancer. Science 1993; 260:810–812.

32. Smith JR, Freije D, Carpten JD, et al. Major susceptibility locus for prostate cancer on chromosome 1 suggested by a genome wide search. Science 1996; 274:1371–1374.

33. Cooney KA, McCarthy JD, Lange E, et al. Prostate cancer susceptibility locus on chromosome 1q: a confirmatory study. J Natl Cancer Inst 1997; 89:955–959.

34. Hsieh CL, Oakley-Garvan I, Gallagher RP, et al. Re: prostate cancer susceptibility locus on chromosome 1q: a confirmatory study. J Natl Cancer Inst 1997; 89:1893–1894.

35. Neuhausen S, Farnham J, Kort E, et al. Prostate cancer susceptibility locus HPC1 in Utah high-risk pedigrees. Hum Mol Genet 1999; 8:2437–2442.

36. Berry R, Schaid DJ, Smith JR, et al. Linkage analyses at the chromosome 1 loci 1q24–25 (HPC1), 1q42.2–43 (PCAP), and 1p36 (CAPB) in families with hereditary prostate cancer. Am J Hum Genet 2000; 66:539–546.

37. Eeles RA, Durocher F, Edwards SM, et al. Linkage analysis of chromosome 1q markers in 136 Prostate cancer families. Am J Hum Genet 1998; 62:653–658.

38. McIndoe RA, Stanford JL, Gibbs M, et al. Linkage analysis of 49 high-risk families does not support a common familial prostate cancer-susceptibility gene at 1q24–25. Am J Hum Genet 1997; 61:347–353.

39. Goode EL, Stanford JL, Chakrabarti L, et al. Linkage analysis of 150 high-risk prostate cancer families at 1q24–25. Genet Epidemiol 2000; 18:251–275.

40. Bergthorsson JT, Johannesdottir G, Arason A, et al. Analysis of HPC1, HPCX, and PCAP in Icelandic hereditary prostate cancer. Hum Genet 2000; 107:372–375.

41. Grönberg H, Isaacs SD, Smith JR, et al. Characteristics of prostate cancer in families potentially linked to the hereditary Prostate cancer 1 (HPC1) locus. JAMA 1997; 278:1251–1255.

42. Xu J, International Consortium for Prostate Cancer Genetics. Combined analysis of hereditary prostate cancer linkage to 1q24–25: results from 772 hereditary prostate cancer families from the International Consortium for Prostate Cancer Genetics. Am J Hum Genet 2000; 66:945–957.

43. Goode EL, Stanford JL, Peters MA, et al. Clinical characteristics of prostate cancer in an analysis of linkage to four putative susceptibility loci. Clin Cancer Res 2001; 7:2739–2749.

44. Carpten J, Nupponen N, Isaacs S, et al. Germline mutations in the ribonuclease L gene in families showing linkage with HPC1. Nature Genet 2002; 30:181–184.

45. Dunsmuir WD, Edwards SM, Lakhani SR, et al. Allelic imbalance in familial and sporadic Prostate cancer at the putative human prostate cancer susceptibility locus, HPC1. CRC/BPG UK Familial Prostate Cancer Study Collaborators. Cancer Research Campaign/British Prostate Group. Br J Cancer 1998; 78:1430–1433.

46. Rokman A, Ikonen T, Seppala EH, et al. Germline alterations of the RNASEL gene, a candidate HPC1 gene at 1q25, in patients and families with prostate cancer. Am J Hum Genet 2002; 70:1299–1304.

47. Casey G, Neville PJ, Plummer SJ, et al. RNASEL Arg462Gln variant is implicated in up to 13 per cent of prostate cancer cases. Nature Genet 2002; 32:581–583.

48. Rennert H, Bercovich D, Hubert A, et al. A novel founder mutation in the RNASEL gene, 471delAAA is associated with prostate cancer risk in Ashkenazi Jews. Am J Hum Genet 2002; 71:981–984.

49. Kotar K, Hamel N, Thiffault I, Foulkes WD. The RNASEZ 471delAAAG allele and prostate cancer in Ashkenazi Jewish men. J Med Genet 2003; 40:e22.

50. Chen H, Griffin AR, Wu YQ, et al. RNASEZ mutations in hereditary prostate cancer. J Med Genet 2003; 40:e21

51. Neuhausen SL, Farnham JM, Kort E, et al. Prostate cancer susceptibility locus HPC1 in Utah high-risk pedigrees. Hum Mol Genet 1999; 8:2437–2442.

52. Berthon P, Valeri A, Cohen-Akenine A, et al. Predisposing gene for early-onset prostate cancer, localized on chromosome 1q42.2–43. Am J Hum Genet 1998; 62:1416–1424.

53. Gibbs M, Chakrabarti L, Stanford JL, et al. Analysis of chromosome 1q42.2–43 in 152 families with high risk of prostate cancer. Am J Hum Genet 1999; 64:1087–1095.

54. Whittemore AS, Lin IG, Oakley-Girvan I, et al. No evidence of linkage for chromosome 1q42.2–43 in prostate cancer. Am J Hum Genet 1999; 65:254–256.

55. Singh R, and the ACTANE Consortium. No evidence of linkage to chromosome 1q42.2–43 in 131 prostate cancer families from the ACTANE Consortium. Br J Cancer 2000; 83:1654–1658.

56. Cancel-Tassin G, Latil A, Valeri A, et al. PCAP is the major known prostate cancer predisposition locus in families from south and west Europe. Eur J Hum Genet 2001; 9:135–142.

57. Gibbs M, Stanford JL, McIndoe RA, et al. Evidence for a rare prostate cancer – susceptibility locus at chromosome 1p36. Am J Hum Genet 1999; 64:776–787.

58. Badzioch M, Eeles R, Leblanc G, et al. Suggestive evidence for a site specific prostate cancer gene on chromosome 1p36. J Med Gen 2000; 37:947–948.

59. Xu J, Zheng SL, Chang B, et al. Linkage of prostate cancer susceptibility loci to chromosome 1. Hum Genet 2001; 108:335–345.

60. Xu JF, Meyers D, Freije D, et al. Evidence for a prostate cancer susceptibility locus on the X chromosome. Nature Genet 1998; 20:175–179.

61. Lange E, Chen H, Brierley K. Linkage analysis of 153 Prostate cancer families over a 30-cM region containing the putative susceptibility locus HPCX. Clin Cancer Res 1999; 5:4013–4020.

62. Peters MA, Jarvik JP, Janer M, et al. Genetic linkage analysis of prostate cancer families to Xq27–28. Hum Hered 2001; 51:107–113.

63. Schleutker J, Matikainen M, Smith J, et al. A genetic epidemiological study of hereditary prostate cancer (HPC) in Finland: frequent HPCX linkage in families with late-onset disease. Clin Cancer Res 2000; 6:4810–4815.

64. Tatvigian SV, Simard J, Teng DHF, et al. A candidate prostate cancer susceptibility gene at chromosome 17p. Nature Genet 2001; 27:172–180.

65. Rebbeck TR, Walker AH, Zeigler-Johnson C, et al. Association of HPC2/ELAC genotypes and prostate cancer. Am J Hum Gen 2000; 67:1014–1019.

66. Suarez BK, Gerhard DS, Lin J, et al. Polymorphisms in the prostate cancer susceptibility gene HPC2/ELAC2 in multiplex families and healthy controls. Cancer Res 2001; 61:4982–4984.

67. Vesprini D, Nam RK, Trachtenberg J, et al. HPC2 variants and screen-detected prostate cancer. Am J Hum Genet 2001; 68:912–917.

68. Rökman A, Ikonene T, Mononen N, et al. ELAC/HPC2 involvement in hereditary and sporadic prostate cancer. Cancer Res 2001; 61:6038–6041.

69. Wang L, McDonnell SK, Elkins DA, et al. Role of HPC2/ELAC2 in hereditary prostate cancer. Cancer Res 2001; 61:6494–6499.

70. Xu J, Zheng SL, Carpten JD, et al. Evaluation of linkage and association of HPC2/ELAC2 in patients with familial or sporadic prostate cancer. Am J Hum Genet 2001; 68:901–911.

71. Meitz JC, Edwards SM, Easton DF, et al. HPC2/ELAC2 polymorphisms and prostate cancer risk: analysis by age of onset of disease. Br J Cancer 2002; 87(8):905–908.

72. Camp N, Tavtigian SV. Meta-analysis of associations of the Ser217Leu and Ala541Thr variants in ELAC (HPC2) and prostate cancer. Am J Hum Genet 2002; 71:1475–1478.

73. Suarez BK, Lin J, Burmester JK, et al. A genome screen of multiplex sibships with Prostate cancer. Am J Hum Genet 2000; 66:933–944.

74. Gibbs M, Stanford JL, Jarvik PG, et al. A genomic scan of prostate cancer families identifies multiple regions of interest. Am J Hum Genet 2000; 67:100–109.

75. Hsieh CL, Oakley-Girvan I, Balise RR, et al. A genome screen of families with multiple cases of prostate cancer: evidence of genetic heterogeneity. Am J Hum Genet 2001; 69:148–158.

76. Berry R, Schroeder JJ, French AJ. Evidence for a prostate cancer susceptibility locus on chromosome 20. Am J Hum Genet 2000; 67:82–91.

77. Bock CH, Cunningham JM, McDonnell SK, et al. Analysis of the prostate cancer susceptibility locus HPC20 in 172 families affected by prostate cancer. Am J Hum Genet 2001; 68:795–801.

78. Cancel-Tassin G, Latil A, Valeri A, et al. No evidence of linkage to HPC20 on chromosome 20q13 in hereditary prostate cancer. Int J Cancer 2001; 93:455–456.

79. Zheng SL, Xu J, Isaacs SD, et al. Evidence for a prostate cancer linkage to chromosome 20 in 159 hereditary prostate cancer families. Hum Genet 2001; 108:430–435.

80. Bergerheim USR, Kunimi K, Collins VP. Deletion mapping of chromosomes 8, 10 and 16 in human prostatic carcinoma. Genes Chromosomes Cancer 1991; 3:215–220.

81. Carter BS, Ewing CM, Ward WS. Allelic loss of chromosomes 16q and 10q in human Prostate cancer. Proc Natl Acad Sci USA 1990; 87:8751–8755.

82. Paris PL, Witte JS, Kupelian PA, et al. Identification and fine mapping of a region showing a high frequency of allelic imbalance on chromosome 16q23.2 that corresponds to a prostate cancer susceptibility locus. Cancer Res 2000; 60:3645–3649.

83. Xu J, Zheng SL, Hawkins GA, et al. Linkage and association studies of prostate cancer susceptibility: evidence for linkage at 8p22-23. Am J Hum Genet 2001; 69:341–350.

84. Xu J, Zheng SL, Komiya A, et al. Germline mutations and sequence variants of the macrophage scavenger receptor 1 gene are associated with prostate cancer risk. Nature Genet 2002; 32:321–325.

85. Seppala EH, Ikonen T, Autio V, et al. Germ-line alterations in MSR1 gene and prostate cancer risk. Clin Cancer Res 2003; 9:5252–5256.

86. Wang L, McDonnell SK, Cunningham JM, et al. No association of germline alteration of MSR1 with prostate cancer risk. Nat Genet 2003; 35:128–129.

87. Ostrander EA, Stanford JL. Genetics of prostate cancer: too many loci, too few genes. Am J Hum Genet 2000; 67:1367–1375.

88. The Prostate 57;2003.

89. Ingles SA, Ross RK, Yu MC, et al. Association of prostate cancer risk with genetic polymorphisms in vitamin D receptor and androgen receptor. J Natl Cancer Inst 1997; 89:166–170.

90. Irvine RA, Yu MC, Ross RK, Coetzee GA. The CAG and GGC microsatellites of the androgene receptor gene are in linkage disequilibrium in men with prostate cancer. Cancer Res 1995; 55:1937–1940.

91. Stanford JL, Just JJ, Gibbs M, et al. Polymorphic repeats in the androgen receptor gene: molecular markers of prostate cancer risk. Cancer Res 1997; 57:1194–1198.

92. Giovannucci E, Stempfer MJ, Krithivas K, et al. The CAG repeat within the androgen receptor gene and its relationship to prostate cancer. Proc Natl Acad Sci USA 1997; 94:3320–3323.

93. Bratt O, Borg A, Kristofersson U, et al. CAG repeat length in the androgen receptor gene is related to age at diagnosis of prostate cancer and response to endocrine therapy, but not to prostate cancer risk. Br J Cancer 1999; 81:672–676.

94. Correa-Cerro L, Wohr G, Haussler J, et al. G. (CAG)nCAA and GGN repeats in the human androgen receptor gene are not associated with prostate cancer in a French German population. Eur J Hum Genet 1999; 7:347–362.

95. Lange EM, Chen H, Brierley K, et al. The polymorphic exon 1 androgen receptor CAG, repeat in men with a potential inherited predisposition to prostate cancer. Cancer Epidemiol Biomarkers Prev 2000; 9:439–442.

96. Miller FA, Stanford JI, Hsu I, et al. Polymorphic repeats in the androgen receptor gene in high-risk sibships. Prostate 2001; 48:200–205.

97. Edwards SM, Badzioch MD, Minter R, et al. Androgen receptor polymorphisms: association with prostate cancer risk, relapse and overall survival. Int J Cancer 1999; 84:458–465.

98. Mononem N, Syrjäkoski K, Matikainen M, et al. Two per cent of Finnish prostate cancer patients have a germ-line mutation in the hormone-binding domain of the androgen receptor gene. Cancer Res 2000; 60:6479–6481.

99. Xue W, Irvine RA, Yu MC, et al. Susceptibility to prostate cancer: interaction between genotypes at the androgen receptor and prostate specific antigen loci. Cancer Res 2000; 60:839–841.

100. Labrie Y, Durocher F, Lachance Y, et al. The human type II 17β-hydroxysteroid dehydrogenase gene encodes two alternatively spliced mRNA species. DNA Cell Biol 1995; 14:849–861.

101. Durocher F, Morissette J, Labrie Y, et al. Mapping of the HSD17β2 gene encoding type II 17b-hydroxysteroid

dehydrogenase close to D16S422 on chromosome 16q24.1-q24.2. *Genomics* 1995; **25**:724–726.

102. Elo JP, Harknen P, Kyllonen AP, *et al.* Loss of heterozygosity at 16q24.1-q24.2 is significantly associated with metastatic and aggressive behaviour of prostate cancer. *Cancer Res* 1997; **57**:3356–3359.

103. Labrie F, Sugimoto Y, Luu-The V, *et al.* Structure of the human type II 5β-reductase gene. *Endocrinology* 1992; **131**:1571–1573.

104. Morissette J, Durocher F, Leblanc J-F, *et al.* Mapping of the steroid 5α-reductase type 2 (*SRD5A2*) gene close to *D2S352* on chromosome 2p22–23 region. *Cytogenet Cell Genet* 1996; **73**:304–307.

105. Ross RK, Bertein L, Lobo RA, *et al.* 5-α-reductase activity and risk of prostate cancer among Japanese and US white and black males. *Lancet* 1992; **339**:887–889.

106. Makridakis N, Ross RK, Pike MC, *et al.* A prevalent missense substitution that modulates activity of prostate steroid 5a-reductase. *Cancer Res* 1997; **57**:1020–1022.

107. Margiotti K, Sangiuolo F, De Luca A, *et al.* Evidence for an association between the *SRD5A* (type II steroid alpha-reductase) locus and prostate cancer in Italian patients. *Dis Markers* 2000; **16**:147–150.

108. Reichardt J, Makridakis N, Pike MC, *et al.* The A49T mutation in the *SRD5A2* gene increases risk for aggressive prostate cancer and prostatic steroid 5-α reductase activity. *Am J Hum Genet* 1997; **61**:A209.

109. Makridakis NM, Ross RK, Pike MC, *et al.* Association of missense substitution in *SRD5A2* gene with prostate cancer in African-American and Hispanic men in Los Angeles, USA. *Lancet* 1999; **354**:975–978.

110. Jaffe JM, Malkowicz B, Walker AH, *et al.* Association of *SRD5A2* genotype and pathological characteristics of prostate tumors. *Cancer Res* 2000; **60**:1626–1630.

111. Feigelson HS, Shames LS, Pike MC, *et al.* Cytochrome *P450c17α* gene (*CYP17*) polymorphism is associated with serum estrogen and progesterone concentrations. *Cancer Res* 1998; **58**:585–587.

112. Lunn RM, Bell DA, Mohler JL, Taylor JA. Prostate cancer risk and polymorphism in 17 hydroxylase (*CYP17*) and steroid reductase (*SRD5A2*). *Carcinogenesis* 1999; **20**:1727–1731.

113. Gsur A, Bernhofer G, Hinteregger S, *et al.* A polymorphism in the *CYP17* gene is associated with prostate cancer risk. *Int J Cancer* 2000; **87**:434–437.

114. Yamada Y, Watanabe M, Murata M, *et al.* Impact of genetic polymorphisms of 17-hydroxylase cytochrome P450 (*CYP17*) and steroid 5alpha-reductase type II (*SRD5A2*) genes on prostate-cancer risk among the Japanese population. *Int J Cancer* 2001; **92**:683–686.

115. Haiman CA, Stampfer MJ, Giovannucci E, *et al.* The relationship between a polymorphism in *CYP17* with plasma hormone levels and prostate cancer. *Cancer Epidemiol Biomarkers Prev* 2001; **10**:743.

116. Wadelius M, Anderson AO, Johanson JE, *et al.* Prostate cancer associated with *CYP17* genotype. *Pharmacogenetics* 1999; **9**:635–639.

117. Habuchi T, Liqing Z, Suzuki T, *et al.* Increased risk of prostate cancer and benign prostatic hyperplasia associated with a *CYP17* gene polymorphism with a gene dosage effect. *Cancer Res* 2000; **60**:5710–5713.

118. Chang B, Zheng SL, Isaacs SD, *et al.* Linkage and association of *CYP17* gene in hereditary and sporadic prostate cancer. *Int J Cancer* 2001; **95**:354–359.

119. Paris PL, Kupelian PA, Hall JM, *et al.* Association between a *CYP34A4* genetic variant and clinical presentation in African American prostate cancer patients. *Cancer Epidemiol Biomarkers Prev* 1999; **8**:901–905.

120. Rebbeck TR, Jaffe JM, Walker AH, *et al.* Modification of clinical presentation of prostate tumors by a novel genetic variant in *CYP3A4*. *J Natl Cancer Inst* 1998; **90**:1225–1229.

121. Murata M, Watanabe M, Yamanata M, *et al.* Genetic polymorphisms in cytochrome *P450* (*CYP*) *1A1*, *CYP1A2*, *CYP2E1*, glutathione S-transferase (*GST*) *M1* and *GSTT1* and susceptibility to prostate cancer in the Japanese population. *Cancer Lett* 2001; **165**:171–177.

122. Thiessen E. Concerning a familial association between breast cancer and both prostatic and uterine malignancies. *Cancer* 1974; **34**:1102–1107.

123. Anderson DE, Badzioch MD. Breast cancer risks in relatives of male breast cancer patients. *J Natl Cancer Inst* 1992; **84**:1114–1117.

124. Tulinius H, Egilsson V, Olafsdottir GH, Sigvaldason H. Risk of prostate, ovarian, and endometrial cancer among relatives of women with breast cancer. *Br Med J* 1992; **305**:855–857.

125. Sellers TA, Potter JD, Rich SS, *et al.* Familial clustering of breast and prostate cancers and risk of postmenopausal breast cancer. *J Natl Cancer Inst* 1994; **86**:1860–1865.

126. Ford D, Easton DF, Bishop DT, *et al.* Risks of cancer in *BRCA1*-mutation carriers. Breast Cancer Linkage Consortium. *Lancet* 1994; **343**:692–695.

127. Breast Cancer Linkage Consortium. Carrier risks in *BRCA2* mutation carriers. *J Natl Cancer Inst* 1999; **91**:1310–1316.

128. Struewing JP, Hartge P, Wacholder S, *et al.* The risk of cancer associated with specific mutations of *BRCA1* and *BRCA2* among Ashkenazi Jews. *N Engl J Med* 1997; **336**:1401–1408.

129. Langston AA, Stanford JL, Wicklund KG, *et al.* Germ-line *BRCA1* mutations in selected men with prostate cancer. *Am J Hum Genet* 1996; **58**:881–884.

130. Lehrer S, Fodor F, Stock R, *et al.* Absence of 185delAG mutation of the *BRCA1* gene and 6174delT mutation of the *BRCA2* gene in Ashkenazi Jewish men with prostate cancer. *Br J Cancer* 1998; **78**:771–773.

131. Wilkens EP, Freje D, Xu J, *et al.* No evidence for a role of *BRCA1* and *BRCA2* mutations in Ashkenazi Jewish families with hereditary prostate cancer. *Prostate* 1999; **39**:280–284.

132. Nastiuk KL, Mansukhani M, Terry MB, *et al.* Common mutations in *BRCA1* and *BRCA2* do not contribute to early-onset prostate cancer in Jewish men. *Prostate* 1999; **40**:172–178.

133. Grönberg H, Åhman A, Emanuelsson M, *et al.* BRCA2 mutation in a family with hereditary prostate cancer. *Genes Chrom Cancer* 2001; **30**:299–301.

134. Sigurdsson S, Thorlacius S, Tomasson J, *et al.* BRCA2 mutation in Icelandic prostate cancer patients. *J Mol Med* 1997; **75**:758–761.

135. Singh R, Eeles RA, Durocher F, *et al.* High risk genes predisposing to prostate cancer development – do they exist? *Prostate Cancer Prostatic Dis* 2000; **3**:241–247.

136. Gayther SA, de Foy KA, Harrington P, *et al*. The frequency of germ-line mutations in the breast cancer predisposition genes *BRCA1* and *BRCA2* in familial Prostate cancer. The Cancer Research Campaign/British Prostate Group United Kingdom Familial Prostate cancer Study Collaborators. *Cancer Res*. 2000; **60**:4513–4518.

137. Edwards SM, Kote-Jarai Z, Meitz J, *et al*. Two per cent of men with early onset prostate cancer harbour germline mutations in the *BRCA2* gene. *Am J Hum Genet* 2003; **72**:1–12.

138. Sinclair CS, Berry R, Schaid D, *et al*. BRCA1 and BRCA2 have a limited role in familial prostate cancer. *Cancer Res* 2000; **60**:1371–1375.

139. Parkin DM, Muir CS, Whelan SL. *Cancer incidence in five continents*, Vol. 6. IARC Press, 1993:971.

140. Hanks GE, Diamond JJ, Krall JM, *et al*. A ten year follow up of 682 patients treated for prostate cancer with radiation therapy in the United States. *Int J Radiat Oncol Biol Phys* 1987; **13**:449–505.

141. Albertson PC. Prostate cancer mortality after introduction of prostate-specific antigen mass screening in the Federal State of Tyrol, Austria. *J Urol* 2002; **168**:880–881.

142. Lalbrie F, Candas B, Cusan L, *et al*. Screening decreases prostate cancer mortality: 1-year follow-up of the 1988 Quebec prospective randomized controlled trial. *Prostate* 2004; **59**:311–318.

143. Roobol MJ, Schroder FH. European Randomized Study of Screening for Prostate Cancer: achievements and presentation. *B J U Int* 2003; **92**(Supp 2):117–122.

144. McWhorter WP, Hernandez AD, Meikle AW, *et al*. A screening study of prostate cancer in high risk families. *J Urol* 1992; **148**:826–828.

145. Catalona WJ, Smith DS, Ratcliff TL, *et al*. Measurement of prostate-specific antigen in serum as a screening test for prostate cancer. *N Engl J Med* 1991; **324**:1156–1161.

146. Catalona WJ, Antenor JA, Roehl KA, Moul JW. Screening for prostate cancer in high risk populations. *J Urol* 2002; **168**:1980–1983.

147. Neuhausen SL, Skolnick MH, Cannon-albright L. Familial prostate cancer studies in Utah. *Br J Urol* 1997; **79**(Supp 1):15–20.

148. Cybulski C, Gorski B, Debniak T, *et al*. NBS1 is a prostate cancer susceptibility gene. *Cancer Res* 2004; **64**:1215–1219.

27

Familial melanoma and its management

ALISA M. GOLDSTEIN AND MARGARET A. TUCKER

INTRODUCTION

Cutaneous malignant melanoma (CMM) is a potentially fatal form of skin cancer whose aetiology is heterogeneous and complex. The incidence of cutaneous malignant melanoma has continued to rise over the past two decades in many regions of the world.[1,2] Data from the Scottish Melanoma Group showed that from 1979 to 1994 the annual age standardized incidence of CMM in Scotland increased significantly from 3.5 to 7.8 per 100 000 per year in men and from 6.8 to 12.3 per 100 000 per year in women. The incidence of melanoma continued to increase significantly in men of all ages during the study but the rate stabilized in women after 1986.[1] In the USA, over the period 1973–1997, the incidence of malignant melanoma among whites increased more than 150 per cent from 6.3 per 100 000 to 16.2 per 100 000, more than that of any other cancer. The overall age-adjusted incidence rate of invasive melanoma for 1990–1997 was 12.4 per 100 000, 14.2 per 100 000 in Whites and 0.8 per 100 000 in blacks. For White men, the overall age-adjusted incidence was 17.4 per 100 000 and for White women 11.9 per 100 000.[2] In Australia, which has the highest incidence of cutaneous melanoma in both men and women, the age-standardized melanoma incidence in 1992–1996 varied with latitude from 33 per 100 000 males and 28 per 100 000 females in Victoria to 63 per 100 000 males and 46 per 100 000 females in Queensland.[3]

Epidemiologic studies of melanoma suggest that exposure to sunlight is the major environmental risk factor, although the exposure–response relationship appears complex with intermittent sun exposure likely to be more important for risk than total lifetime exposure (for a review, see Armstrong and English[4]). The major host factors associated with melanoma are increased numbers of melanocytic naevi, both clinically banal and atypical (dysplastic).[4,5] Clinically dysplastic naevi have been shown to be an independent predictor of melanoma risk in both non-familial and familial melanoma.[5–8] Other host factors implicated in both familial and non-familial melanoma include hair colour, eye colour, extent of freckling and skin type.[9,10] Individuals with blond/fair hair, light eyes, many freckles and an inability to tan are at increased risk of melanoma.

In general, familial melanoma is clinically and histologically indistinguishable from non-familial melanoma. However, differences in age at diagnosis, lesion thickness, and frequency of multiple lesions are generally observed.[11,12] Familial melanoma cases have an earlier age at diagnosis, thinner CMM tumors and a higher frequency of multiple lesions compared to non-familial melanoma patients.

Approximately 5–12 per cent of malignant melanomas develop in individuals with a family history, that is, at least one first-degree relative with CMM,[13–16] often in association with clinically dysplastic or atypical naevi.[17] Some of the familial clusters occur by chance. Others may occur because family members share the same risk factors, such as hair colour, eye colour, freckling and skin type. Familial clustering is greatest in heavily insolated areas, such as Australia, suggesting that clustering may result from both genetic and shared non-genetic factors.[18] Only a subset of familial melanoma patients is likely to have an inherited mutation in a high-risk melanoma susceptibility gene. Although the proportion of such cases is unknown, it is believed to be at least a few per cent.

GENETICS OF MELANOMA

To date, two genes have been strongly implicated in melanoma pathogenesis. The first, *CDKN2A*, encodes two distinct proteins translated, in alternate reading frames (ARFs), from alternatively spliced transcripts. The alpha transcript, comprising exons 1α, 2 and 3, encodes a low-molecular-weight protein, p16, that inhibits the activity of the cyclin D1-cyclin-dependent kinase 4 (CDK4) or 6 (CDK6) complex.[19] These complexes phosphorylate the retinoblastoma protein, allowing the cell to progress through the G1 cell-cycle checkpoint.[19,20] Thus, p16 acts as a tumour suppressor and negatively regulates cell growth by arresting cells at G1. The smaller beta transcript, comprising exons 1β, 2 and 3, specifies the alternative product p14ARF. p14ARF acts via the p53 pathway to induce cell-cycle arrest or apoptosis.[21,22] In contrast, the second identified melanoma susceptibility gene CDK4 acts as an oncogene.[23] Other genetic factors remain to be identified.

CDKN2A

The *CDKN2A* gene is located on chromosome 9p21,[24,25] a region implicated in melanoma from linkage, cytogenetic and loss of heterozygosity studies.[26–32] Germline mutations in *CDKN2A* have been observed in melanoma-prone families from North America, Europe and Australasia. Overall, *CDKN2A* mutations have been observed in approximately 20 per cent (119 out of 579, range <5 per cent to >50 per cent; Table 27.1) of melanoma-prone families from around the world.[33–50] There are few data on the population frequency of *CDKN2A* mutations. In the largest population-based study conducted to date of 482 families in Queensland, Australia, the prevalence of *CDKN2A* mutations was 9 out of 87 (10.3 per cent) in the subgroup of families exhibiting the strongest familial clustering and the overall prevalence in the population was estimated to be 0.2 per cent.[51]

The frequency of *CDKN2A* mutations varies considerably across different geographic areas.[33–51] There are several possible explanations for the divergent frequencies. First, some of the difference may be a chance finding, based on the small numbers of families examined in some studies. Second, the families studied may represent a heterogeneous mix of hereditary and non-hereditary melanoma-prone kindreds. Estimations of frequencies of *CDKN2A* mutations do not always use the same definition of familial melanoma. That is, certain investigations required three or more first-degree relatives with melanoma, others required only two such relatives and still others required only two relatives with CMM not restricted to first-degree. Further, some studies restricted the age at diagnosis in at least one affected family member,

Table 27.1 *Frequency of detected* CDKN2A *mutations*

Characteristic	% of mutations[a]	References
Number of affected first-degree relatives		33–50
2	<5	
≥3	20–40	
>6	>50	
Multiple primary melanoma (MPM)		
No family history	10	43, 58, 57
≥3 affected relatives with MPM in at least one affected	≥32	42, 43, 47
Pancreatic cancer	?	49, 61–64

[a] Confidence intervals for all characteristics are wide and, therefore, estimates are imprecise.

or required an additional neoplastic event, usually either multiple primary melanoma tumours in one or more CMM patients or the occurrence of pancreatic cancer in the family. Third, for some studies, only one melanoma patient per family was examined for a germline *CDKN2A* mutation. Some of the families without mutations may actually have mutations that were not detected because only one patient per family was screened or because the mutation was not revealed by direct sequencing or single-strand conformation polymorphism (SSCP) analysis. Mutations outside the *CDKN2A* coding region that interfere with RNA splicing or expression would not have been detected. In addition, alternative processes linked to transcriptional and/or translational regulation, including methylation, might also inactivate p16.[52] The frequency of such undetected mutations having alternative mechanisms of inactivation is difficult to estimate. Fourth, for many of the studies, the ascertainment event was not well characterized and the families studied are not representative of the underlying population. Finally, the complexity and heterogeneity of CMM, including the identification of founder mutations in different populations and the as yet not identified melanoma susceptibility genes, likely contributed to the divergent frequencies. All of these factors make it difficult to determine the proportion of hereditary melanoma associated with *CDKN2A* mutations.

Most mutations described to date are missense mutations scattered throughout the *CDKN2A* coding region (i.e. exons 1α and 2). A mutation in the 5'-untranslated region (g-34t) and a deep intronic mutation (IVS2-105) have also been described.[53,54] Some mutations have been observed only once (e.g. L62P, L97R), while others have repeatedly been found in different families (e.g. G-34T, M53I, G101W, 113insArg, 225del19). Haplotype analyses of recurrent mutations (113insArg, 225del19, G-34T) in families from the same geographic areas (Sweden, The Netherlands, Canada, respectively) have shown evidence for single genetic origins (i.e. common founders or ancestors[36,38,40,53,55]), rather than mutation hot spots in the *CDKN2A* gene. In addition, haplotype analyses of recurrent mutations from geographically diverse populations have also revealed evidence for common founders for the missense mutations examined (e.g. M53I, G101W, V126D).[50,53,56] To date, only one recurrent mutation has been shown to have multiple origins (23ins24).[56] The 23ins24 mutation, a 24-bp duplication, was hypothesized to have arisen as a result of unequal crossing over between the two 24-bp repeats that occur naturally in the wild-type sequence. This mutation would be more likely to recur because of the inherent instability of the tandem repeat region that produced the 24-bp insertion.[56]

The frequency of detected *CDKN2A* mutations is directly related to the numbers of melanoma patients per family (Table 27.1). The frequency of mutations increases as the number of melanoma cases in the family increases. The frequency of detectable mutations is <5 per cent for families with only two melanoma patients. Mutations have been found in 20–40 per cent of families with three or more affected members. The frequency increases to >50 per cent for families with more than six melanoma cases.[33–50] Two other features increase the chances for detecting mutations: the occurrence of multiple CMM lesions and the presence of pancreatic cancer in a family (Table 27.1). Canadian and American melanoma patients with multiple primary melanoma tumours but without family histories of melanoma were examined to determine whether they had germline mutations in the *CDKN2A* gene. Of 33 unrelated patients with multiple primary melanomas, five (15 per cent, 95 per cent confidence interval 4–27) had disease-related germline *CDKN2A* mutations. In two of these families with mutations, a previously unknown evidence of family history of melanoma was uncovered.[57] Studies from France and Scotland[43,58] have observed similar findings, suggesting that approximately 10 per cent of patients with multiple primary melanoma tumours but without a family history may have germline mutations in the *CDKN2A* gene. In addition, the occurrence of multiple primary melanoma tumours in a patient with a family history of CMM increases the frequency of detecting a CDKN2A mutation.[42,43,47]

Several researchers have investigated whether a familial susceptibility to melanoma also predisposes individuals to an increased risk of other cancers independent of other known family cancer syndromes (e.g. Li–Fraumeni syndrome[59]). Prior to the discovery of *CDKN2A*, these investigations showed inconsistent results. Lynch *et al.* and Bergman *et al.* reported increased risks of gastrointestinal cancers, particularly pancreatic cancer in melanoma-prone families.[60,61] In contrast, Tucker *et al.* and Kopf *et al.* observed no such increased risk.[6,12] The identification of the *CDKN2A* gene may help explain these discrepancies. A follow-up to the Tucker *et al.* study of American melanoma-prone families revealed that the ten families with *CDKN2A* mutations had a significantly increased risk of pancreatic cancer. The risk was increased by a factor of 13 in the prospective period and by a factor of 22 in the entire time interval (i.e. before and after ascertainment of the families). In contrast, the nine families without disease specific *CDKN2A* mutations had no cases of pancreatic cancer.[62] In addition, in the Dutch families,[61] all families with pancreatic cancer had a 19-bp deletion removing nucleotides 225–243 in exon 2 (225del19), named the 'p16-Leiden' mutation.[63] This mutation has been shown to be a Dutch *CDKN2A* founder mutation.[36,55]

Several studies[49,61–64] have now demonstrated an increased risk of pancreatic cancer among *CDKN2A* melanoma-prone families, although the precise risks of pancreatic cancer in *CDKN2A* mutation carriers are unclear. Pancreatic cancer has been observed in *CDKN2A* families with insertions, deletions, missense mutations, splice site alterations, and 5'-untranslated region mutations.[36,38,42,49,50,53] There is little evidence for a direct genotype–phenotype association between pancreatic cancer and specific *CDKN2A* mutations. At present, it is not possible to predict what genotype or phenotype predisposes an individual to pancreatic cancer in *CDKN2A* families. Also, although pancreatic cancer has been observed in the Dutch families with a *CDKN2A* mutation, other large Dutch melanoma-prone families with the p16-Leiden mutation do not have any excess of pancreatic or other cancers.[63] Similar results have been observed in American melanoma-prone families.[50] These results suggest that the inconsistent occurrence of other cancers cannot be explained by the *CDKN2A* mutation itself, but are likely due to the influence of other factors, genetic and/or environmental.[50,58,63]

Breast cancer has been reported to be significantly increased in melanoma-prone families from Sweden with a founder mutation (113insArg).[64] Among families with mutations that affect *p14ARF* and not p16, there may be a different spectrum of tumours, including neural and breast tumours.[65–67] Future studies are needed for these associations to be better understood.

FUTURE STUDIES OF *CDKN2A*

The majority of melanoma-prone families that show strong evidence of linkage to chromosome 9p have *CDKN2A* mutations. However, a subset of these families does not have detectable mutations. Whether these families have non-coding region mutations or alternative mechanisms of inactivation (e.g. methylation) or whether another 9p21 melanoma susceptibility gene(s) located near *CDKN2A* exists will be determined through future studies. Also, the precise relationship between p16 and *p14ARF* has yet to be determined. Studies to evaluate whether mutations that alter both proteins differ from mutations that alter only p16 should help resolve this issue.

CDKN2A mutations confer substantial risk for melanoma.[62] Many mutation carriers, however, do not develop melanoma.[33–50] In addition, unaffected individuals homozygous for a *CDKN2A* mutation have been identified.[36] These studies suggest that other gene(s) and/or environmental factors are involved in the pathogenesis of melanoma and in determining penetrance. In addition, although *CDKN2A* mutations confer increased risk for melanoma, clinicoepidemiologic variables, such as dysplastic or atypical naevi, total numbers of naevi, and solar injury have been shown to further enhance the disease risk among mutation carriers.[68] Future studies should estimate penetrance for melanoma and possibly other tumours, and assess the relationship between *CDKN2A* and modifying genetic and/or environmental factors that may influence disease expression. Finally, population-based studies are needed to determine the frequency of *CDKN2A* mutations around the world.

CDK4

CDK4, a dominant oncogene, is located at chromosome 12q13.[23,69] It consists of eight exons within a 5-kb segment. There is a single 5′-untranslated exon. The initiation codon is located in exon 2, and the stop codon and 3′-untranslated region are contained in exon 8.[70]

To date, co-segregating germline mutations have been detected in only three melanoma-prone families worldwide.[42,70] The Arg24Cys germline mutation was originally identified as a tumour-specific antigen in a human melanoma; the alteration produced a mutated protein that prevented binding of the CDK4 protein to p16.[23] This mutation has been detected in two American melanoma-prone families.[70] Overall, all 12 invasive melanoma patients, 0 of 1 melanoma *in situ* patients, 5 of 13 patients with dysplastic naevi, 2 of 15 unaffected family members and 0 of 10 spouses carried this mutation. In addition, haplotype analysis revealed that these two apparently unrelated families shared the same disease-specific haplotype covering approximately a 5-cM region.[50] The second germline mutation, Arg24His, which occurred in the same codon as the first alteration, has been observed in a single French family.[42] All three melanoma patients in this family carried the mutation or were obligate carriers of the mutation. In addition, five out of seven tested unaffected family members also carried the mutation. The median age of the non penetrant gene carriers is similar to the median age at melanoma diagnosis in this family and, therefore, some of the non-penetrant gene carriers may develop melanoma later in life.

Given the different mechanisms of action of the tumour suppressor *CDKN2A* and the dominant oncogene, *CDK4*, it was hypothesized that clinical characteristics in melanoma patients might differ in these two groups of families. However, comparison of 104 CMM patients from 17 American *CDKN2A* families and the 12 CMM patients from the two American *CDK4* families showed no significant differences in median age at first melanoma diagnosis, number of melanoma tumours or numbers of naevi.[50] This comparison had limited power because of the small numbers of melanoma patients from the *CDK4* families. Direct assessment of *CDK4* families will remain limited because of their rarity.

The original report of a germline *CDK4* mutation evaluated melanoma patients from 10 American and 21 Australian melanoma-prone families, and found only one mutation, Arg24Cys, in two of the American kindreds.[70] Most subsequent studies of *CDK4* have, therefore, either exclusively tested for this alteration[39,41] or limited the evaluation to exon 2 of the *CDK4* gene.[42,46–48,71] Examination of exon 2 led to the identification of the Arg24His germline mutation in the French family.[42] No additional germline mutations have been reported. Given the cumulative evidence, it seems very likely that, although *CDK4* is a melanoma susceptibility gene, it plays an extremely minor role in hereditary melanoma.

Future research

Recently a gene mapping study of 82 predominantly Australian families showed significant evidence for a novel CMM susceptibility locus at chromosome 1p22[72] in a subset of the families; no gene has yet been found.

The search for additional melanoma susceptibility genes will be strongly influenced by the overall frequency of mutations in these genes. For example, if other melanoma susceptibility genes are comparable to the *CDK4* gene in terms of their frequency, they will be extremely difficult to identify. Alternatively, if one or more susceptibility genes have mutations with frequencies similar to what has been observed in *CDKN2A*, identification of these melanoma susceptibility genes will be more likely.

Several candidate genes have been examined for germline mutations. No mutations have been observed in *CDKN2B* (the gene that encodes the p15INK4B proteins and is physically located adjacent to *CDKN2A*);[40,41,73] *CDKN2C* (the gene that encodes the cyclin-dependent kinase inhibitor p18 located on chromosome 1p32);[74] *p19INK4D* (a member of the same INK4 family as p15 and p16);[46] CDK6 (a cyclin-dependent kinase that complexes with cyclin D1 and is inhibited by p16);[75] and *TP53* (a tumour suppressor gene involved in cell-cycle regulation).[74]

Recent studies have indicated that certain variants in the MC1R gene, which recodes the receptor for melanocyte-stimulating hormone (MSN), are associated with an increased risk of melanoma. These variants are also linked to red hair, pale skin and poor tanning response. This is the first low penetrance melanoma susceptibility gene to be identified.

MANAGEMENT OF FAMILIAL MELANOMA

Survival

Survival after early melanoma is very high. Patients diagnosed with melanoma *in situ* have a greater than 99 per cent long-term, disease-free survival. Patients with thin melanoma, defined as lesions <1.5 mm in depth, have a greater than 90 per cent long-term overall survival. In contrast, the 5-year survival rate for thick tumours (>3.5 mm) is only 54 per cent in women and 42 per cent in men.[1,77] In fact, the single most predictive factor for recurrence and long-term prognosis of melanoma is the tumour thickness at the time of diagnosis. Other prognostic factors include regression, level of invasion (Clark), ulceration, anatomic location, radial versus vertical growth phase and sex of the patient.[77]

Aims of management

Early diagnosis of thin lesions is essential to survival following melanoma. It is, therefore, critical to identify individuals at increased risk for melanoma and appropriately screen and manage this high-risk population. There should be two aims in the management of individuals at high risk for melanoma and individuals in melanoma-prone families: (1) prevention of melanoma by reducing risk factors that promote tumorigenesis; and (2) early detection of melanoma by recognizing and biopsying naevi suspicious for melanoma.[78] Clinical follow-up of high-risk patients can lead to the detection of early thin melanomas[6,79,80] and ultimately increased survival.

Who should be screened?

Since familial melanoma is clinically indistinguishable from non-familial melanoma, it is essential for the clinician to obtain a detailed family history from all individuals with melanoma. All first-degree relatives (parents, siblings and children) of individuals with invasive melanoma (or clinically atypical naevi) should be screened. In addition, since individuals with familial melanoma tend to develop multiple primary lesions, they should be followed closely.

Management of high-risk patients

A skilled physician or nurse should examine individuals with melanoma or clinically dysplastic naevi from melanoma-prone families every 3–6 months. The examination should be conducted in a brightly lit room with adequate accessory lighting to allow bright-field illumination of the area being examined. A halogen light source is very effective, because it emits a continuous-spectrum white light. Fluorescent light should be avoided because its discontinuous emission spectrum turns the pink hues of clinically dysplastic naevi to a dull grey.[81] The entire skin surface should be examined, including the scalp, breasts, buttocks, genital area and soles of the feet. Baseline colour photographs, including body overviews, segmental overviews and one-to-one close-ups (with a ruler next to the naevi) of the most atypical naevi should be taken. Close-up photography of selected naevi is an important tool in following such lesions over time.

The indication for surgical removal of a pigmented lesion is the same as in the general population (i.e. suspicion of malignant change).[58] Lesions suspicious for melanoma should be removed by excisional biopsy.[82] In addition, changing naevi that are becoming more abnormal should also be biopsied. Routine or 'prophylactic' removal of non-changing naevi is not recommended. The chances of any one naevus becoming melanoma are slight; biopsying only changing naevi minimizes the amount of surgery. Furthermore, melanomas may occur on previously entirely normal skin.[83]

Management of children

Parents should be taught about the need to protect young children in these families. Complete avoidance of sunburn from the time of birth, and use of sunscreens and protective clothing are strongly recommended. It should be assumed that everyone is at risk and should be protected from the sun. Children should have their first skin examination by age 10 but should be seen by a skilled clinician earlier if they have suspicious lesions.

Education

Family members need to be taught self-examination of the skin, including the scalp, so that they (or a parent, partner, or family member) can examine their naevi monthly. Individuals should look for changes in the signs, shape, colour, elevation, consistency (softening or hardening), and sensation of the naevus itself and the skin surrounding the naevus.[83] The use of clinical photographs greatly aids this task. Patients can observe changes in individual naevi relative to the clinical close-up, as well as identify variation in their naevi from comparison with segmental overviews. Patients should be taught melanoma warning signs and recognition of clinically atypical naevi and melanoma[84] (Table 27.2).

Education of all family members about the need for sun protection is critical. Family members should be taught to avoid peak sun exposure times (e.g. between 10 am and 3 pm), to wear protective clothing, including hats and

Table 27.2 *Warning signs for melanoma: changes in naevi/moles that may signal melanoma*

Large size: usually >5 mm
Shape: irregular border, asymmetric
Surface: scaly, flaky, oozing, bleeding, ulceration, non-healing sore
Colour: multiple colours including tan, brown, white, pink and black; rapid darkening, especially of new areas of black or dark brown, loss of pigmentation (become white or grey), or bleeding of pigment from mole into surrounding skin
Elevation: development of raised areas on a previously flat lesion
Consistency: softening or hardening
Sensation in naevus: unusual sensation in naevus including itchy, painful and tenderness
Sensation in surrounding skin: redness, inflammation

sunglasses, long-sleeved shirts and long trousers, and to use broad-spectrum ultraviolet A and B protective sunscreens. Family members should also be taught to avoid overexposure to the sun, to never sunburn again, and to avoid sunbathing, sun lamps and tanning parlours. Patients should be taught that, during puberty or pregnancy, moles may change and that these changes should be carefully watched.[84]

These guidelines may undergo modification as more data are gathered and more information is learned about the aetiology of melanoma.

MUTATION TESTING

Given that current gaps in the knowledge about the expression of melanoma susceptibility genes in high-risk families and in the general population exist, DNA testing should not be used as a guide to the clinical practice of prevention and surveillance. All individuals considered to be at high risk of melanoma because of the well-established melanoma risk factors should be managed using the same approach.[58,85]

The American Society for Clinical Oncology's statements on genetic testing for cancer susceptibility recommends that this testing be performed only when 'the tests can be adequately interpreted; and the results will influence the medical management of the patient or family member'.[86] The Melanoma Genetics Consortium, comprised familial melanoma research groups from the USA, Europe and Australia, reviewed current information about genetic testing, and concluded that neither of these criteria is currently met for the testing of known melanoma susceptibility genes (i.e. *CDKN2A* and *CDK4*).[58] The consortium, therefore, concluded that it is premature to offer DNA testing outside of defined research protocols, except in rare circumstances and only after careful genetic counselling that adequately addresses the low likelihood of finding mutations, current uncertainties about the penetrance of mutations, the lack of proved efficacy of prevention and surveillance strategies, even for mutation carriers, and the potential benefits and risks of positive and negative results of genetic testing. The consortium will review this advice regularly, in keeping with developments in the field, to maintain a current consensus opinion.[58,85]

KEY POINTS

- Five to twelve per cent of melanomas occur in individuals with a familial predisposition.
- To date, two genes are implicated: *CDKN2A* (tumour suppressor gene; 9p21) and *CDK4* (oncogene; 12q13; rarer and only described in a few families worldwide).
- There is an increased risk of pancreatic cancer in a subset of families with mutations in *CDKN2A*.
- The chance of observing a mutation in *CDKN2A* increases as the number of affecteds in a cluster increases (>50 per cent if >6 cases; <5 per cent if 2 cases), or in multiple melanoma cases (10 per cent without a family history if the case has multiple melanoma).

REFERENCES

1. MacKie RM, Hole D, Hunter JAA, *et al.* Cutaneous malignant melanoma in Scotland: incidence, survival, and mortality, 1979–94. *Br Med J* 1997; **315**:1117–1121.
2. Ries LAG, Eisner MP, Kosary CL, *et al.* (eds) *SEER cancer statistics review, 1973–1997.* Bethesda, MD: National Cancer Institute, 2000.
3. Australian Institute of Health and Welfare (AIHW) and Australasian Association of Cancer Registries (AACR). *Cancer in Australia 1996: incidence and mortality data for 1996 and selected data for 1997 and 1998.* Canberra: AIHW (Cancer Series), 1999.
4. Armstrong BK, English DR. Cutaneous malignant melanoma. In: Schottenfeld D, Fraumeni JF Jr (eds) *Cancer epidemiology and prevention.* New York: Oxford University Press, 1996:1282–1312.
5. Tucker MA, Halpern A, Holly EA, *et al.* Clinically recognized dysplastic nevi: a central risk factor for cutaneous melanoma. *JAMA* 1997; **277**:1439–1444.
6. Tucker MA, Fraser MC, Goldstein AM, *et al.* The risk of melanoma and other cancers in melanoma-prone families. *J Invest Dermatol* 1993; **100**:S350–S355.
7. Halpern AC, Guerry D IV, Elder DE, *et al.* Dysplastic nevi as risk markers of sporadic (nonfamilial) melanoma. *Arch Dermatol* 1991; **127**:995–999.
8. Rousch GC, Norlund JJ, Forget B, *et al.* Independence of dysplastic nevi from total nevi in determining risk for nonfamilial melanoma. *Prev Med* 1988; **17**:273–279.
9. Elwood JM, Whitehead SM, Davidson J, *et al.* Malignant melanoma in England: risks associated with naevi, freckles, social class, hair colour, and sunburn. *Int J Epidemiol* 1990; **19**:801–810.
10. Osterlind A, Tucker MA, Hou-Jensen K, *et al.* The Danish case-control study of cutaneous melanoma. I. Importance of host factors. *Int J Cancer* 1988; **42**:200–206.

11. Barnhill RL, Rousch GC, Titus-Ernstoff L. Comparison of nonfamilial and familial melanoma. *Dermatology* 1992; **184:**2–7.

12. Kopf AW, Hellman LJ, Rogers GS, *et al.* Familial malignant melanoma. *JAMA* 1986; **256:**1951–1959.

13. Greene MH, Fraumeni JF Jr. *The hereditary variant of malignant melanoma.* New York: Grune and Stratton, 1979.

14. Newton JA, Bataille V, Griffiths K, *et al.* How common is the atypical mole syndrome phenotype in apparently sporadic melanoma? *J Am Acad Dermatol* 1993; **29:**989–996.

15. Cutler C, Foulkes W, Brunet J-S, *et al.* Cutaneous malignant melanoma in women is uncommonly associated with a family history of melanoma in first-degree relatives: a case control study. *Melanoma Res* 1996; **6:**435–440.

16. Aitken JF, Youl P, Green A, *et al.* Accuracy of case-reported family history of melanoma in Queensland, Australia. *Melanoma Res* 1996; **6:**313–317.

17. Tucker MA. Individuals at high risk of melanoma. *Pigment Cell* 1988; **9:**95–109.

18. Aitken J, Duffy D, Green A, *et al.* Heterogeneity of melanoma risk in families of melanoma patients. *Am J Epidemiol* 1994; **140:**961–973.

19. Serrano M, Hannon GJ, Beach D. A new regulatory motif in cell-cycle control causing specific inhibition of cyclin D/CDK4. *Nature* 1993; **366:**704–707.

20. Serrano M, Gomez-Lahoz E, DePinho RA, *et al.* Inhibition of ras-induced proliferation and cellular transformation by p16INK4. *Science* 1995; **267:**249–252.

21. Zhang Y, Xiong Y, Yarbrough WG. ARF promotes MDM2 degradation and stabilizes p53: ARF-INK4a locus deletion impairs both the Rb and p53 tumor suppression pathways. *Cell* 1998; **92:**725–734.

22. Pomerantz J, Schreiber-Agus N, Liegeois NJ, *et al.* The Ink4a tumor suppressor gene product, p19Arf, interacts with MDM2 and neutralizes MDM2's inhibition of p53. *Cell* 1998; **92:**713–723.

23. Wolfel T, Hauer M, Schneider J, *et al.* A p16[INK4a] insensitive CDK4 mutant targeted by cytolytic T lymphocytes in a human melanoma. *Science* 1995; **269:**1281–1284.

24. Kamb A, Gruis NA, Weaver-Feldhaus J, *et al.* A cell cycle regulator potentially involved in genesis of many tumor types. *Science* 1994; **264:**436–440.

25. Nobori T, Miura K, Wu DJ, *et al.* Deletions of the cyclin-dependent kinase-4 inhibitor gene in multiple human cancers. *Nature* 1994; **368:**753–756.

26. Cowan JM, Halaban R, Francke U. Cytogenetic analysis of melanocytes from premalignant nevi and melanomas. *J Natl Cancer Inst* 1988; **80:**1159–1164.

27. Dracopoli NC, Alhadeff B, Houghton AN, Old LJ. Loss of heterozygosity at autosomal and X-linked loci during tumor progression in a patient with melanoma. *Cancer Res* 1987; **47:**3995–4000.

28. Petty EM, Gibson LH, Fountain JW, *et al.* Molecular definition of a chromosome 9p21 germ-line deletion in a woman with multiple melanomas and a plexiform neurofibroma: implications for 9p tumor suppressor gene(s). *Am J Hum Genet* 1993; **53:**96–104.

29. Pederson MI, Wang N. Chromosomal evolution in the progression and metastasis of human malignant melanoma. *Cancer Genet Cytogenet* 1989; **41:**185–201.

30. Fountain JW, Karayiorgou M, Ernstoff MS, *et al.* Homozygous deletions within human chromosome band 9p21 in melanoma. *Proc Natl Acad Sci* 1992; **89:**10557–10561.

31. Cannon-Albright LA, Goldgar DE, Meyer LJ, *et al.* Assignment of a locus for familial melanoma, *MLM*, to chromosome 9p13–p22. *Science* 1992; **258:**1148–1152.

32. Nancarrow DJ, Mann GJ, Holland EA, *et al.* Confirmation of chromosome 9p linkage in familial melanoma. *Am J Hum Genet* 1993; **53:**936–942.

33. Hussussian CJ, Struewing JP, Goldstein AM, *et al.* Germline p16 mutations in familial melanoma. *Nature Genet* 1994; **8:**15–21.

34. Kamb A, Shattuck-Eidens D, Eeles R, *et al.* Analysis of the p16 gene (*CDKN2*) as a candidate for the chromosome 9p melanoma susceptibility locus. *Nature Genet* 1994; **8:**22–26.

35. Ohta M, Nagai H, Shimizu M, *et al.* Rarity of somatic and germline mutations of the cyclin-dependent kinase 4 inhibitor gene, *CDK4I*, in melanoma. *Cancer Res* 1994; **54:**5269–5272.

36. Gruis NA, van der Velden PA, Sandkuijl LA, *et al.* Homozygotes for *CDKN2* (p16) germline mutation in Dutch familial melanoma kindreds. *Nature Genet* 1995; **10:**351–353.

37. Liu L, Lassam NJ, Slingerland JM, *et al.* Germline p16[INK4A] mutation and protein dysfunction in a family with inherited melanoma. *Oncogene* 1995; **11:**405–412.

38. Borg A, Johannsson U, Johannson O, *et al.* Novel germline p16 mutation in familial malignant melanoma in southern Sweden. *Cancer Res* 1996; **56:**2497–2500.

39. Fitzgerald MG, Harkin DP, Silva-Arrieta S, *et al.* Prevalence of germ-line mutations in *p16*, *p19ARF*, and *CDK4* in familial melanoma: analysis of a clinic-based population. *Proc Natl Acad Sci USA* 1996; **93:**8541–8545.

40. Platz A, Hansson J, Mansson-Brahme E, *et al.* Screening of germline mutations in the *CDKN2A* and *CDKN2B* genes in Swedish families with hereditary cutaneous melanoma. *J Natl Cancer Inst* 1997; **89:**697–702.

41. Flores JF, Pollock PM, Walker GJ, *et al.* Analysis of the *CDKN2A*, *CDKN2B* and *CDK4* genes in 48 Australian melanoma kindreds. *Oncogene* 1997; **15:**2999–3005.

42. Soufir N, Avril M-F, Chompret A, *et al.* Prevalence of *p16* and *CDK4* germline mutations in 48 melanoma-prone families in France. *Hum Mol Genet* 1998; **7:**209–216.

43. MacKie RM, Andrew N, Lanyon WG, Connor JM. *CDKN2A* germline mutations in UK patients with familial melanoma and multiple primary melanomas. *J Invest Dermatol* 1998; **111:**269–272.

44. Fargnoli MC, Chimenti S, Keller G, *et al.* CDKN2a/p16[INK4a] mutations and lack of p19[ARF] involvement in familial melanoma kindreds. *J Invest Dermatol* 1998; **111:**1202–1206.

45. Yakobson EA, Zlotogorski A, Shafir R, *et al.* Screening for tumor suppressor *p16*(*CDKN2A*) germline mutations in Israeli melanoma families. *Clin Chemistry Lab Med* 1998; **36:**645–648.

46. Newton Bishop JA, Harland M, Bennett DC, *et al.* Mutation testing in melanoma families: *INK4A*, *CDK4*, and *INK4D*. *Br J Cancer* 1999; **80:**295–300.

47. Holland EA, Schmid H, Kefford RF, *et al.* CDKN2A (*p16INK4a*) and *CDK4* mutation analysis in 131 Australian melanoma probands: Effect of family history and multiple primary melanomas. *Genes Chromosom Cancer* 1999; **25:**1–10.

48. Ruiz A, Puig S, Malvehy J, *et al.* CDKN2A mutations in Spanish cutaneous malignant melanoma families and patients with multiple melanomas and other neoplasia. *J Med Genet* 1999; **36:** 490–493.

49. Ghiorzo P, Ciotti P, Mantelli M, *et al*. Characterization of Ligurian melanoma families and risk of occurrence of other neoplasia. *Int J Cancer* 1999; **83**:441–448.

50. Goldstein AM, Struewing JP, Chidambaram A, *et al*. Genotype–phenotype relationships in US melanoma-prone families with *CDKN2A* and *CDK4* mutations. *J Natl Cancer Inst* 2000; **92**:1006–1010.

51. Aitken J, Welch J, Duffy D, *et al*. *CDKN2A* variants in a population-based sample of Queensland families with melanoma. *J Natl Cancer Inst* 1999; **91**:446–452.

52. Merlo A, Herman JG, Mao L, *et al*. 5′ CpG island methylation is associated with transcriptional silencing of the tumour suppressor *p16/CDKN2/MTS1* in human cancers. *Nature Med* 1995; **1**:686–692.

53. Liu L, Dilworth D, Gao L, *et al*. Mutation of the *CDKN2A* 5′ UTR creates an aberrant initiation codon and predisposes to melanoma. *Nature Genet* 1999; **21**:128–132.

54. Harland M, Mistry S, Bishop DT, Newton Bishop J A. A deep intronic mutation in *CDKN2A* is associated with disease in a subset of melanoma pedigrees. *Hum Molec Genet* 2001; **10**:2679–2686.

55. Gruis NA, Sandkuijl LA, van der Velden PA, *et al*. *CDKN2* explains part of the clinical phenotype in Dutch familial atypical multiple-mole melanoma (FAMMM) syndrome families. *Melanoma Res* 1995; **5**:169–177.

56. Pollock PM, Spurr N, Bishop T, *et al*. Haplotype analysis of two recurrent *CDKN2A* mutations in 10 melanoma families: evidence for common founders and independent mutations. *Hum Mutat* 1998; **11**:424–431.

57. Monzon J, Liu L, Brill H, *et al*. *CDKN2A* mutations in multiple primary melanomas. *N Engl J Med* 1998; **338**:879–887.

58. Kefford RF, Newton-Bishop JA, Bergman W, *et al*. Counseling and DNA testing for individuals perceived to be genetically predisposed to melanoma: a consensus statement of the Melanoma Genetics Consortium. *J Clin Oncol* 1999; **17**:3245–3251.

59. Li FP, Fraumeni JF Jr, Mulvihill JJ, *et al*. A cancer family syndrome in twenty-four kindreds. *Cancer Res* 1988; **48**:5358–5361.

60. Lynch HT, Fusaro RM, Kimberling KJ, *et al*. Familial atypical multiple mole melanoma (FAMMM) syndrome: segregation analysis. *J Med Genet* 1983; **20**:342–344.

61. Bergman W, Watson P, deJong J, *et al*. Systemic cancer and the FAMMM syndrome. *Br J Cancer* 1990; **61**:932–936.

62. Goldstein AM, Fraser MC, Struewing JP, *et al*. Increased risk of pancreatic cancer in melanoma-prone kindreds with $p16^{INK4}$ mutations. *N Engl J Med* 1995; **333**:970–974.

63. Bergman W, Gruis N. Correspondence: Familial melanoma and pancreatic cancer. *N Engl J Med* 1996; **334**:471.

64. Borg A, Sandberg T, Nilsson K, *et al*. High frequency of multiple melanomas and breast and pancreatic carcinomas in *CDKN2A* mutation-positive melanoma families. *J Nat Cancer Inst* 2000; **92**:1260–1266.

65. Randerson-Moor JA, Harland M, Williams S, *et al*. A germline selection of *p14ARF* but not *CDKN2A* in a melanoma-neural system tumour syndrome family. *Hum Molec Genet* 2001; **10**:55–62.

66. Rizos H, Puig S, Badenas C, *et al*. A melanoma-associated germline mutation in exon 1β inactivates *p14ARF*. *Oncogene* 2001; **20**:5543–5547.

67. Hewitt C, Wu CL, Evans G, *et al*. Germline mutation of ARF in a melanoma kindred. *Hum Molec Genet* 2002; **11**:1273–1279.

68. Goldstein AM, Falk RT, Fraser MC, *et al*. Sun-related risk factors in melanoma-prone families with *CDKN2A* mutations. *J Natl Cancer Inst* 1998; **90**:709–711.

69. Demetrick DJ, Zhang H, Beach DH. Chromosomal mapping of human *CDK2*, *CDK4*, and *CDK5* cell-cycle kinase genes. *Cytogenet Cell Genet* 1994; **66**:72–74.

70. Zuo L, Weger J, Yang Q, *et al*. Germline mutations in the p16INK4a binding domain of *CDK4* in familial melanoma. *Nature Genet* 1996; **12**:97–99.

71. Harland M, Meloni R, Gruis N, *et al*. Germline mutations of the *CDKN2* gene in UK melanoma families. *Hum Molec Genet* 1997; **6**:2061–2067.

72. Gillanders E, Juo S-HH, Holland EA, *et al*. Localization of a novel melanoma susceptibility locus to 1p22. *Am J Hum Genet* 2003; **73**:301–313.

73. Liu L, Goldstein AM, Tucker MA, *et al*. Affected members of melanoma prone families with linkage to 9p21 but lacking mutations in *CDKN2A* do not harbor mutations in the coding regions of either *CDKN2B* or *p19ARF*. *Genes Chromosomes Cancer* 1997; **18**:1–3.

74. Platz A, Hansson J, Ringborg U. Screening of germline mutations in the *CDK4*, *CDKN2C* and *TP53* genes in familial melanoma: a clinic-based population study. *Int J Cancer* 1998; **78**:13–15.

75. Shennan MG, Badin AC, Walsh S, *et al*. Lack of germline *CDK6* mutations in familial melanoma. *Oncogene* 2000; **19**:1849–1852.

76. Palmer JS, Duffy DL, Box NF, *et al*. Melanocortin-1 receptor polymorphisms and risk of melanoma: is the association explained solely by pigmentation phenotype? *Am J Hum Genet* 2000; **66**:176–186.

77. NIH Consensus Statement: Diagnosis and treatment of early melanoma. *NIH Consensus Development Conference* 1992:10.

78. Tokar IP, Fraser MC, Bale SJ. Genodermatoses with profound malignant potential. *Semin Oncol Nursing* 1992; **8**:272–280.

79. Mackie RM, McHenry P, Hole D. Accelerated detection with prospective surveillance for cutaneous malignant melanoma in high-risk groups. *Lancet* 1993; **341**:1618–1620.

80. Masri GD, Clark WH Jr, Guerry D IV, *et al*. Screening and surveillance of patients at high risk for malignant melanoma result in detection of earlier disease. *J Am Acad Dermatol* 1990; **22**:1042–1048.

81. Crutcher WA, Cohen PJ. Dysplastic nevi and malignant melanoma. *Am Fam Physician* 1990; **42**:372–385.

82. Friedman RJ, Rigel DS, Silverman MK, *et al*. Malignant melanoma in the 1990s: the continued importance of early detection and the role of physician and self-examination of the skin. *Cancer J Clin* 1991; **41**:201–226.

83. Kelly JW, Yeatman JM, Regalia C, *et al*. A high incidence of melanoma found in patients with multiple dysplastic naevi by photographic surveillance. *Med J Aust* 1997; **167**:191–194.

84. National Cancer Institute, NIH, US Department of Health and Human Services. *What you need to know about dysplastic nevi*. NIH Publication no. 91-3133. Bethesda, MD: National Institutes of Health, 1990.

85. Kefford R, Newton Bishop J, Tucker M, *et al*. Genetic testing for melanoma. *The Lancet Oncology* 2002; **3**:653–654.

86. American Society of Clinical Oncology. Statement of the American Society of Clinical Oncology: genetic testing for cancer susceptibility. *J Clin Oncol* 1996; **14**:1730–1740.

28

Familial predisposition to lung cancer

THOMAS A. SELLERS, GLORIA M. PETERSEN AND PING YANG

INTRODUCTION

There can be little doubt that lung cancer is the product of environmental exposures, primarily tobacco but also radioactive ores, heavy metals and petrochemicals. However, the idea that individuals differ in their response to these environmental exposures is at least 40 years old. Recognizing that cigarette smoking was the principal cause of lung cancer, Goodhart[1] noted:

> ... different individuals show wide variation in the type and strength of stimulus needed for a neoplastic reaction so that, although even quite light smokers run a significantly higher risk of lung cancer than nonsmokers, nine out of ten of the heaviest smokers never get it at all.
>
> Personal idiosyncrasy seems to be an important factor in carcinogenesis and this suggests the hypothesis that the population may be genetically heterogeneous for susceptibility to cancer, some individuals being more 'cancer-prone' than others.

This chapter will review the evidence that a familial predisposition, be it genetic, common transmissible environment or both, is involved in the pathogenesis of lung cancer.

CASE REPORTS OF FAMILIAL CLUSTERING OF LUNG CANCER

Published case reports on the familial aggregation of lung cancer are rare: Brisman et al. reported a family in which four of eight siblings had lung cancer,[2] Nagy described a family in which three of 15 siblings were affected[3] and Jones reported the clustering of bronchogenic carcinoma in three of five siblings.[4] Goffman et al. studied two families with over 40 per cent of siblings affected with lung cancer,[5] Joishy et al. reported 58-year-old identical twins who developed alveolar cell carcinoma with nearly synchronous onset[6] and Paul et al. observed three siblings affected with the same histological cell type.[7] Even in the case of a lung malignancy, such as mesothelioma, which is strongly related to asbestos exposure, familial clustering has been reported[8,9] and asbestos exposure among some family members could not be proven. While dramatic case reports such as these may offer a striking clinical impression, they do not constitute sufficient evidence for the role of a genetic effect. In particular, rare familial clusters of a disease with such strong environmental influences may simply represent a chance occurrence.

TWIN STUDIES OF LUNG CANCER

One classic approach to studying genetic and environmental contributions to disease has been the study of twins. The few twin studies that have examined lung cancer concluded that it does not have a compelling genetic basis.[10–13] However, twin studies of common, late-onset cancers are generally difficult to interpret from a genetic perspective because of their low power and because the evidence that genetic effects are usually manifested in younger age of onset.[14] In the study by Braun et al.,[12] which extended the observations of Hrubec and Neel[11] on a cohort of 15 924 pairs of male US military veterans who were twins, only 272 (10 concordant) monozygotic and 378 (21 concordant) dizygotic pairs had at least one twin with lung cancer. This study concluded that genetic factors were not likely to be strongly predictive in male smokers over the age of 50, but it had minimal power to detect a genetic component. No conclusions could be drawn about a genetic contribution to lung cancer under age 50. In the study of over 23 000 Swedish twin pairs by Ahlbom et al.,[13] there was evidence for a familial effect for lung cancer in males but heritability was not significantly different from zero and the number of concordant pairs (four) was small. Most recently, Lichtenstein et al. studied 44 788 pairs from three Scandinavian twin registries and reported a non-significant increase in familial risk for lung cancer, with estimated heritability of 26 per cent (95 per cent confidence interval (CI) 0–49), based upon 314 (18 concordant) monozygotic pairs and 646 (25 concordant) dizygotic pairs.[15] Their heritability estimate for lung cancer was similar to other cancers studied within the same data set, for example, breast cancer (27 per cent), colorectal cancer (35 per cent) and stomach cancer (28 per cent). From his review of the published twin and family data, Risch[14] concluded that, although non-shared environment accounts for a large portion of familial variation in lung cancer (estimated as 62 per cent in the study by Lichtenstein et al.[15] and 71 per cent in the study by Hemminki et al.[16]), the published data were consistent with the conclusion that there is a genetic component in most cancers, including lung cancer.

EPIDEMIOLOGIC STUDIES OF FAMILY HISTORY

The question of whether or not lung cancer clusters in families more often than could be expected by chance alone requires proper epidemiological evaluation, such as selecting a group of patients with lung cancer and a group of cancer-free controls and comparing the frequency with which each group reports a positive family history of the disease. The first landmark study of this type was conducted by Tokuhata and Lilienfeld in 1963.[17] They showed that the occurrence of lung cancer among the parents and siblings of 270 lung cancer patients was three times greater than the frequency among relatives of the patients' spouse. This report remained uncorroborated for over 20 years until the study by Ooi and colleagues in a ten-parish geographic area referred to as the 'lung cancer belt' of southern Louisiana.[18] Studies conducted since these early reports demonstrate a wide range

in the reported frequency of a family history of lung cancer (Table 28.1).[19–31] However, the finding of a statistically significant excess occurrence of lung cancer among relatives of lung cancer cases is, with few exceptions,[32,33] quite consistent. The early studies considered probands regardless of smoking habits. Several recent studies have focused solely on probands who never smoked cigarettes. The magnitude of risk associated with a family history of lung cancer is still evident in these studies[25–28,30] but generally smaller than that observed when probands who smoke are included.

Although the results of early studies on the familial aggregation of cancer led to the prevailing hypothesis that susceptibility to cancer is probably site-specific, most studies of lung cancer have nonetheless examined family history of cancer at any site as a risk factor. Findings have tended to parallel that observed for lung cancer, although the magnitude of the risk elevation is generally lower (Table 28.1). When examined on a site-specific basis, the malignancies observed to be most frequent were usually smoking-associated.[34]

Studies of family history by histologic cell type

Lung cancer can be analysed by cell types, which are often designated as non-small-cell (adenocarcinoma, large-cell, squamous histologies) and small-cell. Adenocarcinoma of the lung demonstrates a weaker association with the use of tobacco products than does lung cancer of small cell, squamous or large-cell histologies. One might, therefore, expect to observe stronger evidence for familial factors in adenocarcinoma of the lung. Most studies that have examined familial risk by histologic type seem to support this hypothesis. Wu et al. studied 336 females with adenocarcinoma of the lung and found that, after adjusting for personal smoking habits, cases were 3.9 times as likely to report a family history of lung cancer than neighbourhood controls.[35] Osann reported a study of females with lung cancer and noted a stronger association of family history of lung cancer with adenocarcinoma (odds ratio; OR 3.0) than with smoking-associated histologies (OR 1.4).[24] Although Lynch et al. observed no association of histology with a family history of lung cancer,[32] they did find that the greatest familial risk of smoking-associated cancers occurred among relatives of patients with adenocarcinoma. When Shaw et al. stratified their cases according to histology,[22] the greatest familial risk was noted for the cases with adenocarcinoma (OR 2.1), but significantly elevated risks were observed for other histologies: squamous (1.9), small-cell (1.7). In contrast to these studies is the report by Sellers et al. of 300 lung cancer patients that the lowest familial risk occurred among those with adenocarcinoma and the highest risk among those with small-cell carcinoma.[36]

Table 28.1 *Case-control studies of family history and lung cancer*

Year of study/ location	Number of cases/ features	Lung cancer family history		Any cancer family history		References
		%	Odds ratio	%	Odds ratio	
1986, Louisiana	336	25.6	3.2	58.3	1.5	18
1986, New Mexico	521	6.9	5.3	31.3	1.6	19
1988, United States	112	7.0	2.8	–	–	20
1988, Saskatchewan	931	9.3	2.0	24.4	1.3	21
1991, Texas	937	26.1	1.8	58.1	1.3	22
1991, Saskatchewan	359	2.6	2.0	13.2	1.2	23
1991, California	217 females	8.2	1.9	41.8	1.8	24
1996, USA	646 females, non-smokers[a]	8.9	1.3	42.2[b]	1.0	25
1996, 1999, Detroit	257 non-smokers[a]	12.5	1.4	57.3	1.32[c]	26–27
1997, Missouri	432 non-smokers[a]; 186 former smokers	13.5	1.3	61.0	1.1	28
1998, Germany	251 ≤age 45;					29
	<45 years	10.0	2.6	33.5	1.2	
	55–69 years	7.0	1.4	35.5	0.9	
1999, New York	437 non-smokers[a]					30
	Father	4.3	1.9	20.2	1.7	
	Brother	6.7	1.8	21.8	1.6	
	Sister	2.8	4.1	25.7	1.7	
2000, Germany	945	7.7	1.7	–	–	31

[a] Patients were lifetime non-smokers.
[b] Prevalence of a positive family history of cancers other than lung cancer.
[c] For the first-degree relatives who never smoked cigarettes.

Ambrosone and colleagues examined family history of cancer at all sites in a much larger sample and observed the greatest familial risks among patients with small-cell and squamous cell histologies.[37] Kunitoh and colleagues published results from a series of nearly 1200 lung cancer cases from Japan.[38] In their series, cases with small-cell carcinoma were most likely to report a family history of lung cancer but the differences were not much greater than that observed for cases with other histologies. Carcinoid tumors of the lung have historically not been well represented in these studies, owing in part to the rarity of the disease. Investigators at MD Anderson reviewed medical records of 86 patients with carcinoid tumors of the lung diagnosed between 1959 and 1994. A family history of cancer was noted in 86 per cent of the medical records, 43 per cent when only first-degree relatives were considered.[39]

What is difficult to reconcile from these studies is the fact that the nature of exposure to cigarettes has not remained constant over time. For example, changes over time in the use of filters, the nicotine content, and the type of tobacco mean that even within a family the bronchial tissues of members may be exposed to quite different chemicals. Some studies suggest that the presentation of different lung cancer histologic cell types is associated with these characteristics of cigarettes.[40,41] Clearly, additional work needs to be done in this area.

Epidemiological studies of families

It is well known that cigarette-smoking habits are familial in nature. That is, children are more likely to smoke if their parents also smoke.[42,43] Therefore, when making comparisons of the prevalence of lung cancer among relatives of lung cancer cases and controls, one must take into consideration the distinct possibility that, unless cases and controls are matched on smoking behaviour, relatives of cases would be more likely to smoke than relatives of controls. The clustering of such behaviours might well explain why lung cancer cases are more likely to have a positive family history of the disease than controls. To date, only four studies have been conducted in which smoking data on the majority of family members were collected.

In the study by Tokuhata and Lilienfeld, the expected number of lung cancer deaths was determined separately by sex, smoking status, age and category of relative (father, mother, brother, sister).[17] The observed number of lung cancer deaths among men who smoked was twofold greater than expected ($p = 0.01$) and fourfold greater than expected among men who did not smoke ($p = 0.02$). There were no cases of lung cancer among smoking female relatives of the index cases. However, among non-smoking female relatives there was a 2.4-fold excess prevalence of lung cancer.

The study by Ooi *et al.* in southern Louisiana also obtained specific exposure data on relatives.[18] Similar to the Tokuhata and Lilienfeld study,[17] the excess risk was evident among non-smokers as well as smokers. The risk to smoking fathers of the cases was increased fivefold, while the risk of lung cancer to non-smoking female relatives of the cases was elevated ninefold. This excess risk could not be explained by age, sex, smoking status, pack-years of tobacco exposure, or a cumulative index of occupational/industrial exposures.

The third study that considered specific environmental measures in family members was not restricted to patients with lung cancer. Since a number of studies had noted a greater-than-normal likelihood of cancer among relatives of lung cancer patients, Sellers and co-workers[44] in southern Louisiana undertook a study to evaluate the familial risk of lung and other cancers among a randomly selected sample of cases with malignancy at any site. An excess of lung cancer was observed among relatives of lung cancer probands (OR 2.5) as well as among relatives of probands with cancers other than lung or breast (OR 1.6). This excess risk was evident even after allowing for each family member's age, sex, frequency of alcohol consumption (<1 vs. ≥ 1 drink per day), pack-years of tobacco consumption and a cumulative index of occupational/industrial exposures.

To more clearly delineate genetic from environmental factors that may underlie familial clusters, Schwartz *et al.* conducted a case-control family study of lung cancer among non-smokers.[26] Non-smoking relatives of lung cancer patients were at 7.2-fold greater risk than relatives of controls. This result was limited to the subset of cases between the ages of 40 and 59 years; no excess risk was evident among non-smoking relatives of cases aged 60–84 years.

In summary, those studies in which specific environmental and lifestyle exposures were determined on individual family members suggest that, even after allowing for the effects of age, sex and smoking, close relatives of lung cancer patients are still at an increased risk for the disease.

MAJOR GENE HYPOTHESES FOR LUNG CANCER

To address the issue of whether the familial aggregation of lung cancer is consistent with an inherited predisposition, one requires a data set in which several family members have been affected, and specific risk factor (level and type of environmental exposures, etc.) and disease information (including age of onset) for individual family members. The statistical determination of whether a major gene may be operative in the pathogenesis of the disease is achieved, in essence, by asking the question: 'Given the pattern of disease observed in these families, the ages of onset and the level of environmental exposure of the affected relatives, what is the most likely explanation?' To date, few attempts to answer this question have been published.

Sellers *et al.*[45] performed a complex segregation analysis of the 337 lung cancer families collected by Ooi *et al.*[18] The probands were identified through death certificates. Next-of-kin identified on the death certificate were contacted to construct pedigrees and obtain contact information to interview family members or their surrogate respondents. Families included the probands, their parents, siblings, offspring and spouses. A total of 4357 family members were studied but, because of missing values on tobacco consumption, only 3276 individuals were included in the analysis. Excluding the probands, there were 86 families (35.6 per cent) with at least one other family member affected with lung cancer (total = 106 lung cancers). Personal tobacco use was directly incorporated into the likelihood calculations. Results of the segregation analysis suggest that three hypotheses could be rejected; environmental ($p < 0.01$), no major-gene ($p < 0.01$) and Mendelian recessive ($p < 0.05$). Although the Mendelian dominant hypothesis could not be rejected ($p = 0.075$), Mendelian co-dominant inheritance provided a significantly better fit to the data ($p > 0.90$). The estimated gene frequency 0.052 implies that approximately 10 per cent of the population can be expected to carry the putative gene. The model further estimates that 28 per cent of the population, regardless of genotype, was susceptible to lung cancer. Based on parameters of the model, it was determined that the gene and its interaction with smoking contributed to 69 per cent, 47 per cent and 22 per cent of lung cancers through the ages of 50, 60 and 70, respectively. While these percentages are quite high, it is important to consider that only 6 per cent of lung cancer is diagnosed before the age of 50, and approximately 22 per cent occur before the age of 60. Therefore, based on these results, the actual number of lung cancers due to inheritance of a major susceptibility gene may be low.

As noted earlier in this chapter, another common approach that has been applied to identify potential genetic influences on a disease with such strong environmental influences is to select probands who are non-smokers. For these individuals, genetic susceptibility may be so high that even passive exposure to side-stream smoke could be sufficient to cause lung cancer. Yang *et al.* performed a complex segregation analysis on 257 families ascertained through non-smoking lung cancer probands.[46] Cases were identified from the Metropolitan Detroit Cancer Surveillance System. Among the 2021 first-degree relatives, 24 males and 10 females were similarly affected. The best explanation for the family clusters was an environmental hypothesis, in apparent contrast to the results obtained by Sellers *et al.*[45] based on families in which

Table 28.2 *Penetrance estimates of lung cancer risk for carriers and non-carriers by smoking status in two published segregation analyses[45,47]*

| Genotype | Cigarette smoking | Age in years | | | Reference |
		50	60	70	
Carrier	No	0.003–0.005[a]	0.009–0.018[a]	0.018–0.042[a]	47
		0.001	0.006	0.031	45
	Yes	0.013–0.020[a]	0.038–0.072[a]	0.072–0.15[a]	47
		0.011–0.052[b]	0.057–0.164[b]	0.171–0.249[b]	45
Non-carrier	No	<0.0001[c]	<0.0001[c]	0.0001[c]	47
		<0.0001	0.0004	0.0024	45
	Yes	<0.0001	0.0001–0.0003	0.0003–0.0008	47
		0.0008–0.0044[b]	0.0048–0.0251[b]	0.0277–0.1060[b]	45

[a] The range betweeen female and male.
[b] The range between 'average' and 'heavy' smokers.
[c] Adjusted for history of passive smoking.

92 per cent of the probands smoked. The analyses were repeated, stratifying the families on age, since the earlier report suggested that the putative gene influenced age at onset.[47] The authors specifically tested the effects of a Mendelian diallelic gene, history of tobacco use, and history of selected chronic lung diseases in families with a proband diagnosed at the age of 60 years or older and in families with a younger proband (i.e. under 60 years of age). In families of older probands, no evidence of a major genetic effect was detected, although a history of both emphysema and tobacco-smoke exposure were found to be significant risk factors. In families of younger probands, however, a Mendelian co-dominant model with significant modifying effects of smoking and chronic bronchitis was found to best explain the observed data.[47]

As shown in Table 28.2, the results of the studies by Sellers *et al.*[45] and Yang *et al.*[47] are remarkably similar. This consistency lends credence to the hypothesis that familial aggregation of lung cancer may reflect an underlying single-gene predisposition. The parameters of these models may, therefore, be considered in efforts to localize the relevant gene or genes using model-based linkage analysis.

EFFECT OF DIFFERENCES IN SMOKING PREVALENCE ON MODELS OF INHERITED SUSCEPTIBILITY

Lung cancer rarely occurs in the absence of environmental exposure. The consequences of this fact on identification of inherited susceptibility are critical. In particular, if lung cancer is the result of a gene–environment interaction, then, in the absence of environmental exposure (i.e. cigarette consumption), an inherited susceptibility to the disease is less likely to be expressed. Sellers *et al.* reasoned that, in the southern Louisiana lung cancer

families, intergenerational differences in the prevalence of the relevant environmental exposures, particularly tobacco, may obscure the true pattern of inheritance of a genetic factor.[48] The probands (index cases) selected for the Louisiana studies on lung cancer were ascertained over a 4-year period (1976–1979) and ranged in age at onset from 32 to 91 years. A potential complicating factor in these analyses is the temporal trend in smoking. In the USA, smoking was uncommon before World War I; after which time there was a dramatic increase in tobacco use. Because of this cohort phenomenon and the wide range in the age of the probands, there was little uniformity in the exposure of the parental generations to the use of tobacco products. The lung cancer families were partitioned into two groups: (1) probands older than age 60 at the time of ascertainment (born before World War I and unlikely to have parents who smoked); and (2) probands younger than age 60 at the time of ascertainment (higher probability of smoking among parents). Of the 337 lung cancer families studied, 106 were ascertained through a proband whose age at death was less than 60 years and 231 through a proband whose age at death was 60 years or greater. Results of the segregation analyses on the early-onset proband families (higher probability of smoking parents) suggested that the pattern of disease was consistent with autosomal dominant transmission of inherited predisposition.[49] In contrast to their earlier publication, the proportion of the population who was susceptible increased from 28 per cent to 60 per cent. In the families ascertained through probands with older ages at onset, there was still evidence for a Mendelian effect but none of the models could be distinguished as providing the best fit.

Although these findings are suggestive of a gene–environment interaction, no direct modelling of such an effect was performed. Gauderman and colleagues analysed the same set of southern Louisiana families utilizing a Markov chain Monte Carlo approach to impute missing values on tobacco use.[50] Evidence for a major gene effect was still observed, but the gene–environment interaction was not statistically significant. Since this approach assumed that the relative increase in lung cancer risk due to a major gene was constant over all ages, and case-control studies tend to suggest that family history is a stronger risk factor at early ages, additional segregation analyses were performed using a variation of the Cox proportional hazards model to allow estimation of age-specific genetic relative risks.[51] After allowing for measures of smoking and gene–environment interactions, the best-fitting hypothesis was that of autosomal dominant transmission with an allele frequency of 0.043. Carrier to non-carrier relative risks were greater than 100 for ages less than 60 years and declined monotonically to 1.6 by age 80.

To more fully resolve the potential confounding effect of intergenerational differences in tobacco exposure on the models of inherited susceptibility, Sellers and colleagues constructed a simulated population of lung cancer families with an underlying autosomal dominant predisposition to lung cancer.[52] The population was constructed, such that tobacco exposure varied over time in a manner consistent with the pattern observed in the USA. A total of 324 families with 380 cases of lung cancer were ascertained and analysed. Curiously, although a dominant model of susceptibility had been simulated, both dominant and co-dominant hypotheses fit the data. These results underscore the potential danger of segregation analysis of complex traits in which exposure to known environmental influences may differ across generations and suggest that inherited susceptibility to lung cancer may in fact be autosomal dominant, a conclusion subsequently reached by Gauderman and Morrison[51] in their analysis of the Louisiana lung cancer data set using a different analytical approach.

IMPLICATIONS OF THE GENETIC MODELS OF LUNG CANCER

Because lung cancer rarely occurs in the absence of tobacco exposure, the results observed by Sellers et al. for the subset of early-onset families (where exposures were more uniform across generations) may be more likely to reflect the true underlying biology.[49] If so, the results suggest a much greater influence of genetic factors in lung cancer pathogenesis than the results obtained when all families were analysed together: the cumulative probability of lung cancer by age 80 for a non-carrier of the gene, at the average level of tobacco consumption, was 2.8×10^{-27}, implying that virtually all lung cancer occurs among gene carriers. In fact, Gauderman and Morrison estimated that more than 90 per cent of lung cancer cases with onset before age 60 would be expected to carry the

high-risk allele.[51] However, the results of studies to date do not suggest that lung cancer is primarily a genetic disease. The cumulative probability that a non-smoking gene carrier develops lung cancer by age 80 was estimated to be only 52 per 100 000 (compared with 2175 per 100 000 for gene carriers who smoked).[49] Thus, the data are more consistent with the hypothesis that a genetic predisposition to lung (and perhaps other smoking-associated cancers)[53] is inherited and that the trait is expressed only in the presence of the major environmental insult: tobacco smoke.

What is currently known about genetic predisposition to lung cancer is based entirely on observational study designs. Thus, it is premature to suggest screening, counselling or education for individuals with a positive family history of lung cancer; the results need to be corroborated by linkage studies. It is also imperative that the results be replicated in other populations, allowing for potentially important risk factors that have not been measured in previous studies (e.g. carotenoid intake, alcohol use, physical activity, passive smoking, radon exposure, occupation). If shown to be correct, however, the existence of a major susceptibility gene for lung cancer would have tremendous public health implications: for the lung cancer-susceptible, smoking would appear to be universally lethal. However, smokers without a family history of lung cancer should not be lulled into a false sense of security. Several studies now suggest that, if parents and siblings have not been challenged by environmental (tobacco) exposure, susceptibility may not have been 'unmasked'. Given the variable age of onset of lung cancer, whether or not a person has a positive family history is a dynamic rather than a static characteristic. It is also important to emphasize that, for the lung cancer non-susceptible, a variety of other disorders are highly likely, especially cardiovascular disease, which accounts for the greatest smoking-related morbidity and mortality.[54]

SUMMARY AND CONCLUSION

The published studies of lung cancer to date suggest that the disease does aggregate in some families, that the clustering does not appear to be entirely the result of shared environmental factors and that the pattern of disease among relatives is consistent with the hypothesis of major gene segregation. There is increasing evidence that the effect of the gene is age-related, with a greater influence among early onset cases. Unfortunately, efforts to locate the major gene(s) predisposing to lung cancer in the human genome, by either traditional parametric or non-parametric linkage methods, have not proven fruitful. This is mainly due to the extreme difficulty in collecting multiplex families that would be informative for analysis. In particular, the high case-fatality and short survival rate from lung cancer makes it rare to identify families with multiple living lung cancer cases. As a result, no published studies of model-based LOD score linkage analysis have yet appeared in the literature, although a number of investigators are actively working in this area. Identification of such a gene (or genes) could have profound implications for prevention, detection and therapy for lung cancer.

NOTE ADDED IN PROOF

The Genetic Epidemiology of Lung Cancer Consortium has recently reported that a locus for familial lung cancer maps to chromosome 6q23-25. Multipoint linkage analysis using a simple autosomal dominant model (as described in this chapter) of 52 families that included 3 or more individuals affected by lung or throat or laryngeal cancer yielded a maximum Heterogeneity LOD score (HLOD) of 2.79. A subset of 23 multigenerational pedigrees with 5 or more affected yielded a multipoint HLOD score of 4.26 at the same position.[55]

KEY POINTS

- Aggregations of lung cancer in families are described.
- No genes have been found to date that explain familial aggregation.
- The use of spiral CT screening is under investigation.

REFERENCES

1. Goodhart G. Cancer-proneness and lung cancer. *Practitioner* 1959; **182**:578–584.
2. Brisman R, Baker RR, Elkins R, Hartmann WH. Carcinoma of lung in four siblings. *Cancer* 1967; **20**:2048–2053.
3. Nagy I. On the observation of bronchial carcinoma in 3 brothers. *Prax Pneumol* 1968; **22**:718–723.
4. Jones FJ. Bronchogenic carcinoma in three siblings. *Bull Geisinger Med Center* 1977; **29**:23–25.
5. Goffman TE, Hassinger DD, Mulvihill JJ. Familial respiratory tract cancer. Opportunities for research and prevention. *JAMA* 1982; **247**:1020–1023.
6. Joishy SK, Cooper RA, Rowley PT. Alveolar cell carcinoma in identical twins. Similarity in time of onset, histochemistry, and site of metastasis. *Ann Intern Med* 1977; **87**:447–450.
7. Paul SM, Bacharach B, Goepp C. A genetic influence on alveolar cell carcinoma. *J Surg Oncol* 1987; **36**:249–252.
8. Dawson A, Gibbs A, Browne K, *et al*. Familial mesothelioma. Details of 17 cases with histopathologic findings and mineral analysis. *Cancer* 1992; **70**:1183–1187.
9. Ascoli V, Scalzo CC, Bruno C, *et al*. Familial pleural malignant mesothelioma: clustering in three sisters and one cousin. *Cancer Lett* 1998; **130**:203–207.
10. Cederlof R, Floderus B, Friberg L. Cancer in MZ and DZ twins. *Acta Genet Med Gemellol* 1970; **19**:69–74.
11. Hrubec Z. Neel JV. Contribution of familial factors to the occurrence of cancer before old age in twin veterans. *Am J Hum Genet* 1982; **34**:658–671.
12. Braun M, Caporaso N, Page W, Hoover R. Genetic component of lung cancer: cohort study of twins. *Lancet* 1994; **344**:440–443.
13. Ahlbom A, Lichtenstein P, Malmström H, *et al*. Cancer in twins: genetic and nongenetic familial risk factors. *J Natl Cancer Inst* 1997; **89**:287–293.
14. Risch N. The genetic epidemiology of cancer: interpreting family and twin studies and their implications for molecular genetic approaches. *Cancer Epidemiol Biomarkers Prev* 2001; **10**:733–741.
15. Lichtenstein P, Holm NV, Verkasalo PK, *et al*. Environmental and heritable factors in the causation of cancer – analyses of cohorts of twins from Sweden, Denmark, and Finland. *N Engl J Med* 2000; **343**:78–85.
16. Hemminki K, Lonnstedt I, Vaittinen P, Lichtenstein P. Estimation of genetic and environmental components in colorectal and lung cancer and melanoma. *Genet Epidemiol* 2001; **20**:107–116.
17. Tokuhata G, Lilienfeld A. Familial aggregation of lung cancer in humans. *J Natl Cancer Inst* 1963; **30**:289–312.
18. Ooi WL, Elston RC, Chen VW, *et al*. Increased familial risk for lung cancer. *J Natl Cancer Inst* 1986; **76**:217–222.
19. Samet JM, Humble CG, Pathak DR. Personal and family history of respiratory disease and lung cancer risk. *Am Rev Respir Dis* 1986; **134**:466–470.
20. Horwitz RI, Smaldone LF, Viscoli CM. An ecogenetic hypothesis for lung cancer in women. *Arch Int Med* 1988; **48**:2609–2612.
21. McDuffie HH, Dosman JA, Klaassen DJ. Cancer, genes and agriculture. *Principles of health and safety in agriculture*. Boca Raton, FL: CRC Press, 1988; 258–261.
22. Shaw GL, Falk RT, Pickle LW, *et al*. Lung cancer risk associated with cancer in relatives. *J Clin Epidemiol* 1991; **44**:429–437.
23. McDuffie HH. Clustering of cancer in families of patients with primary lung cancer. *J Clin Epidemiol* 1991; **44**:69–76.
24. Osann KE. Lung cancer in women: the importance of smoking, family history of cancer, and medical history of respiratory disease. *Cancer Res* 1991; **51**:4893–4897.
25. Wu AH, Fontham ET, Reynolds P, *et al*. Previous lung disease and risk of lung cancer among lifetime nonsmoking women in the United States. *Am J Epidemiol* 1995; **141**:1023–1032.
26. Schwartz AG, Yang P, Swanson GM. Familial risk of lung cancer among nonsmokers and their relatives. *Am J Epidemiol* 1996; **144**:554–562.
27. Schwartz AG, Rothrock M, Yang P, Swanson GM. Increased cancer risk among relatives of nonsmoking lung cancer cases. *Genet Epidemiol* 1999; **17**:1–15.
28. Brownson RC, Alavanja MC, Caporaso N, *et al*. Family history of cancer and risk of lung cancer in lifetime non-smokers and long-term ex-smokers. *Int J Epidemiol* 1997; **26**:256–263.
29. Kreuzer M, Kreienbrock L, Gerken M, *et al*. Risk factors for lung cancer in young adults. *Am J Epidemiol* 1998; **147**:1028–1037.
30. Mayne ST, Buenconsejo J, Janerich DT. Familial cancer history and lung cancer risk in United States nonsmoking men and women. *Cancer Epidemiol Biomarkers Prev* 1999; **8**:1065–1069.

31. Bromen K, Pohlabeln H, Jahn I, *et al*. Aggregation of lung cancer in families: results from a population-based case-control study in Germany. *Am J Epidemiol* 2000; **152:**497–505.

32. Lynch HT, Kimberling WJ, Markvicka SE, *et al*. Genetics and smoking-associated cancers. A study of 485 families. *Cancer* 1986; **57:**1640–1646.

33. Pierce RJ, Kune GA, Kune S, *et al*. Dietary and alcohol intake, smoking pattern, occupational risk, and family history in lung cancer patients: results of a case-control study in males. *Nutr Cancer* 1989; **12:**237–248.

34. Sellers TA, Ooi WL, Elston RC, *et al*. Increased familial risk for non-lung cancer among relatives of lung cancer patients. *Am J Epidemiol* 1987; **126:**237–246.

35. Wu AH, Yu MC, Thomas DC, *et al*. Personal and family history of lung disease as risk factors for adenocarcinoma of the lung. *Cancer Res* 1988; **48:**7279–7284.

36. Sellers TA, Elston RC, Atwood LD, Rothschild H. Lung cancer histologic type and family history of cancer. *Cancer* 1992; **69:**86–91.

37. Ambrosone CB, Rao U, Michalek AM, *et al*. Lung cancer histologic types and family history of cancer. Analysis of histologic subtypes of 872 patients with primary lung cancer. *Cancer* 1993; **72:**1192–1198.

38. Kunitoh H, Sekine I, Kubota K, *et al*. Histologic types of lung carcinoma and related family history of anatomic sites and histologic types of cancers. *Cancer* 1999; **86:**1182–1188.

39. Perkins P, Lee JR, Kemp BL, Cox JD. Carcinoid tumors of the lung and family history of cancer. *J Clin Epidemiol* 1997; **50:**705–709.

40. Thun MJ, Lally CA, Flannery JT, *et al*. Cigarette smoking and changes in the histopathology of lung cancer. *J Natl Cancer Inst* 1997; **89:**1580–1586.

41. McDuffie HH, Klaassen DJ, Dosman JA. Determinants of cell type in patients with cancer of the lungs. *Chest* 1990; **98:**1187–1193.

42. Horn D, Courts F, Taylor R, Solomon E. Cigarette smoking among high school students. *Am J Public Health* 1959; **49:**1497–1511.

43. Silber F, MacMahon B. Cigarette smoking among high school students related to social class and parental smoking habits. *Am J Public Health* 1961; **51:**1780–1789.

44. Sellers TA, Elston RC, Stewart C, Rothschild H. Familial risk of cancer among randomly selected cancer probands. *Genet Epidemiol* 1988; **5:**381–391.

45. Sellers TA, Bailey-Wilson JE, Elston RC, *et al*. Evidence for mendelian inheritance in the pathogenesis of lung cancer. *J Natl Cancer Inst* 1990; **82:**1272–1279.

46. Yang P, Schwartz AG, McAllister AE, *et al*. Genetic analysis of families with nonsmoking lung cancer probands. *Genet Epidemiol* 1997; **14:**181–197.

47. Yang P, Schwartz AG, McAllister AE, *et al*. Lung cancer risk in families of nonsmoking probands: heterogeneity by age at diagnosis. *Genet Epidemiol* 1999; **17:**253–273.

48. Sellers TA, Potter JD, Bailey-Wilson JE, *et al*. Lung cancer detection and prevention: evidence for an interaction between smoking and genetic predisposition. *Cancer Res* 1992; **52:**2694s–2697s.

49. Sellers TA, Bailey-Wilson JE, Potter JD, *et al*. Effect of cohort differences in smoking prevalence on models of lung cancer susceptibility. *Genet Epidemiol* 1992; **9:**261–271.

50. Gauderman WJ, Morrison JL, Carpenter CL, Thomas DC. Analysis of gene-smoking interaction in lung cancer. *Genet Epidemiol* 1997; **14:**199–214.

51. Gauderman WJ, Morrison JL. Evidence for age-specific genetic relative risks in lung cancer. *Am J Epidemiol* 2000; **151:**41–49.

52. Sellers TA, Weaver TW, Phillips B, Altmann M, Rich SS. Environmental factors can confound identification of a major gene effect: results from a segregation analysis of a simulated population of lung cancer families. *Genet Epidemiol* 1998; **15:**251–262.

53. Sellers TA, Chen PL, Potter JD, *et al*. Segregation analysis of smoking-associated malignancies: evidence for Mendelian inheritance. *Am J Med Genet* 1994; **52:**308–314.

54. Doll R, Hill A. Lung cancer and other causes of death in relation to smoking. A second report on the mortality of British doctors. *Br Med J* 1956; **57:**1071–1075.

55. Bailey-Wilson JE, Amos CI, Pinney S, *et al*. A major lung cancer susceptibility locus maps to chromosome 6q23-25. *Am J Hum Genet* 2004; **75:**460–474.

29

Genetic susceptibility to carcinoma of the head and neck, stomach, and pancreas

WILLIAM D. FOULKES, ELSA LANKE, SARAH JEFFERIES AND PIERRE O. CHAPPUIS

INTRODUCTION

Cancers of the head and neck, stomach and pancreas are amongst the commonest cancers in the developing world and not rare in Western countries. Some of these (pituitary, pancreatic endocrine and parathyroid) make up the MEN 1 syndrome. The most important aetiological factors for the former cancers are environmental exposure to tobacco, alcohol and other substances. In a small minority of cases, mendelian inheritance plays an important role. In particular, E-cadherin (*CDH1*), has been found to be mutated in the germline of some individuals with diffuse gastric cancer. Germline *BRCA2* and *CDKN2A* mutations have been identified in those with pancreas cancer, often in families with breast and ovarian cancers, and in the case of *CDKN2A*, cutaneous malignant melanoma. Numerous association studies have focused on polymorphisms in so-called susceptibility genes, such as *GSTM1*, *NAT2* and, more recently, repair enzymes such as *XRCC1*. Overall, this avenue of research has proved to be disappointing and very little consistency has been observed in the results when different populations are studied. Nevertheless, the possibility that, in a non-familial setting, the risk of cancer can be sufficiently accurately characterized to justify preventive intervention remains a major *raison d'être* of genetic research into the aetiology of these cancers. In this chapter, we consider the importance of genetic factors and their possible interaction with non-genetic risk factors at these three sites.

SUSCEPTIBILITY TO SQUAMOUS CELL CARCINOMA OF THE HEAD AND NECK

Epidemiology of squamous cell carcinoma of the head and neck: the role of non-genetic factors

Squamous cell carcinoma of the head and neck (SCCHN) encompasses a group of diseases associated with major morbidity and mortality. It is the fifth most common cancer worldwide and the adjusted incidence of head and neck cancer is increasing in developing countries.[1,2] SCCHN represents a major worldwide health problem, which will worsen if smoking rates in developing countries continue their upward trend.[3] It is clear that the major aetiological agents are tobacco and alcohol exposure.[4,5] In non-drinkers, the effect of smoking is to increase the relative risk (RR) of developing SCCHN from 2-fold to 20-fold. At some sites, the larynx, oral cavity and pharynx, the combined effect of alcohol and tobacco can be multiplicative for cancer risk (RR 2–140).[5] Other risk factors include nutrition, occupation, viral infection and poor dentition.[6,7]

Epidemiology of SCCHN: the role of genetic factors

Until recently, little attention has been paid to possible hereditary factors in SCCHN. There is now increasing epidemiological evidence from case-control studies of SCCHN that a family history of head and neck cancer is a risk factor for this disease. A Dutch matched case-control study gave a RR for SCCHN of 3.5 in association with a family history of upper aerodigestive tract (UADT) cancer and lung cancer.[8] Another study evaluated 754 cases and 1507 age- and sex-matched hospital controls. It showed that the adjusted RR for developing SCCHN in association with a family history of the disease was 3.7 (95 per cent confidence interval (CI) 2.0–6.8).[9] A retrospective cohort study from Montreal showed the adjusted RR for SCCHN in association with a family history of SCCHN was 3.9 (CI 1.1–13.0).[10] Segregation analysis of these data using the SAGE package has shown that a mendelian hypothesis, allowing for covariates (smoking, drinking and age) is not rejected, whereas a purely environmental hypothesis is rejected ($p < 0.025$).[11] Penetrance did not vary by age or sex. The conclusion from this analysis is that it is important to allow for genetic factors in explaining the familial aggregation of SCCHN. Nevertheless, one other large study did not show any evidence for a genetic effect[12] and the true contribution of mendelian genetic factors remains uncertain.

Despite therapeutic advances in the treatment of SCCHN, the overall survival from the disease has remained unchanged over the last 20 years. A contributory factor to this is that patients with successfully treated early-stage SCCHN have a high incidence of second primary cancers of the head, neck and UADT.[13,14] For many cancers, multiple primary cancer in an individual is a sign that there is an increased probability of hereditary predisposition to cancer in that person.[15–17] Individuals with a second primary SCCHN are more likely to have a family history of SCCHN than those with only a single primary (adjusted odds ratios: 7.9 vs. 3.5, $p < 0.009$[10]; 8.9 per cent vs. 2.5 per cent, $p < 0.00001$[17]). Genetic factors may also be important in other UADT cancers: the risk of UADT in those with a family history of oesophageal cancer was eight times that of those without such a family history.[18]

Underlying mechanisms for increased cancer susceptibility

CANCER PREDISPOSITION GENES

CDKN2A (also known as p16/MTS1)

The *CDKN2A* tumour suppressor gene is localized on chromosome 9p21. It encodes a 16 kDa protein that binds to cyclin-dependent kinase (cdk) 4 and 6, inhibiting their association with cyclin D1.[19] The inhibition of the cyclin D1–cdk4/6 complex activity prevents retinoblastoma phosphorylation, leading to the inhibition of the cell-cycle G1/S transition.[19] Genetic alterations involving the 9p21–22 region are common in human cancer and *CDKN2A* is considered to be the target in this region.[20] High frequencies of somatic homozygous deletions and mutations are seen in SCCHN.[21] Germline *CDKN2A* mutations have been shown to predispose to familial melanoma[22,23] and SCCHN has been seen in individuals from melanoma-prone kindreds, where germline *CDKN2A* mutations have been found.[24–26] However, in a series of 40 patients with multiple primary tumours of the head and neck who were not selected for melanoma, no *CDKN2A* germline mutations were observed.[27]

BRCA2

Germline mutations in this gene account for a large proportion of hereditary site-specific breast cancer families. An excessive number of SCCHN cases have been reported in *BRCA2* mutation carriers from several such families. Easton *et al.* reported an excess of laryngeal cancer (RR 7.7) in a large hereditary breast cancer family from Ireland based on two possible carriers.[28] A significant number of cancers of the buccal cavity and pharynx were also observed in a study examining a large series of *BRCA2* families from North America and Europe (RR 2.3, $p = 0.03$).[29] Cancers of the throat and oral cavity were also observed in *BRCA2* carriers in 3 out of 17 French Canadian breast cancer families.[30] Founder mutations have been described within defined ethnic groups, which can facilitate carrier detection, and in a mutation analysis study of 53 French Canadian cases with SCCHN, no founder *BRCA2* mutations (8765delAG, 2816 insA and 6085G > T) were identified.[31] Similarly, no 6174delT mutations were found in 25 Ashkenazi Jewish individuals with SCCHN.

TP53

Squamous cell carcinoma of the head and neck is occasionally featured in the Li–Fraumeni syndrome, which is associated with germline mutations in *TP53*.[32] Germline *TP53* gene mutations have also been found in members of cancer-prone families and individuals with multiple tumours.[33] Among 24 consecutive patients with oral, laryngeal, oropharyngeal and hypopharyngeal squamous cell cancers who developed second cancers in the UADT, 13 had a first-degree relative with cancer and were assessed for germline mutations in the *TP53*.[34] One possibly disease-causing germline mutation was found at codon 197. It has been reported that patients with homozygous arginine alleles at codon 72 of *TP53* were at increased risk of human papillomavirus (HPV)-related cervical cancer.[35,36] These findings have been questioned.[37–40] However, because SCCHN is another cancer where HPV has been implicated, it is possible that this polymorphism could be relevant for the development of SCCHN. No excess of this polymorphism was seen in a study of 163 cases of SCCHN compared with 163 matched controls,[41] although HPV expression status was not determined.

A new development in this area is the observation that this Arg72Pro polymorphism may have unexpected effects on the binding of *TP53* to one of its partners, p73.[42] These authors found that alleles carrying clear disease-associated mutations in *TP53* differed in their ability to transform cells (in co-operation with Ras), depending on whether they carried the Arg or the Pro polymorphism at position 72. It was the commoner (perhaps one could say wild-type) allele, Arg, that enhanced cell transformation. However, in 7 heterozygous individuals who developed SCCHN, only 3 had loss of heterozygosity at the *TP53* locus and, in all three cases, it was the Arg allele that was 'lost'. The Arg allele was no more likely to carry a mutation in *TP53* than was the Pro allele (4 vs. 3). The opposite results were seen for skin cancers and for vulval cancers, where the Arg allele was preferentially mutated and the Pro allele usually lost in the tumours. Thus the true importance of this polymorphism in influencing SCCHN risk remains uncertain.

MUTAGEN SENSITIVITY

Although the predominant cause of SCCHN is exposure to tobacco and alcohol, there is a clear disparity between the number of people who develop tumours and the total number exposed. Differences in carcinogen metabolism and DNA repair due to genetic polymorphisms have been suggested as a possible cause for this variation in susceptibility. Phenotypic assays, such as mutagen sensitivity, host-cell reactivation assays and measurement of DNA repair gene transcript levels have been used to assess risk for SCCHN.[43,44] Mutagen sensitivity is the best documented of these phenotypic assays, which tests whether specific mutagenic agents interfere with chromosome integrity. When used *in vitro*, bleomycin induces single- and double-strand breaks irrespective of cell-cycle status. The number of chromosome breaks per cell in standard lymphocyte cultures has been quantified. This number is not affected by important factors, such as sex, alcohol and tobacco consumption,[45,46] so this assay could be measuring a constitutional component of DNA repair capacity. Rates of chromosomal breakage following *in vitro* exposure to bleomycin in patients with SCCHN are elevated.[47] Rates are highest in those with multiple primary cancers and in those with a positive family history.[48] It is also a feature in younger onset cases.[49] In addition, the rates decrease in cases treated with the differentiating agent 13-*cis* retinoic acid, which has been used successfully in the chemoprevention of second primary tumours.[50,51]

Cloos *et al.* have performed a segregation analysis of bleomycin sensitivity, which showed that this is a heritable characteristic; inheritance of genes is less likely to be affected by bias in the areas previously discussed.[52]

Although the estimate for heritability is sizeable, the group evaluated was heterogeneous, including pedigrees from SCCHN patients who had been successfully treated with no evidence of recurrence for at least 1 year as well as monozygotic twins. Chromatin breaks induced by bleomycin are not random, but occur at fragile sites and may indicate important chromosomal regions in which genes involved in malignant transformation are located. A comparison of breakpoints in tumours with those in lymphocytes may provide insight into the chromosomal instability.

METABOLIC ENZYME POLYMORPHISMS

Individuals may be at increased cancer susceptibility owing to less efficient detoxification of carcinogens, or more efficient activation of co-carcinogens or a failure to maintain adequate DNA repair after carcinogen exposure. Tobacco smoke comprises at least 50 known carcinogens, and polymorphisms in some carcinogen-metabolizing enzyme genes have been well documented in molecular epidemiology studies. The glutathione-*S*-transferases (GSTs) are a family of isoenzymes that catalyse the conjugation of gamma-glutamylcystenylglycine to hydrophobic and electrophilic compounds. These phase II enzymes increase the water solubility of xenobiotic and endogenous substrates, hence allowing their excretion. In addition to their role as catalysts, these enzymes may act as intracellular storage ligands, as they bind hydrophobic compounds.[53] Because of their role in detoxification, these enzymes have been extensively studied with respect to potential population variation and cancer susceptibility. *GSTM1* and *GSTT1* have received most of the attention and will be discussed here. *GSTM1* and *GSTT1* are homozygous null in ~40 per cent and ~15 per cent of the Caucasian population, respectively, although in some isolated populations, nullizygosity for *GSTM1* can reach 100 per cent.[54] A number of different groups have shown that the *GSTM1* null genotype is associated with an increased risk of cancer of the lung, bladder, skin, colon and mesothelium.[55-59] A recent meta-analysis of all studies of bladder cancer confirmed the association (odds ratio (OR) 1.5, 95% CI 1.3–1.8).[60] A similar analysis for lung cancer, while positive, was interpreted as possibly indicating a null effect when publication bias was taken into account (overall OR 1.1, 95% CI 1.0–1.3).[61] Interestingly, one study showed that the null genotype may have its largest effect in lung cancer for those who have smoked less than 40 pack-years.[62] Studies have assessed the risk of SCCHN in relation to *GSTM1* and *GSTT1* null genotype.[63-67] The findings from these studies were that the null phenotype of either enzyme is associated with a slightly increased risk of SCCHN. Some have found an increased risk for SCCHN associated with *GSTT1* nullizygosity in the heaviest smokers.[68,69] On the other hand, Cheng *et al.* demonstrated a significantly elevated risk of disease in patients with both *GSTT1* and *GSTM1* null genotypes (OR 3.6, 95% CI 1.9–6.8).[70] In contrast to previous studies, the highest frequencies of null alleles were seen in those with less exposure to tobacco and alcohol, in younger patients and in those with multiple primary tumours. In an ethnically restricted study, Hamel *et al.* also observed that *GSTT1* nullizygosity is only a risk factor for SCCHN in those with low exposure to tobacco.[71] The largest effect was seen in Ashkenazi Jewish patients.

Cigarette smoke also contains arylamines, which are catalysed by *N*-acetyl transferase (NAT) isoenzymes. *NAT1* is expressed in all tissues and is polymorphic.[72] *NAT2* is expressed in the liver and is highly polymorphic. Polymorphisms in the *NAT2* gene are due to specific point mutations and result in a phenotypic variation: the slow acetylators can be distinguished from the fast acetylators at the DNA level on the basis of restriction enzyme sites or by measuring metabolic activity.[73] It has been shown in retrospective studies that there is an increased risk of bladder cancer among slow acetylators. A meta-analysis gave a pooled OR of bladder cancer associated with slow acetylator status of 1.31 (95% CI 1.1–1.6), suggesting that NAT2 slow acetylator status is associated with a modest increase in risk of bladder cancer.[74] By contrast, there may be an increased risk of colon cancer among fast acetylators.[75] The results for SCCHN have been conflicting. Henning *et al.* assessed *NAT1* and *NAT2* genotypes in 255 patients with laryngeal cancer compared to 510 matched controls.[76] They found that the NAT2 (*)4/(*)4 fast acetylator genotype was a significant risk factor for laryngeal cancer. In contrast, Morita *et al.* did not find an increased risk for fast acetylators but did demonstrate an increased risk for SCCHN (excluding pharyngeal cancers) amongst slow and intermediate acetylators.[77] In summary, there is no consistent evidence in favour of a role for NAT2 polymorphisms in head and neck cancer susceptibility.

Cytochrome P4501A1 metabolizes benzo[a]pyrene in tobacco smoke to its active metabolite. The Ile-Val polymorphism in exon 7 and *Msp*I polymorphism of *CYP1A1* have been studied, and no difference was found between benign and malignant head and neck lesions.[67] However, a study in Japan found a correlation between the Val/Val genotype and increased risk of SCCHN.[77] This may reflect ethnic differences as presence of a *CYP1A1* polymorphism was also correlated with lung cancer in a Japanese population but not in a Caucasian population.[78,79]

In a recent meta-analysis of 4635 cases and 5770 controls, Hashibe *et al.*[80] determined that modest, but statistically significant, increased pooled ORs for SCCHN were observed in association with *GSTM1* (OR 1.32, 95 per cent CI: 1.07–1.62) and *GSTT1* (OR 1.25, 95 per cent CI: 1.00–1.57), but not for *GSTP1* (val 105 allele OR 1.15, 95 per cent 0.86–1.53) or *CYP1A1* (val462 allele OR 0.98, 95 per cent CI: 0.75–1.29). It is unlikely that future single-site studies will refute these findings, but it is fairly clear that this level of risk is unlikely to be of use in clinical practice.

DNA REPAIR MECHANISMS

Some individuals may have increased cancer susceptibility due to defective DNA repair mechanisms. SCCHN is occasionally featured in several inherited cancer syndromes, which have impaired DNA repair mechanisms, including families with hereditary non-polyposis colorectal cancer, Bloom syndrome and ataxia telangectasia.[32,81] Only recently, polymorphisms have been studied in DNA repair genes in the normal population.[82,83] One case-control study has shown an elevated risk for SCCHN associated with polymorphisms in the *XRCC1* gene in patients who had tobacco and alcohol exposure,[84] but the effect was mainly evident on *post hoc* subgroup analysis.

SUSCEPTIBILITY TO GASTRIC CARCINOMA

Descriptive epidemiology of gastric cancer: the role of non-genetic factors

Gastric cancer is one of the commonest cancers in the world but is generally declining in the Western world, probably because of improvements in food quality and refrigeration. The reason for the lower incidence in the Middle East is not known. There are approximately 650 000 new cases of all types of gastric cancer worldwide every year and it is the second largest cause of cancer-related death.[85] More than 95 per cent of cases are adeno carcinoma of the intestinal or diffuse type and, in terms of parts of the stomach, carcinoma of the gastric cardia is increasing in incidence.[2,85] Countries with a high incidence include Japan, China and neighbouring areas, and Central and South America, with a lifetime cumulative incidence in the range of 5–10 per cent. Europe is an intermediate risk area (~2.5 per cent), and North America, the Middle East and Africa are 'low-risk' areas, with cumulative incidences below 1 per cent.[85]

Non-genetic risk factors for gastric cancer include low socioeconomic status, low intake of fruits and vegetables, low levels of antioxidants, consumption of salted, smoked or poorly preserved foods, cigarette smoking and possibly some industrial exposures. Some of these factors lead to conditions that are believed to be precursors of gastric adenocarcinoma. These include chronic atrophic gastritis, intestinal metaplasia, pernicious anaemia, partial gastrectomy for benign disease, *H. pylori* infection, Ménétrier's disease, adenomatous polyps and possibly Barrett's oesophagus.[86–88] Interestingly, in a cohort of nearly 25 000 individuals with duodenal ulcers, the incidence of gastric cancer was lower than expected,[89] supporting both the old data that blood group A is over-represented in those with gastric cancer, whereas for duodenal ulcer, it is group O that is more common[90] and the newer data on *II. pylori* and gastroduodenal disease (see later).

As mentioned, carcinoma of the gastric cardia is increasing, and now accounts for ~30 per cent of all cases of gastric cancer worldwide. It is 3–5 times more common in men than in women, and has similar risk factors as carcinoma of the lower oesophagus. It is particularly associated with gastro-oesophageal reflux disease.[91] While this increase is probably real, it should be noted that part of this increase could have resulted from misclassification.[92]

Epidemiology of gastric cancer: the role of genetic factors

For many years, it has been known that individuals with blood group type A and those with pernicious anaemia have an increased risk of gastric cancer.[90] Interestingly, an interaction between genetic and environmental factors has been identified in that the Lewis(b) blood group antigen mediates *H. pylori* attachment to human gastric mucosa,[93] but how this relates to increased risk for group A individuals is not clear. Pernicious anaemia, which to a certain extent is an inherited disorder and is more common in individuals with blood group A,[90] predisposes to chronic atrophic gastritis and this, in turn, can result in gastric carcinoma.[94]

Following the landmark case studies of Woolf and Isaacson[95] and Maimon and Zinninger,[96] much epidemiological evidence has accumulated over the past 40 years that familial and probably hereditary factors are important in the aetiology of gastric cancer. A number of the most relevant studies are summarized in Table 29.1. Overall, it can be seen that a first-degree family history of gastric cancer is associated with a 2–3 times increased risk for this disease. About 8 per cent of individuals with gastric cancer

Table 29.1 *Epidemiological studies of family history and risk of gastric cancer: selected studies*

Study	Country	Type	GCa cases	Controls (adjusted for)	Relative risk with FH+ of GCa (95% confidence interval)
Macklin[254]	USA	Case-control	167	1429	62 GCa vs. 41.4 expected ($p < 0.05$)
Lehtola et al.[272]	Finland	Case-control	341	2243 (age, sex)	FDR 1.5; intestinal type 1.4; diffuse type 7.0 ($p < 0.005$)
Mecklin et al.[255]	Finland (1963–84)	GCa < 40 years; 94% diffuse type; M = F	32	–	GCa in parents ($p < 0.001$)
Zanghieri et al.[256]	Italy	Case-control	154	154	FDR 3.1; parent ns; sibling 4.3
La Vecchia et al.[257]	Italy	Case-control	628	1766	FDR 2.6 (1.9–3.7)
Kato et al.[258]	Japan (1985–91)	Cohort study	57 (deaths)	9596 (smoking, alcohol, diet)	FDR 1.9 (1.0–3.4)
Palli et al.[259]	Italy	Case-control	116	1623 (nutrient intake)	Parent 1.7 (1.3–2.2); sibling 2.6; ≥2 siblings 8.5
La Vecchia et al.[260]	Italy (1985–93)	Case-control	746	2053	FDR 2.1 (1.5–3.0)
Nagase et al.[261]	Japan	Case-control	136	136	FDR 2.3 (1.1–5.0)
Kikuchi et al.[262]	Japan (1988–92)	GCa < 40 years; 86% diffuse type	108	–	GCa in parents ($p = 0.06$)
Inoue et al.[263]	Japan (1988–95)	Case-referent	995	43 846 (age, smoking, alcohol, diet)	FDR 1.5 (1.3–1.8)
Morita et al.[264]	Japan (1972–95)	Case-control	157 synchronous multiple GCa	157 solitary GCa (smoking, alcohol)	FDR 1.9 (1.1–3.5); ≥2 FDR: 5.1 (1.2–21)
Poole et al.[265]	USA (1959–72)	Case-control nested in CPS-I cohort	494 (females)	(age, race, education, smoking, BMI, number of siblings)	FDR 1.6 (1.1–2.4); parent 1.4; sibling 2.6; ≥2 FDR or <50 years 2.5 (1.4–4.4)

BMI, body mass index; FDR, first-degree relative; FH+, positive family history of cancer; GCa, gastric cancer; ns, not significant.

have some family history of gastric cancer. It appears that the risks are highest if there are only gastric cancers in the family, the histological subtype is diffuse or the location is in the cardia. There is some evidence that the risk of gastric cancer in an offspring is greater when the mother, rather than the father, is affected.

Underlying mechanisms for increased cancer susceptibility

CANCER PREDISPOSITION GENES

CDH1

The most important recent advance in the understanding of inherited susceptibility to gastric cancer came from the work of Reeve and colleagues.[97] They identified three germline mutations in *CDH1*, encoding E-cadherin, in a series of related Maori families with very strong family histories of gastric and other cancers. They then found further mutations in other families, some of which contained cases of lobular breast cancer.[98] Other groups subsequently confirmed their findings and showed that they were not limited to Maori populations, but also suggested that other genes underlying both diffuse and intestinal gastric cancer susceptibility probably do exist (Table 29.2). *CDH1* was an attractive candidate susceptibility gene for gastric cancer because previous work had shown that somatic mutations in this gene were common in diffuse gastric cancer (~50 per cent frequency),[99] whereas they were rare in the intestinal type[99] and abnormalities at the protein, mRNA and DNA level had been observed in human gastric cancer cell lines.[100] These cell lines had growth patterns characteristic of diffuse gastric carcinoma cells. Furthermore, E-cadherin was found to have an important role in the progression from adenoma to carcinoma in an animal model of pancreatic β-cell carcinogenesis.[101] More recently, it has been observed that double heterozygote mice, resulting from a cross between mice null for *CDH1* and mice carrying a disease-causing *Apc* mutation, had a fivefold increase in gastric tumours. Interestingly, the wild-type *CDH1* allele was retained in all cases and immunohistochemical staining remained positive. In humans with hereditary diffuse gastric cancer and *CDH1* mutations, there is rarely loss of heterozygosity (LOH) of the wild type allele. A recent study has shown that instead of LOH, the wild-type allele may be inactivated by methylation of the promoter,[102] leaving little or no normal E-cadherin protein in the gastric cancers.

Other cancers seen in *CDH1* mutation-positive families include colorectal and breast cancer, specifically the lobular subtype. Lobular breast cancers frequently contain somatic mutations in *CDH1*,[103] but germline mutations have not been seen in women with lobular carcinoma *in situ*.[104] It has not been possible to quantify the risk of colorectal cancer or lobular breast cancer in female *CDH1*

mutation carriers, partly because *CDH1* mutations are rare in the population. Nevertheless, risks for both of these cancers are likely to be considerably greater than in the population and increased surveillance from a young age is justified. Unfortunately, lobular breast cancers can be difficult to detect by mammography,[105] so other imaging methods, such as ultrasound and magnetic resonance imaging, are probably indicated.

MLH1, MSH2 and other hereditary non-polyposis colorectal cancer-related genes

Historically, one of the more common extra-colonic cancers seen in hereditary non-polyposis colorectal cancer (HNPCC) was stomach cancer. It has become rare in HNPCC kindreds in the Western world, perhaps mirroring the decrease in incidence of gastric cancer in the general population. It remains an important cause of morbidity and mortality in HNPCC families in those countries where gastric cancer is still a common disease. There have been several reports on the incidence and risk of gastric cancer in HNPCC families.[106–109] In a study from Finland, the lifetime risk of gastric cancer in 40 Amsterdam criteria 1 (AC1) positive families was close to 20 per cent and, among known *MLH1/MSH2* mutation carriers, the RR of gastric cancer was significantly elevated at 19.3 in families with *MSH2* mutations, but only 4.4 (not statistically significant) in *MLH1* families,[108] lending further weight to the idea that the *MSH2*-related phenotype may be broader than *MLH1*.[110] The pathological features of gastric cancers in HNPCC are not especially different from sporadic gastric cancer: the more common intestinal type predominates (79 per cent), *H. pylori* infection is seen in 20 per cent, but high-frequency microsatellite instability (MSI-H) occurs in almost three-quarters of all HNPCC-related gastric cancers.[109] Considering MSI-H as the starting point, it is seen in ~15 per cent of all gastric adenocarcinomas, particularly antral carcinomas[111] and in those with a family history of gastric cancer,[111,112] but is rare in tumours of the cardia.[113] Few of these MSI-H cases are likely to be due to germline *MLH1* or *MSH2* mutations, but instead may form a distinct biological subset, possibly related to hypermethylation of the *MLH1* promoter.[114] Hypermethylation was particularly frequent in MSI-H tumours, whereas it was not common in tumours where only one or two simple sequence length repeats showed abnormality (MSI-L). In colorectal cancer, MSI-H is associated with a better prognosis, even when accounting for stage. In gastric cancer, one study showed that MSI-H cancers were more likely be diploid, have a dense lymphocytic infiltrate and have fewer lymph node metastases.[115] Not surprisingly, this was associated with a better outcome.

Individuals with early-onset intestinal type gastric cancer should be evaluated for a family history of HNPCC-related cancers and, in selected cases, MSI or immunohistochemical analysis of MLH1/MSH2 should be offered.

Table 29.2 *Germline* CDH1 *mutations in gastric cancer families: all reported cases in English literature*

Study	Country	Families	Type of GCa	CDH1 mutation (exon)	Type of mutation	Notes
Guilford et al.[97]	New Zealand (Maori)	>25 deaths from GCa	Early-onset (<40 years) diffuse type	1008G > T (7)	Exon skipping	2 obligate carriers with CRC (30, 74 years). Founder mutations. (Maori)
		6 cases	≡ (<40 years)	2382insC (15)	Frameshift	
		Multiple cases	≡	2095C > T (13)	Nonsense	
Gayther et al.[266]	Europe	18 GCa families: 10 diffuse type + ≥2 FDR; 8 intestinal type + ≥2 FDR;				Large gastric polyposis family (see references 123 and 124) not linked
		9 GCa (45.5 years); 3 gen.	Diffuse	1711insG (11)	Frameshift	
		4 GCa (51 years); 3 gen.	Diffuse	187C > T (3)	Nonsense	
		6 GCa (31 years); 4 gen.	Diffuse	1792C > T (12)	Nonsense	
Richards et al.[267]	UK and Ireland	8 families (≥2 FDR, 1 < 50 years or ≥3 cases)	Diffuse	59G > A (2)	Nonsense	1 mutation carrier with CRC (30 years)
		3 GCa (38 years); 3 gen.	Diffuse	(49-2)A > G (2)	Exon skipping	
		6 GCa (50 years); 2 gen.				
Shinmura et al.[268]	Japan	3632 GCa: 31 families (0.9%) with 'AC for GCa' (59% intestinal type)				Sequence variant carrier was 61-year-old at diagnosis
		1/13 families	Diffuse	185G > T (3)	Gly62Val: polym.?	
Stone et al.[269]	UK	96 sporadic GCa (62 years), 10 GCa with FH+ (53.6 years)		No pathogenic mutation found (CSGE, sequencing)	–	
Guilford et al.[98]		5 GCa	Diffuse	1588insC (11)	Frameshift	Breast cancer of several and unknown histological types seen in family members.
		1 GCa and early-onset breast cancer		70G > T (2)	Nonsense	
				1137 + 1G > A (int. 8)	Exon skipping	
				586G > T (5)	Nonsense	
				190C > T (3)	Nonsense	
				1487del7 (10)	Frameshift	
Keller et al.[270]	Germany	7 GCa families	Diffuse	372delC (3)	Frameshift	1 mutation carrier; metachronous lobular breast cancer and diffuse GCa.
Lida et al.[273]	Japan	14 GCa families	8 at least one diffuse case 6 intestinal only	No pathogenic mutations identified (SSCP)		
Yoon et al.[271]	Korea	5 GCa families	Diffuse	244A > G (6)	Asp > Gly	Point mutations not found in controls.
				487T > C (10)	Val > Ala	

AC, Amsterdam criteria; CRC, colorectal cancer; CSGE, conformation-sensitive gel electrophoresis; FDR, first-degree relative; FH+, positive family history of cancer; GCa, gastric cancer; gen., generations; SSCP, single-strand conformation polymorphism.

Individuals at high risk of stomach cancer could be offered surveillance upper gastrointestinal endoscopy[116] but there are no data to support this management choice.

APC

The most common manifestation of familial adenomatous polyposis (FAP) in the stomach is fundic gland polyps. These hyperplastic lesions are seen in up to 75 per cent of individuals with FAP and in the past have been considered to be exclusively benign lesions. Recent data have suggested that these lesions may not always behave in a benign fashion. In a particularly worrying case report, Zwick *et al.* described the first example of a proven case of gastric adenocarcinoma that arose from a 3.5 cm hyperplastic fundic gland polyp situated on the greater curvature of the stomach.[117] At autopsy, this gland was found to have undergone partial malignant transformation to a high-grade adenocarcinoma, with widespread intra-abdominal metastases. Subsequently, it was reported that fundic gland polyps occurring in FAP are statistically significantly more likely to have increased proliferation, and loss of the normal topographical relationship between Ki-67 and p21^{Cip1}. Dysplasia was also much more common.[118] Therefore, it seems prudent to offer regular upper gastrointestinal endoscopy to all individuals with FAP, not only on the basis of an increased risk of ampullary carcinoma, but also to survey the stomach carefully. Fundic gland polyps have been reported to occur outside the context of FAP.[119,120] While a separate familial disorder may exist (the natural history does appear to differ from that seen in FAP-associated polyps), it is worth recalling that attenuated FAP (AFAP or AAPC) can present with upper intestinal features, including fundic gland polyps.[117,121,122] A case report of a family with FAP limited to the stomach, with gastric cancer developing in four of nine individuals in one generation[123] could represent an atypical presentation of AFAP, but a new genetic entity is perhaps more likely.[124] The family is not linked to the *CDH1* locus.

Despite this renewed interest in fundic gland polyps, the most important precursor of gastric cancer is the adenomatous polyp. In one study, gastric adenomas were only present in those who also had duodenal polyps,[125] whereas in another, they could occur separately.[126] The highest incidence of gastric cancer in FAP, as for HNPCC, is seen in Asian FAP kindreds.[127] The Japanese Polyposis Center has reported a 2 per cent incidence of adenoma-related gastric cancer.[128] The cumulative incidence of adenoma-related gastric cancer among non-Asian FAP cases is much lower (~0.6 per cent).[129–132] This is substantially lower than that observed for ampullary carcinoma.

LKB1/STK11

The causative gene in Peutz–Jeghers syndrome (PJS) is the serine-threonine kinase gene, *LKB1/STK11*. Hamartomatous polyps of the stomach are common in PJS, but gastric cancer is rather uncommon and there have been few reports,[133–136] with several cases originating from high-incidence areas.

DPC4/SMAD4

As detailed in Chapter 24, at least one gene for juvenile polyposis (JP) has been identified. This gene *DPC4/SMAD4* was found to be mutated in several families with JP.[137] It is rare for the stomach to be the only site of juvenile polyps, but cases and families have been reported,[138] and the hamartomatous polyps have been found to develop into frank malignancy in rare cases.[139] In most cases of gastric JP, there are colonic polyps as well. The gastric polyposis has been sufficiently severe in some cases to warrant gastrectomy because of carcinoma or protein-losing enteropathy. As for FAP and HNPCC, the gastric cancer in JP may be more common in Asia than in countries in the Western hemisphere.[140] If families with JP are ascertained solely because of intestinal polyps, a number of different diagnoses are arrived at. These have included Ruvacalba-Myre-Smith (caused by *PTEN* mutations, see below), Gorlin syndrome, caused by *PTCH* mutations (see Chapter 15) and even hereditary haemorrhagic telangiectasia.[141] The risk of gastric cancer in these three conditions has not been precisely estimated but it is likely to be very low.

PTEN

Cowden disease (CD) has been discussed in detail elsewhere (Chapter 12). There have been reports of lower intestinal cancer in CD but gastric cancer is very rare. As in FAP, hyperplastic polyposis appears to be the most common gastric manifestation of CD.[142,143]

BRCA1/2

Gastric cancer is not a common feature of families with either *BRCA1* or *BRCA2* mutations. Nevertheless, in the large Breast Cancer Linkage Consortium study, there was a significant excess (RR 2.6, 95% CI 1.5–4.6) of gastric cancer in the families of known *BRCA2* mutation carriers.[29] Pathological confirmation of the cases was not available in most families. No similar effect was seen for *BRCA1*.[144]

TP53

Li–Fraumeni syndrome (LFS) is often caused by germline mutations in *TP53* but gastric cancer is an uncommon feature of LFS (see Chapter 11). Once again, gastric cancer is more common in Japanese LFS kindreds than in Western families with LFS.[145–149] In some families, the gastric cancers have occurred at very young ages (<25 years).[145,149] It is very difficult to suggest a surveillance plan for LFS: gastric cancer is probably too rare in Western LFS families to justify regular endoscopy.

Other gastric cancer predisposition syndromes

Gastric adenocarcinoma have been reported in two African-American sisters with ataxia telangiectasia

(A-T),[150] but this must be an exceptionally rare manifestation of the tendency towards malignancy in A-T.

There has been a case report of a Portuguese family with autosomal dominant inheritance of hyperplastic polyposis of the stomach, progressing to diffuse gastric carcinoma, with additional family members with chronic atrophic gastritis and intestinal metaplasia.[124] It is not clear how this condition is related to other inherited disorders described above, in particular AFAP, but it appears to be different. No underlying causative mutation has been reported thus far. An Italian family has been described with five cases of gastric cancer over three generations, where all 11 (7M, 4F) siblings in the second generation (three of whom had gastric cancer) were found to have chronic atrophic gastritis and/or intestinal metaplasia.[151] Interestingly, the family diet consisted largely of deep-fried salt-cured pork and alcohol. Fresh vegetables were not consumed.

POLYMORPHISMS IN INFLAMMATION-REGULATING GENES AND *H. PYLORI* SUSCEPTIBILITY

Studies of relatives and co-habitants of patients with gastric dypslasia in high-incidence regions such as China have shown that both genetic and environmental factors are important in the aetiology of pre-cancerous lesions.[152] As discussed above, *H. pylori* infection is associated with an increased risk of gastric cancer.[153–156] If *H. pylori* infection is limited to the antrum, then acid secretion is normal or high, with a risk of duodenal ulcer, whereas extensive infection of the body of the stomach can lead to chronic gastritis, achlorhydria and an increased risk for gastric cancer. *H. pylori* infection is insufficient to cause gastric cancer: infection is common in Africa, but the disease is rare and up to 50 per cent of North Americans are infected but less than 1 per cent of those infected develop gastric cancer.[154] Why some infected individuals develop severe chronic gastritis and others do not is not known, but it is likely that genetic factors are important. In a recent study, almost 70 per cent of the first-degree relatives of gastric cancer cases had evidence of *H. pylori* infection, compared with less than half of the controls.[157] In another study, while there was no difference in *H. pylori* infection rates among relatives of gastric cancer cases and controls, hypochlorhydria and gastric atrophy were very much more common in the case relatives.[158] The common factor could be genetic or non-genetic, but familial. Interleukin 1β (IL-1β) is both a pro-inflammatory cytokine and an inhibitor of gastric acid secretion, which makes it an attractive candidate protein. Interestingly, in the presence of *H. pylori* infection, certain IL-1 genotypes appear to predict both low acid secretion and gastric atrophy among the case relatives.[159] When these gastric atrophy-related alleles were studied in 366 cases of gastric cancer and 429 controls, there was a significant association between the alleles and gastric cancer. For one of the associated alleles, the risk did not vary significantly between heterozygotes and homozygotes. Important supportive evidence for aetiological connections between IL-1β polymorphisms, *H. pylori*, chronic gastritis, hypochlohydria and gastric cancer was provided by studies of the effect of disease-associated IL-1β alleles on IL-1β induction *in vitro*.[159]

METABOLIC ENZYME POLYMORPHISMS

Several studies of the relationship between gastric cancer and polymorphisms in *GSTM1*,[160,161] *GSTT1*,[65,160] *GSTP1*[161] and *CYP2E1*[162] have been carried out, but none have resulted in conclusive findings. The *N*-acetyl transferases *NAT1* and *NAT2* have been implicated in susceptibility to bladder, colorectal and head and neck cancer (see earlier). There does not appear to be an important role for polymorphisms in these genes in the aetiology of gastric cancer.[163] A recent study of the DNA repair gene *XRCC1* suggested that certain genotypes were associated with a twofold increased risk of gastric cancer, particularly of the cardia.[164] However, this conclusion was reached *post hoc* by combining two genotypes and then studying an anatomical subtype. Clearly a study primarily focused on this site will be required. Other studies of *L-myc*[165] and spasmolysin[166] have been negative.

SUSCEPTIBILITY TO PANCREATIC ADENOCARCINOMA

Epidemiology of pancreatic adenocarcinoma: the role of non-genetic factors

Approximately 170 000 new cases of pancreatic cancer occur worldwide yearly.[85] This number represents 2.1 per cent of all cancers and the disease is more prevalent in developed countries. The highest age-adjusted incidence rates are observed in Eastern Europe, Japan and North America, and the lowest age-adjusted incidence rates are seen in Northern and Western Africa, and Southern Asia. The lifetime probability of developing pancreatic cancer in developed countries is approximately 1 per cent.[167] In North America, the incidence rates of pancreatic cancer have remained constant or have declined slightly over the last 25 years. In Japan and in nearly all European countries, the incidence rates of the disease have continued to rise.[168] Pancreatic cancer is the fifth most common cause of cancer-related deaths in both men and women in Western countries, causing more cancer deaths in Canada than brain cancer and melanoma combined.[169] Currently, 80–90 per cent of the tumours are diagnosed at a non-resectable stage and the case:fatality ratio for adenocarcinoma of the cancer is approximately 0.99.[170,171] Numerous epidemiological studies, including descriptive, case-control and cohort studies, investigated a variety of environmental factors suspected to be implicated in the genesis of pancreatic cancer. The only consistent environmental risk factor for pancreatic cancer is cigarette smoking, with an increased relative risk of approximately two (much less than for lung or head and neck cancer).[172] Higher dietary intake of saturated fat, particularly cholesterol, red meat, carbohydrate and salt were associated with an increased risk, and fruits, vegetables and dietary fibre were reported to be protective factors.[173–175] Importantly, alcohol consumption, coffee drinking and exposure to ionizing radiation are no longer considered as significant risk factors for pancreatic cancer. More recently, exposures to certain chemicals, such as metalworking fluids in working environments, have been implicated as risk factors for pancreatic adenocarcinoma.[176] Pre-existing medical disorders, such as pancreatitis, are a risk factor for subsequent pancreatic adenocarcinoma.[177,178] Interestingly, the possibility that some forms of chronic pancreatitis may represent an indolent manifestation of pancreatic cancer has been recently raised.[179]

Both a large cohort study[180] and a meta-analysis of 20 case-control and cohort studies[181] concluded that there was an approximately twofold increase in risk of pancreatic cancer in association with a history of diabetes mellitus. Notably, the RR was still significantly elevated when the history of diabetes mellitus preceded the diagnosis of pancreatic cancer by more than 5 years.

Epidemiology of pancreatic adenocarcinoma: the role of genetic factors

Several case-control studies have showed that there is an increased risk for pancreatic cancer among individuals reporting the diagnosis of any cancer in a close relative.[182–185] Studies have found that the relative risks are in the range of 1.5–4.0 and the risks tend to be largest when more relatives are affected. A recent study of 174 cases and 136 controls from Canada resulted in a RR of 5.0 in association with a family history of pancreatic cancer.[186] Interestingly, the lifetime risk was 12.5 per cent for the relatives of cases who had multiple primary cancers. Clinicoepidemiological results of 84 families with two or more first-degree relatives affected with pancreatic cancer have been compared with 165 families with sporadic pancreatic cancer registered in the National Familial Pancreas Tumor Registry.[187] No difference in the mean age of onset was noted in the 80 familial cases compared to the 132 sporadic cases (65.8 vs. 65.2 years). There was a non-significant increase of second primary cancer among the familial pancreatic cancer index cases and in their first-degree relatives compared to the sporadic cancer group. Overall,

it appears that 3–5 per cent of newly diagnosed pancreatic cancers are familial.

There was a statistically significant excess (RR 1.7) of pancreatic cancer in the male first-degree relatives of Icelandic women with breast cancer.[188] This risk was greater if the proband was diagnosed with breast cancer at less than 45 years of age rather than 45 years or older (2.2 vs. 1.5). A proportion of this risk may be attributed to a founder BRCA2 mutation (999del5) prevalent in the Icelandic population (see later).

Increased risk of pancreatic cancer as a second primary malignancy was reported after testicular cancer (RR 2.2).[189] A previous population-based study showed a significant increased risk after prostate cancer and smoking-related cancers (i.e. lung, head and neck, and bladder cancers) with RR less than 2, except for lung cancer in females (RR 2.5, 95% CI 1.9–3.2).[190] In a study from the Swedish Nationwide Family Cancer Database, a statistically significant increased risk for pancreatic cancer was recorded for offspring from parents affected by stomach, colon and liver cancer.[191] With a father affected by pancreatic cancer, a significant increased risk was noted for melanoma, breast, uterus, lung and liver cancer. It should be noted that, in this study, offspring ages ranged between 15 and 53 years, which is far younger than the mean age of pancreatic cancer diagnosis.

A high risk of pancreas cancer has been shown in patients with hereditary pancreatitis (see later).

Underlying mechanisms for increased cancer susceptibility

CANCER PREDISPOSITION GENES

CDKN2A

Germline mutations in CDKN2A underlie some cases of familial melanoma, with or without dysplastic naevi. The clinical manifestation includes multiple naevi, multiple atypical naevi and multiple malignant melanomas (cutaneous or ocular). Pancreatic adenocarcinoma is probably the second most common cancer in familial melanoma (FM) – sometimes referred to as familial atypical mole-multiple melanoma (FAMMM) syndrome or dysplastic naevus syndrome (DNS), although these three disorders may not be the same. The observed/expected ratio for pancreatic cancer among 200 members of nine melanoma-prone families was 13.4 ($p < 0.001$).[192] Affected family members had an incidence of pancreatic cancer that is 29 times that of the general population.

In several chromosome 9p-linked FM kindreds, a mutation in the cell-cycle inhibitor gene CDKN2A/p16/MTS1 has been found to co-segregate with both melanoma and pancreatic adenocarcinoma.[23] Using an in vitro assay, Goldstein et al. distinguished between FM kindreds with a functionally defective p16 protein and kindreds without defective p16 gene product.[193] An 22-fold excess risk of pancreatic cancer was restricted to those kindreds with impaired p16 function. Independent reports confirmed an increased risk of pancreatic cancer in FM kindreds with identified *CDKN2A* germline mutations.[25,194,195] Following this report, 21 kindreds with familial pancreatic cancer without FM were screened for germline mutations in *CDKN2A* and in the related *CDK4* gene.[196] A germline *CDKN2A* mutation was identified in only one family and one of the affected carriers also had a melanoma. Moreover, it is not completely clear that this missense mutation (Asp145Cys) is disease causing. Lal *et al.* recently screened a series of 38 patients with pancreatic cancer considered as high or intermediate risk, based on their family history for *CDKN2A*, *BRCA1* and *BRCA2* germline mutations.[197] One *CDKN2A* mutation was identified. The same research team have also identified mutations in *CDKN2A* in 2 of 14 individuals with both pancreatic cancer and melanoma,[198] adding further weight to the previously reported association between these cancers.

BRCA1 and BRCA2

Hereditary breast cancer can be site-specific, but in many families other cancers are seen in those who have inherited the at-risk haplotype. Ovarian cancer is seen in excess in most *BRCA1*-linked families.[199] An increased risk for male breast cancer and prostate cancer has been well recognized for *BRCA2* mutation carriers.[200] Pancreatic adenocarcinoma is seen in some breast cancer families, accounted for by *BRCA1*, and more consistently by *BRCA2* mutations.[201,202] Two cases of early-onset pancreatic cancer, where the at-risk haplotype was inherited, were seen in 15 Swedish kindreds with *BRCA1* mutations.[203] Four out of seven families with known *BRCA2* mutations were found to have at least one case of pancreatic cancer,[204] and three of seven breast cancer pedigrees from Iceland contain one or more cases of pancreatic or biliary tract cancer.[205] Most Icelandic breast cancer families can be accounted for by the founder 999del5 mutation in *BRCA2*.[206] Two mutations in *BRCA1* (185delAG, 5382insC) and one mutation in *BRCA2* (6174delT) are common in the Ashkenazi Jewish population. A family history of pancreatic cancer was predictive of the presence of a *BRCA2* mutation in Ashkenazi Jewish families with breast cancer ($p = 0.01$),[207] and there was an association between cancer of the pancreas and ovary in two recent studies.[208,209] In another study, 38 patients with pancreatic cancer from 'intermediate'- or 'high'-risk pedigrees, were screened for *BRCA1/2* mutations. Four were identified: all mutation carriers were Ashkenazi Jewish.[197]

In a mutation screen of a panel of 41 pancreatic adenocarcinomas for *BRCA2* mutations, 4 of the 41 cancers had both a loss of one allele and a mutation in the other allele.[210] Interestingly, three of these mutations were germline (two cases with 6174delT, one case with 2458insT). The study was then enlarged to a series of 214 pancreatic adenocarcinomas for *BRCA2* mutations in the region of the 6174delT mutation. Two additional germline mutations were detected (6174delT and 6158insT). In total, five *BRCA2* germline alterations were identified among the 255 studied specimens. Only one of the five patients with *BRCA2* germline mutation had a relative with breast cancer and one had a relative with prostate cancer. None had a family history of pancreatic cancer. Another study reported the prevalence of the *BRCA2* 6174delT mutation in 39 Jewish individuals with pancreatic cancer.[211] Four germline mutations were identified (10 per cent), and the cumulative risk of pancreatic cancer to age 75 was estimated to be about 7 per cent (95% CI 1.9–19 per cent) in carriers of this mutation, compared to a risk of 0.85 per cent in the general population. All four mutation carriers lacked a family history of breast or pancreatic cancer in any first-degree relatives, and the mean age at diagnosis was 66 years.[211]

STK11/LKB1

Mutations in this serine/threonine kinase gene cause Peutz–Jeghers syndrome. As discussed in Chapter 24, PJS is inherited as an autosomal dominant trait. It is characterized by hamartomatous gastrointestinal polyps and mucocutaneous pigmentation. PJ patients frequently present neoplasms of the colon, stomach, small intestine, breast, ovaries and cervix. Of 31 PJ patients from 13 unrelated kindreds followed from 1973 to 1985, 15 (48 per cent) developed cancer; four had adenocarcinoma of the pancreas, which represents a 100-fold excess of pancreatic cancer compared to the general population.[212] In another study, 16 (22 per cent) of 72 PJ patients developed cancer; of these, there was one case of pancreatic cancer.[213] An adolescent male with PJS has been reported as having died of pancreatic adenocarcinoma[214] and other anecdotal cases of PJ patients developing adenocarcinoma of the pancreas have been reported.[215,216] A germline mutation in *STK11/LKB1* has been identified in the original Dutch family described by Peutz in 1921.[217] Seven of the 22 PJ patients in this kindred died from cancer but no pancreatic cancer was definitively diagnosed. An individual with pancreas cancer and a known *LKB1* mutation was found to have loss of heterozygosity at the PJS locus in the pancreas cancer, but not in an adjacent hamartomatous duodenal polyp.[218]

MLH1, MSH2 AND OTHER HNPCC-RELATED GENES

HNPCC is associated with an increased risk of colorectal cancer and to a lesser extent to cancers of other localizations (i.e. endometrium, stomach, ovary, biliary and urinary tracts, and small intestine). Pancreatic cancer is sometimes included in the tumour spectrum of HNPCC. Lynch *et al.* have described a number of HNPCC kindreds

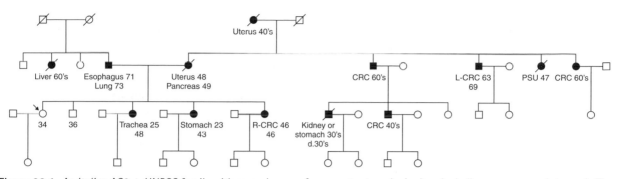

Figure 29.1 *An Italian AC2 + HNPCC family with several cases of cancer at extracolonic sites, including pancreas and stomach. The individual with tracheal cancer at age 25 does not carry the familial* MLH1 *mutation (intron 6 A > G at 545 + 3). We thank Georges Chong, Department of Medicine, SMBD-Jewish General Hospital, Montreal, Quebec, Canada for identifying the mutation and Lidia Kasprzak for working with this family.*

with at least one person diagnosed with pancreatic cancer[219,220] but it is not certain whether the excess number of cases seen is a chance finding, possibly related to ascertainment biases.[221] An investigation of 22 Dutch HNPCC families identified no cases of pancreatic cancer among 148 cancer patients.[222] In a study of 50 Finnish HNPCC kindreds, three of 360 *MLH1* mutation carriers developed pancreatic carcinoma.[223] This is a non-significant excess. No genotype–phenotype correlation, especially regarding the risk for pancreatic cancer, has been established.[224] An example of a family with a germline *MLH1* mutation and a confirmed case of pancreas cancer is shown in Figure 29.1. Interestingly, in this family, there is also a case of gastric cancer and colorectal cancer proven not to be due to the family mutation. Another, perhaps less biased way of looking at this issue is to ascertain individuals with double primary cancers featured in the relevant hereditary syndrome, and estimate the risk of cancer for their first-degree relatives (FDRs). In a study of 964 FDRs of 70 women with invasive cancers of both the endometrium and colorectum,[225] there were eight cases of pancreas observed, but only 2.5 were expected, resulting in a RR of 3.2 (95% CI 1.4–6.3). Interestingly, if the proband had been diagnosed with both cancers at less than 55 years of age, the RR for pancreas cancer in FDRs was 41 (95% CI 11–106) for cases of pancreas cancer diagnosed under 55. The RR was 4.8 (not statistically significant) for those diagnosed with pancreas cancer over 55 years of age. There was no effect on pancreas cancer risk if the proband was diagnosed with both cancers after age 55, suggesting that the risk was limited to families that are likely to carry a mutation in *MLH1* or *MSH2*, as the presence of both endometrial and colorectal cancer at less than 55 years of age is a feature of mutation-positive families.[226]

APC

Familial adenomatous polyposis (FAP) is characterized by the presence of hundreds of colorectal adenomas, which often progress to carcinomas (see Chapter 24).

The disease, which is inherited in an autosomal dominant fashion, is also associated with a number of benign and malignant extracolonic lesions, including, rarely, cancer of the pancreas. A study of 197 FAP pedigrees found a RR of 4.5 (95% CI 1.2–11.4) for pancreatic adenocarcinoma in patients with this syndrome.[227] It is possible that the majority of these cases of pancreatic cancer actually originated in the ampulla. For example, three periampullary carcinoma cases were noted in a recent series of 190 unrelated FAP families, but the statistical significance of the data were not reported.[228]

ATM

Ataxia telangiectasia (A-T) is an autosomal recessively inherited syndrome characterized by progressive cerebellar ataxia, oculocutaneous telangiectasia, cellular and humoral immune deficiencies, and a risk of lymphoproliferative malignancies (see Chapter 13). The causative gene is known as *ATM*. There is an increase in the incidence of cancer in *ATM* homozygotes, including leukaemias, and breast, ovarian and gastric cancers, and, at least for breast cancer, in heterozygotes as well.[229] Oddly, in one study, this increased risk for breast cancer was only seen in the mothers of affected children.[230] A number of studies investigating the incidence of cancer in the relatives of patients with A-T report an association of pancreatic adenocarcinoma with the syndrome. In a study of 110 White families with A-T, seven cases of pancreatic cancer were observed in blood relatives of A-T patients (3.3 cases were expected).[231] Among spouse controls, only one case was observed (1.3 were expected). In a prospective follow-up study of 161 A-T families, six cases of pancreatic cancer were diagnosed in the group formed by adult blood relatives of patients with A-T, and no case was diagnosed in their spouses considered as the control group.[232]

TP53

Adenocarcinoma of the pancreas may also be included in the tumour spectrum of the Li–Fraumeni syndrome

(LFS), but it is rare. In a study of 24 LFS kindreds, one case of pancreatic cancer was seen in each of three families and two cases were seen in a fourth.[233] LFS is often caused by a germline mutation of the tumour suppressor TP53 gene. In a synopsis of 91 families with TP53 germline mutations, half of them fulfilling the diagnostic criteria of the LFS, pancreatic cancer accounted for only 1 per cent of all the 475 tumours registered.[234]

SMAD4/DPC4

Germline mutations in SMAD4/DPC4 were found in five of nine kindreds with juvenile polyposis syndrome[137,235] and cases of pancreatic cancer in the context of juvenile polyposis syndrome have been reported.[236,237] Thus, the SMAD4/DPC4 gene, mapped on chromosome 18q21.1, a tumour suppressor gene predominantly inactivated in pancreatic cancer, is an attractive candidate as a pancreas cancer susceptibility gene.[238] However, to date, germline mutations in SMAD4/DPC4 have not been found in familial pancreatic cancer cases.[239]

Other genes

Hereditary pancreatitis (HP) is inherited as an autosomal dominant disorder with an estimated penetrance of 80 per cent and variable expressivity. HP is clinically characterized by recurrent episodes of acute pancreatitis with an onset usually before 10 years of age, in blood-related family members over two generations. The disease usually progresses to chronic pancreatitis. HP may account for 3–6 per cent of all pancreatitis, and an increased risk for pancreatic cancer is well recognized in this condition, with a prevalence of up to 20 per cent.[240] A more recent epidemiological study of a historical cohort of 246 patients with HP showed a cumulative lifetime risk of developing pancreatic cancer by the age of 70 years of approximately 40 per cent. The mean age of the eight adenocarcinomas in this series was 56.9 years. Interestingly, the lifetime risk rose to 75 per cent with paternal transmission of HP mutation.[241]

Some forms of HP have been attributed to a germline founder mutation (R117H) in the cationic trypsinogen gene (PRSS1/TRY1) mapped on chromosome 7q35.[242] A recent multi-centre study showed that among 112 HP families, 52% probands carried the R122H mutation, 21% had N29I and 4% had A16V. Nineteen percent had no mutation identified.[243] Negative linkage and absence of mutations in PRSS1 in other HP families suggest locus heterogeneity in HP.[244,245]

In patients with idiopathic chronic pancreatitis (ICP), mutations in the cystic fibrosis gene, CFTR have been occasionally identified[246,247] and similarly mutations in the serine protease inhibitor, Kazal type 1 (SPINK1) have been reported in a significant proportion of individuals with ICP: 43% of those with early-onset ICP had either homozygous or heterozygous N34S mutations in SPINK1.[248,249] However, there is very little direct evidence

that mutations in either of these genes specifically predispose to pancreatic cancer.[250,251]

METABOLIC ENZYME POLYMORPHISMS

Little is known about the impact of genetic polymorphisms of metabolic enzymes in pancreas carcinogenesis. A recent case-control study of pancreatic adenocarcinoma conducted in Montreal and Toronto, Canada, found no significant association between GSTM1, GSTT1 and CYP1A1 alleles and the occurrence of pancreatic cancer.[252] A previous study[253] had suggested a borderline effect, so it seems unlikely that these polymorphisms have any important role in pancreatic carcinogenesis.

ACKNOWLEDGEMENT

Work in WDF's laboratory of relevance to this chapter has been funded by the Cancer Research Society.

KEY POINTS

- Head and neck cancer, particularly if associated with multiple primaries, is associated with an increased cancer risk in relatives of upper aerodigestive tract cancer.
- Stomach cancer rarely shows familial aggregation. Helicobacter screening should be considered. Linitus plastica form is associated with mutations in the E Cadherin gene and carriers should be offered prophylactic gastrectomy.
- Familial pancreatic cancer is described. Screening is with MRI and ERPC.

REFERENCES

1. Macfarlane GJ, Boyle P, Evstifeeva TV, et al. Rising trends of oral cancer mortality among males worldwide: the return of an old public health problem. Cancer Causes Control 1994; 5:259–265.
2. Parkin DM, Pisani P, Ferlay J. Estimates of the worldwide incidence of eighteen major cancers in 1985. Int J Cancer 1993; 54:594–606.
3. Liu BQ, Peto R, Chen ZM, et al. Emerging tobacco hazards in China: 1. Retrospective proportional mortality study of one million deaths. Br Med J 1998; 317:1411–1422.
4. Vokes EE, Weichselbaum RR, Lippman SM, Hong WK. Head and neck cancer. N Engl J Med 1993; 328:184–194.
5. Maier H, Dietz A, Gewelke U, et al. Tobacco and alcohol and the risk of head and neck cancer. Clin Invest 1992; 70:320–327.
6. Maier H, Dietz A, Gewelke U, Heller WD. Occupational exposure to hazardous substances and risk of cancer in the area of the

mouth cavity, oropharynx, hypopharynx and larynx. A case-control study. *Laryngorhinootologie* 1991; **70**:93–98.

7. Muscat JE, Wynder EL. Tobacco, alcohol, asbestos, and occupational risk factors for laryngeal cancer. *Cancer* 1992; **69**:2244–2251.

8. Copper MP, Jovanovic A, Nauta JJ, *et al.* Role of genetic factors in the etiology of squamous cell carcinoma of the head and neck. *Arch Otolaryngol Head Neck Surg* 1995; **121**:157–160.

9. Foulkes WD, Brunet JS, Kowalski LP, *et al.* Family history of cancer is a risk factor for squamous cell carcinoma of the head and neck in Brazil: a case-control study. *Int J Cancer* 1995; **63**:769–773.

10. Foulkes WD, Brunet JS, Sieh W, *et al.* Familial risks of squamous cell carcinoma of the head and neck: retrospective case-control study. *Br Med J* 1996; **313**:716–721.

11. De Andrade M, Amos CI, Foulkes WD. Segregation analysis of squamous cell carcinoma of the head and neck: evidence for a major gene determining risk. *Ann Hum Genet* 1998; **62**:505–510.

12. Goldstein AM, Blot WJ, Greenberg RS, *et al.* Familial risk in oral and pharyngeal cancer. *Eur J Cancer* 1994; **30B**:319–322.

13. Gluckman JL, Crissman JD. Survival rates in 548 patients with multiple neoplasms of the upper aerodigestive tract. *Laryngoscope* 1983; **93**:71–74.

14. Day GL, Blot WJ. Second primary tumors in patients with oral cancer. *Cancer* 1992; **70**:14–19.

15. Shah S, Evans DG, Blair V, *et al.* Assessment of relative risk of second primary tumors after ovarian cancer and of the usefulness of double primary cases as a source of material for genetic studies with a cancer registry. *Cancer* 1993; **72**:819–827.

16. Pal T, Flanders T, Mitchell-Lehman M, *et al.* Genetic implications of double primary cancers of the colorectum and endometrium. *J Med Genet* 1998; **35**:978–984.

17. Bongers V, Braakhuis BJ, Tobi H, *et al.* The relation between cancer incidence among relatives and the occurrence of multiple primary carcinomas following head and neck cancer. *Cancer Epidemiol Biomarkers Prev* 1996; **5**:595–598.

18. Morita M, Kuwano H, Ohno S, *et al.* Multiple occurrence of carcinoma in the upper aerodigestive tract associated with esophageal cancer: reference to smoking, drinking and family history. *Int J Cancer* 1994; **58**:207–210.

19. Serrano M, Hannon GJ, Beach D. A new regulatory motif in cell-cycle control causing specific inhibition of cyclin D/CDK4. *Nature* 1993; **366**:704–707.

20. Kamb A, Gruis NA, Weaver-Feldhaus J, *et al.* A cell cycle regulator potentially involved in genesis of many tumor types. *Science* 1994; **264**:436–440.

21. Reed AL, Califano J, Cairns P, *et al.* High frequency of *p16* (*CDKN2/MTS-1/INK4A*) inactivation in head and neck squamous cell carcinoma. *Cancer Res* 1996; **56**:3630–3633.

22. Kamb A, Shattuck-Eidens D, Eeles R, *et al.* Analysis of the *p16* gene (*CDKN2*) as a candidate for the chromosome 9p melanoma susceptibility locus. *Nature Genet* 1994; **8**:23–26.

23. Hussussian CJ, Struewing JP, Goldstein AM, *et al.* Germline *p16* mutations in familial melanoma. *Nature Genet* 1994; **8**:15–21.

24. Yarbrough WG, Aprelikova O, Pei H, *et al.* Familial tumor syndrome associated with a germline nonfunctional *p16INK4a* allele. *J Natl Cancer Inst* 1996; **88**:1489–1491.

25. Whelan AJ, Bartsch D, Goodfellow PJ. Brief report: a familial syndrome of pancreatic cancer and melanoma with a mutation in the *CDKN2* tumor-suppressor gene. *N Engl J Med* 1995; **333**:975–977.

26. Sun S, Pollock PM, Liu L, *et al.* CDKN2A mutation in a non-FAMMM kindred with cancers at multiple sites results in

a functionally abnormal protein. *Int J Cancer* 1997; **73**:531–536.

27. Jefferies S, Edwards SM, Hamoudi RA, *et al.* No germline mutations in *CDKN2A* (p16) in patients with squamous cell cancer of the head and neck and second primary tumours. *Br J Cancer* 2001; **85**:1383–1386.

28. Easton DF, Steele L, Fields P, *et al.* Cancer risks in two large breast cancer families linked to *BRCA2* on chromosome 13q12–13. *Am J Hum Genet* 1997; **61**:120–128.

29. Cancer risks in *BRCA2* mutation carriers. The Breast Cancer Linkage Consortium. *J Natl Cancer Inst* 1999; **91**:1310–1316.

30. Tonin PN, Mes-Masson AM, Futreal PA, *et al.* Founder *BRCA1* and *BRCA2* mutations in French Canadian breast and ovarian cancer families. *Am J Hum Genet* 1998; **63**:1341–1351.

31. Hamel N, Manning A, Black MJ, *et al.* An absence of founder *BRCA2* mutations in individuals with squamous cell carcinoma of the head and neck. *Int J Cancer* 1999; **83**:803–804.

32. Trizna Z, Schantz SP. Hereditary and environmental factors associated with risk and progression of head and neck cancer. *Otolaryngol Clin North Am* 1992; **25**:1089–1103.

33. Wang Q, Lasset C, Sobol H, Ozturk M. Evidence of a hereditary *p53* syndrome in cancer-prone families. *Int J Cancer* 1996; **65**:554–557.

34. Gallo O, Sardi I, Pepe G, *et al.* Multiple primary tumors of the upper aerodigestive tract: is there a role for constitutional mutations in the *p53* gene? *Int J Cancer* 1999; **82**:180–186.

35. Storey A, Thomas M, Kalita A, *et al.* Role of a *p53* polymorphism in the development of human papillomavirus-associated cancer. *Nature* 1998; **393**:229–234.

36. Zehbe I, Voglino G, Wilander E, *et al.* Codon 72 polymorphism of *p53* and its association with cervical cancer. *Lancet* 1999; **354**:218–219.

37. Giannoudis A, Graham DA, Southern SA, Herrington CS. *p53* codon 72 ARG/PRO polymorphism is not related to HPV type or lesion grade in low- and high-grade squamous intra-epithelial lesions and invasive squamous carcinoma of the cervix. *Int J Cancer* 1999; **83**:66–69.

38. Wang NM, Tsai CH, Yeh KT, *et al.* p53 codon 72Arg polymorphism is not a risk factor for carcinogenesis in the chinese. *Int J Mol Med* 1999; **4**:249–252.

39. Yamashita T, Yaginuma Y, Saitoh Y, *et al.* Codon 72 polymorphism of *p53* as a risk factor for patients with human papillomavirus-associated squamous intraepithelial lesions and invasive cancer of the uterine cervix. *Carcinogenesis* 1999; **20**:1733–1736.

40. Ngan HY, Liu VW, Liu SS. Risk of cervical cancer is not increased in Chinese carrying homozygous arginine at codon 72 of *p53*. *Br J Cancer* 1999; **80**:1828–1829.

41. Hamel N, Black MJ, Ghadirian P, Foulkes WD. No association between *p53* codon 72 polymorphism and risk of squamous cell carcinoma of the head and neck. *Br J Cancer* 2000; **82**:757–759.

42. Marin MC, Jost CA, Brooks LA, *et al.* A common polymorphism acts as an intragenic modifier of mutant *p53* behaviour. *Nat Genet* 2000; **25**:47–54.

43. Cheng L, Eicher SA, Guo Z, *et al.* Reduced DNA repair capacity in head and neck cancer patients. *Cancer Epidemiol Biomarkers Prev* 1998; **7**:465–468.

44. Wei Q, Eicher SA, Guan Y, *et al.* Reduced expression of MLH1 and GTBP/MSH6: a risk factor for head and neck cancer. *Cancer Epidemiol Biomarkers Prev* 1998; **7**:309–314.

45. Hsu TC, Cherry LM, Samaan NA. Differential mutagen susceptibility in cultured lymphocytes of normal individuals and cancer patients. *Cancer Genet Cytogenet* 1985; **17**:307–313.

46. Cloos J, Reid CB, Snow GB, Braakhuis BJ. Mutagen sensitivity: enhanced risk assessment of squamous cell carcinoma. *Eur J Cancer Oral Oncol* 1996; **32B**:367–372.

47. Schantz SP, Hsu TC. Mutagen-induced chromosome fragility within peripheral blood lymphocytes of head and neck cancer patients. *Head Neck* 1989; **11**:337–342.

48. Bondy ML, Spitz MR, Halabi S, *et al.* Association between family history of cancer and mutagen sensitivity in upper aerodigestive tract cancer patients. *Cancer Epidemiol Biomarkers Prev* 1993; **2**:103–106.

49. Schantz SP, Hsu TC, Ainslie N, Moser RP. Young adults with head and neck cancer express increased susceptibility to mutagen-induced chromosome damage. *JAMA* 1989; **262**:3313–3315.

50. Trizna Z, Clayman GL, Spitz MR, *et al.* Glutathione S-transferase genotypes as risk factors for head and neck cancer. *Am J Surg* 1995; **170**:499–501.

51. Hong WK, Lippman SM, Itri LM, *et al.* Prevention of second primary tumors with isotretinoin in squamous-cell carcinoma of the head and neck. *N Engl J Med* 1990; **323**:795–801.

52. Cloos J, Nieuwenhuis EJ, Boomsma DI, *et al.* Inherited susceptibility to bleomycin-induced chromatid breaks in cultured peripheral blood lymphocytes. *J Natl Cancer Inst* 1999; **91**:1125–1130.

53. Board P, Coggan M, Johnston P, *et al.* Genetic heterogeneity of the human glutathione transferases: a complex of gene families. *Pharmacol Ther* 1990; **48**:357–369.

54. Board P, Coggan M, Johnston P, *et al.* Genetic heterogeneity of the human glutathione transferases: a complex of gene families. *Pharmacol Ther* 1990; **48**:357–369.

55. Zhong S, Wyllie AH, Barnes D, *et al.* Relationship between the GSTM1 genetic polymorphism and susceptibility to bladder, breast and colon cancer. *Carcinogenesis* 1993; **14**:1821–1824.

56. Nazar-Stewart V, Motulsky AG, Eaton DL, *et al.* The glutathione S-transferase mu polymorphism as a marker for susceptibility to lung carcinoma. *Cancer Res* 1993; **53**:2313–2318.

57. Brockmoller J, Kerb R, Drakoulis N, *et al.* Glutathione S-transferase M1 and its variants A and B as host factors of bladder cancer susceptibility: a case-control study. *Cancer Res* 1994; **54**:4103–4111.

58. Heagerty AH, Fitzgerald D, Smith A, *et al.* Glutathione S-transferase GSTM1 phenotypes and protection against cutaneous tumours. *Lancet* 1994; **343**:266–268.

59. Hirvonen A, Pelin K, Tammilehto L, *et al.* Inherited GSTM1 and NAT2 defects as concurrent risk modifiers in asbestos-related human malignant mesothelioma. *Cancer Res* 1995; **55**:2981–2983.

60. Johns LE, Houlston RS. Glutathione S-transferase mu1 (GSTM1) status and bladder cancer risk: a meta-analysis. *Mutagenesis* 2000; **15**:399–404.

61. Houlston RS. Glutathione S-transferase M1 status and lung cancer risk: a meta-analysis. *Cancer Epidemiol Biomarkers Prev* 1999; **8**:675–682.

62. London SJ, Daly AK, Cooper J, *et al.* Polymorphism of glutathione S-transferase M1 and lung cancer risk among African-Americans and Caucasians in Los Angeles County, California. *J Natl Cancer Inst* 1995; **87**:1246–1253.

63. Katoh T. The frequency of glutathione-S-transferase M1 (GSTM1) gene deletion in patients with lung and oral cancer. *Sangyo Igaku* 1994; **36**:435–439.

64. Jahnke V, Matthias C, Fryer A, Strange R. Glutathione S-transferase and cytochrome-P-450 polymorphism as risk factors for squamous cell carcinoma of the larynx. *Am J Surg* 1996; **172**:671–673.

65. Deakin M, Elder J, Hendrickse C, *et al.* Glutathione S-transferase GSTT1 genotypes and susceptibility to cancer: studies of interactions with GSTM1 in lung, oral, gastric and colorectal cancers. *Carcinogenesis* 1996; **17**:881–884.

66. Jourenkova N, Reinikainen M, Bouchardy C, *et al.* Larynx cancer risk in relation to glutathione S-transferase M1 and T1 genotypes and tobacco smoking. *Cancer Epidemiol Biomarkers Prev* 1998; **7**:19–23.

67. Oude Ophuis MB, van Lieshout EM, Roelofs HM, *et al.* Glutathione S-transferase M1 and T1 and cytochrome P4501A1 polymorphisms in relation to the risk for benign and malignant head and neck lesions. *Cancer* 1998; **82**:936–943.

68. Olshan AF, Weissler MC, Watson MA, Bell DA. GSTM1, GSTT1, GSTP1, CYP1A1, and NAT1 polymorphisms, tobacco use, and the risk of head and neck cancer. *Cancer Epidemiol Biomarkers Prev* 2000; **9**:185–191.

69. Jourenkova-Mironova N, Voho A, Bouchardy C, *et al.* Glutathione S-transferase GSTM1, GSTM3, GSTP1 and GSTT1 genotypes and the risk of smoking-related oral and pharyngeal cancers. *Int J Cancer* 1999; **81**:44–48.

70. Cheng L, Sturgis EM, Eicher SA, *et al.* Glutathione-S-transferase polymorphisms and risk of squamous-cell carcinoma of the head and neck. *Int J Cancer* 1999; **84**:220–224.

71. Hamel N, Karimi S, Hebert-Blouin MN, *et al.* Increased risk of head and neck cancer in association with GSTT1 nullizygosity for individuals with low exposure to tobacco. *Int J Cancer* 2000; **87**:452–454.

72. Weber WW, Vatsis KP. Individual variability in p-aminobenzoic acid N-acetylation by human N-acetyltransferase (NAT1) of peripheral blood. *Pharmacogenetics* 1993; **3**:209–212.

73. Hickman D, Sim E. N-acetyltransferase polymorphism. Comparison of phenotype and genotype in humans. *Biochem Pharmacol* 1991; **42**:1007–1014.

74. Johns LE, Houlston RS. N-acetyl transferase-2 and bladder cancer risk: a meta-analysis. *Environ Mol Mutagen* 2000; **36**:221–227.

75. Grant DM. Molecular genetics of the N-acetyltransferases. *Pharmacogenetics* 1993; **3**:45–50.

76. Henning S, Cascorbi I, Munchow B, *et al.* Association of arylamine N-acetyltransferases NAT1 and NAT2 genotypes to laryngeal cancer risk. *Pharmacogenetics* 1999; **9**:103–111.

77. Morita S, Yano M, Tsujinaka T, *et al.* Genetic polymorphisms of drug-metabolizing enzymes and susceptibility to head and neck squamous cell carcinoma. *Int J Cancer* 1999; **80**:685–688.

78. Hayashi S, Watanabe J, Kawajiri K. High susceptibility to lung cancer analyzed in terms of combined genotypes of P450IA1 and Mu-class glutathione S-transferase genes. *Jpn J Cancer Res* 1992; **83**:866–870.

79. Hirvonen A, Husgafvel-Pursiainen K, Karjalainen A, *et al.* Point-mutational MspI and Ile-Val polymorphisms closely linked in the CYP1A1 gene: lack of association with susceptibility to lung cancer in a Finnish study population. *Cancer Epidemiol Biomarkers Prev* 1992; **1**:485–489.

80. Hashibe M, Brennan P, Strange RC, *et al.* Meta- and pooled analysis of GSTM1, GSTT1, GSTP1, CYP1A1 genotypes and the risk of head and neck cancer. *Cancer Epidemiol Markers Prev* 2003; **12**:1509–1517.

81. Hecht F, Hecht BK. Cancer in ataxia-telangiectasia patients. *Cancer Genet Cytogenet* 1990; **46**:9–19.

82. Broughton BC, Steingrimsdottir H, Lehmann AR. Five polymorphisms in the coding sequence of the xeroderma pigmentosum group D gene. *Mutat Res* 1996; **362**:209–211.

83. Shen MR, Jones IM, Mohrenweiser H. Nonconservative amino acid substitution variants exist at polymorphic frequency in DNA repair genes in healthy humans. *Cancer Res* 1998; **58**:604–608.

84. Sturgis EM, Castillo EJ, Li L, *et al.* Polymorphisms of DNA repair gene *XRCC1* in squamous cell carcinoma of the head and neck. *Carcinogenesis* 1999; **20**:2125–2129.

85. Parkin DM, Pisani P, Ferlay J Estimates of the worldwide incidence of 25 major cancers in 1990. *Int J Cancer* 1999; **80**:827–841.

86. Neugut AI, Hayek M, Howe G. Epidemiology of gastric cancer. *Semin Oncol* 1996; **23**:281–291.

87. Correa P, Chen VW. Gastric cancer. *Cancer Surv* 1994; **19–20**:55–76.

88. Palli D. Epidemiology of gastric cancer: an evaluation of available evidence. *J Gastroenterol* 2000; **35**(Suppl. 12):84–89.

89. Hansson LE, Nyren O, Hsing AW, *et al.* The risk of stomach cancer in patients with gastric or duodenal ulcer disease. *N Engl J Med* 1996; **335**:242–249.

90. McConnell RB. *The genetics of gastrointestinal disorders*, London: Oxford University Press, 1966.

91. Dolan K, Sutton R, Walker SJ, *et al.* New classification of oesophageal and gastric carcinomas derived from changing patterns in epidemiology. *Br J Cancer* 1999; **80**:834–842.

92. Ekstrom AM, Signorello LB, Hansson LE, *et al.* Evaluating gastric cancer misclassification: a potential explanation for the rise in cardia cancer incidence. *J Natl Cancer Inst* 1999; **91**:786–790.

93. Boren T, Falk P, Roth KA, *et al.* Attachment of Helicobacter pylori to human gastric epithelium mediated by blood group antigens. *Science* 1993; **262**:1892–1895.

94. Mosbech J. *Heredit in pernicious anaemia: a proband study of the heredity and the relationship to cancer of the stomach.* Copenhagen, 1953 (quoted in reference 90 above).

95. Woolf CM, Isaacson EA. An analysis of 5 'stomach cancer families' in the state of Utah. *Cancer* 1961; **14**:1005–1016.

96. Maimon SN, Zinninger MM. Familial gastric cancer. *Gastroenterology* 1953; **25**:139–152.

97. Guilford P, Hopkins J, Harraway J, *et al.* E-cadherin germline mutations in familial gastric cancer. *Nature* 1998; **392**:402–405.

98. Guilford PJ, Hopkins JB, Grady WM, *et al.* E-cadherin germline mutations define an inherited cancer syndrome dominated by diffuse gastric cancer. *Hum Mutat* 1999; **14**:249–255.

99. Becker KF, Atkinson MJ, Reich U, *et al.* E-cadherin gene mutations provide clues to diffuse type gastric carcinomas. *Cancer Res* 1994; **54**:3845–3852.

100. Oda T, Kanai Y, Oyama T, *et al.* E-cadherin gene mutations in human gastric carcinoma cell lines. *Proc Natl Acad Sci USA* 1994; **91**:1858–1862.

101. Perl AK, Wilgenbus P, Dahl U, *et al.* A causal role for E-cadherin in the transition from adenoma to carcinoma. *Nature* 1998; **392**:190–193.

102. Grady WM, Willis J, Guilford PJ, *et al.* Methylation of the *CDH1* promoter as the second genetic hit in hereditary diffuse gastric cancer. *Nature Genet* 2000; **20**.10–17.

103. Berx G, Cleton-Jansen AM, Strumane K, *et al.* E-cadherin is inactivated in a majority of invasive human lobular breast cancers by truncation mutations throughout its extracellular domain. *Oncogene* 1996; **13**:1919–1925.

104. Rahman N, Stone JG, Coleman G, *et al.* Lobular carcinoma in situ of the breast is not caused by constitutional mutations in the E-cadherin gene. *Br J Cancer* 2000; **82**:568–570.

105. Holland R, Mravunac M, Hendriks JH, Bekker BV. So-called interval cancers of the breast. Pathologic and radiologic analysis of sixty-four cases. *Cancer* 1982; **49**:2527–2533.

106. Fitzgibbons RJ Jr, Lynch HT, Stanislav GV, *et al.* Recognition and treatment of patients with hereditary nonpolyposis colon cancer (Lynch syndromes I and II). *Ann Surg* 1987; **206**:289–295.

107. Aarnio M, Mecklin JP, Aaltonen LA, *et al.* Life-time risk of different cancers in hereditary non-polyposis colorectal cancer (HNPCC) syndrome. *Int J Cancer* 1995; **64**:430–433.

108. Vasen HF, Wijnen JT, Menko FH, *et al.* Cancer risk in families with hereditary nonpolyposis colorectal cancer diagnosed by mutation analysis. *Gastroenterology* 1996; **110**:1020–1027.

109. Aarnio M, Salovaara R, Aaltonen LA, *et al.* Features of gastric cancer in hereditary non-polyposis colorectal cancer syndrome. *Int J Cancer* 1997; **74**:551–555.

110. Lynch HT, de la Chappelle A. Genetic susceptibility to non-polyposis colorectal cancer. *J Med Genet* 1999; **36**:801–818.

111. Ottini L, Palli D, Falchetti M, *et al.* Microsatellite instability in gastric cancer is associated with tumor location and family history in a high-risk population from Tuscany. *Cancer Res* 1997; **57**:4523–4529.

112. Keller G, Grimm V, Vogelsang H, *et al.* Analysis for microsatellite instability and mutations of the DNA mismatch repair gene *MLH1* in familial gastric cancer. *Int J Cancer* 1996; **68**:571–576.

113. Gleeson CM, Sloan JM, McGuigan JA, *et al.* Widespread microsatellite instability occurs infrequently in adenocarcinoma of the gastric cardia. *Oncogene* 1996; **12**:1653–1662.

114. Fleisher AS, Esteller M, Wang S, *et al.* Hypermethylation of the *MLH1* gene promoter in human gastric cancers with microsatellite instability. *Cancer Res* 1999; **59**:1090–1095.

115. dos Santos NR, Seruca R, Constancia M, *et al.* Microsatellite instability at multiple loci in gastric carcinoma: clinicopathologic implications and prognosis. *Gastroenterology* 1996; **110**:38–44.

116. Burke W, Petersen G, Lynch P, *et al.* Recommendations for follow-up care of individuals with an inherited predisposition to cancer. I. Hereditary nonpolyposis colon cancer. Cancer Genetics Studies Consortium. *JAMA* 1997; **277**:915–919.

117. Zwick A, Munir M, Ryan CK, *et al.* Gastric adenocarcinoma and dysplasia in fundic gland polyps of a patient with attenuated adenomatous polyposis coli. *Gastroenterology* 1997; **113**:659–663.

110. Wu TT, Kornacki S, Rashid A, *et al.* Dysplasia and dysregulation of proliferation in foveolar and surface epithelia of fundic gland polyps from patients with familial adenomatous polyposis. *Am J Surg Pathol* 1998; **22**:293–298.

119. Tsuchikame N, Ishimaru Y, Ohshima S, Takahashi M. Three familial cases of fundic gland polyposis without polyposis coli. *Virchows Arch A Pathol Anat Histopathol* 1993; **422**:337–340.

120. Hizawa K, Iida M, Matsumoto T, *et al.* Natural history of fundic gland polyposis without familial adenomatosis coli: follow-up observations in 31 patients. *Radiology* 1993; **189**:429–432.

121. Gardner RJ, Kool D, Edkins E, *et al.* The clinical correlates of a 3' truncating mutation (codons 1982–1983) in the adenomatous polyposis coli gene. *Gastroenterology* 1997; **113**:326–331.

122. Lynch HT, Smyrk TC, Lanspa SJ, *et al.* Upper gastrointestinal manifestations in families with hereditary flat adenoma syndrome. *Cancer* 1993; **71**:2709–2714.

123. dos Santos JG, de Magalhaes J. Familial gastric polyposis. A new entity. *J Génét Hum* 1980; **28**:293–297.

124. Carneiro F, David L, Seruca R, *et al.* Hyperplastic polyposis and diffuse carcinoma of the stomach. A study of a family. *Cancer* 1993; **72**:323–329.

125. Domizio P, Talbot IC, Spigelman AD, et al. Upper gastrointestinal pathology in familial adenomatous polyposis: results from a prospective study of 102 patients. J Clin Pathol 1990; 43:738–743.

126. Kurtz RC, Sternberg SS, Miller IIII, DeCosse JJ. Upper gastrointestinal neoplasia in familial polyposis. Dig Dis Sci 1987; 32:459–465.

127. Park JG, Park KJ, Ahn YO, et al. Risk of gastric cancer among Korean familial adenomatous polyposis patients. Report of three cases. Dis Colon Rectum 1992; 35:996–998.

128. Utsonumiya J, Maki T, Iwama T. Phenotypic expressions of Japanese patients with familial adenomatous polyposis. New York: Alan Liss, 1990.

129. Jagelman DG, DeCosse JJ, Bussey HJ. Upper gastrointestinal cancer in familial adenomatous polyposis. Lancet 1988; 1:1149–1151.

130. Sarre RG, Frost AG, Jagelman DG, et al. Gastric and duodenal polyps in familial adenomatous polyposis: a prospective study of the nature and prevalence of upper gastrointestinal polyps. Gut 1987; 28:306–314.

131. Gahtan V, Nochomovitz LE, Robinson AM, et al. Gastroduodenal polyps in familial polyposis coli. Am Surgeon 1989; 55:278–280.

132. Offerhaus GJ, Giardiello FM, Krush AJ, et al. The risk of upper gastrointestinal cancer in familial adenomatous polyposis. Gastroenterology 1992; 102:1980–1982.

133. Kyle J. Gastric carcinoma in Peutz–Jeghers syndrome. Scott Med J 1984; 29:187–191.

134. Hizawa K, Iida M, Matsumoto T, et al. Cancer in Peutz–Jeghers syndrome. Cancer 1993; 72:2777–2781.

135. Aideyan UO, Kao SC. Gastric adenocarcinoma metastatic to the testes in Peutz–Jeghers syndrome. Pediatr Radiol 1994; 24:496–497.

136. Foley TR, McGarrity TJ, Abt AB. Peutz–Jeghers syndrome: a clinicopathologic survey of the 'Harrisburg family' with a 49-year follow-up. Gastroenterology 1988; 95:1535–1540.

137. Howe JR, Roth S, Ringold JC, et al. Mutations in the SMAD4/DPC4 gene in juvenile polyposis. Science 1998; 280:1086–1088.

138. Watanabe A, Nagashima H, Motoi M, Ogawa K. Familial juvenile polyposis of the stomach. Gastroenterology 1979; 77:148–151.

139. Sassatelli R, Bertoni G, Serra L, et al. Generalized juvenile polyposis with mixed pattern and gastric cancer. Gastroenterology 1993; 104:910–915.

140. Hizawa K, Iida M, Yao T, et al. Juvenile polyposis of the stomach: clinicopathological features and its malignant potential. J Clin Pathol 1997; 50:771–774.

141. Desai DC, Murday V, Phillips RK, et al. A survey of phenotypic features in juvenile polyposis. J Med Genet 1998; 35:476–481.

142. Hizawa K, Iida M, Matsumoto T, et al. Gastrointestinal manifestations of Cowden's disease. Report of four cases. J Clin Gastroenterol 1994; 18:13–18.

143. Chen YM, Ott DJ, Wu WC, Gelfand DW. Cowden's disease: a case report and literature review. Gastrointest Radiol 1987; 12:325–329.

144. Thompson D, Easton DF. Breast Cancer Linkage Consortium. Cancer incidence in BRCA1 mutation carriers. J Natl Cancer Inst 2002; 94:1344–1345.

145. Horio Y, Suzuki H, Ueda R, et al. Predominantly tumor-limited expression of a mutant allele in a Japanese family carrying a germline p53 mutation. Oncogene 1994; 9:1231–1235.

146. Sameshima Y, Tsunematsu Y, Watanabe S, et al. Detection of novel germ-line p53 mutations in diverse-cancer-prone families identified by selecting patients with childhood

147. Varley JM, McGown G, Thorncroft M, et al. An extended Li–Fraumeni kindred with gastric carcinoma and a codon 175 mutation in TP53. J Med Genet 1995; 32:942–945.

148. Toguchida J, Yamaguchi T, Dayton SH, et al. Prevalence and spectrum of germline mutations of the p53 gene among patients with sarcoma. N Engl J Med 1992; 326:1301–1308.

149. Shiseki M, Nishikawa R, Yamamoto H, et al. Germ-line p53 mutation is uncommon in patients with triple primary cancers. Cancer Lett 1993; 73:51–57.

150. Haerer AF, Jackson JF, Evers CG. Ataxia-telangiectasia with gastric adenocarcinoma. JAMA 1969; 210:1884–1887.

151. Farinati F, Cardin F, Di Mario F, et al. Genetic, dietary, and environmental factors in the pathogenesis of gastric cancer. Study of a high incidence family. Ital J Gastroenterol 1987; 19:321–324.

152. Zhao L, Blot WJ, Liu WD, et al. Familial predisposition to precancerous gastric lesions in a high-risk area of China. Cancer Epidemiol Biomark Prev 1994; 3:461–464.

153. The report of the Digestive Health Initiative SM International Update Conference on Helicobacter pylori. Gastroenterology 1997; 113:S4–S8.

154. Scheiman JM, Cutler AF. Helicobacter pylori and gastric cancer. Am J Med 1999; 106:222–226.

155. Forman D. Helicobacter pylori and gastric cancer. Scand J Gastroenterol Suppl 1996; 215:48–51.

156. Asaka M, Takeda H, Sugiyama T, Kato M. What role does Helicobacter pylori play in gastric cancer? Gastroenterology 1997; 113:S56–S60.

157. Brenner H, Bode G, Boeing H. Helicobacter pylori infection among offspring of patients with stomach cancer. Gastroenterology 2000; 118:31–35.

158. El Omar EM, Oien K, Murray LS, et al. Increased prevalence of precancerous changes in relatives of gastric cancer patients: critical role of H. pylori. Gastroenterology 2000; 118:22–30.

159. El Omar EM, Carrington M, Chow WH, et al. Interleukin-1 polymorphisms associated with increased risk of gastric cancer. Nature 2000; 404:398–402.

160. Katoh T, Nagata N, Kuroda Y, et al. Glutathione S-transferase M1 (GSTM1) and T1 (GSTT1) genetic polymorphism and susceptibility to gastric and colorectal adenocarcinoma. Carcinogenesis 1996; 17:1855–1859.

161. Katoh T, Kaneko S, Takasawa S, et al. Human glutathione S-transferase P1 polymorphism and susceptibility to smoking related epithelial cancer; oral, lung, gastric, colorectal and urothelial cancer. Pharmacogenetics 1999; 9:165–169.

162. Kato S, Onda M, Matsukura N, et al. Genetic polymorphisms of the cancer related gene and Helicobacter pylori infection in Japanese gastric cancer patients. An age and gender matched case-control study. Cancer 1996; 77:1654–1661.

163. Katoh T, Boissy R, Nagata N, et al. Inherited polymorphism in the N-acetyltransferase 1 (NAT1) and 2 (NAT2) genes and susceptibility to gastric and colorectal adenocarcinoma. Int J Cancer 2000; 85:46–49.

164. Shen H, Xu Y, Qian Y, et al. Polymorphisms of the DNA repair gene XRCC1 and risk of gastric cancer in a Chinese population. Int J Cancer 2000; 88:601–606.

165. Shibuta K, Mori M, Haraguchi M, et al. Association between restriction fragment length polymorphism of the L-myc gene and susceptibility to gastric cancer. Br J Surg 1998; 85:681–684.

166. dos Santos SE, Kayademir T, Regateiro F, et al. Variable distribution of TFF2 (Spasmolysin) alleles in Europeans does

not indicate predisposition to gastric cancer. *Hum Hered* 1999; **49**:45–47.

167. Parkin DM. *Cancer incidence in five continents.* Lyon: IARC, 1992.

168. Fernandez E, La Vecchia C, Porta M, *et al.* Trends in pancreatic cancer mortality in Europe, 1955–1989. *Int J Cancer* 1994; **57**:786–792.

169. *Canadian Cancer Statistics 1996.* Ottawa: National Cancer Institute of Canada, 1996; 20–25.

170. Rosewicz S, Wiedenmann B. Pancreatic carcinoma. *Lancet* 1997; **349**:485–489.

171. Yeo CJ, Cameron JL. Pancreatic cancer. *Curr Probl Surg* 1999; **36**:59–152.

172. Boyle P, Maisonneuve P, Bueno de Mesquita HB, *et al.* Cigarette smoking and pancreas cancer: a case control study of the search programme of the IARC. *Int J Cancer* 1996; **67**:63–71.

173. Ghadirian P, Thouez JP, PetitClerc C. International comparisons of nutrition and mortality from pancreatic cancer. *Cancer Detect Prev* 1991; **15**:357–362.

174. Howe GR, Ghadirian P, Bueno de Mesquita HB, *et al.* A collaborative case-control study of nutrient intake and pancreatic cancer within the search programme. *Int J Cancer* 1992; **51**:365–372.

175. Ghadirian P, Baillargeon J, Simard A, Perret C. Food habits and pancreatic cancer: a case-control study of the Francophone community in Montreal, Canada. *Cancer Epidemiol Biomarkers Prev* 1995; **4**:895–899.

176. Calvert GM, Ward E, Schnorr TM, Fine LJ. Cancer risks among workers exposed to metalworking fluids: a systematic review. *Am J Ind Med* 1998; **33**:282–292.

177. Bansal P, Sonnenberg A. Pancreatitis is a risk factor for pancreatic cancer. *Gastroenterology* 1995; **109**: 247–251.

178. Lowenfels AB, Maisonneuve P, Cavallini G, *et al.* Pancreatitis and the risk of pancreatic cancer. International Pancreatitis Study Group. *N Engl J Med* 1993; **328**:1433–1437.

179. Karlson BM, Ekbom A, Josefsson S, *et al.* The risk of pancreatic cancer following pancreatitis: an association due to confounding? *Gastroenterology* 1997; **113**:587–592.

180. Wideroff L, Gridley G, Mellemkjaer L, *et al.* Cancer incidence in a population-based cohort of patients hospitalized with diabetes mellitus in Denmark. *J Natl Cancer Inst* 1997; **89**:1360–1365.

181. Everhart J, Wright D. Diabetes mellitus as a risk factor for pancreatic cancer. A meta-analysis. *JAMA* 1995; **273**:1605–1609.

182. Falk RT, Pickle LW, Fontham ET, *et al.* Life-style risk factors for pancreatic cancer in Louisiana: a case-control study. *Am J Epidemiol* 1988; **128**:324–336.

183. Fernandez E, La Vecchia C, D'Avanzo B, *et al.* Family history and the risk of liver, gallbladder, and pancreatic cancer. *Cancer Epidemiol Biomarkers Prev* 1994; **3**:209–212.

184. Ghadirian P, Boyle P, Simard A, *et al.* Reported family aggregation of pancreatic cancer within a population-based case-control study in the Francophone community in Montreal, Canada. *Int J Pancreatol* 1991; **10**:183–196.

185. Goldgar DE, Easton DF, Cannon-Albright LA, Skolnick MH. Systematic population-based assessment of cancer risk in first-degree relatives of cancer probands. *J Natl Cancer Inst* 1994; **86**:1600–1608.

186. Ghadirian P, Liu G, Gallinger S, *et al.* Family history and the risk of pancreatic cancer. *Int J Cancer* 2002; **97**:807–810.

187. Hruban RH, Petersen GM, Ha PK, Kern SE. Genetics of pancreatic cancer. From genes to families. *Surg Oncol Clin North Am* 1998; **7**:1–23.

188. Tulinius H, Olafsdottir GH, Sigvaldason H, *et al.* Neoplastic diseases in families of breast cancer patients. *J Med Genet* 1994; **31**:618–621.

189. Travis LB, Curtis RE, Storm H, *et al.* Risk of second malignant neoplasms among long-term survivors of testicular cancer. *J Natl Cancer Inst* 1997; **89**:1429–1439.

190. Neugut AI, Ahsan H, Robinson E. Pancreas cancer as a second primary malignancy. A population-based study. *Cancer* 1995; **76**:589–592.

191. Vaittinen P, Hemminki K. Familial cancer risks in offspring from discordant parental cancers. *Int J Cancer* 1999; **81**:12–19.

192. Bergman W, Watson P, de Jong J, *et al.* Systemic cancer and the FAMMM syndrome. *Br J Cancer* 1990; **61**:932–936.

193. Goldstein AM, Fraser MC, Struewing JP, *et al.* Increased risk of pancreatic cancer in melanoma-prone kindreds with *p16INK4* mutations. *N Engl J Med* 1995; **333**:970–974.

194. Gruis NA, van der Velden PA, Sandkuijl LA, *et al.* Homozygotes for *CDKN2* (p16) germline mutation in Dutch familial melanoma kindreds. *Nature Genet* 1995; **10**:351–353.

195. Ciotti P, Strigini P, Bianchi-Scarra G. Familial melanoma and pancreatic cancer. Ligurian Skin Tumor Study Group. *N Engl J Med* 1996; **334**:469–470.

196. Moskaluk CA, Hruban H, Lietman A, *et al.* Novel germline p16(INK4) allele (Asp145Cys) in a family with multiple pancreatic carcinomas. Mutations in brief no. 148. Online. *Hum Mutat* 1998; **12**:70.

197. Lal G, Liu G, Schmocker B, Kaurah P, *et al.* Inherited predisposition to pancreatic adenocarcinoma: role of family history and germ-line *p16, BRCA1,* and *BRCA2* mutations. *Cancer Res* 2000; **60**:409–416.

198. Lal G, Liu L, Hogg D, Lassam NJ, *et al.* Patients with both pancreatic adenocarcinoma and melanoma may harbor germline *CDKN2A* mutations. *Genes Chrom Cancer* 2000; **27**:358–361.

199. Narod SA, Ford D, Devilee P, *et al.* An evaluation of genetic heterogeneity in 145 breast-ovarian cancer families. Breast Cancer Linkage Consortium. *Am J Hum Genet* 1995; **56**:254–264.

200. Easton DF, Steele L, Fields P, *et al.* Cancer risks in two large breast cancer families linked to *BRCA2* on chromosome 13q12–13. *Am J Hum Genet* 1997; **61**:120–128.

201. Simard J, Tonin P, Durocher F, *et al.* Common origins of *BRCA1* mutations in Canadian breast and ovarian cancer families. *Nature Genet* 1994; **8**:392–398.

202. Tonin P, Ghadirian P, Phelan C, *et al.* A large multisite cancer family is linked to *BRCA2. J Med Genet* 1995; **32**:982–984.

203. Johannsson O, Ostermeyer EA, Hakansson S, *et al.* Founding *BRCA1* mutations in hereditary breast and ovarian cancer in southern Sweden. *Am J Hum Genet* 1996; **58**:441–450.

204. Phelan CM, Lancaster JM, Tonin P, *et al.* Mutation analysis of the *BRCA2* gene in 49 site-specific breast cancer families. *Nature Genet* 1996; **13**:120–122.

205. Arason A, Barkardottir RB, Egilsson V. Linkage analysis of chromosome 17q markers and breast-ovarian cancer in Icelandic families, and possible relationship to prostatic cancer. *Am J Hum Genet* 1993; **52**:711–717.

206. Thorlacius S, Olafsdottir G, Tryggvadottir L, *et al.* A single *BRCA2* mutation in male and female breast cancer families from Iceland with varied cancer phenotypes. *Nature Genet* 1996; **13**:117–119.

207. Tonin P, Weber B, Offit K, Couch F, *et al.* Frequency of recurrent *BRCA1* and *BRCA2* mutations in Ashkenazi Jewish breast cancer families. *Nature Med* 1996; **2**:1179–1183.

208. Moslehi R, Chu W, Karlan B, et al. BRCA1 and BRCA2 mutation analysis of 208 Ashkenazi Jewish women with ovarian cancer. Am J Hum Genet 2000; 66:1259–1272.

209. Risch HA, McLaughlin JR, Cole DE, et al. Prevalence and penetrance of germline BRCA1 and BRCA2 mutations in a population series of 649 women with ovarian cancer. Am J Hum Genet 2001; 68:700–710.

210. Goggins M, Schutte M, Lu J, et al. Germline BRCA2 gene mutations in patients with apparently sporadic pancreatic carcinomas. Cancer Res 1996; 56:5360–5364.

211. Ozcelik H, Schmocker B, Di Nicola N, et al. Germline BRCA2 6174delT mutations in Ashkenazi Jewish pancreatic cancer patients. Nature Genet 1997; 16:17–18.

212. Giardiello FM, Welsh SB, Hamilton SR, et al. Increased risk of cancer in the Peutz–Jeghers syndrome. N Engl J Med 1987; 316:1511–1514.

213. Spigelman AD, Murday V, Phillips RK. Cancer and the Peutz–Jeghers syndrome. Gut 1989; 30:1588–1590.

214. Bowlby LS. Pancreatic adenocarcinoma in an adolescent male with Peutz–Jeghers syndrome. Hum Pathol 1986; 17:97–99.

215. Konishi F, Wyse NE, Muto T, et al. Peutz–Jeghers polyposis associated with carcinoma of the digestive organs. Report of three cases and review of the literature. Dis Colon Rectum 1987; 30:790–799.

216. Yoshikawa A, Kuramoto S, Mimura T, et al. Peutz–Jeghers syndrome manifesting complete intussusception of the appendix and associated with a focal cancer of the duodenum and a cystadenocarcinoma of the pancreas: report of a case. Dis Colon Rectum 1998; 41:517–521.

217. Westerman AM, Entius MM, de Baar E, et al. Peutz–Jeghers syndrome: 78-year follow-up of the original family. Lancet 1999; 353:1211–1215.

218. Su GH, Hruban RH, Bansal RK, et al. Germline and somatic mutations of the STK11/LKB1 Peutz–Jeghers gene in pancreatic and biliary cancers. Am J Pathol 1999; 154:1835–1840.

219. Lynch HT, Smyrk T, Kern SE, et al. Familial pancreatic cancer: a review. Semin Oncol 1996; 23:251–275.

220. Lynch HT, Voorhees GJ, Lanspa SJ, et al. Pancreatic carcinoma and hereditary nonpolyposis colorectal cancer: a family study. Br J Cancer 1985; 52:271–273.

221. Watson P, Lynch HT. Extracolonic cancer in hereditary nonpolyposis colorectal cancer. Cancer 1993; 71:677–685.

222. Vasen HF, Hartog Jager FC, Menko FH, Nagengast FM. Screening for hereditary non-polyposis colorectal cancer: a study of 22 kindreds in The Netherlands. Am J Med 1989; 86:278–281.

223. Aarnio M, Sankila R, Pukkala E, et al. Cancer risk in mutation carriers of DNA-mismatch-repair genes. Int J Cancer 1999; 81:214–218.

224. Lin KM, Shashidharan M, Ternent CA, et al. Colorectal and extracolonic cancer variations in MLH1/MSH2 hereditary nonpolyposis colorectal cancer kindreds and the general population. Dis Colon Rectum 1998; 41:428–433.

225. Pal T, Flanders T, Mitchell-Lehman M, et al. Genetic implications of double primary cancers of the colorectum and endometrium. J Med Genet 1998; 35:978–984.

226. Wijnen JT, Vasen HF, Khan PM, et al. Clinical findings with implications for genetic testing in families with clustering of colorectal cancer. N Engl J Med 1998; 339:511–518.

227. Giardiello FM, Offerhaus GJ, Lee DH, et al. Increased risk of thyroid and pancreatic carcinoma in familial adenomatous polyposis. Gut 1993; 34:1394–1396.

228. Wallis YL, Morton DG, McKeown CM, Macdonald F. Molecular analysis of the APC gene in 205 families: extended genotype–phenotype correlations in FAP and evidence for the role of APC amino acid changes in colorectal cancer predisposition. J Med Genet 1999; 36:14–20.

229. Swift M, Chase CL, Morrell D. Cancer predisposition of ataxia-telangiectasia heterozygotes. Cancer Genet Cytogenet 1990; 46:21–27.

230. Olsen JH, Hahnemann JM, Borresen-Dale AL, et al. Cancer in patients with ataxia-telangiectasia and in their relatives in the Nordic countries. J Natl Cancer Inst 2001; 93:121–127.

231. Swift M, Reitnauer PJ, Morrell D, Chase CL. Breast and other cancers in families with ataxia-telangiectasia. N Engl J Med 1987; 316:1289–1294.

232. Swift M, Morrell D, Massey RB, Chase CL. Incidence of cancer in 161 families affected by ataxia-telangiectasia. N Engl J Med 1991; 325:1831–1836.

233. Li FP, Fraumeni JF, Mulvihill JJ, et al. A cancer family syndrome in twenty-four kindreds. Cancer Res 1988; 48:5358–5362.

234. Kleihues P, Schauble B, zur Hausen H, et al. Tumors associated with p53 germline mutations: a synopsis of 91 families. Am J Pathol 1997; 150:1–13.

235. Houlston R, Bevan S, Williams A, et al. Mutations in DPC4 (SMAD4) cause juvenile polyposis syndrome, but only account for a minority of cases. Hum Mol Genet 1998; 7:1907–1912.

236. Stemper TJ, Kent TH, Summers RW. Juvenile polyposis and gastrointestinal carcinoma. A study of a kindred. Ann Intern Med 1975; 83:639–646.

237. Walpole IR, Cullity G. Juvenile polyposis: a case with early presentation and death attributable to adenocarcinoma of the pancreas. Am J Med Genet 1989; 32:1–8.

238. Hahn SA, Schutte M, Hoque AT, et al. DPC4, a candidate tumor suppressor gene at human chromosome 18q21.1. Science 1996; 271:350–353.

239. Moskaluk CA, Hruban RH, Schutte M, et al. Genomic sequencing of DPC4 in the analysis of familial pancreatic carcinoma. Diagn Mol Pathol 1997; 6:85–90.

240. Kattwinkel J, Lapey A, Di Sant' Agnese PA, Edwards WA. Hereditary pancreatitis: three new kindreds and a critical review of the literature. Pediatrics 1973; 51: 55–69.

241. Lowenfels AB, Maisonneuve P, Dimagno EP, et al. Hereditary pancreatitis and the risk of pancreatic cancer. International Hereditary Pancreatitis Study Group. J Natl Cancer Inst 1997; 89:442–446.

242. Whitcomb DC, Gorry MC, Preston RA, et al. Hereditary pancreatitis is caused by a mutation in the cationic trypsinogen gene. Nature Genet 1996; 14:141–145.

243. Howes N, Lerch MM, Greenhalf W, et al. Clinical and genetic characteristics of hereditary pancreatitis in Europe. Clin Gastroenterol Hepatol 2004; 2:252–261.

244. Dasouki MJ, Cogan J, Summar ML, et al. Heterogeneity in hereditary pancreatitis. Am J Med Genet 1998; 77:47–53.

245. Ferec C, Raguenes O, Salomon R, et al. Mutations in the cationic trypsinogen gene and evidence for genetic heterogeneity in hereditary pancreatitis. J Med Genet 1999; 36:228–232.

246. Sharer N, Schwarz M, Malone G, et al. Mutations of the cystic fibrosis gene in patients with chronic pancreatitis. N Engl J Med 1998; 339:645–652.

247. Cohn JA, Friedman KJ, Noone PG, et al. Relation between mutations of the cystic fibrosis gene and idiopathic pancreatitis. N Engl J Med 1998; 339:653–658.

248. Witt H, Luck W, Hennies HC, et al. Mutations in the gene encoding the serine protease inhibitor, Kazal type 1 are

associated with chronic pancreatitis. *Nat Genet* 2000;
25:213–216.

249. Truninger K, Witt H, Kock J, *et al.* Mutations of the serine
protease inhibitor, Kazal type 1 gene, in patients with
idiopathic chronic pancreatitis. *Am J Gastroenterol* 2002;
97:1133–1137.

250. Malats N, Casals T, Porta M, *et al.* Cystic fibrosis transmembrane
regulator (CFTR) DeltaF508 mutation and 5T allele in patients
with chronic pancreatitis and exocrine pancreatic cancer.
PANKRAS II Study Group. *Gut* 2001; **48**:70–74.

251. Teich N, Schulz HU, Witt H, *et al.* N34S, a pancreatitis
associated SPINK1 mutation, is not associated with sporadic
pancreatic cancer. *Pancreatology* 2003; **3**:67–68.

252. Liu G, Ghadirian P, Vesprini D, *et al.* Polymorphisms in
GSTM1, *GSTT1* and *CYP1A1* and risk of pancreatic
adenocarcinoma. *Br J Cancer* 2000; **82**:1646–1649.

253. Bartsch H, Malaveille C, Lowenfels AB, *et al.* Genetic
polymorphism of N-acetyltransferases, glutathione
S-transferase M1 and NAD(P)H:quinone oxidoreductase in
relation to malignant and benign pancreatic disease risk.
The International Pancreatic Disease Study Group.
Eur J Cancer Prev 1998; **7**:215–223.

254. Macklin MT. Inheritance of cancer of the stomach and
large intestine in man. *J Natl Cancer Inst* 1960;
24:551–571.

255. Mecklin JP, Nordling S, Saario I. Carcinoma of the stomach
and its heredity in young patients. *Scand J Gastroenterol*
1988; **23**:307–311.

256. Zanghieri G, Di Gregorio C, Sacchetti C, *et al.* Familial
occurrence of gastric cancer in the 2-year experience of a
population-based registry. *Cancer* 1990; **66**:2047–2051.

257. La Vecchia C, Negri E, Franceschi S, Gentile A. Family history
and the risk of stomach and colorectal cancer. *Cancer* 1992;
70:50–55.

258. Kato I, Tominaga S, Matsumoto K. A prospective study of
stomach cancer among a rural Japanese population: a 6-year
survey. *Jpn J Cancer Res* 1992; **83**:568–575.

259. Palli D, Galli M, Caporaso NE, *et al.* Family history and risk of
stomach cancer in Italy. *Cancer Epidemiol Biomark Prev*
1994; **3**:15–18.

260. La Vecchia C, D'Avanzo B, Negri E, *et al.* Attributable risks for
stomach cancer in northern Italy. *Int J Cancer* 1995;
60:748–752.

261. Nagase H, Ogino K, Yoshida I, *et al.* Family history-related
risk of gastric cancer in Japan: a hospital-based case-control
study. *Jpn J Cancer Res* 1996; **87**:1025–1028.

262. Kikuchi S, Nakajima T, Nishi T, *et al.* Association between
family history and gastric carcinoma among young adults.
Jpn J Cancer Res 1996; **87**:332–336.

263. Inoue M, Tajima K, Yamamura Y, *et al.* Family history and
subsite of gastric cancer: data from a case-referent study in
Japan. *Int J Cancer* 1998; **76**:801–805.

264. Morita M, Kuwano H, Baba H, *et al.* Multifocal occurrence of
gastric carcinoma in patients with a family history of gastric
carcinoma. *Cancer* 1998; **83**:1307–1311.

265. Poole CA, Byers T, Calle EE, *et al.* Influence of a family history of
cancer within and across multiple sites on patterns of cancer
mortality risk for women. *Am J Epidemiol* 1999; **149**:454–462.

266. Gayther SA, Gorringe KL, Ramus SJ, *et al.* Identification of
germ-line E-cadherin mutations in gastric cancer families of
European origin. *Cancer Res* 1998; **58**:4086–4089.

267. Richards FM, McKee SA, Rajpar MH, *et al.* Germline
E-cadherin gene (*CDH1*) mutations predispose to familial
gastric cancer and colorectal cancer. *Hum Mol Genet* 1999;
8:607–610.

268. Shinmura K, Kohno T, Takahashi M, *et al.* Familial gastric
cancer: clinicopathological characteristics, RER phenotype
and germline *p53* and E-cadherin mutations. *Carcinogenesis*
1999; **20**:1127–1131.

269. Stone J, Bevan S, Cunningham D, *et al.* Low frequency of
germline E-cadherin mutations in familial and nonfamilial
gastric cancer. *Br J Cancer* 1999; **79**:1935–1937.

270. Keller G, Vogelsang H, Becker I, *et al.* Diffuse type gastric and
lobular breast carcinoma in a familial gastric cancer patient
with an E-cadherin germline mutation. *Am J Pathol* 1999;
155:337–342.

271. Yoon KA, Ku JL, Yang HK, *et al.* Germline mutations of
E-cadherin gene in Korean familial gastric cancer patients.
J Hum Genet 1999; **44**:177–180.

272. Lehtola J. Family study of gastric carcinoma; with special
reference to histological types. *Scand J Gastroenterol Suppl*
1978; **50**:3–54.

273. Lida S, Akiyama Y, Ichikawa W, *et al.* Infrequent
germ-line mutation of the E-cadherin gene in Japanese
familial gastric cancer kindreds. *Clin Cancer Res* 1999;
5:1445–1447.

PART 5

Psychosocial, ethical and organisational issues

30

The cancer family clinic

ROSALIND A. EELES AND VICTORIA A. MURDAY

WHAT IS THE CANCER FAMILY CLINIC AND WHY IS IT NEEDED?

Until the 1980s, the study of the genetics of cancer was confined to the rarer familial cancer syndromes, such as multiple endocrine neoplasia type 2 and familial polyposis coli. This was restricted to a relatively small number of families. With the advent of the knowledge that at least a small proportion of many of the common cancers is due to an inherited genetic predisposition, the overall numbers of individuals at risk will be large because these cancers are more common. For example, it has been estimated that about 5–10 per cent of breast cancers may occur as a result of the inheritance of a dominant gene.[1] This would equate to 1250 cases of breast cancer per year in the UK occurring in susceptible individuals. This led to the development of cancer family clinics, specializing in the management of families at risk of hereditary cancers.

The functions of the cancer family clinic are to detect whether a family pattern of common cancers is likely to be genetic, diagnose rarer cancer family syndromes, provide cancer risk assessment, keep accurate records according to local Data Protection Acts, link familial data via confidential family registers, provide genetic counselling and genetic testing if appropriate, give advice on early detection and preventative options, and participate in clinical trials of these options. They also have other pivotal roles in the service provision and monitoring: to train other health care professionals so that the appropriate individuals are referred, to guide and support voluntary bodies, monitor the effectiveness and quality of services, provide a resource for research and development, and provide a source of expert advice for purchasers and providers of these services. Increasingly, Cancer Genetics Services are becoming involved in genetic aspects of cancer management as cancer genetics impacts upon cancer care.

ORGANIZATION OF CANCER FAMILY CLINICS

In the UK, the first clinical genetics service was established in 1946 and, currently, the genetics service is organized on a regional basis. The ideal cancer family clinic would be the provision of a specialist clinic with access not only to personnel with experience in genetics, but also to oncological experience, counsellors and psychologists. It is, therefore, likely that these clinics will develop as joint clinics, or with dual-trained staff, serving a regional area.

National registers have been proposed in several countries for recording familial cancers. In France, the French Cooperative Group Network has been formed to coordinate the data collected from such clinics, and has already proved highly effective in identifying families with certain cancer phenotypes for collaborative international research.[2] More recently, a British Family Cancer Network has been instigated. An EU Demonstration project showed that the facilities and structure of the service follow different models throughout Europe with a different skill mix, for example, some countries have adopted the use of genetic counsellors or nurse specialists, while others rely on medical staff to provide the core counselling.[3] In the USA, both medical and genetic counsellors provide the cancer genetic service.

In the UK, the organization of the Cancer Services along the Calman Hine model is easily applied to the Cancer Genetic Services.[4] Cancer centres should have a centralized cancer genetic team. This should involve a core staff of not only geneticists from the regional genetic service, but also oncologists with an interest in cancer genetics, genetic/nurse counsellors, access to psychological services and the necessary administrative staff including those to run the genetic registers.

In addition, there must be the required screening programmes available including staff to provide the screening services and the funding to run them to provide an efficient cancer genetics service. The numbers of individuals requiring screening will vary enormously according to the site being screened. Some of the screening will, therefore, require centralization within the cancer centre, whereas it may be more appropriate for a more devolved screening service structure for screens, such as colonoscopy, which are dependent on intensive clinical staffing.

What is the optimal staffing organization of the clinic?

The individuals at increased risk of cancer due to a genetic predisposition need both genetic and oncological advice. The ideal staffing of such a clinic, therefore, includes a geneticist, oncological specialist (this may be the same person), genetic counsellors (these may be nurses) and psychological support. Data management is important, for maintenance of registers, research and audit. A mechanism is needed for confirming diagnoses from medical records and retrieving death certificates. Such clinics are, therefore, labour intensive. Liaison with a laboratory (preferably linking to or within the regional genetics service) is essential for the storage of blood and tumour samples. The laboratory should participate in a quality assurance scheme and have appropriate accreditation for the country in which it is situated.

Referral patterns

General practitioners (GPs) are increasingly being consulted about genetic risk for cancer. The numbers involved with respect to the common cancers will make it very difficult for all the concerned individuals to be seen in a specialized cancer family clinic, nor indeed do all these people require the specialized services of such a clinic. A key role

of the personnel in these clinics in the next few years will be education of the primary care sector, oncologists and the general public. Nurses are likely to play a large role in many countries and their education is, therefore, very important.[5] Research in the area of cancer genetics is urgently needed to identify the current knowledge and educational needs of the public and their care providers.

Ideally, one would refer potential gene carriers to the clinic but the problem is identifying these individuals. The chance of being a gene carrier rises as the age of cancer diagnosis falls, for example, if female relatives of all cases of breast cancer diagnosed below 50 years were referred to cancer family clinics, this would involve 10 000 new women at risk each year in the UK. This is estimated from the figures that 20 per cent of breast cancer arises in the under-50s (5000 cases/year in the UK) and, on average, each woman has a mother and one sister at risk (A. Howell, personal communication). According to the Claus model,[1] only up to 36 per cent of isolated breast cancers diagnosed under the age of 40 are due to dominant high-risk predisposition genes. The problem is the lack of diagnostic features, which can identify gene carriers from sporadic cases. This may be improved by the recent findings that pathology may help to identify those young-onset cases that are more likely to harbour *BRCA1* germline mutations.[6]

Suggested referral guidelines for a cancer family clinic are shown in Table 30.1. Not all cases where there is a significant predisposition will fall within these groups; conversely, many individuals or families that meet these criteria will not, in fact, have a cancer predisposition. The aim is to provide a simple scheme for ease of referral from GPs and oncology clinics.

The ideal situation would be computer-generated packages, which would provide risk estimates for GPs when

Table 30.1 *Referral guidelines for a cancer family clinic (Modified from Ponder[7])*

The cancers should be through the same genetic lineage, but can be through either the mother or father's side

1 Two or more unusual cancers in the same individual or in close relatives (e.g. brain tumour and sarcoma)
2 Cancer in the context of an associated syndrome (e.g. glioma in neurofibromatosis type I; melanoma in dysplastic naevus syndrome)
3 Clustering of common cancers
   (a) Three or more cancers or the same type or related types in close relatives (e.g. breast/ovary/endometrium/colon/prostate)
   (b) Two cancers of the same type or related types in close relatives where one is diagnosed before age 50 or at any age, if the cancer is relatively rare (e.g. ovary or small bowel)
   (c) A first-degree relative with one of the common cancers diagnosed before age 40 (in the case of prostate, before age 55).

the family history is entered into a desktop computer. This would then advise when an individual should be referred to a cancer family clinic. Some groups are trying to produce such programs.[8] The problem is designing a program that will cater for every possible familial cancer and which is robust enough to ensure unusual families are not missed.

GENETIC COUNSELLING

Genetic counselling is the term that describes the interview that occurs when an individual attends a genetic clinic, although this is only part of what actually happens when a patient visits the clinic. Counselling is important in genetics, and its non-directive nature, offering choices to patients, has been the basis of the practice. This situation is likely to remain until proven preventive options are available for the common cancers. This is likely only to be a matter of time, and then it is possible that this traditional approach will be less prominent and preventive options will be offered in the same way as treatments are offered for clinical disease. Currently, much of the consultation, like any other outpatient appointment, is for diagnosis and management of disease, and this is carried out ordinarily using the history and examination of an affected individual. With genetic disease, it may be the family history that holds the clue to diagnosis and, in a family cancer clinic, diagnosis of a genetic susceptibility to cancer may be largely determined by the family history.

THE FAMILY HISTORY

Establishing the pedigree is an important part of the interview. This is standardized to include the family history of cancer, other diseases, developmental and congenital abnormalities, and a history of miscarriages. The diagnosis of a particular cancer syndrome may be possible from the familial pattern of cancers or associated non-malignant problems. Information about at least first-degree (parents/siblings) and second-degree (grandparents, aunts and uncles) relatives should be requested (preferably also third-degree, such as cousins) and, where appropriate, the family history should be extended as far as possible.[9]

The age at which cancer was diagnosed, the site(s) and the name of the treatment hospital involved should be ascertained. This will allow assessment of risks to relatives and confirmation of diagnosis from hospital records. For example, a common inaccuracy is the diagnosis of ovarian cancer, which can be reported as stomach or uterine cancer. The presence of ovarian cancer in a breast cancer family raises the possibility that *BRCA1* is present and it is, therefore, important to verify abdominal/pelvic cancer histologies.

PEDIGREE CONSTRUCTION

Many cancer family clinics send the counsellee a questionnaire and have the family history available and reviewed before the counsellee is seen in the clinic, where the doctor then simply comments on the pedigree. This saves about 20–30 minutes and can increase the throughput of the clinic. There are advantages and disadvantages of this approach. The family dynamics, which are detected when taking a family history, can be missed and details of the pedigree should be confirmed, since inaccuracies can occur when a client fills out a family history from a questionnaire, or further details may have been ascertained since the questionnaire was completed. However, the advantages are that the information will be more comprehensive, since clients will ask family members about pieces of missing information before the consultation. In addition, diagnoses such as 'womb/ovarian cancer' can be confirmed from medical records or death certificates before the consultation. It has been shown by comparison of family histories from individuals with cancer registry records that abdominal cancers may be misreported up to 17 per cent of the time, and confirmation resulted in a change in screening in about 11 per cent of cases.[10] One example of the expediency of this approach was the case of an individual referred for ovarian cancer screening and cancer risk assessment because of a family history of ovarian cancer in two relatives. The client reported in her questionnaire that one relative had 'stomach cancer' and the other ovarian cancer. Confirmation of the diagnoses by medical records in one case and death certification in the other revealed that only one relative had had ovarian cancer. The counsellee was, therefore, at a lower ovarian cancer risk than she had feared and did not need screening. All this was possible in one consultation, saving time and resources for the counsellee and clinic staff. It should, however, be borne in mind that some people are less able or reticent about filling out forms. It should, therefore, not be made compulsory or some people will not be seen who might have benefited. The role of nurse-led telephone consultations or home visits is important here, although the latter is more time intensive.

For formal computation of pedigrees there are several computer packages that are PC-based (Cyrillic™, Progeny™ Ped-Draw™). There is an attempt to standardize pedigree symbols internationally[11] but, until this occurs, the symbols unique to each centre should be explained in a legend accompanying the pedigree.

RISK ASSESSMENT

Genetic risks have two components: (1) the probability that a particular disorder will occur; and (2) the damage and burden that it will inflict, both on the person that suffers the disease, and their family. The risk of cancer to the individual undergoing counselling is assessed from the family history. This is used to determine the likelihood that there is a cancer-predisposition gene in the family. If the gene involved has been identified, the cancer risks are determined from the genetic epidemiological studies of that gene. If the particular gene has not yet been identified, as is the case in many instances of the common cancers, risk estimates are calculated using the epidemiological studies of risks to relatives of cases with those cancers. There is also an additional component from environment–gene interactions, a relatively unstudied area at present. These will be more clearly defined as further cancer-predisposition genes are identified and genetic epidemiological studies are performed.

As a general rule, the occurrence of the same cancer in three close blood relatives of a family is suggestive that there is a genetic susceptibility, particularly if they were affected at an early age. If there are two close relatives with the same cancer, then the population risk of that cancer is an important guide as to the chance of a genetic susceptibility (i.e. if a cancer is rare, then two cases in a family are less likely to have occurred by chance).

Having a single relative with a particular cancer often does not greatly increase the risk to relatives. The exception to this is if the relative is young or has had multiple primaries or a recognizable cancer syndrome. The risk of bowel cancer in the relatives of a single case illustrates the importance of age at diagnosis (see Figure 30.1).

Some cancer syndromes have phenotypes that can be diagnosed in an individual. Frequently, it is the premalignant phenotype, such as the numerous adenomatous polyps seen in familial adenomatous polyposis (FAP; see Chapter 24).

There is now published information on the risks for relatives of cancer patients, particularly for common cancers, such as breast, colorectal and prostate cancer[1,12,13] (reviewed in Eeles[14]) and these are particularly useful for genetic counselling, permitting visual demonstration of risk assessment to the patient. The likelihood of a genetic susceptibility can be calculated by combining information on the number and age of affected individuals. The risk to the patient will depend upon their relationship to the affected family members and their own age, since the risk will decrease the longer they remain free of disease. An example of such a risk assessment for the kindred is illustrated in Figure 30.2. Table 30.2 shows the method of combining the information by an approximate Bayesian calculation to determine the residual risk for the patient. The prior probability is the chance that the family has a predisposition gene. As II:1 is a daughter of I:2, who is assumed to be a gene carrier, the probability of II:1 having the gene is half of the chance that the cases in the family have a breast cancer predisposition gene (60 per cent/2 = 30 per cent, or 0.3). The posterior probability is the probability that the person in question will have the predisposition gene given all the information available, such as age of the individual, their cancer status (affected/unaffected) and their position in the family. There are difficulties in using these calculations if a significant component of the genetic susceptibility is due to less penetrant genes, since the risk may be underestimated. For instance, in the example given, the residual risk is for the chance of a highly penetrant dominant gene for early-onset breast cancer in the family. There is a possiblility that lower penetrant genes are responsible for the familial cluster.

When a specific diagnosis of cancer susceptibility is possible in a family, then there may be more information

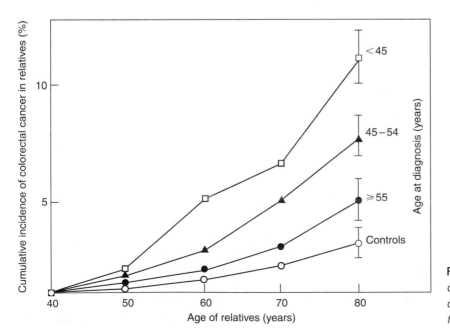

Figure 30.1 *Cumulative risk of colorectal cancer in relatives of a patient diagnosed at various ages. (Reproduced from St John et al.[12])*

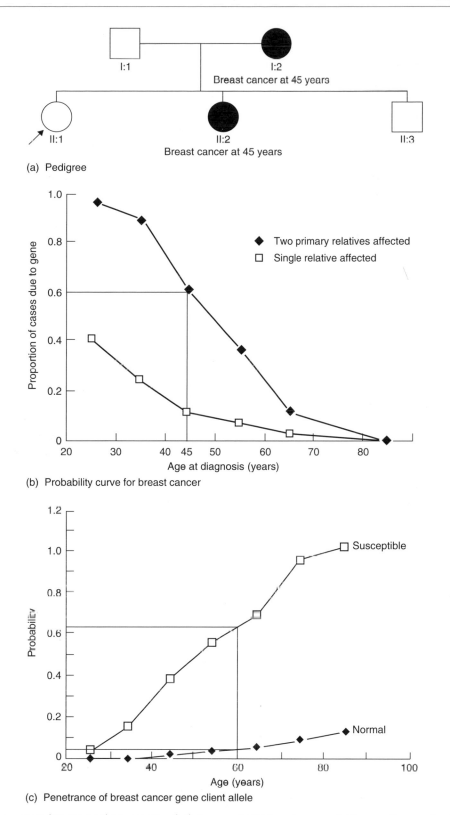

(a) Pedigree

(b) Probability curve for breast cancer

(c) Penetrance of breast cancer gene client allele

Figure 30.2 *(a) The patient (II:1 arrowed) has a mother (I:2) diagnosed with breast cancer at 45 years of age and a sister (II:2) with breast cancer diagnosed at the age of 45 years. (b) The probability that a dominant gene gave rise to the breast cancer in two primary relatives affected is 60 per cent. (c) Since the woman at risk is a sister or daughter of an affected individual, her risk of having the 'gene' is 30 per cent (i.e. half that of the affected relatives). She is 60 years of age, by which age 60 per cent of individuals with the genetic susceptibility will have developed breast cancer. (Actually the true probability that II:1 is a gene carrier is lower than this because the fact that she is unaffected at age 60 slightly reduces the figure from (b). See Table 30.2 for the Bayesian calculation to calculate this.)*

Table 30.2 *Determination of posterior probability of being a gene carrier for client in Figure 30.2*

	Susceptible	Non-susceptible
Prior probability – from Figure 30.2(b)	0.30	0.70
Disease-free at 60 years – from Figure 30.2(c)	0.40	0.96
Posterior probability	$\dfrac{0.3 \times 0.4}{(0.3 \times 0.4) + (0.7 \times 0.96)} = 0.15$	0.85

available, both in terms of the chances of developing cancer and possible non-malignant problems. For instance, if a *BRCA1* mutation is the likely cause of breast cancer in a family, then detailed information is available on the cumulative risk of both ovarian and breast cancer as well as the possibility of other cancers, such as bowel and prostate, for which there may be an increased relative risk in affected individuals (see Chapters 17 and 19). A *BRCA1* mutation may be suspected either from the family structure, a dominant susceptibility to early breast cancer associated with ovarian cancer, or by demonstration of linkage to the *BRCA1* region on chromosome 17, or, best of all, by the demonstration by direct mutation analysis of a cancer-causing mutation in the gene.

RISK PERCEPTION

One of the primary reasons for identifying hereditary cancer is to enable family members to be targeted for advice on risk. This raises the important issue of the process of giving risk information. The uptake of preventive strategies may depend on the individual's perception of risk; for example, Croyle *et al.*[15] have shown that individuals at a perceived increased risk of heart disease were more likely to express their intentions to modify their lifestyle than those at population risk. The understanding and retention of this information may depend on the format in which it is presented and the individual's attitudes to risk. Even with the recent advances in the identification of several cancer-predisposition genes, incomplete penetrance (i.e. not all gene carriers develop cancer, they are, however, at increased risk) means that even known gene carriers still have to comprehend that they are at a certain level of risk and the development of cancer still has an element of uncertainty. Geneticists are still trying to determine the best method for providing information to those at increased risk due to a genetic predisposition.

Risk information is often complex and can be expressed in various ways. It is current practice in genetic counselling clinics and the more recent specialized cancer family clinics, to convey risk information numerically, either as a risk of developing disease per year, or risk by a certain age.[16] The risk value is either given as a percentage risk or a '1 in *x*' value. However, the optimal format for conveying risk information is unknown.

Studies have examined whether women correctly assess their level of risk,[17] but few examine the best way to present genetic information to those who may be at increased risk of familial cancer. It is not clear whether clients understand the rather complex explanations or what they remember of this information. Many women do not remember numerical information. For example, 98 per cent of women attending because of a family history of breast cancer could not remember their percentage annual risk, even when this was given both verbally in the clinic, and by follow-up letter. They were somewhat better at providing feedback on their lifetime risk, but 35 per cent gave an incorrect figure. More importantly, though, they were able to report the category of their risk with reasonable accuracy, even though this information was given in numerical form and not as a risk category. In general, this sample was also unclear about what action to take as a result of this consultation, despite the options being reiterated in a follow-up letter. Some women in this study reported that they did not actually find numerical risk information useful, despite wishing to know their risk status, and being able to report that a risk category, such as high risk, was helpful. Research has shown that audio-tape recording the consultation does not improve recall of risk long term, but does decrease cancer anxiety.[18] The use of a video again does not improve understanding but does increase satisfaction of the consultation. It should be used in conjunction with careful counselling because its use was associated with an increase in general distress, which was not seen with audiotaping.[19]

Green and Brown[20] have suggested that the qualitative aspect of risk is more important than the quantitative aspect, and Sorensen *et al.*[21] suggested that many patients do not remember or understand the genetic information given. Leonard *et al.*[22] claim that 'clients are bad at probabilistic reasoning and find quantitative risk estimates difficult to understand'. However, this finding contrasts with that of Josten *et al.*[23], who report from a cancer family clinic in Wisconsin, USA, that 'clients say that a number gives them boundaries rather than having an ambiguous sense of being high risk'. Interestingly, however, even 5–10 per cent of individuals in this American study did not wish to have numerical risk information. The individual's background information, sociodemographic factors (e.g. educational level) and psychological profile could conceivably alter the optimal method of risk presentation because these can act as barriers to adequate informed consent.[24,25] One study has shown that the sociodemographic factors play a larger part in tailoring counselling style than psychological factors.[26]

Much of the research on risk perception has been done in industrial contexts. Familiarity with the risk has been shown to lower the perception of the risk level. For example, the perception of radiation risk by people living near nuclear power plants is lower than in those not living near to such installations.[27] However, in cancer families, it is possible that a larger cancer burden (the number and age at diagnosis of the cancer cases) may distort the risk above the true level, as is the case in families with cystic fibrosis.[22] Many people in cancer families think erroneously that their risk of developing cancer is 100 per cent and the only uncertainty is the point in time when the disease will occur. Lerman et al.[25] have reported that members of cancer families distort their risk, even when their family history consists of only one affected relative. There is evidence that overestimation of rare events can occur, if the event concerned is salient, for example, a recent cancer diagnosis in a young family member.

The definitions of risk are multidimensional. They consist of the probability of a negatively valued event occurring, the consequences of that event and the possible consequences of a person's behaviour (e.g. preventive actions) upon both these factors.[28] Vlek claims that there are five factors underlying perception of risk.[29] These are: (1) the potential degree of harm or lethality associated with the risk; (2) the controllability through safety/rescue measures (i.e. prevention/early detection); (3) the number of people exposed (this would equate to the cancer burden in the family); (4) the familiarity with the effects of the risk; and (5) the degree of voluntariness of exposure to the risk. Some individuals in our study expressed a wish only to know if they fall into a high, moderate or standard risk category;[30] however, it is unclear what these categories mean to patients. Wilkie assessed the perceived risk of inheriting adult polycystic kidney disease in children of an affected parent, who are at a one in two risk.[31] Although in the same risk category, the perceived risk category was variable, 26 per cent describing a high risk and 53 per cent a medium risk. However, descriptive rather than numerical risk levels may be more easily retained, as has been shown in a study of AFP screening in pregnancy.[32]

There are several reports regarding the perception of risk and the resultant effects on health monitoring behaviours,[20,33,34] some suggesting that those at highest risk have a lower uptake of health preventive measures.

THE FORMAT OF GENETIC RISK INFORMATION

There are several options for the form of presentation of risk information for the risk of developing cancer.

1 Numerical:
- risk per year;
- risk by a certain age;
- 1 in x value or percentage format;
- relative risk corrected for age.
2 General categorization. High/moderate/low risk (many now feel that the latter should be called standard or minimally increased risk as often the risk of common cancers is not a low risk, even in the general population). The problem with this concept is that different individuals and doctors assign the same risk levels to different categories
3 Situation analogy. A situation carrying an equivalent risk without any numerical information (e.g. the chances of picking an ace if one card is chosen blind from a card pack).
4 The risk figure measure:
- risk of developing cancer;
- risk of not developing cancer;
- risk of death from cancer (this is very rarely given in clinics as it is perceived as too distressing).

From studies of lung cancer, there is some evidence that the perceived risk of not developing cancer is different from that of developing the disease.[35] For example, a BRCA1 carrier has a lifetime risk (by age 80) of developing breast cancer of 85 per cent and, therefore, has a 15 per cent chance of not developing the disease. However, many women still believe that this risk level means they will inevitably develop breast cancer by age 80.

Clearly, if cancer family clinics are to provide a useful service, it would be important to ensure that counsellees understand the risk information and advice they are given. Lack of understanding of their risk could impact on their ability to use this information when making decisions about the future management of their health and may also affect their mental health, if cancer-related worries are increased through misunderstanding of information given in the clinic.

MEDICAL HISTORY AND EXAMINATION

It must be established from the history and examination whether the patient is an affected or an at-risk member of the family, and the patient should be questioned on any symptoms indicative of cancer or congenital abnormalities. Initial clinical examination involves looking for any dysmorphic features and congenital anomalies. The skin should be carefully examined, as many cancer syndromes are associated with dermatological features, such as pigmentary abnormalities (e.g. freckles are seen in Peutz–Jeghers syndrome, café au lait patches in neurofibromatosis or Turcot's syndrome, basal cell naevi in

Gorlin's syndrome, etc. Skin tumours, like the epidermoid cysts seen in FAP or keratoacanthomas seen in Muir–Torré or tricholemmas of Cowden's syndrome, can be indicators that the individual is, in fact, a gene carrier without the need for formal DNA genetic testing.

DISCUSSION OF CANCER SUSCEPTIBILITY AND RISKS

After taking a family history the next part of the interview involves communicating to the client the results of the pedigree assessment, risk assessment and clinical examination. If a particular diagnosis is made, then information about that disease is given. Those attending genetic clinics may have a very rudimentary knowledge of genetics, and it is important that they have a simple explanation of Mendelian genetics and how their risk has been assessed. A simple explanation of how cancer develops as a result of somatic genetic events is also sometimes helpful. In this way patients can understand the information they are given. If they are being given empiric risks, then the method by which these figures are derived must be explained. If there are no data, then this must also be discussed and, if the geneticist has a clinical impression that there may be something unusual occurring, but it is no more than a clinical judgement, then this must be made clear. Having a risk figure is useful for the clinician, as this will dictate what options for management are available, but may only be useful to patients if they are put into context, that is, in relation to the population risk of that and other cancers (see earlier). In particular, the age at which they are at greatest risk must be discussed, to enable management choices to be made, as they may affect the timing of prophylactic surgery or screening programmes.

Discussion of possibilities for screening and prevention should follow. Suggested screening protocols are shown in Table 30.3. This is a guide only and differs between different countries and regions. There are now many regional or country-specific guidelines available for management of cancer predisposition (e.g. references 2 and 36–39).

What is known about the value of any particular strategy, including its rationale, is explored. Since some individuals may wish to do nothing, it is important that this is also discussed as an acceptable option, and may be the right decision for some people. In some instances, prophylactic surgery needs to be discussed, but this must be approached with caution, as some patients are frightened or even horrified at the suggestion. They may feel that this is confirmation from the doctor that their risk of cancer is unacceptably high, and may accentuate any fears they may have of the disease and its treatment.

Throughout the interview, it is important to be sensitive to any psychopathology that may be occurring. Frequently, there will have been bereavement due to the premature death of close relatives, particularly a parent. Unresolved bereavement may make it difficult for people to accept their own risks and make decisions on their own management. In addition, patients are sometimes unable to cope with their worries. Referral for formal counselling may resolve these problems. Of particular concern are those individuals who have prophylactic surgery because of excess anxiety but who, while being temporarily relieved, often return at a later date with further cancer phobic symptoms. A psychological assessment and counselling should be mandatory before prophylactic mastectomy.

PREDICTIVE GENETIC TESTING

Direct mutation analysis is now possible for many different cancer susceptibilities (see Chapters 5, 6, 8, 10–12, 19, 24, 25, 27). This allows DNA analysis to be carried out and individuals with a susceptibility gene to be identified before the development of the disease. Owing to genetic heterogeneity (see later), it is important to first identify the specific genetic mutation present in the family. This is determined by testing an *affected* individual in the family (the *diagnostic* genetic test) to find the specific mutation that is present. The unaffected counsellee is then offered a test after full genetic counselling, using a protocol developed initially for Huntington's disease (see later). This is the *predictive* genetic test. Only in this situation is a negative result a true negative, since the disease-causing mutation has been identified in a close affected relative. In rare instances, a test is carried out on an unaffected individual only; for example, where the family is from a founder population and all the affected relatives are deceased or will not give blood for diagnostic testing. In this situation, a negative result for (i) the founder mutations will lower the cancer risk, although not to the level of the general population, or (ii) if a woman is in a family with deceased affected relatives and would decide to have prophylactic surgery, if a deleterious mutation were found, but just continue with screening, if no mutation were found. In this latter instance, part of the counselling session involves the explanation that a negative result may mean that the family is due to another gene other than that being tested and, therefore, the result is not a true negative.

In late-onset genetic disease susceptibilities, there is a consensus view that children (here classified as those aged under 18 years) should not be tested, unless there is to be a therapeutic intervention or change in management. However, some cancer susceptibilities do require screening during childhood; for instance, screening for familial polyposis coli usually starts in early teenage years by sigmoidoscopy. DNA testing before this time will allow half the individuals to avoid having this invasive procedure.

Table 30.3 *Screening protocols (for guidance only; different clinics/countries may have individual minor alterations to these schema)*

Disease	Screen	Age (years)
von Hippel–Lindau Affected	*Annual:* Physical examination Urine testing Direct and indirect ophthalmoscopy Fluorescein angiography 24-hour urinary VMA Renal ultrasound or MRI (CT if multiple cysts in kidneys or pancreas)	11 upwards
	3-yearly: MRI brain	until age 50 (then 5 yearly thereafter)
At-risk relatives	*Annual:* Physical examination Urine testing Direct and indirect ophthalmoscopy Fluorescein angiography 24-hour urinary VMA Renal ultrasound or MRI	5 upwards 5–60 10 upwards until 60 11 upwards 15 until 65
	3-yearly: MRI brain CT kidneys (more frequent if multiple cysts)	15–40 (then 5 yearly until 60) 20–65
	5-yearly: MRI brain	40–60
Familial polyposis Affected	Offer total colectomy with ileorectal anastomosis	Teenager (see below)
	Annual rectal stump screening (if conserved in surgery)	
	Upper gastrointestinal endoscopy 3-yearly (annually if polyps found)	20 upwards
At-risk relatives	Offer genetic analysis if possible	
	Annual sigmoidoscopy: perform colonoscopy when polyps found on sigmoidoscopy and arrange colectomy	11 upwards (polyps are rare before this age) to 40
Gorlin syndrome Affected (at-risk children usually have abnormal skull or spine X-rays by 5 years)	Annual dermatological examination Six-monthly orthopantomogram for jaw cysts Examination of infants for signs of medulloblastoma (some advocate MRI **but not** CT due to radiosensitivity)	Infants upwards
MEN 2	Offer genetic screening if possible – if positive perform prophylactic thyroidectomy	2
	Plasma calcium, phosphate and parathormone Pentagastrin test Thyroid ultrasound Abdominal ultrasound and CT 24-hour urinary VMA	8–70
MEN 1	*5-yearly:* Symptom enquiry (dyspepsia, diarrhoea, renal colic, fits, amenorrhoea, galactorrhoea) Examination Serum calcium Parathormone	5 upwards

(continued)

Table 30.3 *(continued)*

Disease	Screen	Age (years)
	Renal function Pituitary hormones (PL, GH, ACTH, FSH, TSH) Pancreatic hormones (gastrin, VIP, glucagons, neurotensin, somatostatin, pancreatic polypeptide) Lateral skull X-ray for pituitary size and MRI for pituitary adenomas	
Wilms' tumour At-risk individuals	*3 monthly:* Renal ultrasound	Birth to 8 years
	6-monthly: Renal ultrasound	8–12 years
Retinoblastoma (siblings and offspring of affected)	Offer genetic screening if possible Monthly retinal examination without anaesthetic 3-monthly retinal examination under anaesthetic 4-monthly retinal examination under anaesthetic 6-monthly retinal examination without anaesthetic Annual retinal examination without anaesthetic Annual examination for sarcoma	 Birth to 3 months 3 months until 2 years 2–3 years 3–5 years 5–11 years Early teens for life
Li–Fraumeni	Annual breast examination ?MRI (under investigation) Annual examination	18–60 years Lifelong
NF1 Affected	*Annual:* Examination Visual field assessment	Lifelong
NF2 At-risk relatives	Offer genetic screening if possible *Annual:* Examination Ophthalmoscopy for congenital cataracts Annual audiometry Brainstem audiotory-evoked potentials 3-yearly MRI	 Childhood 10–40
HNPCC	1–2-yearly colonoscopy Annual pelvic examination, and ovarian and endometrial ultrasound and CA125. Some units would now add pipelle screening Some screen for other cancers in kindred, such as skin and urothelial malignancy (urine cytology) *Annual:* Mammography:	25 upwards 35 upwards 35 upwards its use depends on the amount of breast cancer in family 35 upwards
Muir–Torré syndrome	As for HNPCC	
Turcot syndrome		
Colon cancer Single relative aged <45 years	5-yearly colonoscopy (3-yearly if polyps are found)	35 upwards
Familial melanoma	*Annual:* Skin examination	Teenager upwards
Breast/ovarian syndrome	Annual mammography	35 upwards or 5 years younger than youngest case (not less than 25; some countries advocate not below 30)

(continued)

Table 30.3 *(continued)*

Disease	Screen	Age (years)
	Annual pelvic transvaginal ultrasound and CA125	30–35 upwards
Familial breast cancer	Annual mammography	35 upwards or 5 years younger than youngest case (not less than 25; some countries advocate not below 30)
Familial ovarian cancer	Annual transvaginal ultrasound and CA125	30–35 upwards
Familial prostate cancer	*Annual:* Serum prostate-specific antigen Digital rectal examination (debate if this is needed)	50 upwards or 5 years younger than youngest case (minimum age 40; exceptionally below this if very index case)
Familial testicular cancer	Regular testicular self-examination	Late teens to 50

ACTH, adrenocorticotrophin; CT, computed tomography; FSH, follicle-stimulating hormone; GH, growth hormone; MRI, magnetic resonance imaging; PL, prolactin; TSH, thyroid-stimulating hormone; VIP, vasoactive intestinal peptide; VMA, vanillyl mandelic acid.

Testing would, therefore, seem entirely reasonable, particularly as preventive treatment by prophylactic surgery has been demonstrated as being a successful cancer prevention. The value of testing for other cancer susceptibilities, where the role of screening and prevention is unknown, is more debatable. Many of the issues that have been discussed at length in relation to testing for other adult-onset genetic diseases, such as Huntington's chorea, where prevention is not possible, are relevant. It has been demonstrated that, using a set protocol for individuals having predictive testing for Huntington's chorea helps to minimize the problems experienced and allows the individual to have time to decide if they really want the test and for what reason.[40] There may be many reasons why individuals may wish to have a predictive test. They may want to know if they have the gene before starting a family or to make plans for their own future. Some wish to make choices concerning prophylactic surgery or participation in screening or chemoprevention studies. Facing a high risk of breast cancer is particularly difficult for some women. Often there have been several deaths from the disease in the family and, since there is often a mother who had died when the patient was only in her teens, the memories can be particularly painful. Since there may already be a great deal of anxiety about the disease, it may be very traumatic to find that the chance of having the gene for early breast cancer is high. It is, therefore, recommended that a formal protocol is followed when offering predictive testing for all cancer predisposition genes.[40]

The genetic testing procedure has several phases. Initially, the pros and cons and accuracy of the test are explained to the patient. These are the differences a positive and negative test result would make to the cancer risk if the gene being tested is indeed the cause of the cancers in the family, the ending of uncertainty, and the provision of more data on which to base decisions about clinical management and lifestyle. Potential disadvantages are psychological morbidity (although many clients are already very anxious) and the insurance implications. In the UK, all results of genetic tests currently have to be declared in the same way as any other medical test, when seeking insurance for policies above a certain value. At present, the insurance companies do not actively request that these tests are performed. In certain instances, testing can be advantageous, since some individuals in families are denied critical illness insurance to cover a cancer diagnosis. A negative test in such individuals may enable them to obtain insurance. There is a concurrent psychological assessment with the first counselling session. The client is then given a period of reflection (usually a minimum of 1 month) to decide whether or not to have the test and, if they decide to proceed, they are seen again to discuss their reasons for wishing to do so. It is only then that the blood sample for testing is collected after written consent. The disclosure session is carefully planned so that the client knows how long they will have to wait for the result and they are advised to bring a supportive person to the consultation when the result is given. Following this, they are seen at suitable intervals to ensure that they are not having any psychological problems.

GENETIC HETEROGENEITY

The number of families that can have predictive testing is limited by the degree of genetic heterogeneity, that is, when more than one locus may cause the same condition.

For instance, approximately one-quarter of large, early-onset breast cancer families tested for linkage to *BRCA1* and *BRCA2* are unlinked, suggesting the possibility of other susceptibility genes. If no mutation is detected, it is difficult to offer molecular testing as the mutation may be present in either *BRCA1* or *BRCA2* but not be detected, or one of the other as yet unidentified genes. Patients are often disappointed that they are unable to have a test. For many cancer predisposition genes, mutation analysis to find the mutation on the diagnostic test is quite labour intensive, particularly when the gene is large and mutations can occur at many different sites within the gene in different families, as is the case with *BRCA1*, and can, therefore, take some time (a matter of months).

KEY POINTS

- The family history is still the cornerstone of cancer predisposition diagnosis, but as genetic analysis and the number of cancer predisposition genes increases, this will be complemented by molecular diagnosis
- Currently, much of cancer genetics is conducted within the genetics services but increasingly cancer genetics is impacting upon oncological practice. This will necessitate the education of oncologists in cancer genetics
- Cancer genetics services should be set up with staff trained in both genetics and oncology, and should incorporate the use of national/international management guidelines, audit and quality assurance. There should be good links with the molecular testing laboratory, which should also comply with national quality assurance guidelines.

REFERENCES

1. Claus EB, Risch NJ, Thompson WD. Genetic analysis of breast cancer in the cancer and steroid hormone study. *Am J Hum Genet* 1991; **48**:232–242.
2. Eisinger F, Alby N, Bremond A, *et al*. Recommendations for the management of women with a genetic risk for developing cancer of the breast and/or the ovary. *Bull Cancer* 1999; **86**:307–313.
3. Hodgson SV, Haites NE, Caligo M, *et al*. A survey of the current clinical facilities for the management of familial cancer in Europe. European Union BIOMED II Demonstration Project: Familial Breast Cancer: audit of a new development in medical practice in European centres. *J Med Genet* 2000; **37**:605–607.
4. *Harper Report: cancer genetic services.* London; HMSO, 1997.
5. Gaff C, Aittomaki K, Williamson R. Oncology nurse training in cancer genetics. *J Med Genet* 2001; **38**:691–695.
6. Lakhani SR, Van De Vijver MJ, Jacquemier J, Anderson TJ, Osin PP, McGuffog L, Easton DF. The pathology of familial breast cancer: predictive value of immunohistochemical markers estrogen receptor, progesterone receptor, HER-2, and p53 in patients with mutations in *BRCA1* and *BRCA2*. *J Clin Oncol* 2002; **20**:2310–2318.
7. Ponder BAJ. Setting up and running a familial cancer clinic. *Br Med Bull* 1994; **50**:732.
8. Emery J, Walton R, Murphy M, Austoker J, Yudkin P, Chapman C, Coulson A, Glasspool D, Fox J. Computer support for interpreting family histories of breast and ovarian cancer in primary care: comparative study with simulated cases. *BMJ* 2000; **321**:28–32.
9. Harper PS. In: *Practical genetic counselling*, 3rd edn. Wright, Butterworth & Co, 1988; 3–17.
10. Douglas FS, O'Dair LC, Robinson M, Evans DG, Lynch SA. The accuracy of diagnoses as reported in families with cancer: a retrospective study. *J Med Genet* 1999; **36**:309–312.
11. Bennett, RL, Steinhaus, KA, Uhrich, SB. *et al*. Recommendations for standardized human pedigree nomenclature. *Am J Hum Genet* 1995; **56**:745–752.
12. St John DVB, McDermott FT, Hopper VL, *et al*. Cancer risks in relatives of patients with common colorectal cancer. *Ann Intern Med* 1993; **118**:785–790.
13. Murday VA, Slack J. Inherited disorders associated with colorectal cancer. *Cancer Surv* 1989; **8**:139–159.
14. Eeles RA, the UK Familial Prostate Study Co-ordinating Group & the CRC/BPG UK Familial Prostate Cancer Study Collaborators. Genetic predisposition to prostate cancer. *Prostate Cancer Prostatic Dis* 1999; **2**:9–15.
15. Croyle RT, Sun L-C, Louie TH. Psychological minimization of cholesterol test results: moderators of appraisal in college students and community residents. *Health Psychol* 1993; **12**:503–507.
16. Kelly PT. Informational needs of individuals and families with hereditary cancers. *Semin Oncol Nurs* 1992; **8**:288–292.
17. Evans DGR, Burnell LD, Hopwood P, Howell A. Perception of risk in women with a family history of breast cancer. *Br J Cancer* 1993; **67**:612–614.
18. Watson M, Duvivier V, Wade-Walsh M, *et al*. Family history of breast cancer: what do women understand and recall about their genetic risk? *J Med Genet* 1998; **35**:731–738.
19. Cull A, Miller H, Porterfield T, *et al*. The use of videotaped information in cancer genetic counseling: a randomised evaluation study. *Br J Cancer* 1998; **77**:830–837.
20. Green CIA, Brown RA. Counting lives. *J Occup Accidents* 1978; **2**:55.
21. Sorensen JR, Swazey JP, Scotch NA. Reproductive past, reproductive futures: genetic counselling and its effectiveness. *Birth defects: original article series*, 17, 4. New York, 1981:1–19.
22. Leonard C, Chase G, Childs B. Genetic counselling, a consumer's view. *N Engl J Med* 1972; **287**:433–439.
23. Josten DM, Evans AM, Love RR. The cancer prevention clinic: a service program for cancer-prone families. *J Psychosoc Oncol* 1985; **3**:5–20.
24. Merz JF, Fisdhoff B. Informed consent does not mean rational consent. *J Legal Med* 1990; **11**:321–350.
25. Lerman C, Daly M, Masny A, Balshem A. Attitudes about genetic testing for breast–ovarian cancer susceptibility. *J Clin Oncol* 1994; **12**:843–850.

26. Lobb EA, Butow PN, Meiser B, *et al.* Tailoring communication in consultations with women from high risk breast cancer families. *Br J Cancer* 2002; **87**:502–508.

27. Guedeney C, Mendel C. *L'Angoisse atomique et les centres nucleaires.* Paris: Payot, 1973.

28. Evers-Kiebooms C, Cassiman JJ, Van der Ilerghe H, d'Ydewalle G. (eds) *Genetic risk, risk perception and decision making.* New York: Alan R. Liss, Inc, 1987.

29. Vlek C. Risk assessment, risk perception and decision making about courses of action involving genetic risk: an overview of concepts and methods. *March Dimes Birth Defects Found* 1987; **23**:171–207.

30. Watson M, Lloyd S, Davidson J, *et al.* The impact of genetic counseling on risk perception and mental health in women with a family history of breast cancer. *Br J Cancer* 1999; **79**:868–874.

31. Wilkie PA. *Genetic counselling and adult polycystic kidney disease. Patients' knowledge, perceptions and understanding.* PhD thesis, Stirling University, 1992.

32. Chase GA, Faden RR, Holtzman NA, *et al.* Assessment of risk by pregnant women: implications for genetic counseling and education. *Soc Biol* 1986; **33**:57–64.

33. Kash KM, Holland JC, Halper MS, Miller DC. Psychological distress and surveillance behaviors of women with a family history of breast cancer. *J Natl Cancer Inst* 1991; **84**:24–30.

34. Polednak AP, Lane DS, Burg MA. Risk perception, family history and use of breast cancer screening tests. *Cancer Detect Prevent* 1991; **15**:257–263.

35. McNeil BJ, Pauker SC, Sox HG Jr, Tversky A. On the elicitation of preferences for alternative therapies. *N Engl J Med* 1982; **306**:1259–1262.

36. Vasen HF, Haites NE, Evans DG, *et al.* Current policies for surveillance and management in women at risk of breast and ovarian cancer: a survey among 16 European family clinics. European Familial Breast Cancer Collaborative Group. *Eur J Cancer* 1998; **34**:1922–1926.

37. Moller P, Evans G, Haites N, *et al.* Guidelines for follow-up of women at high risk for inherited breast cancer: consensus statement from the Biomed 2 Demonstration Programme on Inherited Breast Cancer. *Dis Markers* 1999; **15**:207–211.

38. Eccles DM, Evans DGR, Mackay J, on behalf of the UK Cancer Family Study Group. Guidelines for a genetic risk based approach to advising women with a family history of breast cancer. *J Med Genet* 2000; **37**:203–209.

39. Dunlop MG. British Society for Gastroenterology: Association for Coloproctology for Great Britain & Ireland. Guidance on gastrointestinal surveillance for hereditary non-polyposis colorectal cancer, familial adenomatous polyposis, juvenile polyposis and Peutz-Jeghers syndrome, and guidance on large bowel surveillance for people with two first degree relatives with colorectal cancer or one first degree relative diagnosed with colorectal cancer under 45 years. *Gut* 2002; **51**(Suppl 5):v 21–27 and v 17–20.

40. Tyler A, Ball D, Craufurd D, on behalf of the United Kingdom Huntington's Disease Prediction Consortium. Presymptomatic testing for Huntington's Disease in the United Kingdom. *Br Med J* 1992; **304**:15934.

31

Psychological issues in cancer genetics

KATHRYN M. KASH, MARY KAY DABNEY AND SUSAN K. BOOLBOL

INTRODUCTION

It was over 10 years ago that the first gene was identified as being a likely candidate for breast cancer predisposition.[1] Prior to this time, Lynch and colleagues[2] had begun looking at families in which there was a preponderance of breast cancer and ovarian cancer. Since that time two major breast–ovarian cancer susceptibility genes have been cloned and sequenced, namely, the *BRCA1* and *BRCA2* genes for hereditary breast and/or ovarian cancer (HBOC).[3,4] In addition, other major cancer susceptibility genes have been cloned and sequenced, including the *APC* gene for familial adenomatous polyposis (FAP)[5] and the *MLH1, MSH2, MSH6, PMS1* and *PMS2* genes for hereditary non-polyposis colon cancer (HNPCC).[6,7] These scientific advances offer new opportunities for members of families with several relatives with various cancers to discover whether or not they carry a genetic mutation and subsequently have an increased risk of developing cancer.

Approximately 205 000 new cases of breast cancer will be diagnosed this year in the USA, with an estimated 44 000 women dying of the disease.[8] Although only 5–10 per cent of all breast cancers are thought inherited,[1,2] women with family histories of the disease are being targeted for genetic testing. The picture for ovarian cancer is somewhat different. Ovarian cancer is the fifth leading cause of cancer in women in the USA, with an estimated 25 200 occurring each year, and it is the fifth leading cause of cancer deaths in women, with a total of 14 500 deaths each year.[8] Ovarian cancer is frequently called 'the silent killer', as there are few patient complaints, and

non-specific signs or symptoms of the disease until it is diagnosed. Because ovarian cancer is diagnosed at later stages, the cure rate is significantly lower than if detected at an earlier stage. This can take an emotional toll on the woman with ovarian cancer as well as other family members.

Given the high breast cancer rate, the deadly nature of ovarian cancer, and the preponderance of media attention to breast and ovarian cancer susceptibility genes, many women want to have genetic testing without understanding the full ramifications of the decision-making process. The focus of this chapter will be on the consequences of genetic testing for breast and ovarian cancers in both the research and clinical settings. We will discuss genetic testing for breast and ovarian cancer susceptibility, describe optimal genetic counselling, present the latest prevention strategies for breast and ovarian cancers, and summarize the interactions between genetic testing and psychological distress throughout the chapter.

CANCER GENETIC TESTING AND PSYCHOLOGICAL DISTRESS

Early studies of women at high risk for cancer

Prior to genetic testing for cancer susceptibility genes being available on a clinical basis, there were studies done looking at the interest in genetic testing, and the emotional distress of individuals at risk for breast and ovarian cancer. These women and men were the most likely to be mutation carriers of BRCA1/2.

Initially studies were conducted to investigate the screening behaviours of women who were at high risk for breast cancer because of their strong family histories of the disease. The first study was done by Kash and colleagues[9] and reported on adherence to screening in high-risk women. The investigators found that, in 217 high-risk women, 94 per cent had age-appropriate mammograms, only 69 per cent had appropriate clinical breast examinations by a physician or nurse practitioner, and a small number (40 per cent) performed monthly breast self-examinations (BSE). Increased anxiety significantly predicted poor adherence to both clinical breast examination and BSE. In addition, 27 per cent of these women were suffering clinical psychological distress. Lerman and colleagues also conducted a study looking at adherence to screening guidelines.[10] The authors found that the more intrusive thoughts about breast cancer a woman had, the less adherence to mammography guidelines. The concern raised by these early studies was that adherence to screening was not higher but lower, and predicted by women's anxiety levels and intrusive thoughts of cancer.

A large sample of women at risk for breast cancer was used to investigate knowledge and attitudes about genetic testing and psychological distress.[11] A total of 1007 women, who were part of a national high-risk registry, from rural and urban areas of the USA completed a questionnaire regarding genetic testing, psychological distress and health beliefs. Anxiety played a major role in this study and was breast cancer specific.[12] The predictors of willingness to undergo genetic testing were:

1 fewer negative aspects of testing ($p < 0.0001$);
2 more positive aspects of testing ($p < 0.0001$);
3 greater anxiety about breast cancer ($p < 0.0005$);
4 greater the perception of risk ($p < 0.0001$);
5 less formal education ($p < 0.01$);
6 less knowledge of genetic testing ($p < 0.01$).

Thus, it appears that women who seek testing are more anxious and may have poorer decision-making skills. Distressed individuals may be more vulnerable to adverse psychological consequences upon learning their positive (or negative) genetic status. Women who are distressed, have poor knowledge of genetic testing and a greater perception of being a gene carrier may suffer negative psychological sequelae.

Over 70 per cent of women in this study overestimated their risk for developing breast cancer. A woman's perception of her risk is frequently overestimated, despite genetic counselling. It has been our experience that perception of risk varies from time to time depending on the cancer status of family members, current events in their lives, information received from professionals, as well as the latest from the print and Internet media. Thus, we think of risk perception as a 'moving target' in that it can be influenced by various factors and change. Accurate risk communication and information as well as information about prevention and screening options are necessary to help women make appropriate decisions about genetic testing. It is clear from the data above that the more knowledge that women have, the less likely they are to undergo genetic testing. All women need to be educated regarding the appropriate use of genetic testing.

There were two studies looking at the short-term effects in distress following genetic testing for BRCA1/2. Lerman and colleagues[13] reported interim data from a prospective cohort study of members of several HBOC families. At baseline and 1 month follow-up, all carriers, non-carriers and decliners of BRCA1 testing scored in the normal ranges on these measures. However, non-carriers exhibited significant decreases in depressive symptoms and role impairment, and marginally significant decreases in sexual impairment, as compared to carriers and decliners. In a second outcome study of BRCA1 testing, Croyle and colleagues[14] reported on the short-term (1–2 week) impact of testing on general distress and breast cancer-specific distress in high-risk women. Although BRCA1 carriers did not demonstrate increases in general distress, they did report significantly higher post-test levels of intrusive thoughts. In a follow-up study, Lerman and colleagues found that decliners were more depressed, from 26 per cent at baseline, to 47 per cent at 6 months.[15] While these studies indicated some negative psychological impact of testing on carriers and decliners, and improvement in non-carriers, long-term studies were indicated as the next step in trying to determine if there is a lasting impact of genetic testing on distress, and what are the best ways to help individuals cope with their risk or gene mutation status.

Impact of genetic testing

What have we learned from research about the impact of genetic testing on decision-making, emotional distress and family communication about testing? Armstrong and colleagues[16] examined the factors involved in decision-making about genetic testing and found that those who had testing were more likely to:

1 have a family history;
2 be of Ashkenazi Jewish descent;
3 want information about cancer risk for other family members (siblings, etc.);
4 want information about ovarian cancer risk;
5 be less concerned about employment or insurance discrimination.

Other studies looking at decision-making about preventive strategies versus surveillance measures and ways to improve decision-making will be discussed later in this chapter.

One of the main reasons women give for obtaining genetic testing is to learn the risks for other family members, including their siblings and children. Tercyak and colleagues[17] queried a small number of children of women who had breast–ovarian cancer. They found that the children had average levels of distress and cancer worries. Their suggestion is that children with high distress have increased cancer worries and need more attention when learning the gene mutation status of the parent. Close familial relationships foster good communication among family members. However, in some families there is alienation prior to genetic testing and already distant relationships become more strained. Hughes and colleagues[18] studied the process and content of family communications. They found that women who were BRCA1/2 gene mutation positive communicated their results to significantly more sisters than women who received uninformative results did. Women who are gene mutation positive need emotional support and advice about the medical decisions that need to be made. Women who receive uninformative results continue to have uncertainty about their risk and may not want to discuss the information with anyone. They also found that women who did not share test results had emotionally distant relationships.

In terms of emotional distress associated with genetic testing, there are a few studies but with varying results. Dorval and colleagues[19] looked at 41 (34 gene mutation-negative and 7 gene mutation-positive) individuals pre- and post-testing for BRCA1 carrier status. They were queried as to their anticipated reactions to genetic testing results, imagining first that they were gene mutation negative and then they were gene mutation positive. The findings were that affected BRCA1 carriers have higher levels of anger and worry than they anticipated. In addition, those who underestimated the subsequent emotional distress had an increase in psychological distress 6 months later. While the number who were gene-mutation positive was small, this is similar to Tercyak and colleagues,[20] who found that post-testing there was greater distress in those with a positive gene mutation status. Coyne and colleagues questioned the validity of the psychological distress measures being used. He used standard psychiatric diagnostic measures and found that women enrolled in a hereditary breast ovarian registry showed 'average' levels of distress.[21] Perhaps measuring distress in cancer-prone families needs newer ways that are genetic testing specific.[22] These would seem to be more appropriate for this population. One study[23] of both affected ($n = 186$) and unaffected ($n = 93$) individuals seeking genetic testing saw no adverse effects on distress among affected or unaffected individuals. However, unaffected gene mutation negative individuals showed less cancer-specific distress at 6 months.

It appears that psychological or emotional distress may be less than anticipated, thus reducing the need for extensive psychological counselling.

GENETIC COUNSELLING

Our clinical cancer genetics programme instituted a protocol for cancer susceptibility testing several years ago. Specifically, this protocol requires that all individuals interested in pursuing such testing participate in a genetic counselling consultation with a genetic counsellor prior to testing. Prior to the first genetic counselling session, a form is completed to assist the counsellor in preparing for the session. Among the items on this form is the woman's risk perception for being a gene mutation carrier as well as developing breast and ovarian cancer, reasons for genetic counselling and testing, as well as current screening methods. The responses are discussed in the genetic counselling session. A family history of all cancers is obtained from the individual seeking genetic counselling and testing. For the most part, individuals without a personal or family history of breast, ovarian or any cancer are not appropriate candidates for BRCA1/2 gene testing. Whenever possible, a confirmatory diagnosis of cancer should be obtained. It is possible for individuals to falsify their histories of cancer to obtain risk-reducing surgery (mastectomies). Thus, there are certain times when the genetic counsellor may be suspicious about the reported family history of cancer. If there is a prolonged survival from an early-onset breast or ovarian cancer, inconsistent information about the age or diagnosis of the person with cancer, a lack of detailed information about close relatives or a psychiatric history in the family, then further investigation is warranted. Additionally, test results are only disclosed during a follow-up consultation with the genetic counsellor. During the genetic counselling consultation, the genetics of breast and ovarian cancer, the nature of BRCA1 and BRCA2 genes, cancer risks associated with a mutation in either the BRCA1 or BRCA2 genes, the risk of carrying a mutation in either the BRCA1 or BRCA2 genes based on her personal and family history of cancer, the risks, benefits and limitations of genetic testing, medical management of her unaffected breast (if a personal history of breast cancer), and cancer-screening recommendations are discussed in detail.

If a woman is Ashkenazi Jewish with breast and/or ovarian cancer, and has a family history of either disease, she is more likely to carry two common mutations in BRCA1 (called 185delAG and 5382insC) and one common mutation in BRCA2 (called 6174delT), owing to a phenomenon called founder effect. Collectively, these three mutations have been shown to have a frequency of approximately 1 in 40 to 1 in 50 (or 2–2.5 per cent) in the general Ashkenazi Jewish population. These mutations are thought to account for most of the breast and ovarian cancer risk associated with inherited mutations in the BRCA1 and BRCA2 genes in Ashkenazi Jewish women.

If after the consultation, a woman agrees to have her blood drawn, she must read and sign the consent form. A blood sample is taken and sent to a clinical laboratory in Utah. Women are told that the results would be ready in 3–5 weeks. Once we receive them, the woman is contacted by telephone to set up a time to come in to discuss her test results in detail. The information presented in the first session is very complex and may need to be repeated again during a second discussion, as some individuals cannot recall all of the information and need cognitive reinforcement.[24–26]

When the genetic counsellor feels it is necessary, a psychologist may participate in the genetic counselling process. From a psychological perspective, there are factors to be considered in the process. One is the motivation for genetic testing. Is the individual seeking testing because they need certainty in order to make medical decisions? This is one of the best reasons to undergo testing. However, many individuals are highly anxious, have misinformation, or are pressured from family members and seek genetic testing. It is important to ascertain any problems as they may interfere with the individual's capacity for providing informed consent as well as impeding good decision-making.

SCREENING AND PREVENTION STRATEGIES FOR BREAST AND OVARIAN CANCER

The identification of breast and ovarian cancer predisposition genes, BRCA1 and BRCA2, has allowed women who are at a 50–85 per cent lifetime risk of developing breast cancer and a 15–65 per cent lifetime risk of developing ovarian cancer to be identified.[27] Options for carriers of BRCA1/BRCA2 mutations fall into one of three categories: early and frequent surveillance, chemoprevention and prophylactic or risk-reducing surgery.[28] We use the term 'risk-reducing' rather than 'prophylactic' as there is a small chance of a cancer occurring at a later date. Since the occurrence of and the prevention options for breast and ovarian cancer are different, the psychological issues associated may be distinct for each disease.

Breast cancer options

SURVEILLANCE

For decades, the best ways to ensure secondary prevention of breast cancer have been screening. While the data has been conflicting regarding the efficacy of breast self-examination, the three recognized methods of screening for breast cancer include mammography (yearly over the age of 40 for all women), clinical breast examination (annually for women at average risk and semi-annually for women at high risk over the age of 25) and BSE (monthly for all women beginning by age 18–21). There has been research indicating that high levels of distress interfere with mammography,[10] clinical breast examination[9] and BSE.[9] Women who report distress around screening issues should be counselled and educated regarding the efficacy of these methods. For women who are carriers of a BRCA1 or BRCA2 gene mutation, a Consensus Statement from the Cancer Genetics Studies Consortium[28] has established recommendations. These guidelines include mammography, clinical breast examination and BSE in a stepped-up fashion for these women. At one family cancer clinic, the investigators screened 128 women who were BRCA1/2 gene mutation carriers with annual mammogram and 6-month clinical breast examinations, and taught them BSE.[29] More breast cancers were detected than expected in the carrier group during the 3-year follow-up. This study demonstrates that screening, when followed, is effective. In the Kash et al. study above, women reported that, if they had a gene mutation, they would be more likely to follow screening guidelines. However, evidence indicates that women who are most distressed would need help in coping with distress and adhering to the guidelines. Studies indicated that younger women who are BRCA1/2 gene mutation carriers do not follow the guidelines for mammography.[30,31] Perhaps this is because the sensitivity of mammography for women under 35 years of age is limited.[32] Ways to increase surveillance for gene mutation carriers need further investigation.

CHEMOPREVENTION

Chemoprevention studies have been limited to the use of tamoxifen (hormonal therapy) in a large randomized controlled study. The National Surgical Adjuvant Breast and Bowel Project (NSABP) in the USA found that the risk of invasive breast cancer was significantly reduced by 55 per cent in women who took tamoxifen in a placebo-controlled trial.[33] However, two other trials in the UK and Italy found no significant effects of tamoxifen.[34] There may be confounding factors, such as the use of hormone replacement therapy (HRT) in the UK and Italian studies, and the use of risk-reducing surgery of oophorectomy in the Italian sample. In clinic settings in the USA, women at high risk are being offered tamoxifen even though there are some side effects (hot flashes, vaginal dryness, etc.) that interfere with quality of life and adverse consequences (pulmonary emboli, endometrial cancer, etc.) that can be potentially life threatening. There are reports in our clinic from young women that they go

both ovaries. As far back as the early 1980s, risk-reducing surgery has been recommended to decrease the occurrence of ovarian cancer.[54] In 1995, a National Institutes of Health Consensus Development Panel recommended risk-reducing oophorectomy for women who are *BRCA1* and *BRCA2* gene mutation carriers, after they have finished their childbearing years.[55] While this may be a reasonable alternative to the uncertainty of ovarian cancer screening, it is not an option for women in the general population. In addition, bilateral oophorectomy is risk-reducing surgery and does not guarantee 100 per cent effectiveness, as a small number of women may develop peritoneal carcinomatosis.[54,56] A risk-reducing bilateral salpingo-oophorectomy can be done laparoscopically as long as adequate margins are obtained. A recent paper by Kauff *et al.* suggests that bilateral oophorectomy reduces the incidence of both ovarian and breast cancers in women who are *BRCA1/2* gene mutation carriers.[57] A very interesting study by Grann *et al.* estimated both the survival benefits and quality-adjusted survival of women who are *BRCA1/2* gene mutation carriers undergoing eight preventive strategies. They found that there was a greater survival benefit for risk-reducing strategies over surveillance. The best overall survival was from mastectomy and oophorectomy, but the best quality-adjusted survival was for tamoxifen and oophorectomy.[58] Women would prefer to keep their breasts and remove their ovaries while using hormonal therapy.

Research studies have examined the psychological issues of participating in an Ovarian Cancer Registry[59] or a Family Risk Assessment Program,[60] the psychological impact of being screened for familial ovarian cancer,[60–63] and the predictors of psychological distress among women at increased risk for ovarian cancer[64] or women who are attending an ovarian cancer screening program.[63] One study found that screening for ovarian cancer increased anxiety when a false positive was found on ultrasonography and anxiety decreased in those who were true negatives.[61] Another study found that CA-125 screening increased as both the number of relatives affected with ovarian cancer and cancer worries increased.[62] A third study found that one-third of women attending a screening clinic for high-risk women were above the cut-off point for depression and 16 per cent were above the cut-off point for anxiety. Those who minimized their risk had no anxiety and only 16 per cent were clinically depressed.[63]

The same suggestion for risk-reducing surgery for breast cancer applies to ovarian cancer. All women seeking risk-reducing surgery by removing their ovaries should have a consultation with a gynaecologic surgeon, a genetic counsellor and a psychologist. Women should take time (sometimes months) to consider this option for the prevention of ovarian cancer. The implications for childbearing should be carefully considered. Perhaps risk-reducing surgery for ovarian cancer should only be offered to women who are over the age of 40 or childbearing age.

Psychological consultation for risk–reducing surgery

One of the roles for psychiatry and psychology in the field of genetics is to provide consultation to women who are considering risk-reducing surgery. Since these procedures impact on a woman's sense of self-esteem, her sexuality and childbearing ability, a full and thorough discussion of all the nuances is warranted. The purpose of the consultation is to assist women with appropriate decision-making in respect to gene mutation status and perceived risk, impact on the family, key steps and certainty of decision-making, and the motivating factors for risk-reducing surgery. The first step is to determine if there is a previous psychiatric history. This includes past and present mental health, current mental health status, and premorbid personality and life events. Levels of anxiety and depression are crucial and, if too high, may interfere with decision-making. The next step is to determine her perception of risk for developing cancer, her perception of the management options and her perception of disease outcome, should it develop. The focus shifts then to current life events as well as family communication patterns. This is frequently the time when the psychologist learns of 'secrets' or lack of knowledge about the family. This information is important in order to look at the social support and coping strategies of a woman. If there is little or no support, and the woman feels socially isolated, than services or some type of intervention may be necessary. How a woman copes with other issues that arise in her life will tell you how she will handle the stress associated with genetic testing. If the woman uses active coping for life events or a perceived threat versus using behavioural disengagement, then it is more than likely that she will handle genetic testing well. A discussion of the risk-reducing strategies is necessary as well as any age guidelines, side effects, intimacy issues, etc. This consultation usually takes about one and a half hours and the woman is asked to bring her spouse, partner, friend or significant other in order to help with recall of information, increase communication within families, and offer support.

SUMMARY

Perhaps the most serious limitation of genetic testing is that state-of-the-art preventive and surveillance strategies do not match the test information. To receive positive test results when there is no adequate treatment can be tragic. Since the inception of genetic testing for cancer susceptibility, there have been great strides made in trying to find the optimal ways to decrease risk for breast and ovarian cancer in *BRCA1/2* gene mutation carriers. Genetic testing results can have a profound impact, not only on the individual, but also on the entire family. The option of risk-reducing surgery should only be considered if the family or personal history of cancer has been verified and is not fictitious, if a genetic test result is not pending, and if the risk-reducing surgery is the woman's own choice. Studies indicated that at times family communications are poor, emotional distress is high, and anxiety and worry about cancer interfere with good decision-making. Going forward, studies of tailored and targeted interventions that improve personal choices about surveillance and risk-reducing surgery are essential.

KEY POINTS

- Genetic testing for cancer susceptibility genes has a profound impact on the lives of everyone within a family.
- Perception of risk is frequently a 'moving target'.
- Women need clear, accurate information in order to consider genetic testing.
- Anxiety and worry may interfere with the decision-making process.
- Those who decline genetic testing may be at risk for psychological distress.
- Gene mutation carriers may not adhere to current recommendations for surveillance or risk-reducing surgery.
- The long term psychological impact of genetic testing is unknown in carriers and non-carriers of gene mutations.
- Psychological evaluation is essential prior to any risk-reducing surgery.

REFERENCES

1. Hall JM, Lee MK, Morrow J, *et al*. Linkage analysis of early onset familial breast cancer to chromosome 17q21. *Science* 1990; **250**:1684–1689.
2. Lynch HT, Harries RE, Guirgis HA, *et al*. Familial association of breast/ovarian cancer. *Cancer* 1978; **41**:1543–1549.
3. Miki Y, Swensen J, Shattuck-Eidens D, *et al*. A strong candidate for the breast and ovarian cancer susceptibility gene *BRCA1*. *Science* 1994; **266**:66–71.
4. Wooster R, Bignell G, Lancaster J, *et al*. Identification of the breast cancer susceptibility gene *BRCA2*. *Nature* 1995; **378**:789–792.
5. Leppert M, Burt R, Hughes JP, *et al*. Genetic analysis of an inherited predisposition of colon cancer in a family with a variable number of adenomatous polyps. *N Engl J Med* 1990; **322**:904–908.

6. Nicolaides NC, Papadopoulos N, Liu B, *et al*. Mutations of two PMS homologues in hereditary nonpolyposis colon cancer. *Nature* 1994; **271**:75–78.
7. Peltomäki P, Aaltonen LA, Sistonen P, *et al*. Genetic mapping of a locus predisposing to human colorectal cancer. *Science* 1993; **260**:810–812.
8. American Cancer Society. *Cancer facts and figures: 2002*. New York: American Cancer Society 2002.
9. Kash KM, Holland JC, Halper MS, Miller DG. Psychological distress and surveillance behaviors of women with a family history of breast cancer. *J Natl Cancer Inst* 1992; **84**:24–30.
10. Lerman C, Daly M, Sands C, *et al*. Mammography adherence and psychological distress among women at risk for breast cancer. *J Natl Cancer Inst* 1993; **85**:1074–1080.
11. Kash KM, Ortega-Verdejo K, Dabney MK, *et al*. Psychological aspects of genetic breast cancer. *Semin Surg Oncol* 2000; **18**:333–338.
12. Kash KM, Jacobsen PB, Holland JC, *et al*. An instrument to measure breast cancer anxiety. *Psychosom Med* 1996; **58**:45.
13. Lerman C, Narod S, Schulman K, *et al*. *BRCA1* testing in hereditary breast–ovarian cancer families: a prospective study of patient decision-making and outcomes. *JAMA* 1996; **275**:1885–1892.
14. Croyle RT, Smith K, Botkin J, *et al*. Psychological responses to *BRCA1* mutation testing. Preliminary findings. *Health Psychol* 1997; **16**:63–72.
15. Lerman C, Hughes C, Lemon SJ, *et al*. What you don't know can hurt you: Adverse psychologic effects in members of *BRCA1*-linked and *BRCA2*-linked families who decline genetic testing. *J Clin Oncol* 1998; **16**:1650–1654.
16. Armstrong K, Calzone K, Stopfer J, *et al*. Factors associated with decisions about clinical *BRCA1/2* testing. *Cancer Epidemiol Biomarkers Prev* 2000; **9**:1251–1254.
17. Tercyak KP, Peshkin BN, Streisand R, Lerman C. Psychological issues among children of hereditary breast cancer gene (*BRCA1/2*) testing participants. *Psycho-Oncol* 2001; **10**:336–346.
18. Hughes C, Lerman C, Schwartz M, *et al*. All in the family: evaluation of the process and content of sisters' communication about *BRCA1* and *BRCA2* genetic results. *Am J Med Genet* 2002; **107**:143–150.
19. Dorval M, Patenaude AF, Schneider KA, *et al*. Anticipated versus actual emotional reactions to disclosure of results of genetic tests for cancer susceptibility: findings from *p53* and *BRCA1* testing programs. *J Clin Oncol* 2000; **18**:2135–2142.
20. Tercyak KP, Lerman C, Peshkin BN, *et al*. Effects of coping style and *BRCA1* and *BRCA2* test results on anxiety among women participating in genetic counselling and testing for breast and ovarian cancer risk. *Health Psychol* 2001; **20**:217–222.
21. Coyne JC, Benazon NR, Gaba CG, *et al*. Distress and psychiatric morbidity among women from high-risk breast and ovarian cancer families. *J Consult Clin Psychol* 2000; **68**:864–874.
22. Cella D, Hughes C, Peterman A, *et al*. A brief assessment of concerns associated with genetic testing for cancer: the multidimensional impact of cancer risk assessment (MICRA) questionnaire. *Health Psychol* 2002; **21**:564–572.
23. Schwartz MD, Peshkin BN, Hughes C, *et al*. Impact of *BRCA1/BRCA2* mutation testing on psychologic distress in a clinic-based sample. *J Clin Oncol* 2002; **20**:514–520.

24. Evans DGR, Blair V, Greenhalgh R, *et al*. The impact of genetic counseling on risk perception in women with a family history of breast cancer. *Br J Cancer* 1994; **70**:934–938.

25. Lloyd S, Watson M, Waites B, *et al*. Familial breast cancer: a controlled study of risk perception, psychological morbidity and health beliefs in women attending for genetic counseling. *Br J Cancer* 1996; **74**:482–487.

26. Watson M, Duvivier V, Walsh MW, *et al*. Family history of breast cancer: what do women understand and recall about genetic risk? *J Med Genet* 1998; **35**:731–738.

27. Claus EB, Schildkraut J, Iverson ES Jr, *et al*. Effect of *BRCA1* and *BRCA2* on the association between breast cancer risk and family history. *J Natl Cancer Inst* 1998; **90**:1824–1829.

28. Burke W, Daly M, Garber J, *et al*. Recommendations for follow-up care of individuals with an inherited predisposition to cancer: *BRCA1* and *BRCA2*. *JAMA* 1997; **277**:997–1003.

29. Brekelmans CTM, Seynaeve C, Bartels CCM, *et al*. Effectiveness of breast cancer surveillance in *BRCA1/2* gene mutation carriers and women with high familial risk. *J Clin Oncol* 2000; **19**:924–930.

30. Lerman C, Hughes C, Croyle RT, *et al*. Prophylactic surgery decisions and surveillance practices one year following *BRCA1/2* testing. *Prev Med* 2000; **31**:75–80.

31. Peshkin BN, Schwartz MD, Isaacs C, *et al*. Utilization of breast cancer screening in a clinically based sample of women after *BRCA1/2* testing. *Cancer Epidemiol Biomarkers Prev* 2002; **11**:1113–1118.

32. Beam CA, Layde PM, Sullivan DC. Variability in the interpretation of screening mammograms by US radiologists. *Arch Intern Med* 1996; **156**:209–213.

33. Fisher B, Costantino JP, Wickerman DL, *et al*. Tamoxifen for the prevention of breast cancer: report of the national surgical adjuvant breast and bowel project P-1 study. *J Natl Cancer Inst* 1998; **90**:1371–1388.

34. Eeles R, Powles TJ. Chemoprevention options for *BRCA1* and *BRCA2* mutation carriers. *J Clin Oncol* 2000; **18**:93s–99s.

35. King MC, Wieand S, Hale K, *et al*. Tamoxifen and breast cancer incidence among women with inherited mutations in *BRCA1* and *BRCA2*: National Surgical Adjuvant Breast and Bowel Project (NSABP-P1) Breast Cancer Prevention Trial. *JAMA* 2001; **286**:2251–2256.

36. Chlebowski RT, Col N, Winer EP, *et al*. American Society of Clinical Oncology Technology Assessment of Pharmacologic interventions for breast cancer risk reduction including tamoxifen, raloxifene, and aromatase inhibition. *J Clin Oncol* 2002: **20**:3328–3343.

37. Hartmann LC, Schaid DJ, Woods JE, *et al*. Efficacy of bilateral prophylactic mastectomy in women with a family history of breast cancer. *N Engl J Med* 1999; **340**:77–84.

38. Rebbeck TR, Levin AM, Eisen A, *et al*. Breast cancer risk after bilateral prophylactic oophorectomy in *BRCA1* mutation carriers. *J Natl Cancer Inst* 1999; **91**:14759.

39. Stefanek ME. Bilateral prophylactic mastectomy: issues and concerns. *Monogr Natl Cancer Inst* 1995; **17**:37–42.

40. Frank TS, Manley SA, Olopade OI, *et al*. Sequence analysis of *BRCA1* and *BRCA2*: correlation of mutations with family history and ovarian cancer risk. *J Clin Oncol* 1998; **16**:2417–2420.

41. Meijers-Heijboer H, van Geel B, van Putten WLJ, *et al*. Breast cancer after prophylactic bilateral mastectomy in women with a *BRCA1* or *BRCA2* mutation. *N Engl J Med* 2001; **345**:159–164.

42. Julian-Reynier C, Eisinger F, Moatti JP, Sobol H. Physicians' attitudes towards mammography and prophylactic surgery for hereditary breast/ovarian cancer risk and subsequently published guidelines. *Eur J Hum Genet* 2000; **8**:204–208.

43. Matloff ET, Shappell H, Brierley K, *et al*. What would you do? Specialists' perspective on cancer genetic testing, prophylactic surgery and insurance discrimination. *J Clin Oncol* 2000; **18**:2484–2492.

44. Holtzman NA, Bernhardt BA, Doksum T, *et al*. Education about *BRCA1* testing decreases women's interest in being tested. *Am J Hum Genet* 1996; **59**:A56.

45. Meiser B, Butow P, Friedlander M, *et al*. Intention to undergo prophylactic bilateral mastectomy in women at increased risk of developing hereditary breast cancer. *J Clin Oncol* 2000; **18**:2250–2257.

46. Stefanek ME, Helzlsouer KJ, Wilcox PM, Houn F. Predictors of and satisfaction with bilateral prophylactic mastectomy. *Prev Med* 1995; **24**:412.

47. Borgen PI, Hill ADK, Tran KN, *et al*. Patient regrets after bilateral prophylactic mastectomy. *Ann Surg Oncol* 1998; **5**:603–606.

48. Frost MH, Schaid DJ, Sellers TA, *et al*. Long-term satisfaction and psychological and social function following bilateral prophylactic mastectomy. *JAMA* 2000; **284**:319–324.

49. Jacobs I, Davies AP, Bridges J, *et al*. Prevalence screening for ovarian cancer in postmenopausal women by CA 125 measurement and ultrasonography. *Br Med J* 1993; **306**:1030–1034.

50. Einhorn N, Bast R, Knapp R, *et al*. Long-term follow-up of the Stockholm screening study on ovarian cancer. *Gynecol Oncol* 2000; **79**:466–470.

51. van Nagell JR, DePriest PD, Reedy MB, *et al*. The efficacy of transvaginal sonographic screening in asymptomatic women at risk for ovarian cancer. *Gynecol Oncol* 2000; **77**:350–356.

52. Hoskins WJ. Prospective on ovarian cancer: why prevent? *J Cell Biochem* 1995; **23**:189–199.

53. Narod S, Risch H, Moslehi R, *et al*. Oral contraceptives and the risk of hereditary ovarian cancer. *N Engl J Med* 1998; **339**:424–428.

54. Tobacman JK, Tucker MA, Kase R. Intra-abdominal carcinomatosis after prophylactic oophorectomy in ovarian-cancer-prone families. *Lancet* 1982; **2**:795–597.

55. NIH Consensus Conference. Ovarian cancer: screening, treatment, and follow-up. NIH Consensus Development Panel on Ovarian Cancer. *JAMA* 1995; **273**:491–497.

56. Piver MS, Jishi MF, Tsukada Y, *et al*. Primary peritoneal carcinoma after prophylactic oophorectomy in women with a family history of ovarian cancer. *Cancer* 1993; **71**:2651–2655.

57. Kauff ND, Satagopan JM, Robson M, *et al*. Risk-reducing salpingo-oophorectomy in women with a *BRCA1* or *BRCA2* mutation. *N Engl J Med* 2002; **346**:1609–1615.

58. Grann VR, Jacobson JS, Thomason D, *et al*. Effect of prevention strategies on survival and quality-adjusted survival of women with *BRCA1/2* mutations: an updated decision analysis. *J Clin Oncol* 2002; **10**:2520–2529.

59. Green J, Murton F, Statham H. Psychosocial issues raised by a familial ovarian cancer registry. *J Med Genet* 1993; **30**:575–579.

60. Daly M, Lerman C, Grana G, *et al*. Psychologic outcomes of participation in a cancer risk program (Abstract). *American Society of Preventive Onc*ology, 19th Annual Meeting, 8th March, 1995.

61. Wardle FJ, Collins W, Pernet AL, *et al*. Psychological impact of screening for familial ovarian cancer. *J Natl Cancer Inst* 1993; **85:**653–657.

62. Schwartz MD, Lerman C, Miller SM, *et al*. Coping disposition, perceived risk, and psychological distress among women at increased risk for ovarian cancer. *Health Psychol* 1995; **14:**232–236.

63. Erlick Robinson G, Rosen BP, Bradley LN, *et al*. Psychological impact of screening for familial ovarian cancer: reactions to initial assessment. *Gynecol Oncol* 1997; **65:**197–205.

64. Schwartz MD, Lerman C, Daly M, *et al*. Utilization of ovarian cancer screening by women at increased risk. *Cancer Epidemiol Biomarkers Prev* 1995; **4:**267–273.

32

The ethics of testing for cancer-predisposition genes

D. GARETH R. EVANS AND PATRICK J. MORRISON

INTRODUCTION

The recent advances in molecular genetics have uncovered new ethical dilemmas in cancer genetics as vexed and almost certainly more complex as in the disease which has provoked the most debate; Huntington disease. Many genes that predispose to cancer have no effect until well into adult life and, as with Huntington disease, important issues arise about predictive tests in fetal, childhood and adult life. Unlike Huntington disease, there are sometimes options that may prevent or at least alter the course to the end result (cancer). Nonetheless, there are hereditary cancers where little or no effective screening or treatment is possible, even when presymptomatic testing shows an individual to carry a cancer-predisposing gene. Many of the lessons that have been learnt from study of Huntington disease can be applied to predictive testing for cancer predisposition genes.[1]

CANCER-PREDISPOSITION GENES AND TESTING IN CHILDHOOD

For the purposes of this chapter, we have divided these genes into those in which there is an identifiable phenotype (at least in a proportion of cases) and those in which there is no phenotype, only the end result of a particular cancer. In phenotypic conditions, the diagnosis can be made in a single individual, whereas in many cancer syndromes, a clear familial aggregation is required for diagnosis. In recessive conditions, such as Bloom's or ataxia-telangiectasia, the phenotype is usually clinically evident without predictive testing. This may also be the case in neurofibromatosis type 1 when the pigmentary disturbance and neurofibromas are nearly always expressed by 5 years of age,[2] and the need for predictive testing is thus minimal. However, in familial adenomatous polyposis (FAP), neurofibromatosis type 2 (NF2) and von Hippel–Lindau disease (vHL), the phenotype is variable and diagnostic features may not be present until well into adult life.[3–5] In such conditions, individuals at 50 per cent prior risk are usually screened for signs that may require mild (indirect ophthalmoscopy with mydriasis, magnetic resonance imaging (MRI) scanning of the brain) to considerable invasiveness (sigmoidoscopy/colonoscopy). Some of these tests could be described as being to the benefit of at-risk individuals in that they might find premalignant adenomatous polyps (FAP), vestibular schwannomas (NF2) or retinal angiomas (vHL), which could be treated and prevent further disability. Others such as congenital hypertrophy of the retinal pigment epithelium (CHRPE in FAP), posterior lenticular opacities (NF2) and pancreatic cysts (vHL) would merely indicate that person had inherited the mutated gene without there being any immediate clinical benefit to the individual. Unlike many DNA-predictive tests, these clinical predictions do not give the same level of reassurance if they are favourable. Performing these tests has not been subjected to anywhere near the same ethical scrutiny as DNA-predictive tests. Clinicians undertake such tests and clients who have them should be fully aware of the genetic implications of a mutation-positive test. It is all too easy, for example, to send a client to a busy ophthalmology clinic where they are casually told that they have the FAP gene because CHRPE are found without adequate and immediate back-up in terms of follow-up and genetic counselling.

There is, therefore, a right *not* to know. While it may be argued that individuals at risk of one of the conditions with a phenotype (Table 32.1) are benefited in that there is something that can be done for their condition, it may be many years before they require any intervention. In the same way as the vast majority of geneticists would not perform a predictive test on a child at risk of Huntington disease,[6] even in the phenotypic conditions, there are ages at which even apparently non-invasive tests, such as ophthalmoscopy, should not be used. For instance, very few geneticists in the UK would advocate DNA testing of a 1-year-old child with a 50 per cent risk of FAP because the cancer risk at this age is minimal and the psychological problems for the parent/child relationship are considerable. It would, as suggested above, be all too easy to forget that a simple eye test may have the same predictive value.

However, most of the phenotypic cancer-predisposing conditions to some extent may result in tumour formation in childhood, and this decides when screening should be offered both to detect potentially harmful tumours and also to identify 'benign' disease markers (e.g. CHRPE). Table 32.2 shows the probable earliest reported instance

Table 32.1 *Cancer-predisposition genes*

	Inheritance
Identifiable phenotype	
Familial adenomatous polyposis	AD
Gorlin syndrome	AD
Neurofibromatosis (1 and 2)	AD
Multiple endocrine neoplasia (1 and 2)	AD
von Hippel–Lindau	AD
Ataxia telangiectasia (*ATM*)	AR
Bloom syndrome	AR
Xeroderma pigmentosa	AR
Dysplastic naevus syndrome (*TP16*)	AD
No phenotype	
Hereditary non-polyposis colorectal cancer (*MSH2, MLH1*, etc.)	AD
BRCA1	AD
BRCA2	AD
E-Cadherin (gastric)	AD
Li–Fraumeni	AD
AT carrier	AD

AD, autosomal dominant; AR, autosomal recessive.

Table 32.2 *Implications of various dominant cancer syndromes in childhood*

Disease	Tumours	Probable earliest tumour	Risk in childhood	Recommended start of screening
Familial adenomatous polyposis	Adenomas	First year	80%	10–16 years
Bowel cancer	?4 years, 7 years	<1%		
Neurofibromatosis 2	Schwannomas, meningiomas	First year (meningioma)	30%	Birth
von Hippel–Landau	Haemangioblastoma, renal carcinoma	1–2 years (retinal)	15%	5 years
Multiple endocrine neoplasia (MEN 1)	Parathyroid, insulinoma, gastrinoma	5 years	5%	5 years
Multiple endocrine neoplasia (MEN 2A)	Medullary thyroid cancer, parathyroid, phaeochromocytoma	3 years	2.5%	3–4 years
Multiple endocrine neoplasia (MEN 2B)	As in MEN 2A, except parathyroid	1 year	<50%	Birth
Li–Fraumeni	Sarcoma (bone/soft tissue), adrenal, breast cancer, gliomas	First year	30%	First year
Breast cancer (BRCA1)	Breast and ovary, prostate carcinoma, colon	>16 years	<0.1%	30 years
Breast cancer (BRCA2)	Breast and ovary, prostate carcinoma, male breast	>16 years	<0.1%	30 years
Hereditary non-polyposis colorectal cancer	Colorectum, endometrium, ovary, gastric, ureter	>16 years	<0.1%	25–30 years

of a cancer or other harmful neoplasm for each condition, and the overall risk in childhood.

In the UK, most centres offering DNA tests would build these into the initial work-up for the disorder. For instance, if screening was commenced at 12 years for FAP, the DNA test would be offered in conjunction with ophthalmoscopy and dental screening. Nevertheless, there are families in which huge pressure is exerted by the parents to have the DNA test earlier. In deciding when to use a DNA test, one should assess the balance between benefit and damage to the *child*, and not the potential for relief of anxiety in the parents. If a screening programme starts at 12 years of age with sigmoidoscopy or colonoscopy, there is a clear benefit for 50 per cent of children who are shown by DNA tests not to have the mutated gene, as they will have to undergo fewer, if any, invasive tests. In contrast, at 1 year of age, the potential for benefit is unclear, while there is potential for harm, particularly if one child in the family is stigmatized from infancy as 'affected' and another is 'unaffected'. Nonetheless, colorectal cancer has been reported even under the age of 10 years and hepatoblastoma is also a potential risk in infancy with little possibility of effective screening. In balancing these various difficulties, most centres in the UK would still offer the DNA tests at the time of initial screening and most parents with sympathetic counselling will accept this timing of the test. Earlier testing may well be offered in occasional families where an individual clinician deems this to be psychologically beneficial.

The situation in the USA is fundamentally different; where in some centres testing in infancy is the norm. Indeed, at the Leeds Castle Polyposis Meeting in Copenhagen (1993), the consensus was that ethical decisions on timing should be discussed in each country, as it would be impossible to impose a single international policy.

Timing of the DNA tests in the other conditions in which there is a distinctive recognizable phenotype again depends on weighing up the benefits (Table 32.3). It could be argued that DNA testing does not differ from other tests, which are also predictive (cataracts at birth in NF2, high calcitonin in MEN2A or 2B at 4 years of age). It could also be argued that, if the clinical investigations are non-invasive, there is no harm to the unaffected child of delaying DNA testing until a time at which they can participate in the decision. Because some conditions may occur in childhood, clinical screening and repeated hospitalization of children unnecessarily could be avoided by early DNA testing, if they are found not to have the gene. So-called non-invasive tests, such as MRI scans, can actually be very traumatic and, if necessary, require a general anaesthetic to keep a child still. Repeated blood tests are also unpleasant for children. While the debate should not really be centred on cost, there is the potential cost saving of *not* performing expensive screening on

Table 32.3 *Guidelines for timing of DNA-predictive tests*

Disease	Age in years of:		
	Earliest screen	Intensive screening	DNA testing
Familial adenomatous polyposis	10	16	10–16
Neurofibromatosis 2	Birth	10–12	Birth, or 10, or 18+
von Hippel–Landau	5	15	5, or 15, or 18+
Multiple endocrine neoplasia (MEN 1)	5	5	5 or 18+
Multiple endocrine neoplasia (MEN 2A)	3–4	3–4	3–4 or 18+
Multiple endocrine neoplasia (MEN 2B)	1	1	Birth
Li–Fraumeni	First year	None yet agreed	Birth ?? 18+
Breast cancer (BRCA1/2)	30	30	18+
Hereditary non-polyposis colorectal cancer	25–30	25–30	18+
E-Cadherin	20–25	20–25	18+

those who do not have the gene. Overall, most centres in the UK would, therefore, offer the tests at the time of the initial screen. However, even using commencement of screening can be troublesome. It is important to examine newborn infants for cataracts in NF2 as these may threaten vision.[3] Nonetheless, only 10 per cent of individuals present in the first decade when screening can be confined to a simple annual physical examination.[7] More intense screening for vestibular schwannomas (acoustic neuromas) with brainstem-evoked responses or MRI scans should probably commence at puberty and detects the great majority of mutation carriers by 16 years of age.[8] Should we, therefore, delay DNA testing until 16 years of age or an age at which the individual can make a decision for themselves. While the MRI scan is a predictive test, it has an immediate benefit in diagnosing a tumour, which can be managed optimally. The DNA test will only say that the individual carries the normal or abnormal gene when tumours, particularly in late-onset families, may not arise for decades. In NF2 there is a possible argument for testing at any age including birth but equally that individual may have no features of the condition until they are 40. The decision on timing of DNA-predictive testing could, therefore, be left to the individual clinician treating each NF2 family on its own merits (age at onset, etc.). Our own experience in three genetic centres shows a very high uptake for presymptomatic childhood testing in NF2, FAP and vHL.[9]

Non-phenotypic cancer syndromes

The debate about testing in childhood is potentially easier where the risk of a child being affected is close to zero. This is the case in hereditary non-polyposis colorectal cancer (HNPCC) and in those that carry a mutation in *BRCA1* or *BRCA2*. There are few potential benefits of testing an 8-year-old girl for the *BRCA1* gene, as she will have little risk until she is 30 years old. It could be argued that there is a potential for prevention by hormonal manipulation (delay of puberty, early first pregnancy), but these are unproven in dominant cancer syndromes and are highly contentious. Gene therapy administered in childhood may one day help prevent cancer in these families but, as this is not yet possible, there can be little benefit to a child in having a predictive test for the *BRCA1* gene. Therefore, the situation is similar to that for Huntington disease.[10] Many adults would prefer to live with the relative uncertainty (40–45 per cent risk) of whether they were going to develop breast cancer rather than be faced with an 80–90 per cent lifetime risk in the absence of definitive preventative or curative measures.[11,12] Nonetheless, in some Northern European countries the uptake of testing for *BRCA1* is around 40–50 per cent in women at risk of a known family mutation and >50 per cent of these opt for prophylactic surgery.[13,14] Recent evidence from a study of prophylactic mastectomy showing a 90 per cent risk reduction even in high-risk individuals is likely to increase uptake of this measure.[15]

GENETIC AND OTHER SCREENING FOR COMMON CANCERS

All of the conditions described so far have the potential benefit of early detection of tumours by screening at risk individuals. With benign tumours, this allows optimal management and may be life-saving; with cancers there is a real hope of improving morbidity and mortality. Screening programmes for the phenotypic conditions are well established and have been shown to be beneficial.[3,5,16–18] The situation is less clear with common cancer predisposition. In the USA and some other countries, population screening is advocated for bowel and breast cancer from a relatively early age. Screening for breast cancer is now accepted in the UK only after 50 years,[19] with no general acceptance for the bowel at any age. However, targeted screening is offered by many for breast,[20] bowel[21] and ovary.[22] While the benefits of early screening in breast cancer are still not clear even in high-risk groups, evidence of benefit is now emerging for colorectal cancer.[23,24]

It is not the purpose of this chapter to define whether a screening programme is suitable for a specific condition. However, when discussing predictive testing the nature of screening for a specific disorder is relevant. Negative screening at a particular age, may in itself substantially reduce the risk of that individual having inherited the family gene fault.[3,5,18] Alterations in an established screening programme, dependent on the result of a DNA test, may also need to be discussed. This may involve more active screening with a bad predictive outcome, or relaxing or stopping screening altogether in those at low risk. Individuals who are accustomed to being screened for a condition for which there is still a relatively high population risk (breast, bowel or ovarian cancer) may wish to continue as before. The efficacy of any screening programme also needs to be made clear to someone considering undergoing a predictive test. It is unlikely that many women at 40 per cent risk of breast cancer would accept prophylactic mastectomy even when it is readily available[13] but, faced with an 80 per cent risk, would they still be happy with a screening programme which is yet to be proven beneficial? Positive DNA predictive tests may substantially alter the current practice of screening. This has already led to early thyroidectomy before thyroid disease in MEN 2,[25] and may well lead to prophylactic colectomy and greater uptake of prophylactic mastectomy in familial bowel and breast cancer.

ADULT DNA PREDICTIVE TESTS

The right to know

Many ethicists argue that it is every individual's right to know any information relevant to themselves, particularly if others (health care workers) are already party to it.[26] There are various reasons why someone may want to know if they have inherited the family gene fault.[27]

1 to make decisions concerning having children;
2 to have certainty;
3 to plan appropriate action (prophylactic surgery);
4 to inform children and/or partner;
5 to make provisions for the future;
6 to help science.

Where a predictive test is possible in adulthood and when this is of physical or probable psychological benefit to an individual, the test should be offered after adequate counselling.

However, there are instances when an individual's 'right to know' may interfere with another individual's 'right not to know'.[28] Such a situation would occur if someone whose grandparent had a cancer predisposing syndrome wanted a test when their relevant parent who was still clinically unaffected did not (so-called '25 per cent risk' testing[29]). In this situation, the autonomy of one individual is in conflict with another. The situation is simpler when there is real physical benefit in knowing that they have the gene fault. For instance, denial of a predictive test in FAP could be extended to denying endoscopic screening as, if this were positive, it too would inform the unwilling parent of their genetic status. Clearly, where there is a clear clinical benefit, the wishes of the offspring should prevail. The converse of this is in a condition where no treatment was possible, such as Huntington disease, where it is now very easy to do a simple DNA predictive test, which may be of marginal benefit to an adult offspring, but a devastating and unwanted blow to the parent, if positive.[28] Therefore, the clinician must weigh up the conflicts in autonomy to decide whether it is appropriate to offer tests in these circumstances. In future, these decisions may involve the advice of medical ethicists.

DISCLOSURE

Another contentious area is the disclosure of information to an individual in a family who is at risk, when the affected individual specifically does not want this to happen. Again, the ethicist would argue that it is the duty of people in this situation to inform their relatives.[26] If the clinician were to disclose the information, this would be a breach of confidentiality. However, there is also a possibly stronger duty to the at-risk individual who could have a life-saving procedure denied them by lack of this knowledge. Already physicians have been sued for not making family members aware in conditions like MEN 2.[30] In the UK and USA, the right to privacy can certainly be overruled and geneticists may need to take reasonable steps to ensure that a relative is informed of their risks.[31] Privacy laws are stricter in many European countries and direct approaches to relatives by medical services is often forbidden. DNA tests may further complicate the issue as it may be necessary to use the DNA sample from the unwilling affected relative either in linkage analysis or in a mutation study, to allow a predictive test on the at risk relative. Although the at-risk individual may have a right to important relevant clinical information, do they also have the right to specific information from their unwilling relatives DNA?[32]

Disclosure may take another form, for instance, a child and his/her adoptive parents hearing of genetic disease in the biological family. This may be quite common in cancer-predisposing syndromes because either the nature of the predisposition or the disease itself does not arise until later in the natural parent. After adequate consultation with social services, disclosure of the likely genetic predisposition and with it the possibility of DNA tests may well be indicated.[33]

THE RIGHT *NOT* TO KNOW

We have already pointed out potential areas of conflict in families, when the right of one individual to know may conflict with the right of a relative not to know. This has been described with regard to testing in childhood and also when an offspring's result would reveal a parent's genotype. However, there are several other reasons why a DNA-predictive test may be refused:[11,12,27]

1 because a positive result would be too difficult to live with/could not cope with a bad result;
2 the test does not predict when the disease will appear;
3 preference to live in uncertainty;
4 fear of increasing the risk to children;
5 problems at work and with insurance;
6 a positive result would impose too great a burden on partner/family;
7 negative tests generate guilt feelings in sibling relationships;
8 reluctance to give up screening if mutation negative.

All of these reasons are applicable to a DNA-predictive test for cancer predisposition, although, unlike Huntington disease, screening and prophylactic surgery may prevent the disease. However, Li–Fraumeni syndrome poses almost identical quandaries to Huntington disease. Li–Fraumeni syndrome causes malignancies, which may appear in childhood or more commonly in adult life. The range and number of tumours and sites make screening or removal of all at-risk tissues impossible.[34] While early diagnosis may allow cure of a particular primary cancer, many go on to develop further primaries and 90 per cent will have developed a malignancy by 50 years of age.[34] A decision to opt for a predictive test in Li–Fraumeni should, therefore, be preceded by counselling as is advocated for Huntington disease.[35,36]

After counselling, most people at risk of Huntington disease (which is effectively untreatable at present) do not opt for a predictive test.[37–39] The uptake of Huntington disease testing in the UK is around 18 per cent.[39] In contrast, for conditions like FAP, predictive testing is more acceptable because there are clear benefits which follow knowledge about one's genetic status.[9] This gives a differential of 18 per cent uptake for Huntington disease to 90 per cent for FAP in adults in the same health region.[9] However, many people with predisposition to cancers for which screening or treatment is of arguable benefit may not want to know. Although those working in the cancer genetic field may have the impression that there is enthusiasm for predictive tests, one should be cautious because in the early stages, as with Huntington disease, a highly motivated self-referred population volunteers itself. Such tests offered on a less selected or population basis will prove less acceptable. Many people may also be happy to be screened for their 40 per cent risk of a cancer and prefer to continue with screening rather than have a predictive test. In a similar way to the work with Huntington disease, it is important that the effects of counselling and predictive testing on the psychological well-being of each individual is carefully studied.[38] Follow-up of 'favourable' test results is also important because even here there may be an adverse reaction based upon the well recognized 'survivor syndrome'.[38] We are beginning to see this in our own practice, particularly with sisters who have different *BRCA1/2* results. Nonetheless, overall, with careful counselling there do not appear to be any particularly adverse effects from presymptomatic testing for cancer predisposition.[9,12]

Prenatal testing

It is not yet clear what level of demand there will be for prenatal testing in the cancer-predisposing syndromes. Some work has been done on type 1 neurofibromatosis suggesting that, in spite of couples expressing an interest in prenatal tests, few would contemplate termination.[40] This is reflected in the fairly low uptake of these tests when offered.[41,42] It is likely that decisions will depend on the experience within the particular family. The severity of the condition combined with the perceived benefits of screening and treatment in the particular couple will likely predict the uptake.

Prenatal testing again touches on the rights of minors not to know should a positive test not be followed by termination. In Huntington disease, a prenatal test is usually offered only if the couple intend to terminate if the test result is unfavourable.[6] When the prenatal test is limited to 'exclusion', the 25 per cent risk to the fetus may be reduced to a very low risk or the same risk as the parent (50 per cent). When, subsequently, the parent develops, for example, early-onset breast cancer, this would imply the fetus also carried the gene and the child would carry the burden of knowledge through life. Prenatal tests should usually only be undertaken if there is a clear wish to terminate high-risk pregnancies or, in the future, when this will allow early intervention, which will be beneficial to the resultant child.

Research samples

Ethical problems arise in connection with samples taken for research, which are subsequently used for prediction. Individuals at risk of a cancer syndrome may be tested as part of research into linkage in families or have blood taken 'for research' when attending family history clinics for screening. If individuals in these circumstances are fully aware of the possible outcome of this research, then there may not be a problem when a predictive 'result' is arrived at. However, many will be unaware of the implications of a gene-positive test result. It is unwise to store DNA on 'at-risk' individuals unless informed consent is given, or the samples are anonymously coded and used for research purposes only.[43] Blood from unaffected relatives adds little information in late-onset disease unless specific questions

about non-penetrance are being asked. In this situation, the gene defect is known and the at-risk relative should be approached again for sampling on the understanding that the sample will be coded and there will be no result, or that there will be a proper predictive test with attendant counselling. Ideally, informed consent should be obtained with the first sample when there will be no need for a repeat.

Testing without specific consent

It is important to distinguish between screening for existing disease and genetic screening with its implications for the individuals and for relatives. A predictive test may be done incidentally while in hospital for related or even unrelated problems.[1] For example, a woman undergoing a laparoscopy for an ovarian cyst found on scan, may have blood taken for the biomarker CA125 but a request may be made for DNA diagnosis too. This is not appropriate without informed consent and appropriate genetic counselling.

The extreme sensitivity of the polymerase chain reaction test raises the prospect of illicit testing,[26] as it is now possible to perform DNA tests on saliva samples. These could, for example, be carried out on residual traces on a glass someone had just drunk from, or also from semen analysis and other body fluids. Employers and others could thus obtain information about the genetic status of unsuspecting individuals.

Population screening

A major aim of a population screen would be to identify the up to 50 per cent of new germline mutations, which occur in many cancer predisposition syndromes.[2,3] At present, population screening for cancers by genetic tests is impractical, although it is an area for potential problems in the future. Population screening is impractical because of the variety of mutations within any of the cancer-predisposition genes. There is no simple test, or small number of tests, which could be performed on each gene on a population basis. There are nonetheless exceptions to this, as 2–2.5 per cent of individuals of Ashkenazi Jewish origin carry one of three mutations in the *BRCA1* and *BRCA2* genes.[44] Once more, informed consent would be mandatory should population screening for cancer predisposition become possible.

Insurance

There is also the problem of insurance. Common cancer predisposition can only be classified as dominant in a very few families. Insurance companies are currently unlikely to load or refuse the policy as they would for someone whose parent has Huntington disease.[45] However, if the results of a test in childhood showed an inherited fault in the BRCA1 gene, this may (depending on the legal situation in each country) have to be disclosed on an insurance application leading to refusal or heavy loading. The implications of genetic testing on personal insurance has received extensive attention in the medical and lay press.[45–48] In the UK, the main concern is about the consequences of such testing on the eligibility for life assurance.[48,49] Insurance companies are not currently asking for DNA tests as they do for HIV tests but may do so in the future. Indeed, the industry is aware of the potential usefulness of such tests for life assurance underwriting.[50] As in Huntington disease, if the genetic nature of the condition is well-enough defined, individuals may be unable to obtain insurance because they are at 50 per cent risk, irrespective of DNA tests.[45] This may prompt those at risk to request testing in the hope that their 50 per cent prior risk will be reduced to the point of being able to obtain insurance. However, this has not been found to be a particularly important reason for opting for a test.[51] Nonetheless, we are aware of at least one woman who has tested positive for BRCA1 whose weighted premiums have been reduced to normal after prophylactic mastectomy and oophorectomy.

Insurance companies are understandably concerned about the possibility that someone who receives a high-risk result will obtain a policy with a high pay out either for life insurance or 'dread disease'. They are also concerned about competition from other companies if they were not to discriminate and, therefore, have to increase payments to ordinary risk individuals. Nonetheless, they want to avoid unnecessary discrimination and any attendant adverse publicity, which may lead to stricter legislation.

In the USA and other countries without national health services, the main concern is about health insurance, where a positive predictive test would have great relevance, although predictive genetic tests are rarely able to determine the time at which someone will become ill. In the USA, most health insurance is purchased on a group basis by employers, and the unemployed or low income groups are often not insured. There is no obligation on an employer to insure a high-risk employee who would raise their costs. Thus, 31–36 million people in the USA have no health insurance.[51] President Clinton in February 2000, signed an executive order forbidding the USA federal government from using genetic information in employment decisions.[52] Eventually, national legislation in the USA is likely in order to prevent discrimination. Indeed, this has been proposed for some time.[52,53] In the interim, 28 states have already introduced fairly restrictive legislation,[53] including the recent Massachusetts law, which prohibits genetic discrimination by employers and health insurance agents.[54] Interestingly, there does not appear to be any advantage taken of the gap in those states without

laws. Indeed, there is little evidence of discrimination in obtaining health insurance in the USA for presymptomatic individuals.[53] Nonetheless, health insurers are unwilling to pay for testing of, for instance, BRCA1, with only 15 per cent covering the costs,[54] and this is likely to increase if the tests are targeted in the high-risk situation, such as a family with a known mutation.[55] Unless more is done to encourage insurers, they may not to be prepared to pay for, for example, an FAP predictive test, thus denying those on lower incomes the opportunity for testing in the first place. Further work in the USA has also shown that insurance industry's fears about adverse selection may be groundless. Women testing positive for BRCA1 mutations did not take out higher levels of life insurance.[56]

Currently, the UK is the only country that has taken the active decision to allow the insurance industry to regulate itself.[48,57] While this currently allows policies up to £500 000 of life insurance associated with a mortgage on a property not to be assessed for genetic reasons, and up to £300 000 for critical illness and other health cover, there is evidence that the industry have ignored their own guidelines.[57]

The UK government established a genetics and insurance advisory committee (GAIC) in April 1999 in an attempt to validate genetic tests proposed by the Association of British Insurers (ABI). The ABI is the major regulating body for the insurance companies in the UK, and had listed matrices of autosomal dominant, autosomal recessive and X-linked recessive diseases for potential validation. Initially, a list of around 30 tests was drafted and then shortened to eight autosomal dominant diseases. Adult polycystic kidney disease was then dropped as a test, as ultrasound scanning was found to be reliable and easier to institute than a genetic test. The list of seven conditions included Huntington disease, multiple endocrine neoplasia (MEN 2), breast cancer (BRCA1/2 genes), FAP, Alzheimer disease, hereditary motor and sensory neuropathy (HMSN) and myotonic dystrophy. The list was never openly published, but interestingly, the majority of these tests were familial cancers.[57]

The first condition for validation, Huntington disease, was approved by GAIC in October 2000 as reliable and relevant for the purposes of life insurance policies. The insurance companies accepted this ruling and disclosed that they would not use tests, which were not received for approval by GAIC by the end of 2000. Two more conditions were submitted and are currently being processed: early-onset familial Alzheimer disease and hereditary breast–ovarian cancer. HNPCC applications are planned in the near future. Regrettably, the insurance companies took the view that, although they had withdrawn other tests including the cancers FAP and MEN 2, as they felt genetic testing by middle age was not going to add much to family history and clinical examination, they refused to allow the results of negative (i.e. not carrying a family mutation) tests, which would have been advantageous in securing normal rates in those penalized by family history of these diseases.[58] Although there was a large amount of public opposition to the first approval of Huntington disease by GAIC, the role of GAIC has been useful in that it forced the ABI to consider the topic seriously, rather that its previous view that no problem existed. It also put the onus on insurers to produce facts and a case to submit evidence to GAIC regarding reliability and, for just these reasons, five of the eight tests were dropped.

The approval of Huntington disease for mortgage-related life insurance was followed by two significant events. The Human Genetics Commission (HGC; a statutory government body that advises on ethical social and legal aspects of genetics) published a consultation on public opinion on several issues in December 2000 and showed that there was strong opposition to the use of genetic test results by insurance companies.[59] This was confirmed in a MORI opinion survey published by the HGC in March 2001,[60] which concluded that the level of public concern over the issue required a response. This information coincided with the new House of Commons Committee on Science and technology report[61] also in March 2001, which was severely critical of the insurance companies. This led the HGC to publish a statement in May 2001 recommending interim recommendations on the use of genetic information in insurance.

The UK government response to both the House of Commons select committee report and the HGC interim recommendations was published on 23rd October 2001.[62] The Government and the ABI announced a joint 5-year moratorium on the use of genetic test results by insurers (Table 32.4). The moratorium applies to life insurance policies up to £500 000 and critical illness, long-term care insurance and income protection up to £300 000 for each type of policy.[58] In policy applications above these limits, the insurance industry may use genetic test results where these tests have been approved by GAIC. Legislation has not been introduced; however, independent monitoring of the ABI code of conduct will take place possibly through an enhanced role for GAIC in monitoring both insurance compliance and customer complaints. It is also to review the composition of the GAIC committee with extension of its membership. The moratorium has not been extended to use of family history data and the whole moratorium will be reviewed after 3 years. The use of negative test results is encouraged by the insurer, subject to confirmation in most cases, by a geneticist of the relevance of the result.

Ironically it is, therefore, in the UK, which has extensive national health cover but no firm legislation, where insurance discrimination is most evident. In Europe, where most countries have restrictive legislation, there is little evidence of discrimination.[57,63] Although in Norway,

Table 32.4 *UK Government and Association of British Insurers (ABI) agreed moratorium on genetic testing and insurance, October 2001*

1 There will be a moratorium on the use of genetic test results by insurers, for 5 years.
2 It will apply to life insurance policies up to £500 000 and critical illness, long-term care insurance and income protection up to £300 000 for each type of policy.
3 In applications above these limits, the insurance industry may use genetic test results where these tests have been approved by the Genetics and Insurance Advisory Committee (GAIC).
4 Legislation has not been introduced; however, independent monitoring of the ABI code of conduct will take place through an enhanced role for GAIC in monitoring both insurance compliance and customer complaints.
5 The moratorium has not been extended to use of family history data.
6 The moratorium will be reviewed after 3 years.
7 The use of negative test results in obtaining normal premiums is encouraged by the insurer subject to confirmation in most cases by a geneticist of the relevance of the result.

there is evidence of increased premiums for HNPCC but not for *BRCA1/2*.[64]

The duty of the clinician is to ensure that there are no untoward pressures on an individual to accept or refuse genetic tests and classification, perhaps legalisation or state indemnity may be required. Insurance matters are a legitimate concern during the process of pretest counselling and most UK centres now routinely mention this.

CONCLUSIONS

The purpose of this chapter has been to highlight the ethical issues that arise in connection with DNA predictive tests. The duty of the clinician/counsellor is first of all to do no harm (non-maleficence).[28] The secondary aim is for the test to be of some benefit (beneficence). Clearly each cancer predisposition syndrome will have to be considered on its own merits with counselling on the implications of testing in pregnancy, childhood and, indeed, at any age for the individual and family requesting, or being offered testing. A full support service should be in place with follow-up not only of unfavourable but also good predictive results.

KEY POINTS

- Genetic testing is now possible for most high-risk cancer-predisposing genes.
- Simple non-DNA-screening tests can be as predictive as a genetic test in presymptomatic diagnosis.

- Syndromic genetic predisposition can be diagnosed in a single individual on the association of disease features (e.g. familial adenomatous polyposis).
- Non-syndromic predisposition requires genetic testing, such as for breast cancer with *BRCA1/2* or *TP53*.
- Presymptomatic genetic testing should only be carried out with informed consent after at least two counselling sessions.
- Clients undergoing genetic testing need to be informed of the possible insurance implications.
- Clinicians need to be aware of the possible conflicts in disclosure between patient privacy rights and the rights of an individual to know he/she is at risk.
- The primary consideration in genetic testing as in all other medicine is 'first do no harm'.

REFERENCES

1. Harper P. Ethical issues in genetic testing for Huntington's disease: lessons for the study of familial cancers. *Dis Markers* 1992; **10**:185–188.
2. Huson SM, Harper PS, Compston DAS. Von Recklinghausen neurofibromatosis. *Brain* 1988; **111**:1355–1381.
3. Evans DGR, Huson S, Donnai D, *et al.* A clinical study of type 2 neurofibromatosis. *Q J Med* 1992; **84**:603–618.
4. Evans DGR, Guy SP, Armstrong J, *et al.* Non penetrance and late appearance of polyps in families with familial adenomatous polyposis. *Gut* 1993; **34**:1389–1393.
5. Maher ER, Iselius L, Yates JRW, *et al.* Von Hippel Lindau disease: a genetic study. *J Med Genet* 1991; **28**:443–447.
6. Turner D. Ethical considerations in the social context of Huntington disease. *Dis Markers* 1992; **10**:171–183.
7. Evans DGR, Huson SM, Donnai D, *et al.* A genetic study of type 2 neurofibromatosis: II Guidelines for genetic counselling. *J Med Genet* 1992; **29**:847–852.
8. Evans DGR, Newton V, Neary W, *et al.* Use of MRI and audiological tests in pre-symptomatic diagnosis of type 2 neurofibromatosis. *J Med Genet* 2000; **37**:944–947.
9. Evans DGR, Maher ER, Macleod R, *et al.* Uptake of genetic testing for cancer predisposition. *J Med Genet* 1997; **34**:746–748.
10. Watson M, Murday V, Lloyd S, *et al.* Genetic testing in breast/ovarian cancer (*BRCA1*) families. *Lancet* 1995; **346**:583.
11. Lerman C, Narod S, Shulman K, *et al.* BRCA1 testing in families with hereditary breast-ovarian cancer: a prospective study of patient decision making and outcomes. *JAMA* 1996; **275**:1885–1892.
12. Binchy A, Evans DGR, Eng C, *et al.* Factors influencing decisions on whether to proceed with predictive testing for breast/ovarian cancers. *J Med Genet* 1995; **32**:140.
13. Meijers-Heijboer EJ, Verhoog LC, Brekelmans CTM, *et al.* Presymtomatic DNA testing and prophylactic surgery in families with a BRCA1 or BRCA2 mutation. *Lancet* 2000; **355**:2015–2020.
14. Lalloo F, Baildam A, Brain A, *et al.* Preventative mastectomy for women at high risk of breast cancer. *Eur J Surg Oncol* 2000; **26**:711–713.
15. Hartmann LC, Schaid DJ, Woods JE, *et al.* Efficacy of bilateral prophylactic mastectomy in women with a family history of breast cancer. *N Engl J Med* 1999; **340**:77–84.
16. Ponder BAJ, Coffey R, Gagel RF. Risk estimation and screening in families of patients with medullary thyroid carcinoma. *Lancet* 1988; **I**:397–401.
17. Morrison PJ. Genetic aspects of familial thyroid cancer. *CME Bull Oncol* 2000; **2**:7–12.
18. Burn J, Chapman P, Delhanty J, *et al.* The UK Northern Region Genetic register for familial adenomatous polyposis coli: use of age of onset, congenital hypertrophy of the retinal pigment epithelium, and DNA markers in risk calculation. *J Med Genet* 1991; **28**:289–296.
19. *Breast cancer screening: Forrest report.* London: HMSO, 1988.
20. Eccles DM, Evans DGR, Mackay J. Guidelines for managing women with a family history of breast cancer. *J Med Genet* 2000; **37**:203–209.
21. Dunlop MG. Screening for large bowel neoplasms in individuals with a family history of colorectal cancer. *Brit J Surg* 1992; **79**:488–494.
22. Bourne TH, Campbell S, Reynolds KM. Screening for early familial ovarian cancer with transvaginal ultrasonography and colour flow imaging. *Br Med J* 1993; **306**:1025–1029.
23. Mandel JS, Bond JH, Church TR. Reducing mortality from colorectal cancer by screening for faecal occult blood. *N Engl J Med* 1993; **328**:1365–1371.
24. Jarvinen JH, Mecklin J-P, Sistonen P. Screening reduces colorectal cancer rate in hereditary nonpolyposis colorectal cancer (HNPCC) families. *Gastroenterology* 1995; **108**:1405–1411.
25. McNally D, Campbell WJ, Sloan JM, *et al.* Thyroidectomy for medullary carcinoma in MEN 2a: positive genetic screening as the sole indicator for surgery. *U Med J* 1997; **66**:134–135.
26. Harris J. The use of information (autonomy and confidentiality). *Dis Markers* 1992; **10**:195–198.
27. Wolff G, Walter W. Attitudes of at risk persons for Huntington disease toward predictive genetic testing. *Birth Defects OAS* 1992; **28**:119–126.
28. de Wert G. Predictive testing for Huntington disease and the right not to know, some ethical reflections. *Birth Defects OAS* 1992; **28**:133–138.
29. Benjamin CM, Lashwood A. United Kingdom experience with presymptomatic testing of individuals at 25 per cent risk for Huntington's disease. *Clin Genet* 2000; **58**:41–49.
30. Rothenberg KH. Breast cancer, the genetic 'Quick fix' and the Jewish community. *Health Matrix* 1997; **7**:97–124.
31. ASHG statement: Professional disclosure of familial genetic information. *Am J Hum Genet* 1998; **62**:474–483.
32. *Committee on the ethics of gene therapy. Report.* London: HMSO, 1992.
33. Evans G. Ethical issues: the geneticist's viewpoint. *Dis Markers* 1992; **10**:199–203.
34. Varley J, Evans DGR, Birch JM. Li–Fraumeni syndrome – a molecular and clinical review. *Br J Cancer* 1997; **76**:1–14.
35. Craufurd D, Kerzin-Storrer L, Dodge A, Harris R. Uptake of presymptomatic predictive testing for Huntington's disease. *Lancet* 1989; **ii**:603–605.
36. Ethical issues policy statement on Huntington's disease molecular genetic predictive test. *J Med Genet* 1990; **27**:34–38.

37. Craufurd D, Harris R. Ethics of predictive testing for Huntington's chorea: the need for more information. *Br Med J* 1986; **293**:249–251.

38. Demyttenaere K, Evers-Kiebooms G, Decruyenaere M. Pitfalls in counselling for predictive testing in Huntington disease. *Birth Defects OAS* 1992; **28**:105–111.

39. Harper PS, Lim C, Craufurd D. Ten years of presymptomatic testing for Huntington's disease: the experience of the UK Huntington's disease prediction consortium. *J Med Genet* 2000; **37**:567–571.

40. Benjamin CM, Colley A, Donnai D, *et al.* Neurofibromatosis type 1 (NF1): knowledge, experience and reproductive decisions of affected individuals and families. *J Med Genet* 1993; **30**:567–574.

41. Upadhyaya M, Fryer A, MacMillan J, *et al.* Prenatal diagnosis and presymptomatic detection of neurofibromatosis type 1. *J Med Genet* 1992; **29**:180–183.

42. Simpson SA, Harper PS. United Kingdom Huntingdon Disease Prediction Consortium. Prenatal testing for Huntington disease: experience within the UK 1994–1998. *J Med Genet* 2000; **38**:333–335.

43. Harper PS. Research samples from families with genetic disease: a proposed code of conduct. *Br Med J* 1993; **306**:1391–1394.

44. Struewing JP, Hartge P, Wacholder S. The risk of cancer associated with specific mutations of BRCA1 and BRCA2 among Ashkenazi Jews. *N Engl J Med* 1997; **336**:1401–1408.

45. Harper PS. Insurance and genetic testing. *Lancet* 1993; **341**:224–227.

46. Ostrer H, Allen W, Crandall LA, *et al.* Insurance and genetic testing: where are we now? *Am J Hum Genet* 1993; **52**:565–577.

47. Pokorski RJ. Insurance underwriting in the genetic era. *Am J Hum Genet* 1997; **60**:205–216.

48. Morrison PJ. Implications for genetic testing for insurance in the UK. *Lancet* 1998; **352**:1647–1648.

49. Morrison PJ. Genetic testing and insurance in the United Kingdom. *Clin Genet* 1998; **54**:375–379.

50. Brett P, Fischer EP. Effects on life insurance of genetic testing. *The Actuary* 1993; **10**:11–12.

51. Tyler A, Morris M, Lazarou L, *et al.* Presymptomatic testing for Huntington's disease in Wales 1987–90. *Br J Psychiatr* 1992; **161**:481–488.

52. Josefson J. Clinton outlaws genetic discrimination in federal jobs. *Br Med J* 2000; **320**:168.

53. Hall MA, Rich SS. Laws restricting health insurers' use of genetic information: impact on genetic discrimination. *Am J Hum Genet* 2000; **66**:293–307.

54. Anon. Private matters, public affairs. *Nature Genet* 2000; **26**:1–2.

55. Schoonmaker MM, Bernhardt BA, Holtzman NA. Factors influencing health insurers' decisions to cover new genetic technologies. *Int J Technol Assess Health Care* 2000; **16**:178–189.

56. Zick CD, Smith KR, Mayer RN, Botkin JR. Genetic testing, adverse selection, and the demand for life insurance. *Am J Med Genet* 2000; **93**:29–39.

57. Morrison PJ, Steel CM, Vasen HFA, *et al.* Insurance implications for individuals with a high risk of breast and ovarian cancer in Europe. *Dis Markers* 1999; **15**:159–165.

58. Morrison PJ. Insurance, genetic testing and familial cancer: recent policy changes in the United Kingdom. *U Med J* 2001; **70**:79–88.

59. Human Genetics Commission. *Whose hands on your genes? A discussion document on the storage, protection and use of personal genetic information.* London: Department of Health, November 2000.

60. Human Genetics Commission. *Public attitudes to human genetic information. Peoples panel quantitative study conducted for the human genetics commission.* London: Department of Health, February 2001.

61. *Genetics and Insurance. Fifth report of the Science and technology committee.* House of Commons, HC174. London: HMSO, March 2001.

62. *Government response to the report from the House of Commons Science and Technology Committee: genetics and insurance.* London: Department of Health, UK. October 2001.

63. Morrison PJ, Steel CM, Nevin NC, *et al.* Insurance considerations for individuals with a high risk of breast cancer in Europe: some recommendations. *CME Hung J Gynaecol* 2000; **5**:272–277.

64. Norum J, Tranebjaerg L. Health, life and disability insurance and hereditary risk for breast and colorectal cancer. *Acta Oncol* 2000; **39**:189–193.

Index

Compiled by Indexing Specialists (UK) Ltd (www.indexing.co.uk). *Italic* page numbers refer to graphs and illustrations